Maternity Nursing

An Introductory Text

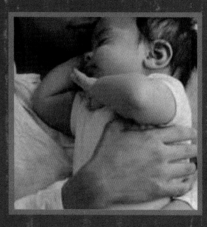

Gloria Leifer, RN, MA, CNE
Professor, Obstetric and Pediatric Nursing
Riverside City College
Riverside, California

11th Edition

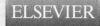ELSEVIER

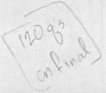
120g3
cn final

ELSEVIER
SAUNDERS

3251 Riverport Lane
St. Louis, Missouri 63043

MATERNITY NURSING: AN INTRODUCTORY TEXT, 11 ed.   ISBN: 978-1-4377-2209-3

Notices

Knowledge and best practice in this field are constantly changing. As new research and experience broaden our understanding, changes in research methods, professional practices, or medical treatment may become necessary.

Practitioners and researchers must always rely on their own experience and knowledge in evaluating and using any information, methods, compounds, or experiments described herein. In using such information or methods they should be mindful of their own safety and the safety of others, including parties for whom they have a professional responsibility.

With respect to any drug or pharmaceutical products identified, readers are advised to check the most current information provided (i) on procedures featured or (ii) by the manufacturer of each product to be administered, to verify the recommended dose or formula, the method and duration of administration, and contraindications. It is the responsibility of practitioners, relying on their own experience and knowledge of their patients, to make diagnoses, to determine dosages and the best treatment for each individual patient, and to take all appropriate safety precautions.

To the fullest extent of the law, neither the Publisher nor the authors, contributors, or editors, assume any liability for any injury and/or damage to persons or property as a matter of products liability, negligence or otherwise, or from any use or operation of any methods, products, instructions, or ideas contained in the material herein.

Library of Congress Cataloging-in-Publication Data
Leifer, Gloria.
    Maternity nursing : an introductory text / Gloria Leifer. – Eleventh ed.
        p. ; cm.
    Includes bibliographical references and index.
    ISBN 978-1-4377-2209-3 (pbk. : alk. paper) 1. Maternity nursing. I. Title.
    [DNLM: 1. Maternal-Child Nursing. 2. Perinatal Care–methods. 3. Pregnancy
    Complications–nursing. 4. Pregnancy. WY 157.3]
    RG951.B87 2012
    618.2–dc23
                                                                    2011018052

Vice President and Publisher: Loren Wilson
Executive Editor: Teri Hines Burnham
Developmental Editor: Tiffany Trautwein
Publishing Services Managers: Deborah Vogel and Hemamalini Rajendrababu
Project Managers: Brandilyn Tidwell and Maria Bernard
Book Designer: Karen Pauls

Printed in Canada

Last digit is the print number: 9 8 7 6 5

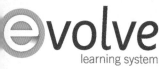
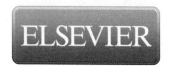
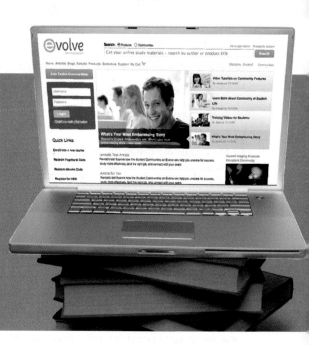

Evolve Student Resources

☀ ANIMATIONS

Chapter 2
Breasts
Female External Genitalia
Female Reproductive Ducts
Male External Genitalia
Menstrual Cycle
Ovarian Cycle
Ovarian Cyst
Ovarian Torsion
Ovaries
Ovulation
Spermatogenesis
Spermatozoa

Chapter 3
Fertilization to Implantation
Fetal Circulation
Fetal Development, First Trimester
Fetal Development, Second Trimester
Fetal Development, Third Trimester
Function of the Placenta
Maternal-Fetal Circulation
Oogenesis
Pregnancy Stages, Trimesters
Sex Determination

Chapter 7
Birth or Parturition
Fetal Hypoxia
Membrane Rupture
Normal Delivery
Placental Delivery

Chapter 13
Abruptio Placentae
Bleeding Complications
Ectopic Pregnancy
Placenta Previa
Rh Compatibility
Seizure in Pregnancy
Sickle Cell Anemia
Type 1 Diabetes
Type 2 Diabetes

Chapter 14
Breech Delivery, Arms
Breech Delivery, Face

Breech Presentation Examination
Breech Presentation with Sonogram
Cesarean Section
Postterm Pregnancy
Shoulder Dystocia
Umbilical Cord Prolapse

Chapter 20
Breast Cancer
Breast Cancer Metastasis
Pelvic Inflammatory Disease

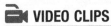 VIDEO CLIPS

Chapter 4
Breast
Chest Wall

Chapter 5
Abdomen Fundal Height

Chapter 6
Fetal Lie
Position
Presentation

Chapter 7
Fetal Heart Rate
Leopold First
Leopold Second
Leopold Third
Leopold Final
Normal Delivery

Chapter 9
Auscultation: Breath Sounds, Anterior Chest—Female Neonate
Auscultation: Heart, Anterior Chest—Female Neonate
Evaluation: Babinski Reflex—Male Infant
Evaluation: Cremasteric Reflex—Male Neonate
Evaluation: Cry—Female Neonate
Evaluation: Head Circumference—Male Neonate
Evaluation: Legs, Symmetry and Length—Male Neonate
Evaluation: Moro Reflex—Male Neonate
Evaluation: Motor Development—Male Infant
Evaluation: Motor Development (Sitting)—Male Infant
Evaluation: Plantar Grasp—Male Neonate
Evaluation: Rooting and Sucking Reflexes—Male Neonate

Inspection and Palpation: Genitalia (Supine Position)—Male Neonate

Inspection and Palpation: Head and Hair—Male Neonate

Inspection: Buttocks—Male Neonate

Inspection: Ear Canal—Male Infant

Inspection: External Eye—Male Neonate

Inspection: External Genitalia—Female Neonate

Inspection: Eye Alignment—Male Infant

Inspection: Head—Male Neonate

Inspection: Male Genitalia—Male Neonate

Inspection: Male Genitalia, Circumcision—Male Neonate

Inspection: Neck, Posterior—Male Neonate

Inspection: Oropharynx, Teeth, and Tongue—Female Infant

Inspection: Range-of-Motion, Upper Extremities—Male Neonate

Inspection: Tongue—Male Infant

Motor Development—Male Infant

Palpation: Abdomen—Male Neonate

Palpation: Femoral Pulses—Male Neonate

Palpation: Male Breasts (Spine Position)—Male Neonate

Percussion: Chest and Abdomen—Male Neonate

Chapter 14
Cesarean Section

PATIENT TEACHING PLANS IN ENGLISH AND SPANISH

Bathing Your Infant

Breastfeeding Your Infant

Breast Self-Exam

CALCULATORS

Body Mass Index (BMI)

Body Surface Area

Fluid Deficit

Glasgow Coma Scale

IV Dosage

Units Conversion

RESOURCES IN EVERY CHAPTER

Answers and Rationales for Review Questions for the NCLEX® Examination

Answer Guidelines for Critical Thinking Questions

Concept Map Creator

Fluids and Electrolytes Tutorial

Glossary with Pronunciations in English and Spanish

ADDITIONAL RESOURCES

Nutrient Requirements for Pregnancy

Sequence for Donning and Removing Personal Protective Equipment (PPE)

Standard Precautions and Body Substance Isolation Precautions

SKILLS PERFORMANCE CHECKLISTS

7-1 Auscultating Fetal Heart Rate
7-2 Determining Manual Fetal Heart Rate
7-3 Applying an External Fetal Monitor
7-4 Determining Contractions by Palpation
7-5 Performing Leopold's Maneuvers
7-6 Testing for the Presence of Aminotic Fluid (Nitrazine Paper Test)
7-7 Cleansing the Perineum Before Delivery
7-8 Administering Intramuscular Injections to the Newborn
7-9 Administering Eye Ointment to the Newborn
7-10 Assisting with an Emergency Birth
9-1 Taking the Axillary Temperature
9-2 Measuring the Fontanelles
10-1 Providing Umbilical Cord Care
10-2 Weighing and Measuring the Newborn
10-3 Bathing the Newborn
10-4 Suctioning with a Bulb Syringe
10-5 Swaddling the Newborn
11-1 Breastfeeding Techniques
11-2 Bottle Feeding the Infant
12-1 Assessing and Massaging the Uterine Fundus
12-2 Assessing Lochia
12-3 Assessing the Perineum
12-4 How to Perform Perineal Care
12-5 Assisting with a Sitz Bath
13-1 Blood Pressure Measurement During Pregnancy
13-2 Modification of Standard Cardiopulmonary Resuscitation (CPR) for Pregnant Women
14-1 Testing for the Presence of Amniotic Fluid (Nitrazine Paper Test)
15-1 Gavage Feeding
15-2 Kangaroo Care
16-1 Detecting Jaundice in the Newborn
16-2 Applying a Urine Collection Bag to a Newborn
19-1 How to Use a Male Condom Effectively
19-2 How to Use a Diaphragm Effectively
20-1 Breast Self-Examination

Dedicated to the memory of

Sarah Masseyaw Leifer
Nurse, Humanitarian, and Mother

And

Daniel Peretz Hartston
Pediatrician, Husband, and World Traveler

To the honor of

Barnet,
Heidi, Paul, and Ruby,
Amos, Gina, and Spencer,
Eve, David, Zoe, Elliot, and Ian

*Who remind me of the excitement and joys of parenthood
and the marvels of grandparenthood.*

Acknowledgments

A dedicated team effort is required to create and update a dynamic and useful textbook that will serve the student in a fast-paced LVN/LPN program and also provide the broad foundation necessary to enable application of concepts in an advanced LPN/LVN-to-ADN ladder program.

I am grateful to each member of the team who helped achieve the scope of revision of this text. This teamwork ensured the inclusion of the latest information essential for students to provide quality family care in the obstetric setting with critical thinking skills and cultural sensitivity. Readers, reviewers, practitioners, educators, and students provided many comments and suggestions that reinforced the preservation of unique aspects of this text, including the clarity of presentation that is so valuable to English as a second language (ESL) students with limited English proficiency. Their suggestions inspired the addition of many illustrated skills and techniques unique to the maternal-newborn specialty, supported by clear color photographs and drawings to enhance text content.

The enormous task of updating and adding essential new information while containing text size and cost was facilitated by the cooperation and dedication of the Elsevier editorial staff. Ilze Rader and Terri Wood, former nursing editors, will always be gratefully remembered for originally encouraging me concerning the joys of writing and introducing me to the Elsevier family. Teri Hines Burnham, the Executive Editor, met with me personally and challenged me to new heights of creative production. Tiffany Trautwein, the Developmental Editor, evidenced a commitment to excellence and detail and provided seamless communication, guidance, and support throughout the publication process. Brandi Tidwell, the Project Manager, provided me with editing advice and technical support and maintained the ongoing oversight necessary for the success of this project. Karen Pauls designed a book that was attractive to the eye and easy to read. Each member of the Elsevier team maintained close contact with me and each other, resulting in a seamless and successful product.

I would also like to thank those who personally enabled me to experience the joys of parenthood and grandparenthood while encouraging me to remain focused on this project. Heidi and Paul Epstein, Barnet Hartston, Eve and David Fleck, and Amos and Gina Hartston taught me how to survive the anxieties of parenthood, and my grandchildren, Zoe, Elliot, Ian, Ruby, and Spencer, contributed to the text as photographic models and also helped me develop insight and sensitivity to the role of a grandparent in the modern-day extended family.

The informal assistance of the staff of Loma Linda University Medical Center in Loma Linda, California; Riverside County Regional Medical Center in Moreno Valley, California; and the Southern California Kaiser Permanente Medical Center in Fontana, California, helped me to achieve the goals of this project.

Finally, and most important, I would like to thank my nursing students, past and present, from Fordham School of Nursing in New York City, Hunter College of the City University of New York, California State College in Los Angeles, and Riverside City College in Riverside, California, for helping me apply and redefine concepts of teaching and learning, thus enabling the creation of a text that will promote enthusiastic participation in the learning process and serve as both a learning tool and a professional resource.

Gloria Leifer Hartston

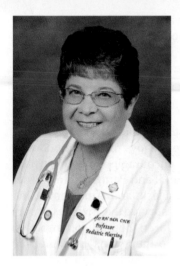

Professor Gloria Leifer embarked on her nursing career in 1958 and soon identified a special interest in teaching and curriculum development. She obtained a Master's degree in the Art of Teaching Maternal-Child Nursing from Columbia University in New York in 1968 and entered postmaster's study at Columbia University, specializing in curriculum development in nursing.

She taught obstetric and pediatric nursing at Hunter College of the City University of New York for 7 years until her marriage to a pediatrician brought her to California where she continued to teach obstetric and pediatric nursing at California State University at Los Angeles. For several years, she traveled extensively to developing countries with her pediatrician husband and studied patterns and problems related to obstetrics and pediatrics. She obtained a Radio Class license as a Ham Radio operator and attended classes at the Department of Homeland Security Training Center at College Station, Texas.

Her recent professional presentations include *Hospital Response to Mass Casualties* with renowned speaker and Israeli physician Itimar Ashkenazi, MD, and *Utilizing Learning Experiences within Our Environment* in conjunction with her development and planting of a "poison garden" and "allergy-free garden" on the campus of Riverside City College, which was designed for student and community health education.

She served as a consultant for the National Council of State Boards of Nursing as an Item Writer for the NCLEX® Examination for several years. For her teaching excellence, she received the coveted Caring Spirit Award, sponsored by Professional Hospital Supply, Johnson & Johnson, Inland Valley Hospitals, and the Press Enterprise newspaper. She is listed in the Strathmore *Who's Who in Nursing* and in *Who's Who in American Nursing* from the Society of Nursing Professionals.

Publications include Leifer, G. (1966). Symposium on the nurse and the ill child. *Nursing Clinics of North America, 1*(1), 1-121; Leifer, G. (1967). Rooming in despite complications. *The American Journal of Nursing, 67*(10), 2114-2120; Leifer, G., & Brown, M. (1997). Pediatric codes: A cheat sheet. *RN Journal, 60*(4), 30-35; Leifer, G. (2001). Hyperbaric oxygen therapy. *The American Journal of Nursing, 101*(8), 26-35; *Principles and Techniques in Pediatric Nursing* (published by W.B. Saunders from 1965 until 1982), which won a Book of the Year award from *The American Journal of Nursing*; and three textbooks currently published by Elsevier, including *Growth and Development Across the Lifespan: A Health Promotion Focus; Introduction to Maternity & Pediatric Nursing;* and *Maternity Nursing: An Introductory Text.* She has also written several chapters concerning reproductive health in *Medical-Surgical Nursing: Concepts & Practice* by Susan C. deWit.

Professor Leifer is a Certified Nurse Educator (CNE) and a full-time professor of obstetric and pediatric nursing at Riverside City College in Riverside, California.

Ancillary Contributors and Reviewers

ANCILLARY CONTRIBUTORS

Laura Bevlock Kanavy, RN, BSN, MSN
Instructor, Practical Nursing Program
Career Technology Center of Lackawanna
 County
Scranton, Pennsylvania
*Answers and Rationales for Review Questions for the
 NCLEX® Examination*
Study Guide

Trena L. Rich, RN, PHN, MSN, APRN, CIC
Director, Quality Assurance
Patient Care Center

Western University of Health Sciences
Pomona, California
*PowerPoint Slides with Audience Response System
 Questions*
TEACH Instructor Resource

Laura Travis, MSN, BSN, RN
Health Careers Coordinator
Tennessee Technology Center at Dickson
Dickson, Tennessee
Test Bank

REVIEWERS

Janis A. Baker, RN, BSN
Lead Instructor
Valley Baptist School of Vocational Nursing
Harlingen, Texas

Terry Bichsel, RN, BSN
Instructor, Allied Health Department
Moberly Area Community College
Moberly, Missouri

Miranda Burford, RN, BSN, MPH
Supervisor of Health Services
Lompoc Unified School District;
Director, Vocational Nursing Program
Lompoc Unified Adult Education
Lompoc, California

Katina M. Camp, RN
Instructor, Practical Nursing
Nursing and Allied Health
Southeast Arkansas College
Pine Bluff, Arkansas

Erin Hahs, RN
Nursing Instructor
Valley Baptist School of Vocational Nursing
Harlingen, Texas

Laura Bevlock Kanavy, RN, BSN, MSN
Instructor, Practical Nursing Program
Career Technology Center of Lackawanna County
Scranton, Pennsylvania

Donna Murry, RN, BS, MEd
Formerly Program Coordinator and Assistant
 Professor of Nursing
South Plains College
Plainview, Texas

Kendra S. Seiler, RN, MSN
Associate Professor, Nursing Division
Rio Hondo College
Whittier, California

Allison St. Clair, RN, MSN
Coordinator, Nursing
Summers County School of Practical Nursing
Hinton, West Virginia

Laura Travis, MSN, BSN, RN
Health Careers Coordinator
Tennessee Technology Center at Dickson
Dickson, Tennessee

LPN/LVN Advisory Board

Karin M. Allen, BSN, RN
Coordinator, Practical Nurse Program
Hutchinson Community College
McPherson, Kansas

Tawne D. Blackful, RN, MSN, MEd
Supervisor of Health Services and School Nurse
Lawrence Hall Youth Services
Chicago, Illinois

Barbara Carrig, BSN, MSN, APN
LPN Nurse Program Coordinator, Academic/Clinical
    Instructor
Passaic County Technical Institute
Wayne, New Jersey

Mary-Ann Cosagarea, RN, BSN
Practical Nursing Coordinator
Portage Lakes Career Center
W. Howard Nicol School of Practical Nursing
Uniontown, Ohio

Dolores Cotton, MSN, RN
Practical Nursing Coordinator
Meridian Technology Center
Stillwater, Oklahoma

Phyllis Del Mastro, RN, MSN
Corporate Director, Nursing
Porter and Chester Institute
Rocky Hill, Connecticut

Laurie F. Fontenot, BSN, RN
Department Head, Health Services Division
Acadiana Technical College – C.B. Coreil Campus
Ville Platte, Louisiana

Shelly R. Hovis, RN, MS
Director, Practical Nursing
Kiamichi Technology Centers
Antlers, Oklahoma

Janet M. Kane, RN, MSN
Director of Nursing
NewCourtland Education Center
Philadelphia, Pennsylvania

Patty Knecht, MSN, RN
Director of Practical Nursing
Center for Arts and Technology–Brandywine Campus
Coatesville, Pennsylvania

Joe Leija, MS, RN, DON
Director of Nursing, Vocational Nursing
RGV Careers
Pharr, Texas

Hana Malik, MSN, FNP-BC
Family Nurse Practitioner
Take Care Health Systems
Villa Park, Illinois

Barb McFall-Ratliff, MSN, RN
Director of Nursing, Program of Practical Nurse
    Education
Butler Technology and Career Development Schools
Hamilton, Ohio

Toni L.E. Pritchard, BSN, MSN, EdD
Allied Health Professor, Practical Nursing Program
Central Louisiana Technical College – Lamar Salter
    Campus
Leesville, Louisiana

Barbra Robins, BSN, MSN
Program Director
Leads School of Technology
New Castle, Delaware

Fleur de Liza S. Tobias-Cuyco, BSc, CPhT
College Dean, Director of Student Affairs,
    and Instructor
Preferred College of Nursing
Los Angeles, California

To the Instructor

ABOUT THE TEXT

The 11th edition of *Maternity Nursing: An Introductory Text* is designed to enable the LPN/LVN to provide safe, effective, and comprehensive nursing care to mothers, newborns, and their families in diverse settings; and to provide a broad foundation of knowledge, skills, concepts and practices. In years past, completion of the LPN/LVN program was considered a terminal certificate, but today many LPN/LVN programs are considered "ladders" into the associate degree nursing (ADN) program. Most LPN/LVN-to-ADN ladder programs do not include additional content classes or clinical practice in the specialty of maternal/newborn nursing, and this text will enable the graduate to apply advanced concepts to the broad foundation that it provides.

This edition builds upon the strong foundation of earlier editions. Some content has been condensed and streamlined to improve the flow and minimize repetition. Essential new content has been added to maintain a comprehensive presentation in an easy to read format. Emphasis remains focused on the role of the nurse in providing knowledgeable, safe, and evidenced-based patient care while using clinical critical thinking skills in common patient care situations. Information in the text includes the scientific basis of health promotion, illness prevention and dysfunction, and related nursing actions using the nursing process. Effective communication, unique obstetric skills, culturally specific nursing care, and patient teaching are highlighted throughout the text.

This text is also designed to bridge the gap between the classroom and the clinical arena by presenting current facts, concepts, and principles that promote learning through comprehension rather than memorization. With wellness of the mother and newborn, goals of *Healthy People 2020*, the Joint Commission's National Patient Safety Goals and Quality, and Safety Education for Nurses (QSEN) at its core, this text also provides a detailed understanding of health problems and disease processes related to maternity and newborn care and women's health. Some of the key teaching and learning features of this text are as follows:

- Childbearing is presented as a normal process and is followed by complications and their implications for preventive and therapeutic nursing care.
- The mother and newborn and the nuclear and extended family are portrayed as the patient.

- The nurse's role as a member of the multidisciplinary health care team is emphasized.
- Preventive nursing care in the community and complementary and alternative therapies are included with patient teaching suggestions and techniques that promote effective self-care.
- The nursing process is integrated throughout the text along with clinical pathways and care plans, which help the student apply the nursing process in the clinical arena.
- The integrated health care delivery system, which includes traditional and nontraditional products and practices requiring critical thinking in the daily nursing plan of care, is addressed.
- Past traditions are correlated with modern trends to inspire nurses to be prepared for rapid changes that will affect future care.
- Special attention to the learner with limited proficiency in English is provided by clear definitions of medical terminology and detailed, clear explanations of physiologic processes, medical and nursing interventions, and preventive techniques.
- In-depth concepts of maternal-newborn care are provided in a clear, readable format with an array of tables, figures, and special features (see pp. xiii-xiv) that enhance learning and retention.
- Key Concepts at the end of each chapter foster effective review for the practitioner who plans to reenter the specialty of maternal-newborn nursing.
- Review Questions for the NCLEX® Examination and Critical Thinking Questions are included in each chapter with Answers, Rationales, and Answer Guidelines available for the student on Evolve.
- Each chapter offers credible Online Resources for students to use to enhance their knowledge and critical thinking skills.
- Detailed, step-by-step Skills are presented throughout and include several icons that symbolize common steps for any skill in any area of general medical-surgical nursing—checking the order, introducing yourself, identifying the patient, performing hand hygiene, and so forth (see p. xiii).
- A complete updated bibliography and reference guide to provide the evidence-based source of the information contained in the text as well as sources to increase depth of information.

- A Multilingual Glossary of Symptoms (Appendix D) helps the student to communicate in 14 different languages with non-English speaking patients.

LPN THREADS

The 11th edition of *Maternity Nursing: An Introductory Text* shares some feature and design elements with other Elsevier LPN/LVN textbooks. The purpose of these *LPN Threads* is to make it easier for students and instructors to use the variety of books required by the relatively brief and demanding LPN/LVN curriculum. The following features are included in the *LPN Threads*.

- A **reading level evaluation** is performed on every manuscript chapter during the book's development to increase the consistency among chapters and ensure the text is easy to understand.
- The **full-color design, cover, photos,** and **illustrations** are visually appealing and pedagogically useful.
- **Objectives** (numbered) begin each chapter and provide a framework for content and are especially important in providing the structure for the TEACH Lesson Plans for the textbook.
- **Key Terms** with phonetic pronunciations and page number references are listed at the beginning of each chapter. Key terms appear in color in the chapter and are defined briefly, with full definitions in the **Glossary.** The goal is to help the student reader with limited proficiency in English to develop a greater command of the pronunciation of scientific and nonscientific English terminology.
- A wide variety of **special features** relate to critical thinking, clinical practice, health promotion, safety, patient teaching, complementary and alternative therapies, communication, home health care, delegation and assignment, and more. Refer to the To the Student section of this introduction on pp. xiii to xiv for descriptions and examples of features from the pages of this textbook.
- **Critical Thinking Questions** presented at the ends of chapters and with Nursing Care Plans give students opportunities to practice critical thinking and clinical decision-making skills with realistic patient scenarios. Answers are provided on the Evolve website.
- **Key Points** at the end of each chapter correlate to the objectives and serve as a useful chapter review.
- A full suite of **Instructor Resources** is available on the Evolve website, including TEACH Lesson Plans, Lecture Outlines, PowerPoint Slides, Test Bank, Image Collection, and Open-Book Quizzes.
- In addition to consistent content, design, and support resources, these textbooks benefit from the advice and input of the **Elsevier LPN/LVN Advisory Board (see p. x).**

TEACHING AND LEARNING PACKAGE

FOR THE INSTRUCTOR

The comprehensive and free *Evolve Resources with TEACH Instructor Resource* include the following:

- **Test Bank** with approximately 700 multiple-choice and alternate-format questions with topic, step of the nursing process, objective, cognitive level, NCLEX® category of client needs, correct answer, rationale, and textbook page reference.
- **TEACH Instructor Resource** with Lesson Plans, Lecture Outlines, and PowerPoint slides—with Audience Response System questions embedded—that correlate each text and ancillary component.
- **Image Collection** that contains all the illustrations and photographs in the textbook.
- **Answer Keys** for Open-Book Quizzes and the Study Guide.

FOR THE STUDENT

The *Evolve Student Resources* include the following assets:

- **Animations** depicting anatomy, physiology, and procedures.
- **Answers and Rationales** for Review Questions for the NCLEX® Examination.
- **Answer Guidelines** for Critical Thinking Questions.
- **Audio Glossary** with pronunciations in English and Spanish.
- **Calculators** for determining body mass index (BMI), body surface area, fluid deficit, Glasgow coma score, IV dosages, and conversion of units.
- **Fluids and Electrolytes Tutorial.**
- **Patient Teaching Plans** in English and Spanish.
- **Skills Performance Checklists** for all Skills in the textbook.
- **Video clips** of patient assessment, vaginal birth, and cesarean birth.

The in-text *Study Guide* is a valuable supplement to help students understand and apply the content. *Multiple Choice* questions, *Clinical Situation* case studies with critical thinking questions, and *Group Internet Activities* provide students with various learning tools for reinforcement and exploration of text material. The Study Guide includes text page number references for each question, and an Answer Key is provided for instructors on the Evolve website.

To the Student

READING AND REVIEW TOOLS

- **Objectives** introduce the chapter topics.
- **Key Terms** are listed with page number references; and difficult medical, nursing, or scientific terms are accompanied by simple phonetic pronunciations. Key terms are considered essential to understanding chapter content and are defined within the chapter. Key terms are in color the first time they appear in the narrative and are briefly defined in the text, with complete definitions in the Glossary.
- Each chapter ends with a *Get Ready for the NCLEX® Examination!* **section** that includes: (1) **Key Points** that reiterate the chapter objectives and serve as a useful review of concepts; (2) a list of **Additional Resources** including the Study Guide, Evolve Resources, and Online Resources; (3) an extensive set of **Review Questions for the NCLEX® Examination** with answers located in Appendix G and Answers and Rationales on Evolve; and (4) **Critical Thinking Questions** with Answer Guidelines located on Evolve.
- A complete **Bibliography and Reader References** in the back of the text cite evidence-based information and provide resources for enhancing knowledge.

CHAPTER FEATURES

Skills are presented in a logical format with *purpose,* relevant *illustrations,* and clearly defined and numbered nursing *steps.* Each Skill includes icons that serve as a reminder to perform the basic steps applicable to *all* nursing interventions:

 Check orders.

 Gather necessary equipment and supplies.

 Introduce yourself.

 Check patient's identification.

 Provide privacy.

 Explain the procedure/intervention.

 Perform hand hygiene.

 Don gloves (if applicable).

It is essential that you understand the importance of these steps and know when to perform them. The actions that these icons represent must be considered before performing any intervention; however, you must use critical thinking and consider agency protocol to determine the specific supplies and equipment you may need and decide when it is necessary to don gloves.

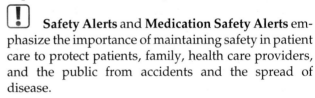

Nursing Care Plans, developed around specific case studies, include nursing diagnoses with an emphasis on patient goals and outcomes and questions to promote **critical thinking.**

Safety Alerts and **Medication Safety Alerts** emphasize the importance of maintaining safety in patient care to protect patients, family, health care providers, and the public from accidents and the spread of disease.

Health Promotion boxes emphasize healthy lifestyle choices, preventive behaviors, and screening tests.

Medication tables provide quick access to information about medications commonly used in maternity nursing care.

Cultural Considerations explore select specific cultural preferences and how to address the needs of a culturally diverse patient and family.

Nutrition Considerations provide important nutrition information for infants and women before pregnancy, during pregnancy, and while breastfeeding.

Patient Teaching boxes help develop awareness of the vital role of patient and family teaching in health care today.

(Continued)

Communication boxes focus on strategies for therapeutic communication.

Legal and Ethical Considerations present pertinent information about the legal issues and ethical dilemmas that may face the practicing nurse.

Memory Joggers provide easy-to-remember mnemonics and acronyms for recalling specific information.

Did You Know? boxes present interesting—and sometimes surprising—facts related to maternity nursing care.

Evidence-Based Practice boxes present research evidence and highlight its influence on nursing care.

Animations depicting anatomy, physiology, and procedures available on Evolve are referenced with icons in the margins where applicable.

Video clips portraying patient assessment, vaginal birth, and cesarean birth available on Evolve are referenced with icons in the margins where applicable.

Contents

APPENDIXES

chapter

Contemporary Maternity Care, Family, and Cultural Considerations

1

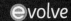

Objectives

1. Define key terms listed.
2. Compare two current birth settings for women.
3. Review how technology and research have influenced maternal-infant care.
4. Discuss the Human Genome Project in relation to the development of gene therapy.
5. Contrast a nursing care plan with a clinical pathway.
6. Identify the role of the nurse in the community-based setting.
7. State the influence of the federal government on maternity care.
8. List two reasons that statistics are important in maternal-infant care.
9. Discuss how standards of care influence nursing.
10. Explain evidence-based practice.
11. Recall three major components of communication.
12. Recognize the importance of documentation.
13. Illustrate the HIPAA rights of patients.
14. Discuss the five steps in the nursing process.
15. Define *critical thinking* and illustrate its use in nursing and in test taking.
16. Discuss how examining one's own culture can affect the care of a patient during the labor and delivery process.
17. Contrast defining characteristics of four family types.
18. Contrast complementary and alternative health care with conventional health care.
19. Illustrate the role of the nurse in alternative or complementary health care.

Key Terms

alternative therapies (p. 14)
birthing centers (p. 2)
certified nurse-midwives (p. 3)
clinical pathways (p. 3)
collaborative care (p. 3)
complementary therapies (p. 14)
critical thinking (p. 9)
culture (p. 11)
documentation (p. 8)
evidence-based practice (p. 8)

family (p. 13)
integrative health care (p. 14)
managed care (p. 3)
maternity nursing care (p. 1)
nursing care plans (p. 9)
nursing process (p. 9)
Quality and Safety Education for Nurses (QSEN) (p. 7)
standards of care (p. 5)
variances (p. 4)

MATERNITY NURSING CARE

DEFINITION AND GOALS

Maternity nursing care is viewed as the care, support, instruction, and health promotion given by the nurse to the expectant woman, partner, and family during pregnancy, during labor, and after birth (the postpartum period). Maternity nursing is unique in that, for 9 months of pregnancy through birth, the caregiver's attention is focused almost equally on two people: the expectant mother and the fetus or newborn infant. In principle and practice, maternity nursing emphasizes the integrity of the family unit and considers childbearing to be a normal physiologic process. Wellness is an overriding concern, with symptoms and complications being treated if they occur.

The strength of a society rests on the health of its mothers, infants, and families. The nurse's investment in health promotion during the childbearing process can make a significant difference, not only for women and their infants, but also for society.

The goal of maternity nursing care is for the expectant woman's pregnancy, labor, and birth to be as uneventful (normal) as possible, with the additional goal of ensuring the well-being of the newborn infant. In addition, most health care consumers want a satisfying, family-centered, and meaningful experience that meets their needs and expectations. More specific goals of maternity nursing care are found in Box 1-1.

Box 1-1   Goals of Maternity Nursing Care

- Ensure the health of the woman during pregnancy, labor, birth, and the postpartum period.
- Help the expectant woman view pregnancy, labor, and birth as normal physiologic processes.
- Provide adequate support to make pregnancy a positive, gratifying experience.
- Provide adequate instruction to the expectant woman during pregnancy, labor, birth, and the postpartum period.
- Be sensitive to the expectant woman's social, spiritual, and economic needs.
- Assist in the early detection of deviations from the normal process of fetal development and maternal health.
- Encourage the parent-newborn attachment process.

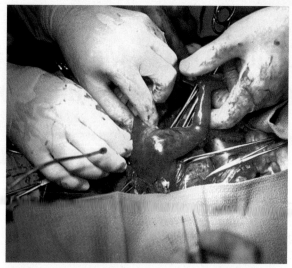

FIGURE 1-1 Fetal surgery can be performed to correct a congenital defect before birth. Fetal surgery usually does not result in a scar at the incision site.

CURRENT TRENDS

Birth Settings

Health care consumers expect their childbirth experience to occur in "natural" surroundings. To meet this expectation, many hospitals have developed modified birth settings. The most common is the labor, delivery, and recovery (LDR) room, where normal birth and recovery take place in one setting. The woman may be transferred to a postpartum unit, but the newborn will usually remain with her. Some hospitals offer rooms in which women can remain throughout the postpartum experience (a labor, delivery, recovery, and postpartum [LDRP] room). In these settings, the family is encouraged to stay with the mother overnight, and nursing and medical care is available if an emergency arises. In addition, breastfeeding is encouraged, and the mother and father (or partner) are encouraged to bond with the new infant.

Freestanding birthing centers are an alternative for parents seeking a homelike atmosphere. Some of these settings have conveniences, such as a kitchen for family members, but many freestanding birthing centers do not have adequate technology and medical care readily available if complications to the mother or fetus arise.

Federal legislation has been passed that enables women who have a vaginal birth to stay in the birth facility for 24 to 48 hours and women who have a cesarean birth to stay for 72 hours. Home births in the United States represent only a small number of births because malpractice insurance for midwives attending home births is expensive and difficult to obtain. Many midwives have moved their practice to hospitals or birthing centers.

Technology and Maternity Care

Technologic advances such as high-flow oxygen ventilation machines, 3-D ultrasonography, and genetic testing have enabled many infants to survive who years ago might have died. Intrauterine fetal surgery is being performed on a more routine basis (Figure 1-1), and

high-risk prenatal clinics and neonatal intensive care units (NICUs) provide care that the at-risk fetus and preterm infant need to survive. Chromosomal studies and biochemical engineering have made the identification of congenital anomalies and genetic counseling available to families who are at high risk for particular conditions. Cord blood, which is rich in stem cells, can be taken from a newborn at birth. This blood can be banked or stored for later use if certain disorders arise.

Human Genome Project

The Human Genome Project is an international effort to identify and "map" all genetic material present in the human body. The genes responsible for diseases such as cystic fibrosis, fragile X syndrome, and breast cancer have been isolated and identified. The findings of the Human Genome Project may enable gene therapy to replace missing genes or alter defective genes, thus eliminating the cause of many genetic disorders. The technique of inserting new or replacement genes into the human body has been developed, but social issues still need to be resolved before it becomes a routine medical practice.

Gender Selection

Gender selection itself is not a new practice. Pregnancies have been terminated when the sex of the fetus was not the "right one," and some newborns have been abandoned or killed if they were not of the desired sex. The ability to determine and select the sex of the fetus before conception places an end to inhumane practices, but the impact on the population and society needs to be more fully researched. Gender selection of the fetus can be accomplished by sperm separation. For example, sperm carrying the Y chromosome can be identified and used for the fertilization of an ovum to produce a male child. A couple may desire a child of a specific sex to avoid passing on a genetic disorder that affects a specific sex only or because the couple already has several children of one sex and now wants a child of the opposite sex. Moral and ethical issues abound with this technology.

Global Genetics Therapy

According to the World Health Organization (WHO), more than 7 million children throughout the world are born annually with severe genetic disorders or birth defects, with 90% occurring in developing countries (Callister, 2006). It is known that specific cultural and ethnic groups and specific geographic locations are associated with specific genetic disorders. For example, persons of African, Greek, Italian, and Middle Eastern ancestries may be at risk for inherited thalassemia, a type of anemia. The African ethnic group may be at increased risk for sickle cell anemia, and the Ashkenazi Jewish population may be at increased risk for inherited Tay-Sachs disease. Preconception genetic testing can reduce the occurrence of these genetic disorders, and, in the near future, gene therapy may be able to treat many genetic defects. Newborn screening is already standard procedure in most countries. The integration of genetics in general health care worldwide is a goal of the international health organizations. The WHO is helping develop standards and regulations to deal with the social and ethical issues, including informed consent and confidentiality.

Providers of Maternity Care

Maternal-newborn health care professionals include certified nurse-midwives (CNMs); registered professional nurses who have completed an advanced program approved by the American College of Nurse-Midwives; and **nurse practitioners,** registered nurses who have completed a master's program, including the area of women's health, and are certified by a national credentialing organization, such as the American Nurses Credentialing Center (ANCC). **Obstetricians/gynecologists** are licensed physicians who have completed a residency program that specializes in the diseases related to women and the care of pregnant women and their fetuses throughout pregnancy, labor, childbirth, and the postpartum period. **Pediatricians** are licensed physicians who have completed a residency program that specializes in pediatrics and are responsible for the diagnosis, treatment, and well-being of infants and children. **Neonatologists** are pediatricians who have received additional preparation, training, and board certification in the care of neonates (newborns from birth to age 28 days).

Several other health care professionals may assist in maternal-infant health care and in meeting the family's needs. **Geneticists** may provide testing and counseling for families at risk for genetically determined disorders.

Social workers may be asked to find assistance for families in financial need. **Dietitians** may educate the family about nutrition and infant feeding. **Lactation specialists** help new mothers initiate breastfeeding.

Together, all of these health care providers work toward collaborative care. Collaborative care involves working together cooperatively, sharing the responsibilities for solving problems, and making decisions about patient care. The focus is on multidisciplinary care, which may include a licensed practical nurse/licensed vocational nurse (LPN/LVN), registered nurse, physician, nutritionist, and social worker. Collaboration among the health care team, the patient, and the family can increase the satisfaction among all participants, facilitate the provision of appropriate health care, and assist in meeting patient goals. As a part of this team, the nurse is a key member in making referrals to appropriate resources.

Health Care Delivery Systems

It is estimated that 15.9% of the U.S. gross domestic product was spent on health care in 2010. Thus, there has been concerted effort by the government, insurance companies, hospitals, and health care providers to control the ever-increasing costs of health care. One way that insurance companies and institutions have attempted to control these costs is through the use of diagnosis-related groups (DRGs), which is the basis of financial compensation through Medicare, in which a fixed amount of money is determined in advance for providing necessary services for specifically diagnosed conditions. If the hospital spends more on a patient than the specific diagnosis allows, the hospital typically absorbs the excess cost. If the hospital spends less than what is allowed for a patient with a specific diagnosis, the hospital usually keeps the profit. This type of plan provides incentives to decrease the average length of stay in the hospital, thereby reducing the cost of service.

Managed Care. Some health insurance companies have examined the cost of health care and instituted a health care delivery system called managed care. Examples of managed care organizations are **health maintenance organizations (HMOs),** which provide total health care for members. Most of the cost savings come from efforts to reduce hospitalization days and hospital admissions. **Preferred provider organizations (PPOs)** contract with a network of providers (physicians and hospitals) to provide services at a discounted rate to members. Patients may use non-PPO providers, but they must pay those expenses out of pocket. Monthly payment premiums are required in managed care health plans.

Clinical Pathways. Clinical pathways are also known as care paths, care maps, case management plans, coordinated care plans, clinical guidelines, and outcome management. Clinical pathways are maps of collaborative care given by the interdisciplinary health care team. The pathways are designed from evidence-based standards of care concerning the expected progress and timelines for specific patient diagnoses. This approach provides research-based care rather than tradition-based care. Clinical pathways include independent nursing assessments, teaching, and interventions; medical orders given by physicians or other health care providers, such as nurse practitioners; and recommendations by nutritionists, social workers, or other community agencies involved in the patient's care. These pathways also provide information regarding the patient's expected progress each day.

By stating the specific care and progress of a patient within a specified timeline that is related to a planned outcome, health care providers can clearly identify and address any deviations. These deviations from the expected timelines are called variances. If the patient's progress is slower than expected or the outcome (goal) is not achieved within the set timeline, a negative variance occurs, and the length of stay in the hospital may be increased. Identification of variances helps nurses reorganize the care plan to meet individual patient needs.

The use of clinical pathways improves the quality of care and reduces hospitalization time. Clinical pathways are an essential component of managed care that promotes coordination of the health care team, resulting in high-quality patient care delivered in a more cost-effective time frame. The nurse documents the care on the clinical pathway and reports any variances to the charge nurse or physician. Selected examples of clinical pathways are presented in chapters concerning postpartum care, newborn care, and breastfeeding.

Community-Based Nursing

Nursing care within the community and in the home is not a new concept in maternal-child nursing. The work of Lillian Wald, founder of the Henry Street Settlement in New York City, brought home health care to poor children. Margaret Sanger's work as a public health nurse provided care for poor pregnant women and was the seed for the development of today's Planned Parenthood programs. The community is now one of the major health care settings for all patients, and the challenge is to provide safe, caring, cost-effective, high-quality care to mothers, infants, and families. This challenge involves the nurse as a patient advocate in influencing the government, businesses, and the community to recognize the need for supporting preventive care of maternal-infant patients, thereby ensuring a healthy population for the future.

The nurse must work with the interdisciplinary health care team to identify needs within the community and to create cost-effective approaches to comprehensive preventive and therapeutic care. The nurse's

role as an educator within the community is facilitated by the use of schools, churches, health fairs, Internet websites, and the media. Some registered nurses are branching out into the community as private practitioners, such as lactation consultants for new mothers. The nursing care plan is expanding to become a family care plan because the nurse provides care to the patient in the home. Creativity, problem solving, coordination of multidisciplinary caregivers, case management, assessment, and referral are just some of the essential skills required of a nurse providing community-based care to maternal-infant patients.

Preventive care is only one aspect of current and future home care and community-based nursing. Therapeutic care is also provided in the home setting, and the nurse must educate the family concerning monitoring, care, and need for professional referral when necessary. Specialized care such as fetal monitoring of high-risk pregnant women, apnea monitoring of high-risk newborns, diabetic glucose monitoring, heparin therapy, and total parenteral nutrition can be safely accomplished in the home setting, often with computer or telephone accessibility to a nurse case manager (see Chapter 18).

The home health care team, as advocated by the American Academy of Pediatrics Committee on Children with Disabilities, includes a pediatrician; licensed nurses; occupational, physical, and respiratory therapists; speech therapists; home teachers; social workers; and home health aides. The American Academy of Home Care Physicians has expressed a medical commitment to the concept of home care for the future.

Specific Government Influences in Maternal-Infant Care

Government involvement in maternal-newborn care is designed to reduce maternal and infant morbidity and mortality rates. The National Institutes of Health (NIH) supports and provides funds for maternity research and education. The Title V amendment of the Public Health Service Act established maternity-infant care centers in public clinics. Title XIX of the Medicaid program provides care for indigent women. The Center for Family Planning provides contraception information, and the Women, Infants, and Children (WIC) program provides supplemental food and education for those in need. The Medicaid program assists in funding care for eligible women and children who cannot afford to pay health insurance premiums.

Senators, representatives, and others in the federal government designed a health care reform plan to reduce the cost of health care while making it more accessible to all. Nurses are involved in the health care reform movement as patient advocates to ensure that the patient receives high-quality care. Health insurance plays an important role in health care delivery. However, having health insurance has not always assured access to appropriate care because the insurance company often had to approve the expenditure before the test or care was provided. Those families who cannot afford health insurance often did not seek preventive health care, such as prenatal care, infant immunizations, and well-baby checkups. This can lead to a number of undiagnosed or improperly treated health conditions. These types of problems are dealt with as health care reform evolves.

The Heath Care Reform Bill of 2010 expanded coverage to millions of Americans who were previously uninsured. Some provisions were immediately effective in 2010, some will be effective in 2012, and all provisions will be fully effective by 2014. Children will not be denied insurance because of preexisting conditions and can stay on their parents' policy until age 26. Payment for the plan will come from a Medicare payroll tax on investment income and some unearned income by 2012 and a special 3.8% tax on individuals earning more than $200,000. In 2018, an excise tax will be paid by insurance companies with high-end health care plans.

Healthy People 2020. *Healthy People 2020* is the U.S. contribution to the WHO's Health for All plan. National health objectives are periodically developed and published in a document titled, *Healthy People*. Each document is a decade-long action agenda with goals to improve the health of all Americans. *Healthy People 2020* (U.S. Department of Health and Human Services [USDHHS], 2010) establishes national health goals and identifies the greatest preventable threats to our nation's health. The two main goals identified for 2020 are to (1) increase years of healthy life and (2) eliminate health disparities. These broad goals are supported by four subgoals, which are to (1) promote healthy behaviors, (2) protect health, (3) provide access to high-quality health care, and (4) strengthen community prevention and provide access to care.

The USDHHS has developed national objectives covering all areas of health and the environment. *Healthy People 2020* focuses on population-based health planning and stresses the importance of improving the public health infrastructure. State health departments must assess their residents' health status and the existing resources and provide this information to the USDHHS. The state and local communities use this information to develop action plans that contribute to families' and individuals' behaviors and lifestyles to achieve and maintain healthy lives. See Chapter 18 for a detailed listing of *Healthy People 2020* goals relating to maternal-newborn care.

Statistics Important to Maternal and Newborn Care. Health professionals need to obtain information about the way maternity care is given and the outcomes of maternal and newborn care. One way they can do this is by looking at statistics (Table 1-1). In the United States, it is a legal requirement in all 50 states and the District of Columbia to have a birth certificate completed for every infant born alive. The birth certificate is registered with the local government, and a state report is ultimately sent to the National Office of Vital Statistics. These statistics are important because they depict the health status of the nation's women and children. This information helps the government allocate resources to various identified needs. The outcomes of pregnancies in different states and counties can be compared; these outcomes generally show that maternal and infant mortality rates fall when the overall health of the people improves. Current statistics show that health care improvement must be directed toward having healthy babies (Box 1-2).

Standards of Care

Standards of care establish minimum criteria for competent nursing care. They are designed to protect the public and are used to judge the quality of care provided. Legal interpretation of actions within the standards of care is based on what a reasonable nurse with similar education and work experience would do in like circumstances. Sources that have provided standards of care include the American Nurses Association (ANA); the ANA Divisions of Practice; and organizations such as the Association of Women's Health, Obstetric and Neonatal Nurses (AWHONN). The Joint Commission (TJC) (formerly the Joint Commission on Accreditation of Healthcare Organizations [JCAHO]) and federal and state governments establish minimum standards that hospitals must meet to receive accreditation, licensing, funding, and approval to continue providing patient care.

National Patient Safety Goals. National Patient Safety Goals (NPSGs) established by the Joint Commission are updated annually and include:
- Ensure accurate patient identification with a minimum of two identifiers, such as name and date of birth.
- Ensure effective communication among caregivers and a timely report of critical test results.
- Improve the safety of medication labeling with name, expiration date, strength, etc.
- Reduce health–care-associated infections. Use the Centers for Disease Control and Prevention (CDC) hand hygiene guidelines.
- Provide medication reconciliation protocols.
- Identify patients at risk for falls and self-harm.
- Use universal protocol for preventing wrong patient, site, or procedure for surgery.
- Use list of "do not use" abbreviations.
- Encourage active patient involvement.
- Prevent pressure ulcers.
- Have organizations identify safety risks inherent in their patient population.

| Table 1-1 | Birth Rate Statistics in the United States, 2002 to 2006 |

AREA	LIVE BIRTHS 2006	LIVE BIRTHS 2002	INFANT MORTALITY 2005	EARLY PRENATAL CARE 2002-2004	LOW BIRTH WEIGHT 2003-2006
Alabama	63,235	58,599	8.96	83.7	10.35
Alaska	10,991	9,939	6.45	80.2	6.02
Arizona	102,475	87,889	6.69	76.5	7.05
Arkansas	40,973	37,833	8.29	81.1	9.04
California	562,431	529,420	5.22	87.0	6.71
Colorado	70,750	68,289	6.27	79.5	9.04
Connecticut	41,807	42,613	5.53	88.1	7.74
Delaware	11,998	11,151	9.00	85.6	9.31
District of Columbia	8,529	7,622	9.22	76.8	11.06
Florida	236,882	205,541	7.4	No data	8.59
Georgia	148,619	133,664	8.35	84.2	9.27
Hawaii	18,982	17,424	6.67	82.7	8.23
Idaho	24,184	20,936	6.12	No data	6.65
Illinois	180,583	180,197	7.53	85.3	8.40
Indiana	88,674	85,367	7.87	81.2	8.10
Iowa	40,610	36,674	5.40	88.7	6.92
Kansas	40,964	40,328	7.12	87.0	7.28
Kentucky	58,291	54,216	6.79	No data	8.86
Louisiana	63,399	64,841	9.79	84.5	11.02
Maine	14,151	13,558	5.87	87.9	6.58
Maryland	77,478	73,381	8.0	83.4	9.17
Massachusetts	77,769	80,844	4.89	89.8	7.77
Michigan	127,476	129,951	8.02	85.9	8.28
Minnesota	73,559	68,213	4.78	86.1	6.43
Mississippi	46,069	41,512	10.74	84.4	11.62
Missouri	81,388	74,368	7.63	88.2	8.12
Montana	12,506	11,033	6.35	83.8	7.02
Nebraska	26,733	25,166	5.89	83.2	6.97
Nevada	40,085	32,392	5.86	75.6	8.11
New Hampshire	14,380	14,439	5.02	No data	6.65
New Jersey	115,006	114,913	5.44	79.8	8.19
New Mexico	29,937	27,715	6.13	69.1	8.38
New York	250,091	257,940	6.02	No data	8.11
North Carolina	127,841	117,084	8.58	84.3	9.07
North Dakota	8,622	7,677	6.35	86.4	6.49
Ohio	150,590	148,486	7.82	87.8	8.51
Oklahoma	54,018	50,341	7.86	77.6	7.92
Oregon	48,717	45,094	5.68	81.1	6.09
Pennsylvania	149,082	140,898	7.30	No data	8.20
Rhode Island	12,379	12,682	6.20	90.2	8.12
South Carolina	62,271	54,501	9.03	No data	10.15
South Dakota	11,917	10,843	7.18	78.0	6.71
Tennessee	84,345	77,534	8.87	No data	9.35

Table 1-1 Birth Rate Statistics in the United States, 2002 to 2006—cont'd

AREA	LIVE BIRTHS 2006	LIVE BIRTHS 2002	INFANT MORTALITY 2005	EARLY PRENATAL CARE 2002-2004	LOW BIRTH WEIGHT 2003-2006
Texas	399,012	368,481	6.45	81.1	8.07
Utah	53,499	49,244	4.92	79.9	6.68
Vermont	6,509	6,392	5.37	89.8	6.57
Virginia	107,817	99,701	7.50	85.4	8.23
Washington	86,848	79,152	53.9	No data	6.13
West Virginia	20,928	20,404	7.73	85.9	9.16
Wisconsin	72,335	68,455	6.34	84.9	6.93
Wyoming	7,670	6,520	6.95	85.5	8.71

Data from Health, United States (2007) with chart book on trends in the health of Americans and *National Vital Statistics Report 52(19)*. Retrieved May 9, 2009, from www.cdc.gov/nchs/data/hus/hus06trend.pdf.

Box 1-2 Maternal-Infant Statistics

Birth rate: Number of live births in 1 year per 1000 population
Infant mortality rate: Number of deaths of infants younger than 1 year per 1000 live births
Maternal mortality rate: Number of maternal deaths per 100,000 live births that occur as a direct result of pregnancy (including the 42-day postpartum period)
Neonatal mortality rate: Number of deaths of infants younger than 28 days per 1000 live births per year
Perinatal mortality rate: Number of fetal deaths (20 weeks' gestation or more) and number of neonatal deaths per 1000 live births per year
Fetal mortality rate: Number of fetal deaths (fetuses weighing 500 g [1 lb] or more) per 1000 live births per year
Stillbirth: A newborn who, at birth, demonstrates no signs of life, such as breathing, heartbeat, or voluntary muscle movements

The Institute of Medicine (IOM) established Quality and Safety Education for Nurses (QSEN) competencies for nurses, which are the basis of nursing knowledge, skills, and attitudes taught in schools of nursing. The broad competencies include patient-centered care, teamwork and collaboration, evidence-based practice, safety, and informatics. Details can be accessed at www.qsen.org (NLN, 2008).

The emergence of technology in the hospital setting is thought to promote patient safety, and technologic tools are being integrated into the nursing process. Information technology improves communication between caregivers and prevents medication errors (The Joint Commission, 2010). Electronic health records starting in the prenatal ambulatory care setting provide a continuum of care record that is easily accessible at any point in the perinatal cycle by any member of the multidisciplinary health care team. A computerized

medication reconciliation process and an "intelligent IV pump" can reduce medication errors and are in current use at many hospitals. Caution must be taken not to override any computerized system without proper authorization. Some common acronyms used in information technology are shown in Box 1-3.

Nurses are also responsible for practicing according to the accepted standards of their state, and nursing actions must meet the nurse practice acts of that state. The California Board of Vocational Nursing and Psychiatric Technicians (BVNPT) and the National Federation of Licensed Practical Nurses (NFLPN) are examples of organizations for LPNs/LVNs that describe their role in clinical practice today. All nurses should familiarize themselves with their state's nurse practice acts.

Although some standards are not legally based, they carry important legal significance. A nurse who fails to provide the expected standards of care invites legal allegations of negligence or malpractice. The intent of standards of care, care plans, critical pathways, and written procedures is to provide a measure against which a nurse can compare his or her practice, assess patients' responses, and compile the required documentation that the appropriate care was provided, thus minimizing any legal and ethical problems that may arise.

Box 1-3 Acronyms Used in Information Technology

ADE: Adverse drug event
ADU: Automated drug-dispensing unit
BCMA: Bar code medication administration
CPOE: Computerized provider order entry (physician's order)
EHR: Electronic health record
EMAR: Electronic medication administration record
POC: Point of care
PRBC: Pump readable bar code

Legal and Ethical Considerations

Documentation

For legal purposes, if the nurse does not document an intervention, then the intervention was not done!

Evidence-Based Practice. Evidence-based practice refers to the use of research data in the design of a care plan. AWHONN standards of practice in the care of women and newborns include an evidence-based approach to practice. Nursing journals publish the results of studies about nursing practice. Evidence from these research studies is the basis of modifications in the approach to care, procedures, and practices. The *Cochrane Pregnancy and Childbirth Group* disseminates reviews of current clinical research in maternal and child care.

Communication

Effective communication is an important nursing skill that is essential in promoting positive interpersonal relationships. Communication is the process of exchanging ideas, beliefs, thoughts, and feelings; it involves both verbal and nonverbal language. Nonverbal language can be conveyed through symbols, actions, gestures, smiles, frowns, or body postures.

Three major components of communication are listening, observation, and documentation. A good listener can provide reassurance and respect. Through observation of words and nonverbal language, the nurse can pick up subtle cues of how the patient perceives the nurse-patient relationship and mutual exchange of ideas. Therapeutic communication is a skill that is learned through practice. This level of communication requires the nurse to be open-minded, honest, and nonjudgmental. Reporting is a form of oral communication among health care workers that can summarize the status and care of patients. Status reports are usually given at the end of each shift to ensure smooth continuity of care. Oral reporting enhances documentation found in the individual patient's chart but does not replace it.

SBAR. SBAR is a technique of structured communication between health care team members that is designed to reduce errors of miscommunication, improve patient safety, and provide a more concise method of communicating to other health care providers about the patient's condition. This structured technique of communication can be used at the shift change report, during the transfer of patients, or during the reporting of a critical change of condition to the health care provider. It includes:

Situation: Patient identification, vital signs, and nursing concerns

Background: Patient's mental status, skin condition, oxygen needs, and updated medications and critical laboratory values list

Assessment: Description of nursing assessment of the patient

Recommendations: Health care provider's response to the report received

The SBAR communication tool is in compliance with The Joint Commission Patient Safety Goals and is currently used in many hospitals across the country.

Documentation. Documentation in nursing is the written communication of nursing care in the form of charting, recording, and reporting. Nursing notes and flow sheets may be used. Standardized nursing notes are becoming more common in hospital settings, especially in a 24-hour flow sheet format. Computerized documentation in the form of clinical record systems is also used. Documentation is important because it verifies nursing interventions, patient responses, and the involvement of the multidisciplinary health care team in the provision of patient care. Accurate and detailed documentation helps identify whether standards of care are met and often provides a basis of legal protection for the nurse when quality of care is challenged.

Patient Privacy and HIPAA Rights. Patient privacy is protected by federal law and regulated by accrediting agencies. The Privacy Act of 1974 required that a patient's consent be obtained before any identifying information such as a name, Social Security number, or diagnosis is disclosed from the medical records. The Health Insurance Portability and Accountability Act of 1996 (HIPAA) required more detailed protection of patient privacy. The Joint Commission also requires that strict standards be adhered to concerning the patient's right to privacy (TJC, 2010).

Names of patients must not be posted where they are visible to the public. This includes placing card inserts on newborn bassinettes that contain the infant's name, sex, and personal information when the newborn nursery has a viewing window available to the public. Nurses must not discuss patients outside of the hospital or in elevators, and information on written care plans taken out of the hospital by nursing students must not contain patients' identifying information. All patients have a right to privacy, and the nurse must protect that right.

 Legal and Ethical Considerations

Confidentiality

HIPAA regulations mandate that the names and personal information of patients be kept in a secure and private place. Nurses and other health care personnel must maintain strict confidentiality concerning all patient information. The 2009 HITECH addition to the regulations includes the management of access to electronic medical records.

THE NURSING PROCESS

The nursing process is a method that applies patient and nursing responses based on a structured problem-solving approach to a clinical situation. It provides a way to use clinical judgment to recall facts and apply the information to meet individual needs of patients or provide a method of comprehensive nursing care. Nursing care plans that use the nursing process are included in many chapters in this book, and nursing diagnoses approved by NANDA International (NANDA-I) are found on the inside back cover of this book. A nursing diagnosis differs from a medical diagnosis (Table 1-2). Terminology common to nursing is listed in Box 1-4. The nursing process follows five steps that have been internationally accepted (Nursing Care Plan 1-1):

1. **Assessment:** Collecting objective and subjective patient data
2. **Diagnosis:** Identifying problems or potential problems, validating them through a process called **critical thinking,** and grouping them as **nursing diagnoses**
3. **Planning:** Planning care for the problems that were identified, which are stated in specific, individualized, measurable goals
4. **Implementation:** Carrying out specific interventions necessary to achieve the desired outcomes or goals (putting the plan into action)
5. **Evaluation:** Determining how well the plan worked and, if necessary, modifying the plan accordingly to meet the goals and outcomes

CRITICAL THINKING

Nurses have job-specific knowledge and skills they incorporate into their daily nursing practice by applying thought. *General thinking* involves random or

Table 1-2	**Comparison of Medical and Nursing Diagnoses**

MEDICAL DIAGNOSIS	POSSIBLE NURSING DIAGNOSIS
Acquired immunodeficiency syndrome	*Imbalanced nutrition: less than body requirements* related to anorexia and evidenced by weight loss
Gestational diabetes mellitus	*Deficient knowledge* related to gestational diabetes mellitus (GDM) and its effects on pregnant woman and fetus: manifested by crying, anxiety
Cystic fibrosis	*Ineffective airway clearance* related to mucus accumulation; manifested by rales, fatigue

Data from *Nursing Diagnoses—Definitions and Classification 2009–2011.* © 2009, 2007, 2005, 2003, 2001, 1998, 1996, 1994 NANDA International. Used by arrangement with Wiley-Blackwell Publishing, a company of John Wiley and Sons, Inc.

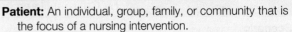

Box 1-4	**Common Terms Used in Nursing**

Patient: An individual, group, family, or community that is the focus of a nursing intervention.

Nursing activity: An action that implements an intervention to assist the patient toward a desired outcome. (A series of activities may be needed to implement an intervention.)

Nursing diagnosis: A clinical judgment about a patient's response to an actual or potential health problem. (The nursing diagnosis provides the basis for selecting nursing interventions to achieve an outcome for which the nurse is accountable.*)

Nursing intervention: Any treatment or nursing activity based on clinical judgment and knowledge that a nurse performs to achieve a specific outcome for the patient, including direct or indirect patient care or community or public health activities.

Scope of practice: Legal authority to perform specific activities related to health care or health promotion. (These activities require substantial knowledge or technical skill. Specific activities are listed by individual states' nurse practice acts; nurses must practice within these limitations. For example, an LPN/LVN cannot perform surgery; that activity is within the scope of a medical doctor.)

*Data from *Nursing Diagnoses—Definitions and Classification 2009–2011.* © 2009, 2007, 2005, 2003, 2001, 1998, 1996, 1994 NANDA International. Used by arrangement with Wiley-Blackwell Publishing, a company of John Wiley and Sons, Inc.

Based on specific situation, what could be going on, scientific data

memorized thoughts. An example of general thinking would be memorizing the steps in a clinical procedure or skill. *Critical thinking,* however, is purposeful, goal-directed thinking based on scientific evidence rather than assumption or memorization.

The way a nurse solves the problems of a patient is not always found in a textbook or in class lectures. Sometimes the nurse must consider factors that are specific to the individual patient or affected by an individual situation. For example, the cultural background of the patient or the age of the patient influences the effectiveness of a given intervention. If the problem is a protein deficiency, and the nurse selects the intervention to teach the importance of meat in the diet, the intervention will be ineffective and will not have a positive outcome if this patient is a vegetarian, because meat will not be eaten. Thus, critical thinking must enter the picture for optimum nursing care to be provided. Critical thinking entails applying creativity and ingenuity to solve a problem: combining basic standard principles with data specific to the patient. The basic steps in preparing a care plan involve critical thinking.

Evidence-based practice starts when the nurse uses the best evidence obtained from current, valid, published research. When the nurse combines that information with his or her critical thinking process and experiences and patient needs, it is then possible to plan

Nursing Care Plan 1-1 | **Care of Childbearing Families Related to Potential or Actual Stress Caused by Cultural Diversity**

Scenario

A 22-year-old woman, para 0 gravida 1, is admitted to the labor room in active early labor. Her partner is with her, and they do not speak English.

Selected Nursing Diagnosis

Impaired verbal communication related to language barriers

Expected Outcomes	Nursing Interventions	Rationales
Patient will have an opportunity to share information and will state she understands what is explained to her.	Arrange for a family or staff member interpreter as needed.	Interpreter can provide support for woman and help lessen her anxieties. Poor communication can result in time delays, errors, and misunderstandings of intent.
	Clearly define instructions in woman's language of origin.	A shared language is necessary for communication to take place.
	Provide written instructions in woman's language whenever possible.	Patient can review written instructions at a less stressful time. In some cases, it is necessary to determine whether person can read.
	Explain the use and purpose of all instruments and equipment, along with the effects or possible effects on the mother and fetus.	Education of family reduces anxiety and provides family with a sense of control.
	Provide opportunities for clarification and questions.	Learning takes time; repetition of important material promotes learning. Nurse can determine woman's understanding of information and clarify misconceptions.

Selected Nursing Diagnosis

Compromised family coping related to isolation, different customs, attitudes, or beliefs

Expected Outcomes	Nursing Interventions	Rationales
Family members will state that they feel welcome and safe in the environment provided.	Encourage orientation visit to the maternity unit before delivery.	Families who have clear, accurate information can better participate in labor and delivery. Viewing the delivery setting before using it decreases anxiety about the unknown.
	Inform families about routines, visiting hours, significant persons who can assist in labor and delivery, and location of newborn after delivery.	Families have different expectations of the health care system. They may hesitate to ask questions because of shyness or fear of "losing face."
	Determine and respect practices and values of family and incorporate them into nursing care plans as much as possible.	Clarification of culturally specific values and practices will avoid misunderstanding and conflict with the nurse's value system. Nursing care plans promote organization of care and communication among staff members.

Critical Thinking Questions

1. The extended family of a patient in the labor room requests permission to stay with the patient and the husband throughout labor. How should you respond?
2. A patient admitted to the labor room refuses to let a male physician perform a vaginal examination. What should be the nursing role?

safe, effective nursing care for the patient. Two nursing journals that focus on evidence-based practices in maternal and child health are the *Journal of Obstetric, Gynecologic & Neonatal Nursing* (JOGNN) and the *American Journal of Maternal/Child Nursing* (MCN).

An example of critical thinking would be modifying the steps in a clinical procedure or skill so that the individual patient's needs are met, and the basic principles of the skill are not violated. With critical thinking, *problem solving* is effective and *problem prevention* occurs. General thinking can occur naturally, but critical thinking is a skill that must be learned.

Because critical thinking is an active process, the regular use of critical thinking can assist in moving general information into long-term memory and can increase creativity. Critical thinking skills help the nurse adapt to new situations that occur every day and aid in clinical decision-making about care. Critical thinking can improve the care that nurses give to patients, improve test scores (through critical thinking about a scenario in the question), and improve working conditions by enabling the nurse to analyze and find creative ways to improve existing policies and practices (Box 1-5).

The Nursing Process and Critical Thinking

The nursing process (assessment, diagnosis, outcomes identification, planning, implementation, and evaluation) is a tool for effective critical thinking. When a nurse uses the nursing process in critical thinking, a clinical judgment can be made that is specific to the data collected and the clinical situation. In every clinical contact, a nurse must identify actual and potential problems and make decisions about a plan of action that will result in a positive patient outcome, know the reason the actions are appropriate, differentiate between those problems that the nurse can handle independently and those that necessitate contacting other members of the health care team, and prioritize those actions.

Differentiating between actions that can be carried out independently and those requiring collaboration with other health care providers is based on the *scope of practice* of the LPN or LVN. The scope of practice of the LPN/LVN is published by the state board of nursing.

Using Critical Thinking to Improve Test Scores

Attending class, reading the text, and studying are the basis of learning, and the evaluation of learning is achieved by testing. Weekly tests evaluate short-term learning. Final examinations evaluate long-term learning or retention of learning. Retained learning is subject to later recall and therefore is most useful in nursing practice after graduation from nursing school. Recalling facts that have been retained is what makes critical thinking in nursing practice possible. For a nurse to recognize or analyze abnormal findings, the normal findings must be recalled and used for comparison. An intervention can then be formulated.

Box 1-5	The Process of Critical Thinking

1. Identify the problem.
2. Differentiate fact from assumption.
3. Check reliability and accuracy of data.
4. Determine what is relevant and irrelevant.
5. Identify possible conclusions or outcomes.
6. Set priorities or goals.
7. Evaluate the response of the patient.

Using critical thinking in studying involves the following:
1. *Understanding* facts before trying to memorize them
2. *Prioritizing* information to be memorized
3. *Relating* facts to other facts (clusters, patterns, and groups)
4. *Using all five senses* to study (read, write, draw, listen to tapes, and see pictures of symptoms)
5. *Reviewing* before tests
6. *Reading critically* (identifying key concepts and using critical thinking) when working with sample questions during study

CULTURE

Culture is the body of socially inherited characteristics that one generation can hand down or tell to the next generation. It is shaped by values, beliefs, norms, and practices that are shared by persons of the same background. Culture guides thoughts and actions and becomes a patterned expression of what we are. As these expressions or traditions are passed down from one generation to the next, they become cultural values that are preferred behaviors. To understand why patients respond as they do, a nurse must assess their cultural background.

The United States is a culturally diverse nation. It is estimated that by the year 2020, 40% of school-age children will be from nonwhite ethnic groups. Just as variations are seen among cultures, variations exist within each culture. These variations often are related to social and economic factors and to education level. Attitudes about pregnancy and the sex of the child vary among cultures. In general, Hispanics and many Native Americans view pregnancy as a natural and desirable experience. In these cultures, children are desired. Some cultures put a high priority on having a son, and the woman who gives birth to a son receives a higher status within the family. This is noticeably true in traditional Chinese families. Among Hispanics and other groups, having children is evidence of the male's virility and manliness. In some cultures, the grandmother is expected to play a role in caring for the newborn.

The effect of different cultures and individuality on health care delivery challenges nurses to reevaluate expectations of others. Nurses must first develop a *cultural awareness*, which is an understanding of the reasons that patients respond as they do related to cultural practices; and develop a *cultural sensitivity* to recognize practices and values that differ from their own; and only then can nurses develop **cultural competence**, that is, use skills and knowledge necessary to understand and appreciate cultural differences, and be able to adapt clinical skills and practices as necessary. Nurses who are interacting with expectant families from a different culture or ethnic group can provide culturally sensitive nursing care by critically examining their own cultural beliefs; identifying biases, attitudes, and prejudices; learning practices of major cultures; and recognizing that ultimately it is the woman's right to make her own health care choices (Table 1-3). Issues related to culture are integrated in nursing care plans that appear throughout this book.

Table 1-3 Examples of Cultural Beliefs and Practices: Pregnancy, Birth, Postpartum, and Newborn Care*

PREGNANCY	DURING BIRTH	POSTPARTUM PERIOD, NEWBORN CARE
Hispanic/Latin American		
Pregnancy is usually desired soon after marriage. Cool air motion is thought dangerous during pregnancy. Food cravings that are not satisfied are thought to cause birthmarks. Milk is avoided because it is thought to cause large babies with difficult labor. Massage is given to aid fetus into favorable position. Pregnant woman lies on back to protect baby. Pelvic examination by male caregiver is unacceptable and frightening. Herbs are used to treat common discomforts. Permission of grandparents may be required before treatment.	In lower economic class, presence of grandmother is preferred over presence of husband. After birth of baby, mother's legs are brought together to prevent air from entering womb (uterus). Some still use lay midwife. Loud behavior is common during labor.	They believe in hot-cold balance of health. Currents of air are thought dangerous (keep warm). Diet may be restricted to special foods; hot or warm beverages preferred after birth. Bathing is permitted after several days. During recovery, grandmother cares for mother. Baby is usually breastfed after third day (colostrum considered dirty). Infant is given olive oil or castor oil for passage of meconium. Male newborn is often uncircumcised. Female newborn's ears are frequently pierced. Newborn is firmly swaddled in blankets. Belly band is used to prevent umbilical hernia. Fontanelles may be manipulated if newborn is ill.
Asian		
Pregnancy is perceived as a normal process. Sour and spicy foods may be avoided. Soy sauce may be avoided to prevent dark-skinned baby. Rice is main food. Female health care provider is preferred. Alcohol is not allowed. Physical activities are not limited (except carrying heavy loads). Daily baths are taken to produce a clean baby. Sitting in doorways is avoided because of fear labor will be complicated. Eye contact is avoided as a sign of respect. Herbs and folk medicine are used for discomforts.	Father usually does not actively participate. Mother labors in silence; she must not cry out because it would embarrass family. They may wrap white yarn around wrist of newborn to "lock the soul in."	They believe in hot-cold balance of health. Room must be warm; heat lost during birth needs to be replaced; may request space heater under bed. Many women are vegetarians. Lactose deficiency or intolerance is common. Birth of boy is preferred over girl. They may ask to take placenta home to dispose of it (a ritual carried out in Korea, Philippines, China, and Thailand). Touching head of newborn may be considered offensive to a Southeast Asian family; Hmong believe it is bad luck to praise newborn. They may swaddle newborn even in hot weather.
Middle Eastern		
Friends and family expect to be present during hospital stay. Family may fulfill obligation with demanding behavior. Touching is limited to members of the same sex. Man's permission is needed when family member requires health care. Future is left to the will of God; thus prenatal care may not be sought; they may have home cures such as herbs, hot and cold foods. Pork, intoxicants, and illicit drugs are avoided. Modesty is important.	Pain is expressed privately, except during labor and birth, when pain may be expressed vehemently.	They breastfeed newborns. Only parents are allowed to touch the baby's head.

Table 1-3	Examples of Cultural Beliefs and Practices: Pregnancy, Birth, Postpartum, and Newborn Care*—cont'd	
PREGNANCY	**DURING BIRTH**	**POSTPARTUM PERIOD, NEWBORN CARE**
African American		
Pregnancy is considered state of wellness. Lower-income group may be passive about prenatal care until a crisis develops. Strong kinship bond exists with extended family. They may treat illness with home remedies. Old wives' tales include the following: reaching up above head will cause cord to strangle baby; having picture taken during pregnancy will cause a stillbirth; emotional fright will mark baby. Mother may have cravings for food nutrients and non-nutrients, mustard or turnip greens, or pica (laundry starch, clay).	Mothers have varied emotional responses; some appear stoic to avoid showing weakness. Emotional support is often provided by women, usually own mother. Women often report to labor unit in advanced labor. Muslim women oppose use of analgesia for labor. Premature rupture of membranes is considered harmful (called *dry labor*).	Mothers are afraid of spoiling baby. Baby crying excessively may be seen as behaving in a "bad way." Emphasis is placed on feeding baby ("A good mother is one whose baby eats well"). Oil is put on baby's head and skin. Belly band is often used to prevent umbilical hernia. Clothing for newborn tends to be excessive. Muslim women, if possible, breastfeed their newborns.
Native American		
They are family oriented. Herbs are used to treat ailments. Traditionally, society is matriarchal. Food preferences vary among tribes; milk is not commonly desired. Two-visitor rule often has no meaning to them. Mothers have below-recommended intake of calcium, iron, and vitamins. They are not time oriented; do not see importance of clocks (important for taking medications and follow-up care). Native healing ceremonies and healing practices are common.	They do not see need to limit visitors. Relatives often come to hospital to care for woman.	Infant mortality rate is high. Newborn birth rate is less than average. They may want to carry newborn on papoose board.

*Many of these cultural beliefs and customs reflect the traditional culture and may not be currently practiced. These lists are intended to serve as guidelines while discussing cultural beliefs with women and their families.

FAMILY

FAMILY TYPES

A family is defined by the U.S. Census Bureau as a group of two or more people who reside together and who are related by blood, marriage, or adoption (U.S. Census Bureau, 2004). This definition is workable for gathering comparative statistics; however, it is limited when assessing a family for health purposes because families can and do contain unmarried couples. Some define the family in a much broader content as "two or more people who live in the same household, share a common emotional bond, and perform certain interrelated social tasks" (Levine, Carey, & Crocker, 1999, p. 119). Nurses must be aware of and respect family types and values that differ from their own. Box 1-6 presents family types, along with some of their defining characteristics.

THE ROLE OF THE FAMILY IN HEALTH CARE DELIVERY

The role of the family in self-care and health care has influenced the way health care is provided in the United States. Since the 1960s, parents began to expect to be part of the decision-making process and questioned routine care that excluded family members. Fathers waited in waiting rooms for news that their child was born. The father's presence in the labor and delivery room is now the norm. Visiting hours are liberal, and contact with the newborn is encouraged. It has been demonstrated that informed parents can make wise decisions about their own care during pregnancy, birth, and delivery if they are adequately educated and given professional support.

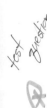

Test question

Box 1-6 Family Types

Nuclear: Husband, wife, and their biologic children living together

Blended or reconstituted: A combination of two families with children from one or both families

Cohabitating: An unmarried couple living together (they may have their own children, children from previous marriages, or adopted children.)

Communal: Several families living together who share responsibilities of work and child care

Extended: More than one generation, expanded to include relatives outside of the nuclear family (e.g., grandparents, aunts, uncles, and their families)

Same-sex: A gay or lesbian couple with or without children (children may be adopted, from previous relationships, or artificially conceived.)

Single-parent: Never married, divorced, separated, or widowed male or female who has at least one child

Stepparent: A person who has married a man or woman who has at least one child

COMPLEMENTARY AND ALTERNATIVE THERAPIES

Alternative therapies for health problems are treatments not typically recommended by health care providers and differ from conventional or mainstream remedies. Alternative therapy does not rely on evidence-based practice, and some therapists are not state or nationally licensed or certified.

Complementary therapies are nontraditional methods used in conjunction with conventional therapy. The body is thought to have a self-healing ability that can be aided by complementary and alternative therapies commonly used alone or sometimes integrated with standard medical practice. Although nurses do not advocate or discourage the use of specific health care practices, knowledge of various types of complementary and alternative medicine (CAM) therapies can aid the nurse in identifying the reason the individual is using them and in recognizing a contraindication or interaction with traditional medicine that may have been prescribed.

Alternative and complementary therapies in health care are not new. The use of herbs and oils, therapeutic touch, and the treatment of forms of energy within the human body have existed for years. The shift toward self-care has increased the use of unconventional therapies. Today, community-based nurses will encounter some **alternative health care practices** involving patients who want increasing control over their health problems, wish to be a part of the decision-making process, and want to incorporate these practices in their care. **Integrative health care** involves the use of both CAM treatments and traditional allopathic medicine tailored to meet individual needs in a safe, least invasive, and most cost-effective manner (Rakel, 2007). The NIH National Center for Complementary and Alternative Medicine has classified alternative medicine into major categories. An overview of alternative and complementary health care practices is discussed in Chapter 21.

Get Ready for the NCLEX® Examination!

Key Points

- Changes in childbirth practices have created a more homelike and family-centered approach to maternity care.
- Advances in technology have increased neonatal survival rates.
- Technology in the hospital setting can promote patient safety.
- The Human Genome Project identifies genetic materials present in the body. Inserting missing genes or replacing defective genes may be a way to eliminate genetic disorders.
- Major efforts by government, insurance companies, and health care providers to control health care costs have resulted in a decreased length of patients' hospital stays.
- Managed care is a health care delivery system designed to reduce health care costs.
- Nursing care plans and clinical pathways provide a basis for critical thinking and judgment that guide patient care toward positive outcomes.

- Home- and community-based nursing includes preventive care and therapeutic management.
- Statistics provide information about the outcomes of maternal-newborn care.
- Standards of care establish minimum criteria for competent nursing care. Legal interpretation of actions based on standards of care determine what nurses are expected to do.
- Evidence-based practice is the use of research data in the design and implementation of a care plan.
- Effective communication is an important nursing skill with three main components: listening, observing, and documenting.
- Documentation can facilitate continuity of care, which can enhance patient outcomes and minimize legal problems.
- The patient's right to privacy is protected by HIPAA; nurses must protect these rights.
- Culture is an organized structure that guides behavior for a particular group. It is shaped by values, beliefs, and practices shared by persons of the same background.

- There are many different family types. A family can be defined as two or more people who share a common emotional bond and relate to each other with specific patterns of behavior.
- Critical thinking is purposeful, goal-directed thinking based upon scientific evidence rather than on assumption or memorization.
- Evidence-based practice occurs when the nurse uses the best evidence obtained from current, valid published research combined with critical thinking concerning patient needs.
- Alternative and complementary therapies include unconventional ways to heal the body and are becoming acceptable to a larger percentage of the population. Although nurses do not advocate or discourage the use of these therapies, they should be knowledgeable about them.

Additional Learning Resources

SG   Go to your Study Guide on pages 473–474 for additional Review Questions for the NCLEX® Examination, Critical Thinking Clinical Situations, and other learning activities to help you master this chapter content.

evolve   Go to your Evolve website (http://evolve.elsevier.com/Leifer/maternity) for the following FREE learning resources:
- Animations
- Answer Guidelines for Critical Thinking Questions
- Answers and Rationales for Review Questions for the NCLEX® Examination
- Concept Map Creator
- Glossary with pronunciations in English and Spanish
- Patient Teaching Plans
- Skills Performance Checklists and more!

 Online Resources
- www.ahcpr.gov
- www.cdc.gov/nchs
- www.cochrane.org
- www.dol.gov/ebsa/newsroom/fsnmhafs.html
- www.genome.gov/e/si
- www.georgetown.edu/research/gucdc/nccc
- www.healthcare.gov
- www.ihi.org/IHI/Topics/PerinatalCareGeneral/emergingcontent/perinatalSBARtools.htm
- www.jointcommission.org
- www.nln.org/aboutnln/positionstatement/index.htm
- www.npsf.org
- www.qsen.org

Review Questions for the NCLEX® Examination

1. Federal legislation has been passed that enables women who have a cesarean birth to stay in the birth facility for:
   1. 24 hours
   2. 48 hours
   3. 72 hours
   4. 96 hours

2. Individuals at increased risk for inherited Tay-Sachs disease are those in the:
   1. Ashkenazi Jewish population
   2. African American population
   3. Hispanic population
   4. Greek population

3. The founder of the Henry Street Settlement in New York City, which brought home health care to poor children, was:
   1. Margaret Sanger
   2. Florence Nightingale
   3. Lillian Wald
   4. Jean Watson

4. Place the 5 steps of the nursing process in the correct order.
   1. Assessment   *Assessment*
   2. Evaluation   *Diagnosis*
   3. Planning   *Planning*
   4. Diagnosis   *Implementation*
   5. Implementation *Evaluation*

5. Several families living together who share responsibilities of work and child care are called a(n):
   1. Communal family
   2. Cohabitating family
   3. Nuclear family
   4. Extended family

6. Complementary therapies can be described by which characteristic(s)? *(Select all that apply.)*
   1. New in health care
   2. Nontraditional
   3. Involve implementation of experimental medications
   4. Should neither be advocated nor discouraged by the nurse
   5. Used in conjunction with conventional therapy

Critical Thinking Questions

1. You are going to interview someone whose background differs from your own. You will ask this patient about her health beliefs and practices that might influence her pregnancy, childbirth, and care of the infant. If you use this interview for future teaching, what self-assessment might you need to consider after the interview?

2. You are scheduling an interview with an unmarried pregnant girl and her parents. You want to identify how the parents plan to assist their daughter during her pregnancy and childbirth, as well as in caring for the grandchild. What questions are essential to ask in the interview? What self-assessment will you need to consider before beginning the interview?

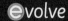
Reproductive Anatomy and Physiology

Objectives

1. Define key terms listed.
2. Discuss puberty in the developing male and female.
3. Identify the female external reproductive organs.
4. Describe the female internal reproductive organs.
5. Describe the influence of hormones on the female reproductive process.
6. Explain the menstrual and ovarian cycles.
7. Discuss the functions of the uterus.
8. Identify the bones that make up the pelvis.
9. Identify the male organs of reproduction.
10. Review the functions of the male hormone testosterone.
11. Explain the physiology of the sex act in the male and female.

Key Terms

diagonal conjugate (DĪ-ăg-ĕn-ŭl KŎN-jŭ-gĭt, p. 21)
fimbriae (fim'bre-ə, p. 20)
follicle-stimulating hormone (FSH) (FŎL-lĭ-kŭl STĬ-mū-lā-tĭng HŌR-mōn, p. 26)
luteinizing hormone (LH) (LŪ-tĕ-nī-zĭng HŌR-mōn, p. 26)
ovulation (ŏv-ū-LĀ-shŭn, p. 20)

oxytocin (ŏks-ē-TŌ-sĭn, p. 22)
perineum (pĕ-rĭ-NĒ-ŭm, p. 18)
prostate gland (PRŎS-tāt glănd, p. 26)
rugae (ROO-jē, p. 18)
testosterone (tĕs-TŎS-tĕ-rōn, p. 25)

Human reproduction is a complex and fascinating process. The male and female reproductive systems functioning together produce a new life. For an understanding of how human reproduction is possible, knowledge of the structural features and functions of various organs is needed.

PUBERTY

Before puberty, male and female children appear very much alike except for their genitalia. Puberty involves changes in the whole body and the psyche as well as in the expectations of society toward the individual.

Puberty is a period of rapid change in the lives of boys and girls during which the reproductive systems mature and become capable of reproduction. Puberty begins when the secondary sex characteristics appear (e.g., pubic hair). Puberty ends when mature sperm are formed or when regular menstrual cycles occur. This transition from childhood to adulthood has been identified and often celebrated by various rites of passage. Some cultures have required demonstrations of bravery, such as hunting wild animals or displays of self-defense. Ritual circumcision is another rite of passage in some cultures and religions. In the United States today, some adolescents participate in religious ceremonies such as bar or bat mitzvah or confirmation, but for others, these ceremonies are unfamiliar.

The lack of a "universal rite of passage" to identify adulthood has led to confusion for some contemporary adolescents in many industrialized nations.

THE MALE

Male hormonal changes normally begin between 10 and 16 years of age. Outward changes become apparent when the size of the penis and testes increases and there is a general growth spurt. Testosterone, the primary male hormone, causes the boy to grow taller, become more muscular, and develop secondary sex characteristics such as pubic hair, facial hair, and a deep voice. The voice deepens but is often characterized by squeaks or cracks before reaching its final pitch. Testosterone levels are constant, not cyclic like female hormones, although levels may decrease with age to 50% of peak levels by age 80 years. Nocturnal emissions ("wet dreams") may occur without sexual stimulation. These emissions usually do not contain sperm.

THE FEMALE

The first outward change of puberty in females is the development of breasts. The first menstrual period **(menarche)** occurs 2 to 2½ years later (ages 11 to 15 years). Female reproductive organs mature to prepare for sexual activity and childbearing. The female experiences a growth spurt, but hers ends earlier than the male's. Her hips broaden as her pelvis assumes the wide basin shape needed for birth. Pubic and axillary hair appears. The quantity varies, as it does in males.

FEMALE REPRODUCTIVE SYSTEM

EXTERNAL GENITALIA: VULVA

The female external reproductive organs consist of the mons pubis, which is covered with pubic hair; two paired folds of tissue, called the *labia majora* and *labia minora*, which surround a space called the vestibule; the vaginal opening; the fourchette; the perineum; the clitoris; and glandular structures (Figure 2-1). Collectively these structures are known as the *vulva.*

Mons Pubis

The mons pubis is formed at the upper margin of the symphysis pubis and is shaped like an inverted triangle. It is located over the two pubic bones of the pelvis. This structure is composed of fatty tissue lying beneath the skin and, from puberty on, is covered with varying amounts of pubic hair. The mons pubis surrounds delicate tissue and protects it from injury.

Labia Majora and Labia Minora

The labia majora are two folds of fatty tissue that form the lateral boundaries of the vulva. They are covered with coarse skin and pubic hair on the outer aspect and are smooth and moist on the inner aspect, where the openings of numerous small glands are found. The labia are analogous to the scrotum in the male. Just inside the labia majora are two smaller folds of skin called the labia minora that meet at the fourchette above the anus. This area is also known as the *obstetric perineum.* It is often the site of lacerations during childbirth.

When the labia majora are separated, the labia minora are exposed. The labia minora are soft folds of skin that are rich in sebaceous glands. The labia minora are moist and are composed of erectile tissue containing loose connective tissue, blood vessels, and involuntary muscles. The functions of the labia minora are to lubricate and waterproof the vulvar skin and to provide bactericidal secretions that help prevent infections.

Clitoris

The clitoris is a small, sensitive structure that, like the penis, is composed of erectile tissue, nerves, and blood vessels; it is covered at its tip with very sensitive tissue. It exists primarily for female sexual enjoyment. Partially hidden at the upper end of the labia, the clitoris may seem to be the opening to an orifice and may be mistaken for the opening to the urethra. In addition, the clitoris secretes a cheese-like substance from the sebaceous glands, which is called *smegma.* The odor of smegma may be sexually stimulating to the male.

Vaginal Vestibule

The vaginal vestibule is a boat-shaped depression enclosed by the labia minora and is visible when the labia minora are separated. The vestibule contains the vaginal opening, or **introitus,** which is located between the external and internal genitalia. At the vaginal introitus, there is a thin, elastic, mucous membrane called the **hymen.** The hymen may be broken by the use of tampons, strenuous physical activity, or sexual intercourse. A broken hymen does not prove the loss of virginity.

The vestibule contains the openings of five structures that drain into it: the urethral meatus, Skene's ducts, and the ducts from Bartholin's glands that are located on each side of the vagina. These glands secrete yellowish mucus that lubricates the vagina, particularly during sexual arousal. Skene's glands are located just inside the urethra and are part of the vestibule. The vestibule ends with the formation of the fourchette.

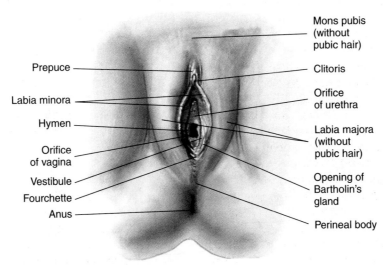

FIGURE 2-1 **Female external genitalia.** The obstetric perineum lies between the vaginal orifice and the anus.

When the nurse is preparing to do a urinary catheterization, he or she cleanses this area of the vestibule.

Perineum

The perineum is the region of the genital area that lies between the vagina and the anus. Because of its location, it plays an important role in the birth process. It is composed of the levator ani muscles, the deep perineal muscles, and the external genitalia muscles. These muscles function as supports to the pelvic organs. The pudendal arteries, veins, and nerves supply the muscles, fascia, and skin of the perineum.

The perineum is supported during the delivery of the infant's head and shoulders because it stretches significantly during the infant's birth and may tear. An **episiotomy** (incision) in the perineal area may be performed to prevent tears in the underlying muscles or tissues; the episiotomy is repaired (sutured) immediately after delivery. Pelvic weakness or painful intercourse (dyspareunia) may result if this tissue does not heal properly.

INTERNAL REPRODUCTIVE ORGANS

The internal female organs of reproduction are the ovaries, fallopian (uterine) tubes, uterus, and vagina (Figure 2-2).

Vagina

The vagina is a curved tube leading from the uterus to the external opening at the vestibule. It lies between the urinary bladder and the rectum. Because it meets at a right angle with the cervix, the anterior wall is about 2.5 cm (1 inch) shorter than the posterior wall, which varies from 7 to 10 cm (approximately 2.8 to 4 inches). It consists of muscle and connective tissue and is lined with epithelial tissue, which contains folds called rugae. These folds allow the vagina to stretch considerably during childbirth. The epithelial cells lining the vagina show cyclic changes related to circulating estrogens, progestins, and androgens. Doderlein's bacilli, which are normally present in the vagina, act on glycogen from the epithelial cells to produce lactic acid. This maintains the acidity of the vagina and is the reason that the vagina is resistant to most infections. A change in the pH of the vagina, which can be caused by frequent douching, antimicrobial therapy, or deodorant tampons, can increase the vagina's susceptibility to invading pathogens. The cyclic changes in the vagina related to age and changing pH are shown in Figure 2-3. The vagina functions as:

1. A passageway of the uterus through which the uterine secretions and menstrual flow escape

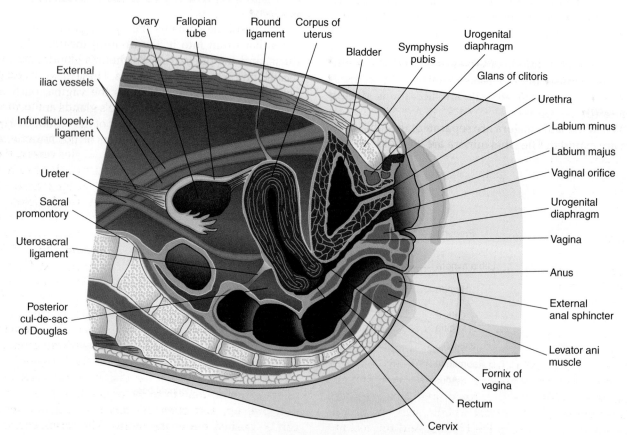

FIGURE 2-2 Internal female reproductive organs with woman lying supine.

	Estrogen	Epithelium	Glycogen	pH	Flora
Newborn	+	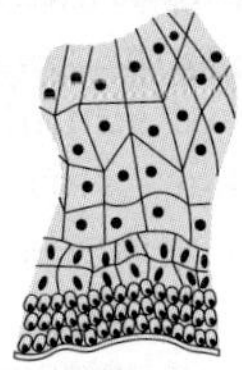	+	Acid 4-5	Sterile ↓ Doderlein's bacilli Secretion abundant
Month-old child	−	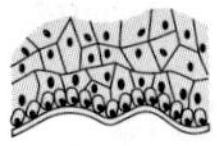	+	Alkaline >7	Sparse, coccal, and varied flora Secretion scant
Puberty	Appears	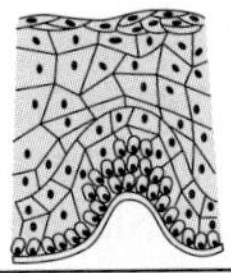	− → +	Alkaline ↓ Acid	Sparse, coccal ↓ Rich bacillary
Mature	++	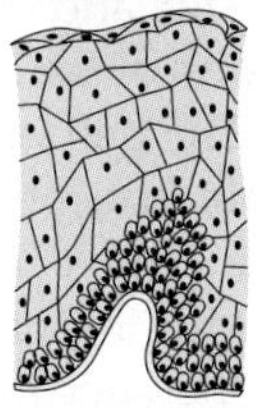	+	Acid 4-5	Doderlein's bacilli Secretion abundant
Postmenopause	+ → −	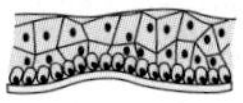	−	Neutral or alkaline 6 to >7	Varied Dependent on level of circulating estrogen Secretion scant

FIGURE 2-3 Cyclic changes in the vagina related to age.

2. A female organ of copulation (sexual intercourse), allowing sperm to enter the uterus
3. Part of the birth canal

Vulvovaginal glands, called *Bartholin's glands*, provide lubrication to the vaginal introitus during sexual arousal but are typically not visible. After puberty, the vagina maintains a normal acidic pH of 4 to 5. Excessive use of vaginal sprays, douches, or deodorant tampons can alter the pH of the vagina and its self-cleansing properties, thus increasing the risk of infection.

Uterus

The uterus (womb) is a hollow, pear-shaped, muscular organ. It is approximately 2.5 cm (1 inch) thick, 5 cm (2 inches) wide, and 7.5 cm (3 inches) long. During pregnancy, the uterus can stretch and enlarge considerably. The weight of the nonpregnant uterus is approximately 75 g (2.5 oz); it increases to approximately 907 g (2 lbs) during pregnancy. During pregnancy, the uterus increases in vascularity, which allows sufficient blood supply for its growth, and can stretch and enlarge to a considerable size. After pregnancy, it returns almost entirely to its former weight, size, and shape. The uterus lies between the bladder and the rectum. It is supported by two important pairs of ligaments,

the **round** and **broad ligaments.** During pregnancy, these ligaments become stretched, frequently causing discomfort.

The uterus is divided into three parts: (1) the **fundus,** the upper rounder portion; (2) the **corpus** (body), the middle portion, which plays an important role in menstruation and pregnancy; and (3) the **cervix,** the lower portion, which is a tubular structure that projects into the vagina and provides an outlet for menstrual blood and a passageway for the delivery of a fetus.

The fundus and corpus of the uterus are made up of three layers: (1) the **perimetrium,** the outer layer that envelops the uterus; (2) the **myometrium,** the middle layer, which is a thick muscular layer; and (3) the **endometrium,** the inner mucous membrane layer. The endometrium is functional during menstruation and implantation of the fertilized ovum. During menstruation and after delivery, the cells of the endometrium are sloughed off. The myometrium contains muscle fibers that are arranged in the longitudinal, transverse, and oblique directions—a network that offers extreme strength to the organ. It is able to thin out, pull up, and open the cervix so that the fetus can be pushed out of the uterus. The cervix consists of a cervical canal with an internal opening near the uterine corpus, called the **internal os,** and an opening into the vagina, called the **external os.** The cervix is known for its elasticity. The mucosal lining of the cervix has four functions: (1) providing lubrication for the vagina, (2) acting as a bacteriostatic agent, (3) providing an alkaline environment to shelter the sperm from the acidic vagina, and (4) producing a mucous plug in the cervical canal during pregnancy.

The following are the three functions of the uterus:
1. Menstruation: The uterus sloughs off of the endometrium or lining of the uterus.
2. Pregnancy: The uterus supports the fetus and allows the fetus to grow.
3. Labor and birth: The uterine muscles contract, and the cervix dilates during labor to expel the fetus.

☀ Fallopian Tubes

The fallopian tubes (uterine tubes or oviducts) extend laterally from the uterus, one to each ovary. They are small, narrow, and approximately 10 cm (4 inches) long. The tubes carry the ovum from the ovary to the uterus by the peristaltic action (contractions) of cilia, or hairlike projections found in the lining of the tubes. Extending from the ends of the fallopian tubes are small, fingerlike projections called fimbriae. Their movements sweep the ovum into the tube, after which the ovum travels to the uterus. It takes approximately 5 days for the ovum to travel the 10 cm from the ovary to the uterus. Fertilization of an ovum with sperm normally takes place in the outer third of the fallopian tube.

The four functions of the fallopian tubes are to provide:
1. A passageway in which sperm meet the ovum
2. A site of fertilization, usually the outer third of the tube
3. A safe, nourishing environment for the ovum or zygote (fertilized ovum)
4. A means of transporting the ovum or zygotes to the corpus of the uterus

☀ Ovaries

The ovaries in the female and the testes in the male are similar in embryologic origin. The ovaries are two small, almond-shaped organs located on each side of the uterus. They are the female gonads, or sex glands. Approximately 2 million ova (eggs) are present at birth. Many ova degenerate until puberty, when a few thousand remain. During the course of a woman's reproductive life, only about 400 ova mature enough to be fertilized.

During the reproductive years, the ovaries act in concert with the uterus. Saclike structures are in various stages of maturity; as they mature, they are called **follicles.** During each menstrual cycle, one follicle matures into what is called a **graafian follicle,** which contains the ovum that is released each month during ovulation.

Estrogen, secreted by the ovary, stimulates the development of secondary sexual characteristics, such as the breasts. **Progesterone** is responsible for preparing and maintaining the lining of the uterus for implantation of the ovum. Any remaining ova after the climacteric (menopause) will not respond to hormonal stimulation to mature.

The ovaries have two main functions:
1. The development, maturation, and later expulsion of the ovum (i.e., ovulation)
2. The secretion of hormones, chiefly estrogen and progesterone

PELVIS

The female bony pelvis has the unique functions of supporting and protecting the pelvic contents, as well as forming a relatively fixed passage through which the fetus travels during the birth process. Therefore, its size and shape are important factors in the mechanisms of labor and birth.

The pelvis is made up of four bones: the two innominate bones (hip bones), the sacrum, and the coccyx. The pelvis resembles a basin or bowl; its two sides are the innominate bones, and its back is composed of the sacrum and coccyx. The four bones are lined with fibrocartilage and held tightly together by ligaments. These bones are joined in the front by the symphysis pubis and in the back by the sacroiliac joints and the sacrococcygeal joint (Figure 2-4).

The innominate bones result from the fusion of the **ilium,** the **ischium,** and the **pubis.** The two ilia form the upper part of the pelvis, known as the **false pelvis.** The **ischial spines,** sharp projections that form the posterior border of the ischium, are important landmarks and represent the shortest distance (diameter) of the pelvic cavity. The spines can be palpated during a vaginal examination and are used to determine how far the fetal head has descended into the birth canal. The ischium is a heavy bone below the ilium that forms the lower part of the innominate bone. Its protuberance, the **ischial tuberosity,** is the part on which the body rests while in a sitting position. The pubis is the part of the innominate bone that forms the front of the pelvis. It consists of two pubic bones that unite to form a joint, called the **symphysis pubis,** a rounded arch under which the fetal head must pass as it emerges from the birth canal.

Pelvic Divisions

The pelvic cavity is divided into two sections, the false pelvis and true pelvis. The **linea terminalis** is an imaginary line that separates the pelvis into the true pelvis and false pelvis. The false pelvis is the portion above the pelvic brim (upper portion) and has little obstetric significance. However, it does support the growing uterus during pregnancy and directs the presenting fetal part (usually the head) into the true pelvis near the end of pregnancy. The **true pelvis** (the lower part)

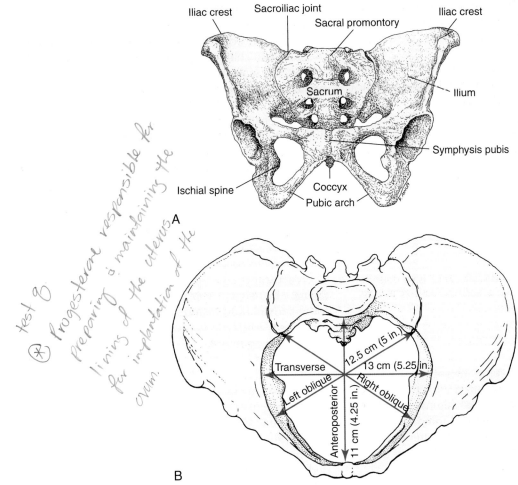

test 9
(X) Progesterone responsible for preparing & maintaining the lining of the uterus for implantation of the ovum.

FIGURE 2-4 **A,** Female pelvis, anterior view. **B,** Four important pelvic inlet diameters are the anteroposterior, the transverse, and the right and left oblique diameters.

consists of the inlet, pelvic cavity, and outlet and is most important during birth.

Pelvic Measurements

The bony circumference of the true pelvis is made up of the sacrum, the coccyx, and the lower part of the innominate bones. This area determines the size and shape of the pelvis, which must be adequate for passage of the baby during labor and birth. For convenience, three imaginary flat surfaces crossing the pelvis have traditionally been described: the plane of the pelvic inlet, the plane of the (shortest dimensions) midpelvis, and the plane of the outlet. The diameter of the midpelvis (bordered posteriorly by the sacrum, laterally by the ischial spines, and anteriorly by the symphysis pubis) can be most accurately measured by an x-ray examination. Because x-rays are potentially hazardous to the fetus, their use is all but obsolete. An evaluation of adequacy may be based on the prominence of the ischial spines and the degree of convergence of the sidewalls. The outlet is a clinical measurement made by palpating the distance between the ischial tuberosities.

This diameter is shortened when the pubic arch is narrow; therefore, the pubic arch is assessed for curvature or for the type of pelvis. A magnetic resonance imaging (MRI) pelvimetry may be indicated when there is high suspicion for labor dystocia.

A clinical measurement used to predict pelvic size is the diagonal conjugate. The diagonal conjugate is the distance from the lower margin of the symphysis pubis to the sacral promontory (Figure 2-5). The examiner measures this diameter by placing two fingers in the woman's vagina and touching the sacral promontory. The optimal distance for most women is 11.5 cm (4.5 inches). This procedure may be part of the prenatal examination and may be uncomfortable for the patient. The woman should be prepared for the pelvic examination by being instructed to empty her bladder beforehand and to take deep breaths during the examination.

Pelvic Types

The four basic pelvic types are (1) **gynecoid,** or normal female-type pelvis, which is round; (2) **android,** or male-type pelvis, which has a heart-shaped outlet;

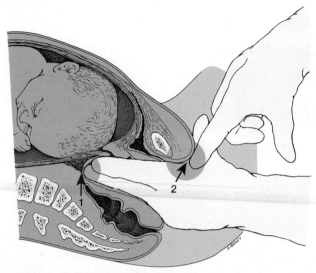

FIGURE 2-5 Measuring the diagonal conjugate, which is the distance from the lower margin of the symphysis pubis to the sacral promontory. The true obstetric conjugate can be estimated by subtracting 1.5 to 2 cm (0.6 to 0.8 inches).

(3) **anthropoid,** which has a long anteroposterior outlet; and (4) **platypelloid,** which has a wide transverse outlet and is not favorable to a vaginal delivery (Figure 2-6). The gynecoid pelvis is adapted for childbirth. Its inlet, cavity, and outlet are in better proportion; the pubic arch is wide; and the coccyx is more movable than in the android pelvis.

ENDOCRINE SYSTEM AND FEMALE REPRODUCTION

The Normal Menstrual Cycle

A woman's reproductive life has a definite beginning and ending; it begins at puberty and ends at menopause, or climacteric. Puberty is when reproduction

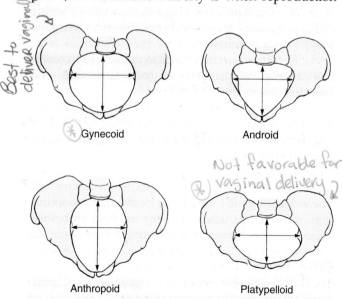

Best to deliver vaginally →

Gynecoid   Android

Not favorable for vaginal delivery

Anthropoid   Platypelloid

FIGURE 2-6 Four basic types of pelvis.

becomes possible and other events such as breast development, growth of pubic and axillary hair, and menstruation occur. During the female reproductive years, cyclic changes occur in the ovaries and in the uterus. These changes can be considered as two interrelated cycles: the menstrual cycle and the ovarian cycle (Table 2-1).

The menstrual cycle is a predictable event that normally occurs monthly. The typical monthly menstrual cycle is influenced by ovarian follicle maturation, ovulation, and corpus luteum formation and ends with menstrual bleeding (Figure 2-7). The changes that occur in the uterus depend on the changes occurring simultaneously in the ovaries. In this unique pattern of events, the development of the endometrium occurs at the precise time of the month that the release of a mature ovum occurs.

Ovulation occurs 14 days before the beginning of the next menstrual cycle, and the ovum remains fertile for approximately 24 hours. The sperm can survive up to 5 days. Fertilization most often occurs in the first few hours after ovulation.

Breasts

The breasts, or mammary glands, are considered accessory organs of reproduction because of their functional role in producing milk to feed and nourish the infant (Figure 2-8). The process is called **lactation.** The nipple, in the center of the breasts, is surrounded by a pigmented areola, which darkens during pregnancy. Montgomery's glands (also known as Montgomery's tubercles) are small sebaceous glands in the areola that secrete a substance that lubricates and protects the breasts during lactation (when the infant sucks). Beginning at the nipple, each breast is divided into 10 to 20 branchlike structures called **lobes,** which can be visualized as a treelike structure. They are separated by adipose (fatty) and fibrous tissue. Branching off from each lobe are 20 to 40 **lobules;** each lobule branches further, dividing into 20 to 80 saclike structures, called **alveoli.** These saclike structures have a lining that contains tiny secretory cells, called **acini,** which secrete milk. Surrounding the alveolar cells are contractile cells, called **myoepithelial cells,** which contract the alveolus and eject milk into the reservoir, called the **lactiferous ducts.** It is from these ducts that the infant, by sucking, gets milk through the nipple.

During pregnancy, high levels of estrogen and progesterone produced by the placenta inhibit milk secretion. After the expulsion of the placenta, there is an abrupt change in estrogen and progesterone levels. This allows a hormone, called **prolactin,** to be released from the anterior pituitary gland when the infant sucks. Prolactin stimulates the acini cells to produce milk. Infant suckling also stimulates the release of the hormone oxytocin from the posterior pituitary gland. **Oxytocin**

Table **2-1** The Female Reproductive Cycle	
PHASE	**CHARACTERISTICS**
Menstrual Cycle (Occurs When Ovum is Not Fertilized, Approximately 14 Days After Ovulation)	
Menstrual phase (days 1 5)	Endometrium is shed. Estrogen levels are low. Cervical mucus is scanty, viscous, and opaque.
Proliferative phase (days 6-14)	Endometrium thickness increases. Estrogen levels increase. Cervical mucus increases in elasticity, is called **spinnbarkeit,** and shows ferning pattern (indicates ovulation). Cervical mucus is more favorable to sperm.
Secretory phase (days 15-26)	Estrogen levels decrease and progesterone dominates. Endometrial cells become thicker, dilated, and tortuous. Glycogen is secreted by endometrial glands in preparation for the fertilized ovum.
Ischemic phase (days 27-28)	Both estrogen and progesterone levels fall as the corpus luteum degenerates. Spiral arteries undergo vasoconstriction, causing a deficiency of blood necessary for the endometrium. Blood pools and escapes through the endometrial surfaces (beginning of next menstrual phase).
Ovarian Cycle	
Follicular phase (days 1-14)	Ovarian follicle (ovum) matures under the influence of two hormones: FSH and LH. Follicle secretes estrogen, which accelerates maturation, and moves toward surface of ovary and is called *graafian follicle*. Estrogen produced affects the uterine lining (endometrium). Graafian follicle ruptures, and ovulation occurs with a surge of LH.
Luteal phase (days 15-28)	After the rupture of the follicle, the ovum enters the fallopian tube and travels to the uterus; corpus luteum develops under LH influence and produces high levels of estrogen and progesterone. Increased estrogen and progesterone levels suppress the growth of other follicles. If fertilization does not occur, the corpus luteum atrophies, LH levels fall, and estrogen and progesterone levels decrease.

FSH, Follicle-stimulating hormone; *LH,* luteinizing hormone.

stimulates the contraction of the myoepithelial cells, which causes the ejection of milk from the alveoli into the ductal system (see Chapter 11).

The size of the breasts depends on the amount of fatty tissue deposited in the breasts. Breast size does not indicate the amount of milk the breasts will produce.

MALE REPRODUCTIVE SYSTEM

The male reproductive system includes the testes, glands, and ducts, which are internal structures, and the penis and scrotum, which are external structures (Figure 2-9).

☀ EXTERNAL MALE GENITALIA

Penis
The penis is the male organ of copulation (sexual intercourse) and is part of the urinary system. The penis is made up of three columns of erectile tissue covered by thick skin that is freely movable. Two of the columns, the **cavernous bodies,** contain blood spaces, which when empty cause the penis to be limp (flaccid). When emotional or sexual stimulation occurs, these spaces fill with blood and the penis becomes engorged

(swollen), considerably enlarged, and erect. The third column of erectile tissue, the spongy layer, lies beneath the cavernous bodies. Through it passes the urethra from the urinary bladder. The head of the penis is composed of an enlarged portion of spongy tissue, which forms a cap called the **glans penis.** Covering the glans is the loosely fitting skin, called the **prepuce,** or foreskin. The foreskin is sometimes removed by circumcision for hygienic, religious, or cultural reasons. The penis has the following functions:
1. It provides a passageway for urine to exit the body.
2. It deposits sperm in the female's vagina to fertilize an ovum.

Scrotum
The scrotum is the wrinkled, pigmented pouch of skin, muscle, and fascia that lies beneath the penis and outside of the abdominal cavity. It is divided into two sacs, with each sac containing one testis (testicle), the epididymis, and a portion of the spermatic cord. Because the sperm require a temperature slightly lower than normal body temperature for development and maintenance, when the body temperature is high,

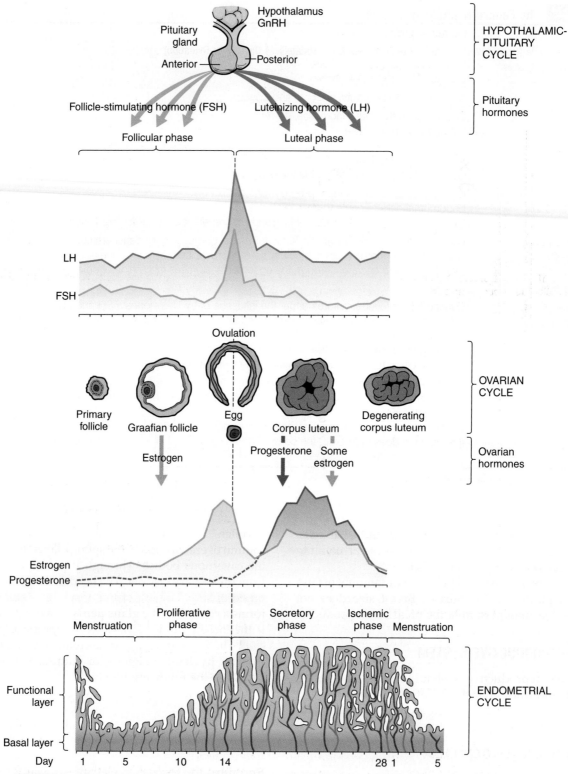

FIGURE 2-7 Menstrual cycle: hypothalamic-pituitary, ovarian, and endometrial. *GnRH,* Gonadotropin-releasing hormone.

the muscles of the scrotum relax, dropping the testes away from the body. Conversely, when exposed to low temperatures, the muscles of the scrotum are stimulated to contract and bring the testes close to the body for warmth.

INTERNAL MALE STRUCTURES

Testes

The testes are two oval-shaped glands approximately 5 cm (2 inches) long and 2.5 cm (1 inch) wide, located within the scrotal sac. They correspond to

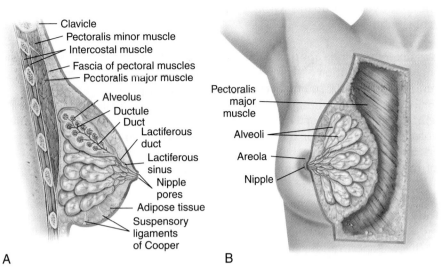

FIGURE 2-8 **The female breast. A,** Side view. Each lobule is drained by a lactiferous duct that leads to the nipple. **B,** Anterior view with internal structures. Glandular tissue is less prominent in the nonlactating breast.

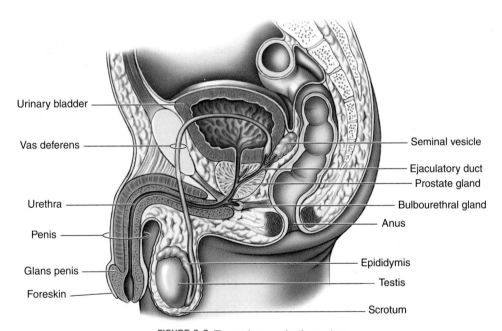

FIGURE 2-9 The male reproductive system.

the ovaries of the female. Each testis contains specialized tissue arranged in coiled tubes, called **seminiferous tubules,** where the **spermatozoa** (sperm) are produced. Between the small tubes is a small group of interstitial (Leydig's) cells that produce the male sex hormone testosterone. This hormone is responsible for the masculine characteristics of the male body. Some of the seminal fluid, or **semen,** in which the spermatozoa are transported, is also produced in the tubules in the testes. The two principal functions of the testes are to manufacture sperm cells

(spermatogenesis) and to secrete male hormones (androgens).

Within the testes is an elaborate ductal system. The tubelike path in each testis includes the epididymis, the vas deferens, and the seminal vesicles.

Epididymis. The testes open into the epididymis, a small coiled tube that, if stretched to its full extent, is approximately 6 m (20 feet) long. It becomes the vas deferens and is the excretory duct of each testis that provides a reservoir for the sperm. Sperm may be maintained within the epididymis for up to 3 weeks as they mature and become motile.

Vas Deferens. The vas deferens, a tube approximately 45 cm (18 inches) long, is a continuation of the epididymis. It ends by joining the duct of the seminal vesicle to form the ejaculatory duct. It carries the sperm from each testis to the urethra. The peristaltic activity of the muscles is responsible for the passage of the sperm along the vas deferens to the ejaculatory duct. A vasectomy, or severing of the vas deferens, is a means of male birth control.

Ejaculatory Duct. The ejaculatory duct is found at the base of the prostate gland and opens into the prostate portion of the urethra. It ejects sperm and seminal fluid into the urethra.

Accessory Glands

The accessory glands produce secretions for the following purposes:

1. Nourish the sperm
2. Protect the sperm from the acidic environment of the woman's vagina
3. Enhance movement (motility) of the sperm

Seminal Vesicles. The seminal vesicles are two saclike structures at the base of the urinary bladder. Their glandular lining produces a thick, milky secretion that forms much of the ejaculated semen. This secretion is thought to provide nourishment and protection for the sperm. The ducts of the seminal vesicles join the vas deferens to form the ejaculatory ducts, which empty into the urethra.

Prostate Gland. The prostate gland is a chestnut-sized structure that surrounds the urethra, just below the urinary bladder. During ejaculation, it contracts along with the vas deferens and seminal vesicles. It adds a thin, milky, alkaline fluid to the semen. The alkalinity of the fluid contributes to fertilization of an ovum. It helps neutralize the relatively acidic fluid of the vas deferens and the acidic environment of vaginal secretions, thereby enhancing sperm motility and life span.

Bulbourethral Glands (Cowper's Glands). The bulbourethral glands are approximately the size of a pea and are situated by the prostate gland on each side of the urethra. These glands secrete mucus into the urethra to serve as a lubricant and to supply alkaline fluid to the semen.

ENDOCRINE SYSTEM AND MALE REPRODUCTION

As in the female, many changes occur in the male at puberty. At roughly 10 years of age, the testes, prostate gland, seminal vesicles, and penis begin to enlarge as part of the general adolescent growth spurt. Pubic and axillary hair and hair on the upper lip and chin appear, and the larynx enlarges. By age 15 years (range, 9 to 17 years), boys are physically able to produce and ejaculate sperm.

During puberty, the pituitary gland begins to release follicle-stimulating hormone (FSH) and luteinizing hormone (LH) (interstitial cell-stimulating hormones). FSH helps in the production of spermatozoa. LH acts on the interstitial Leydig's cells of the testes to release androgens, the most significant of which is testosterone.

Testosterone hormonal functions include:

1. Developing the penis, scrotum, prostate gland, and seminal vesicles
2. Developing male secondary sex characteristics
3. Helping bones and muscles become thicker and longer
4. Enlarging the larynx, causing a lower voice
5. Enhancing the production of red blood cells

SPERMATOGENESIS

The formation of sperm (spermatogenesis) begins at puberty and continues throughout a male's life. A sperm's fertile life is estimated to be up to 5 days after ejaculation. Sperm are much smaller than ova. Sperm cells resemble tadpoles in shape, with oval heads and long tails. During each ejaculation, approximately 300 million sperm are deposited into the vagina. Only a few sperm achieve proximity to the ovum. Typically, only one sperm penetrates and fertilizes the ovum released at ovulation. Immediately after one sperm enters the ovum, a physiologic change takes place in the outer surface of the ovum that prevents entry of additional sperm. Presumably, this change occurs in response to a substance released from the cytoplasm of the ovum.

PHYSIOLOGY OF THE SEX ACT

The sexual response occurs in the following phases:

1. Excitement: Heart rate and blood pressure increase; nipples become erect.
2. Plateau: Skin flushes, erection occurs, and semen in the male appears on head of penis.
3. Orgasm: Involuntary muscle spasms of rectum, vagina, and uterus occur in the female; ejaculation occurs in the male.
4. Resolution: Engorgement resolves; vital signs return to normal.

PHYSIOLOGY OF THE MALE SEX ACT

The male psyche can initiate or inhibit the sexual response. The massaging action of intercourse on the glans penis stimulates sensitive nerves that send impulses to the sacral area of the spinal cord and to the brain. The parasympathetic nerve fibers cause the relaxation of penile arteries, which fill the cavernous sinuses in the shaft of the penis so that the penis becomes firm and elongated (erection). The same nerve impulses cause the urethral glands to secrete mucus to aid in lubrication for sperm motility. The sympathetic nervous system then stimulates the spinal nerves to contract the vas deferens and cause expulsion of the sperm into the urethra (emission). Contraction of the muscle of the prostate gland and seminal vesicles also expels prostatic and seminal fluid into the urethra, contributing to the flow and motility of the sperm. The nerves in the sacral region of the spinal cord aid in expelling semen from the urethra (ejaculation). The period of emission and ejaculation is called *male orgasm.*

Within minutes, erection ceases (resolution), the cavernous sinuses empty, penile arteries contract, and the penis becomes flaccid. Sperm can reach the woman's fallopian tube within 5 minutes and can remain viable in the female reproductive tract for 4 or 5 days. Of the millions of sperm contained in the ejaculate, a few thousand reach each fallopian tube but only one typically fertilizes the ovum. The sphincter in the base of the bladder closes during ejaculation so that sperm does not enter the bladder and urine cannot be expelled.

PHYSIOLOGY OF THE FEMALE SEX ACT

The female psyche can initiate or inhibit the sexual response. Local stimulation by massage to the breasts, vulva, vagina, and perineum creates sexual sensations. The sensitive nerves in the glans of the clitoris send signals to the sacral areas of the spinal cord, and these signals are transmitted to the brain. Parasympathetic nerves from the sacral plexus return signals to the erectile tissue around the vaginal introitus, dilating and filling the arteries and resulting in a tightening of the vagina around the penis. These signals stimulate the Bartholin's glands at the vaginal introitus to secrete mucus that aids in vaginal lubrication. The parasympathetic nervous system causes the perineal muscles and other muscles in the body to contract. The posterior pituitary gland secretes oxytocin, which stimulates the contraction of the uterus and dilation of the cervical canal. This process (orgasm) is believed to aid in the transport of the sperm to the fallopian tubes. (This process is also the reason why sexual abstinence is advised when there is a high risk for miscarriage or preterm labor.)

After orgasm, the muscles relax (resolution). The egg lives for only 24 hours after ovulation; therefore, sperm must be available during that time if fertilization is to occur.

Get Ready for the NCLEX® Examination!

Key Points

- Human reproduction requires an interaction between the reproductive organs, the central nervous system, and the endocrine system (pituitary, hypothalamus, ovaries, and testes).
- The female reproductive system consists of external and internal organs. The ovaries are where the female sex cells (ova) are formed. The fallopian tubes capture the ovum (egg) and transport it to the uterus, which provides an implantation site for the fertilized ovum (blastocyst). The lowest part of the uterus, the cervix, provides an opening into the vagina, which is a passageway from the cervix to the external genitalia. The vagina provides a passage for the discharge of menstrual blood and, during birth, a way for the fetus to be delivered outside of the body.
- The myometrium (middle muscular uterine layer) is functional in pregnancy and labor. The endometrium (inner uterine layer) is functional in menstruation and in the implantation of a fertilized ovum.
- There are four basic pelvis shapes, but women often have a combination of characteristics. The gynecoid pelvis is the most favorable for vaginal birth.
- The female reproductive system maintains a complex cycle known as the menstrual cycle. This cycle involves the ovaries and the uterus in the process of preparing for

conception, making changes in the uterine lining to support the embryo if conception occurs, and shedding the uterine (endometrial) lining through the process of menstruation if pregnancy does not occur.
- The breasts, or mammary glands, are generally considered part of reproduction because of their functional relation, that is, secreting milk (lactation).
- The male reproductive system consists of external and internal organs. The testes are where the male sex cells and male sex hormones are formed. There is a series of continuous ducts through which spermatozoa are transported outside of the male's body. Secretions are produced for sperm nutrition, survival, and movement. The penis serves as the male reproductive organ for sexual intercourse.
- Testosterone is the principal male hormone. Estrogen and progesterone are the principal female hormones. Testosterone secretion continues throughout a man's life, but estrogen and progesterone secretions are very low after a woman reaches the climacteric.
- The formation of sperm (spermatogenesis) begins at puberty and continues throughout life. A sperm is smaller than an ovum. Usually, only one sperm fertilizes a single ovum (egg) released at ovulation.
- The psyche can initiate or inhibit the sexual response.

Additional Learning Resources

SG Go to your Study Guide on page 475 for additional Review Questions for the NCLEX® Examination, Critical Thinking Clinical Situations, and other learning activities to help you master this chapter content.

evolve Go to your Evolve website (http://evolve.elsevier.com/Leifer/maternity) for the following FREE learning resources:
- Animations
- Answer Guidelines for Critical Thinking Questions
- Answers and Rationales for Review Questions for the NCLEX® Examination
- Concept Map Creator
- Glossary with pronunciations in English and Spanish
- Patient Teaching Plans
- Skills Performance Checklists and more!

 Online Resources
- www.aap.org
- www.ornl.gov/hgmis
- www.visibleembryo.com

Review Questions for the NCLEX® Examination

1. The first outward change of puberty in females is:
    1. Appearance of pubic and axillary hair
    2. Menarche
    3. Development of breasts
    4. Broadening of the hips

2. The acidic pH of the vagina is maintained by:
    1. The Bartholin's glands
    2. Frequent douching
    3. Doderlein's bacilli
    4. Circulating estrogens, progestins, and androgens

3. Spermatogenesis begins:
    1. During fetal life
    2. At birth
    3. At puberty
    4. During the excitement phase of the male sexual response

4. During what phase of the male sex act does flushing of the skin occur?
    1. Excitement
    2. Plateau
    3. Orgasm
    4. Resolution

5. Sperm can remain viable in the female reproductive tract for approximately:
    1. 1 week
    2. 4-5 days
    3. 24 hours
    4. 5 minutes

6. The vaginal vestibule contains what structure(s)? *(Select all that apply.)*
    1. Labia minora
    2. Vaginal opening
    3. Skene's ducts
    4. Urethral meatus
    5. Perineum

7. Fallopian tubes provide what function(s)? *(Select all that apply.)*
    1. Site of implantation for the fertilized ovum
    2. Passageway in which sperm meet the ovum
    3. Secretion of hormones
    4. Site for development and maturation of the ovum
    5. Means of transporting the ovum to the corpus of the uterus

8. Indicate the order in which the typical monthly menstrual cycle occurs by numbering the following 1 *(first)* to 4 *(last)*.
    2 Ovulation
    3 Corpus luteum formation
    1 Ovarian follicle maturation
    4 Menstrual bleeding

Critical Thinking Questions

1. A community high school teacher has asked you, a student nurse, to explain to students in a biology class the function of the male and female reproductive systems. What issues would you need to consider in planning your discussion?

2. Explore how a pregnant woman might feel about changes in her body caused by the anatomic and physiologic adaptations of the uterus and breasts during pregnancy.

chapter

3

Fetal Development

*e*volve

http://evolve.elsevier.com/Leifer/maternity

Objectives

1. Define key terms listed.
2. Define *chromosome* and state the number in each human body cell.
3. Compare a gene and a chromosome.
4. Explain how the sex of an individual is determined.
5. Describe human fertilization and implantation.
6. Discuss fetal development.
7. Explain the development and function of the placenta.
8. Review the functions of amniotic fluid and the umbilical cord.
9. Diagram fetal circulation to circulation after birth.
10. Discuss multifetal pregnancy, and compare two types of twins.

Key Terms

age of viability (p. 37)
amnion (ĂM-nē-ŏn, p. 32)
blastocyst (BLĂS-tō-sĭst, p. 31)
chorion (KŌ-rē-ŏn, p. 32)
chorionic villi (KŌ-rē-ŏn-ĭk VĬL-ī, p. 33)
chromosomes (KRŌ-mō-sōmz, p. 29)
conception (p. 31)
decidua (də-sidū-ə, p. 31)
deoxyribonucleic acid (DNA) (dē-ŎK-sē-rī-bō-nū-KLĀ-ĭk, p. 29)
dizygotic (p. 37)
ductus arteriosus (DŬK-tŭs ăhr-TĒR-ē-Ō-sŭs, p. 35)
ductus venosus (vĕn-Ō-sŭs, p. 35)
embryonic period (ĕm-brē-ŎN-ĭk, p. 32)
fertilization (p. 30)
foramen ovale (fŏrā-mĕn ō-VĂL, p. 35)

gametes (GĂM-ētz, p. 30)
gametogenesis (găm-ĕ-tō-JĔN-ĕ-sĭs, p. 30)
genes (jēnz, p. 29)
hydramnios (hī-DRĂM-nē-ŏs, p. 33)
implantation (p. 31)
meiosis (mī-Ō-sĭs, p. 30)
mitosis (mī-TŌ-sĭs, p. 30)
monozygotic (p. 37)
morula (MŌR-ū-lă, p. 31)
multifetal pregnancy (p. 37)
oligohydramnios (ol-ĭgō-hī-DRĂM-nē-ŏs, p. 33)
placenta (plăSĔN-tă, p. 33)
teratogenic agents (p. 31)
trophoblasts (TRŌF-ō-blăsts, p. 31)
Wharton's jelly (p. 35)
zygote (ZĪ-gōt, p. 31)

GENETICS

At birth, the human body consists of many millions of cells, but life begins with a single cell. The first cell of a new human being is formed by the fusion of a sperm from the male and an ovum from the female. Genetic codes are programmed into the new individual's cells by deoxyribonucleic acid (DNA).

DNA is viewed as spiral-shaped strands found in the nucleus of all human cells. Figure 3-1 shows the relationships of the cell, nucleus, chromosome, genes, and DNA. DNA is the master protein that controls the development and functioning of all cells.

Genes are programmed to use DNA through specific codes of instructions from four molecules: adenine (A), thymine (T), cytosine (C), and guanine (G). A single mistake in a code or variation in the genetic sequence means a cell may make the wrong amount or type of protein, which can disrupt the cell's function and lead to changes that may have serious effects on the developing organism. These mistakes can lead to mutations or disease. Defects within the cell's DNA code are the root of many inherited disorders. The master blueprint for a person's characteristics is determined by genes in chromosomes, which are located within the nucleus of each body cell.

CHROMOSOMES

Chromosomes are threadlike, spiral structures found within the nucleus of each cell. Chromosomes are made up of long chains or building blocks of DNA that

INSIDE THE CELL

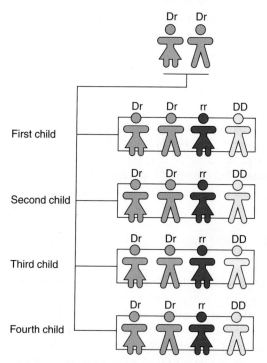

Cell   Nucleus   Chromosome   DNA   Gene (Segment of DNA)

FIGURE 3-1 Inside the cell: cell, nucleus, chromosome, DNA, and gene.

control heredity. Chromosomes occur in pairs; one member of the pair is supplied by the mother and the other by the father. Each cell in the human body contains 46 chromosomes, or 22 arranged pairs, known as *autosomes* (body chromosomes), and one pair of gametes, or "sex cells," which determine the sex of the fetus. Each chromosome is composed of genes, which are defined as segments of DNA that control heredity. A gene can be described as a single bead, and a chromosome is like a string of beads.

CELL DIVISION AND GAMETOGENESIS

The division of a cell begins in its nucleus, which contains the gene-bearing chromosomes. The two types of cell division are mitosis and meiosis.

Mitosis is a continuous process by which the body grows and develops and dead body cells are replaced. In this type of cell division, each daughter cell contains the same number of chromosomes as the parent cell. The 46 chromosomes in a body cell are called the **diploid** number of chromosomes. The process of mitosis in the sperm is called **spermatogenesis,** and in the ovum is called **oogenesis** (the development of an oocyte into an ovum).

Meiosis is a different type of cell division in which the reproductive cells undergo two sequential divisions. During meiosis, the number of chromosomes in each cell is reduced to half, or 23 chromosomes, each with one sex chromosome only. This is called the **haploid** number of chromosomes. This process is completed in the sperm before it travels toward the fallopian tube and in the ovum after ovulation if fertilized. At the moment of fertilization (when the sperm and ovum unite), the new cell contains 23 chromosomes from the sperm and 23 chromosomes from the ovum, thus returning to the diploid number of chromosomes (46); traits are therefore inherited from both the mother and the father. The formation of gametes by this type of cell division is called gametogenesis.

As soon as fertilization occurs, a chemical change in the membrane around the fertilized ovum prevents penetration by another sperm.

GENES

Each gene (a segment of the DNA chain) is coded for inheritance. The coded information carried by the DNA in the gene is responsible for individual traits, such as eye and hair color, facial features, and body shape. Genes carry instructions for **dominant** and **recessive** traits. Dominant traits usually overpower recessive traits and are passed on to the offspring. If only one parent carries a dominant trait, 50% of the offspring will have that dominant trait. If *each* parent carries a recessive trait, there is a chance that one of the offspring will display that trait (Figure 3-2).

Key

- ■ Person has disorder
- ▨ Person carries one gene for disorder but does not have disorder
- □ Person has no disorder and does not carry one gene for disorder

FIGURE 3-2 This figure shows how a disorder carried as a recessive trait can be passed on to offspring when each parent is a carrier of that recessive trait. (D) represents a dominant gene, and (r) represents a recessive gene.

SEX DETERMINATION

The sex of an individual is determined at the time of fertilization. It depends on the type of spermatozoon that penetrates the ovum (egg). The spermatozoon (sperm cell) has an X or Y chromosome, whereas the female ovum always contains the X chromosome. When the spermatozoon with an X factor unites with the ovum, a female (XX) will result. When an ovum is fertilized with a spermatozoon that contains the Y factor, a male (XY) will result. Because the father may contribute either a Y- or X-bearing sperm, it is the male sperm that is responsible for determining the sex of the embryo (Figure 3-3).

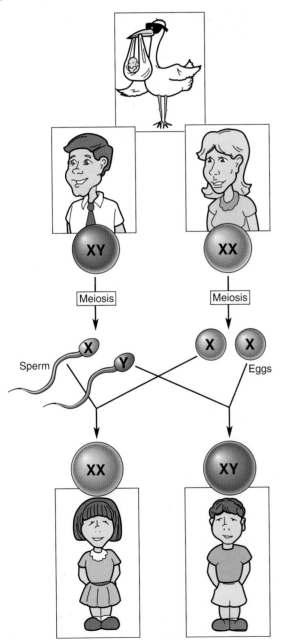

FIGURE 3-3 Sex determination at the time of conception. If an X chromosome from the man unites with an X chromosome from the woman, the child will be female (XX). If a Y chromosome from the man unites with an X chromosome from the woman, the child will be male (XY).

BEGINNING OF EMBRYONIC DEVELOPMENT

FERTILIZATION

Conception is the union of the egg and sperm, also known as *fertilization*. Fertilization normally takes place in the outer third of the uterine (fallopian) tube. Approximately 300 million spermatozoa are deposited into the vagina at ejaculation. Most of the sperm remain in the vagina and within the cervical mucus in the endometrium. After a single sperm enters the ovum, a membrane forms that prevents the entry of more sperm. The ovum can be fertilized for approximately 6 to 24 hours after its release from the ovary, whereas sperm are viable for up to 5 days after ejaculation and their entrance into the female genital tract. At fertilization, the nucleus of the sperm and the nucleus of the ovum unite to form a zygote.

[?] Did You Know?

Life Expectancy of Ovum and Sperm

Although the ovum lives and can be fertilized for 6 to 24 hours after ovulation, the sperm can live for up to 5 days after ejaculation.

IMPLANTATION

The zygote begins a rapid series of cell divisions while traveling down the fallopian tube toward the uterus. Within approximately 3 days, cell division results in a solid mass of 16 cells, called a morula. The morula cells continue to multiply as the morula floats free in the uterine cavity for another 3 or 4 days. Large cells tend to mass at the periphery of the morula ball, leaving a fluid space surrounding an inner cell mass. At this stage, the formed structure is termed a blastocyst. The cells in the outer ring are known as trophoblasts. At this time, the blastocyst contains various components: (1) a fluid-filled cavity; (2) the trophoblast (outer wall), which later will become the **placenta;** and (3) an inner cell mass, which will form the **embryo.** The trophoblast cells secrete enzymes that permit them to invade the thickened uterine lining, or endometrium (decidua). During implantation (the cell mass typically takes root in the upper segment of the uterus), trophoblastic cells provide nutrition for the embryo from nutrients carried in the maternal blood. The trophoblastic layer (which later forms the chorion) of blastocyst cells begin to mature rapidly (Figure 3-4). As early as the twelfth day, miniature villi, or rootlike projections, reach out from the layer of cells into the uterine endometrium. These projections (**chorionic villi**) extend from the chorion into the endometrium.

During the stages of development that immediately follow implantation, teratogenic agents such as drugs, viruses, or radiation may exert profound and

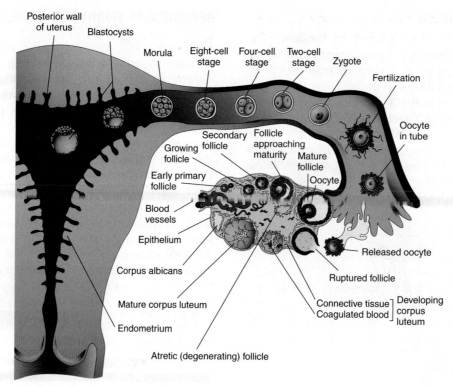

FIGURE 3-4 **Ovulation and fertilization.** Ovulation occurs; the egg is caught by the fimbriae and is guided into the fallopian tube, where fertilization occurs. The zygote continues to multiply (but not grow in size) as it passes through the fallopian tube and implants into the posterior wall of the uterus at approximately 7 days.

damaging effects on the developing embryo. The embryonic period of development is from the second to the eighth week after conception, when most of the basic organ structures are formed. From the eighth week until birth, this developing human being is called a **fetus** (Box 3-1).

EMBRYONIC CELL DIFFERENTIATION

During the second and third weeks after conception, three cell layers form: the **ectoderm, mesoderm,** and **endoderm.** These cell layers become all of the tissues and organs of the embryo. Each germ layer has specific characteristics (Box 3-2). The differentiated cells stay attached by a body stalk, which later forms the umbilical cord by day 14. Small spaces soon form the **amniotic cavity.** This hollow space will eventually surround the developing embryo and fetus like a protective, transparent sac.

FETAL MEMBRANES AND AMNIOTIC FLUID

The two membranes, called the *chorion* and the *amnion,* begin to form at the time of implantation. The amnion, the inner membrane, protects the developing embryo. It forms a cavity in which the embryo or fetus floats, suspended in amniotic fluid. The amnion expands to accommodate the growing fetus. The chorion is the

---

Box 3-1 | **Fetal Development**

Zygote: From fertilization to the second week; then the blastocyst stage lasts 2 or 3 days
Embryo: Between the second and eighth weeks of gestation
Fetus: From the ninth week of gestation to birth

Box 3-2 | **Structures Derived from Three Germ Cell Layers**

ECTODERM
- Outer layer of skin
- Oil glands and hair follicles of skin
- Nails and hair
- External sense organs
- Mucous membrane of mouth and anus

MESODERM
- True skin
- Skeleton
- Bone and cartilage
- Connective tissue
- Muscles
- Blood and blood vessels
- Kidneys and gonads

ENDODERM
- Lining of trachea, pharynx, and bronchi
- Lining of digestive tract
- Lining of bladder and urethra

outer membrane that encloses the growing amnion. As the fetus grows, the amnion expands until the chorion and the amnion fuse together to become the amniotic sac, or "bag of waters." The amniotic sac contains a clear, slightly straw-colored liquid, called the **amniotic fluid**. This fluid consists of 98% water and contains traces of protein, glucose, fetal lanugo (hair), fetal urine, and vernix caseosa (a cheesy material that covers the fetal skin). Examination of the amniotic fluid for diagnostic purposes (amniocentesis) is discussed in Chapter 5. Most amniotic fluid appears to be derived from the maternal blood. Later, the fetus also adds to the fluid by excreting urine into it. Some amniotic fluid is swallowed by the fetus and is subsequently absorbed by its gastrointestinal tract. The amount of amniotic fluid present at term varies from 800 to 1000 mL. The presence of more than 2 L is called hydramnios (excessive fluid). An excess of amniotic fluid is associated with malformations of the fetal central nervous system and the gastrointestinal tract. An amount of amniotic fluid that is less than 300 mL is oligohydramnios, and it is associated with renal abnormalities. The functions of the amniotic fluid are listed in Box 3-3.

PLACENTA

The placenta is a remarkable fetomaternal organ that consists of both fetal and maternal sections. This organ permits the exchange of materials carried in the bloodstream between the mother and the embryo or fetus (Figure 3-5).

The placenta formation begins at the outer layer of the blastocyst, called the *trophoblastic cells*. These cells proliferate and develop the chorionic villi (projections that become the major site of exchange between maternal and fetal circulation). These villi penetrate the decidua (lining of the uterus). The maternal vessels dilate around the villi and form sinuses that become the intervillous spaces. The chorionic villi float freely in a pool of maternal blood and divide repeatedly to form complex treelike structures in which each villus becomes a branch. Some villi attach themselves to the endometrial maternal tissue, anchoring the zygote

(fertilized egg) to the endometrium (lining of the uterus). The placental villi can be likened to the roots of plants submerged in a bowl of water in that they absorb nourishment from the water that surrounds them. The maternal blood circulates slowly, enabling it to be transferred across the membrane of the villi, absorbing nutrients and oxygen and excreting waste. Minimum uteroplacental circulation begins early, approximately 17 days after conception. As gestation continues, the intervillous spaces grow larger and become separated by a series of partitions or segments. In the mature placenta, there are as many as 30 separate segments, called **cotyledons.** Approximately 100 maternal arterioles supply the mature placenta to provide enough blood for gas and nutrient exchange. The rate of uteroplacental blood flow increases from 50 mL/min at 10 weeks to 500 to 600 mL/min at term. The maternal and fetal circulatory systems are separate, with an occasional break in one of the smaller chorionic villi, allowing some mixing of fetal and maternal blood products.

PLACENTAL FUNCTIONS

The placental functions include protection, nutrition, respiration, excretion, and hormone production.

Placental Transfer

Placental transport or transfer involves movement of gases, nutrients, waste materials, drugs, and other substances across the placenta from maternal to fetal circulation or from fetal to maternal circulation. Transfer can be modified by maternal nutritional status, exercise, and disease. Transfer can be increased by maternal hyperglycemia and decreased by reduced uteroplacental blood flow.

Immunologic Functions

Immunologic functions of the placenta include protection of the fetus from pathogens and prevention from rejection by the mother. The placenta allows most viruses, some bacteria, pollutants, and most drugs to cross the placental membrane. In general, blood cells are too large to cross unless there is a placental leak (break), which would allow them to enter fetal circulation, or the reverse (fetal cells entering maternal circulation). Because of this, prenatal $Rh_o(D)$ immune globulin (RhoGAM) is given to Rh-negative women at 28 weeks' gestation to prevent Rh isoimmunization (see Chapter 13). Some substances (e.g., drugs and pollutants) that circulate in the maternal bloodstream can be teratogenic and can harm the fetus. Because some prescribed drugs for medical conditions may be harmful to the fetus, the woman should consult her health care provider before taking them.

Box 3-3 Functions of Amniotic Fluid

- Allows the embryo or fetus to move about freely
- Prevents the amnion from adhering to the embryo or fetus
- Cushions the embryo or fetus against injury from external sources
- Maintains a constant temperature surrounding the embryo or fetus
- Provides fluid homeostasis for the embryo or fetus
- Prevents umbilical cord compression

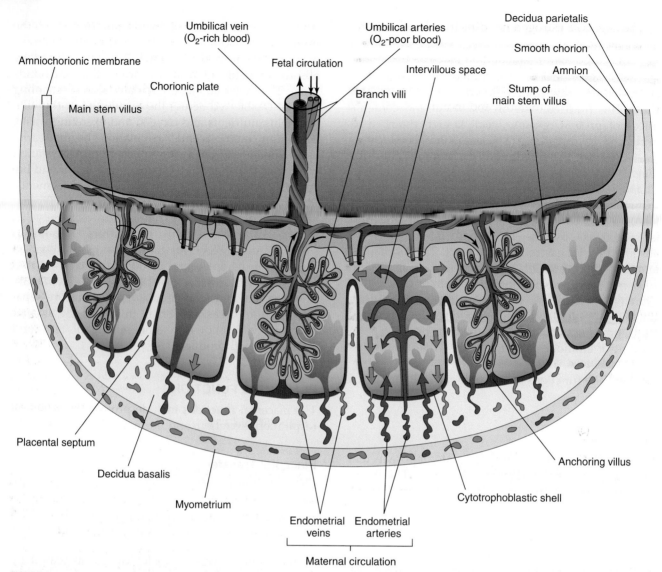

FIGURE 3-5 **Placental circulation.** The blood of the fetus flows through the umbilical arteries into the fetal capillaries in the villi and then back to the fetal circulation through the umbilical vein. Maternal blood is transported by the uterine spiral arteries to the intervillous space, and it leaves by the uterine veins to return to the maternal circulation. Metabolic and gaseous exchange occurs as the blood flows slowly around the villi. *Fetal and maternal blood do not mix together.*

Placental Blood Flow

Placental blood flow can be reduced if the uterine artery is constricted because of certain maternal diseases, such as hypertension. Substances that can cross the placental barrier and harm the fetus are alcohol, nicotine, carbon monoxide, and some prescription and recreational drugs. Uterine contractions will decrease the amount of blood flow to the intervillous spaces because the spiral arterioles travel through the myometrium. Therefore, the uterus should be monitored for relaxation between contractions. Position change from supine to side-lying position will increase the blood flow.

Placental Hormones

Four hormones are produced by the placenta: progesterone, estrogen, human chorionic gonadotropin (hCG), and human placental lactogen (hPL).

Progesterone. Progesterone is first produced by the corpus luteum and later by the placenta. It has the following functions during pregnancy:
- Maintain the uterine lining for implantation of the zygote
- Reduce uterine contractions to prevent spontaneous abortion
- Prepare the glands of the breasts for lactation
- Stimulate testes to produce testosterone, which aids the male fetus in developing the reproductive tract

Estrogen. Estrogen has the following important functions during pregnancy:
- Stimulate uterine growth
- Increase the blood flow to uterine vessels
- Stimulate the development of the breast ducts to prepare for lactation

The effects of estrogen not directly related to pregnancy include:
- Increased skin pigmentation (such as the "mask of pregnancy")
- Vascular changes in the skin and the mucous membranes of the nose and mouth
- Increased salivation

UMBILICAL CORD

The lifeline linking the fetus with the placenta is the umbilical cord. It extends from the umbilicus (navel) of the fetus to the placenta. Within the cord are two umbilical arteries and one umbilical vein. The cord is embedded in Wharton's jelly, a thick substance that is a physical buffer to prevent kinking of the cord and interference with circulation.

In contrast to the pattern of circulation after birth, the umbilical arteries carry deoxygenated blood, and the umbilical vein carries oxygenated blood. Blood from the fetus flows through the umbilical arteries to the placenta, where it releases carbon dioxide and other waste products. The umbilical vein carries oxygen and nutrients from the placenta to the fetus (Figure 3-6).

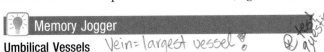

Memory Jogger
Umbilical Vessels

An easy way to remember the number and types of umbilical vessels is to use the mnemonic *AVA*, which stands for *Artery, Vein, Artery.*

CIRCULATION BEFORE AND AFTER BIRTH

Embryonic Circulation
The developing fertilized ovum derives nutrition first from its own cytoplasmic mass and then from the decidua (the thickened lining of the uterus) by the activity of the trophoblastic cells. At approximately the fourth week, the embryo gains circulation and nourishment from the yolk sac. Later, the fetus relies on circulation of oxygenated blood from chorionic villi in the placenta through the umbilical vein.

Fetal Circulation
After the fourth week of gestation, blood circulation through the placenta to the fetus is well established (Figure 3-7). Because the fetus does not breathe, and

the liver does not have to process most waste products, several physiologic diversions in the prebirth circulatory route are needed. The three fetal circulatory shunts are as follows:
1. Ductus venosus, which diverts some blood away from the liver as it returns from the placenta
2. Foramen ovale, which diverts most blood from the right atrium directly to the left atrium, rather than circulating it to the lungs
3. Ductus arteriosus, which diverts most blood from the pulmonary artery into the aorta

Circulation Before Birth
Oxygenated blood enters the fetal body through the umbilical vein. About half of the blood goes to the liver through the portal sinus, with the remainder entering the inferior vena cava through the ductus venosus. Blood in the inferior vena cava enters the right atrium, where most passes directly into the left atrium through the foramen ovale. A small amount of blood is pumped to the lungs by the right ventricle. The rest of the blood from the right ventricle joins that from the left ventricle through the ductus arteriosus. After circulating through the fetal body, blood containing waste products is returned to the placenta through the umbilical arteries (Table 3-1).

Circulation After Birth
Fetal shunts are not needed after birth once the infant breathes and blood is circulated to the lungs. The foramen ovale closes because pressure in the right side of the heart falls as the lungs become fully inflated and there is now little resistance to blood flow. The infant's blood oxygen level rises, causing the ductus arteriosus to constrict. The ductus venosus closes when the flow from the umbilical cord stops (Table 3-2).

Closure of Fetal Circulatory Shunts. The foramen ovale closes functionally (temporarily) within 2 hours after birth and permanently by age 3 months. The ductus arteriosus closes functionally within 15 hours and closes permanently in about 3 weeks. The ductus venosus closes functionally when the cord is cut and closes permanently in about 1 week. After permanent closure, the ductus arteriosus and ductus venosus become ligaments.

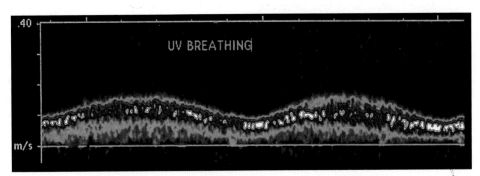

FIGURE 3-6 An ultrasound of the umbilical cord showing circulation.

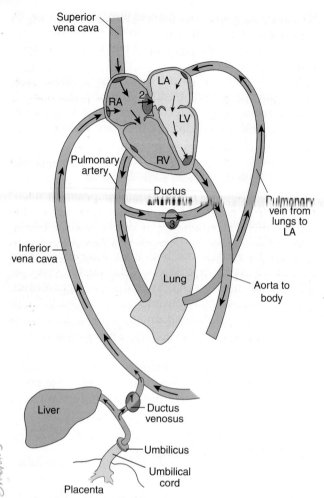

FIGURE 3-7 **Fetal circulation.** Three shunts exist to allow most blood from the placenta to bypass the fetal lungs and liver: ductus venosus (*1*), foramen ovale (*2*), and ductus arteriosus (*3*). *LA*, Left atrium; *LV*, left ventricle; *RA*, right atrium; *RV*, right ventricle.

Table 3-1	Structures in Fetal Circulation
STRUCTURE	**DESCRIPTION**
Placenta and vessels	Vessels necessary for oxygenation and exchange of waste products.
Umbilical vein	One vein that carries oxygenated blood from the placenta to the fetus.
Umbilical arteries	Two arteries that carry deoxygenated blood from the fetus to the placenta
Foramen ovale	Opening between the right and left atria of the heart
Ductus arteriosus	Fetal blood vessel connecting the pulmonary artery and the aorta
Ductus venosus	Fetal blood vessel connecting the umbilical vein with the inferior vena cava

Because they are functionally closed rather than permanently closed, some conditions may cause the foramen ovale or ductus arteriosus to reopen after birth. A condition that impedes full lung expansion (e.g., respiratory distress syndrome) can increase the resistance to blood flow from the heart to the lungs, causing the

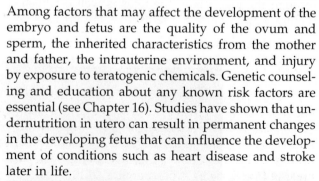

Table 3-2	Circulatory Changes After Birth
CIRCULATORY FEATURE	**CHANGES**
Umbilical vessels	The umbilical vessels are clamped and cut; to receive oxygen, the infant must use the lungs.
Lungs	Aeration occurs; blood is circulated through the lungs.
Pattern of blood flow	Blood flow pattern changes from fetal to newborn as the infant begins to breathe.
Circulation to lungs	As the infant inflates the lungs, pressure is released from the lungs' blood vessels.
Line of least resistance	As the blood vessels open in the lungs, blood is no longer diverted through ductus arteriosus; rather, following the line of least resistance, blood enters the vessels leading to the lungs.
Increased pressure	The change in blood flow increases pressure in the left atrium, which causes the foramen ovale to close.
Heart functions with two separate pumps	The right side of the heart receives deoxygenated blood and pumps it to the lungs; the oxygenated blood is directed to the left side of the heart, where it is pumped through the aorta to other parts of the body.
Ductus arteriosus	The ductus arteriosus functionally closes; therefore, deoxygenated blood cannot mix with oxygenated blood.
Ductus venosus	The ductus venosus functionally closes, and the blood flows through the portal system (the liver).

foramen ovale to reopen. Similar conditions often reduce the blood oxygen levels and can cause the ductus arteriosus to remain open. See Chapter 16 for further discussion of newborn congenital cardiac problems. Details concerning the onset of respirations and the changes in body functions in the newborn are discussed in Chapter 9.

FETAL DEVELOPMENT

Among factors that may affect the development of the embryo and fetus are the quality of the ovum and sperm, the inherited characteristics from the mother and father, the intrauterine environment, and injury by exposure to teratogenic chemicals. Genetic counseling and education about any known risk factors are essential (see Chapter 16). Studies have shown that undernutrition in utero can result in permanent changes in the developing fetus that can influence the development of conditions such as heart disease and stroke later in life.

The fetus develops in an orderly fashion. Developmental milestones exist in fetal growth and

test * must avoid intercourse for a pregnant women @ risk for preterm labor!

Fetal Development   CHAPTER **3**   37

development as they do in growth and development after birth. The three basic developmental stages include the *zygote* (conception to second week), the *embryo* (second to eighth weeks), and the *fetus* (ninth week to birth). By the second week after fertilization, the *ectoderm, endoderm,* and amnion begin to develop. By the third week, the *mesoderm* and neural tube form, and the primitive heart begins to pump. At this time, the mother may first recognize she may be pregnant. Neural tube defects can be prevented by folic acid supplements, which are very important during the first few weeks of pregnancy. By the end of the seventh week, the beginnings of all major fetal organs and systems are present. At first, the functions of most organs are minimal; however, by the end of 9 months, the fetus is prepared structurally, functionally, and metabolically for extrauterine life.

 Nutrition Considerations

Folic Acid Supplementation

Folic acid supplements can prevent most neural tube defects such as spina bifida. Because it is possible for a neural tube defect to occur before the woman knows she is pregnant, early prenatal care and good nutrition for all women during the childbearing years are important.

The most critical time for fetal development is the first 8 weeks; this is called the **organogenesis period.** In addition, each organ has a critical period when insults, such as teratogenic agents (agents in the environment that cause damage to the developing fetus), can easily cause physical and functional defects (Figure 3-8). The potential for harm caused by maternal malnutrition, chronic and acute diseases, and teratogens, such as drugs, continues until birth. Teaching the pregnant woman about maintaining her health, avoiding teratogens, and protecting her unborn infant is an important nursing responsibility. The growth of the fetus is limited by the nutrients and oxygen received from the mother.

 Health Promotion

Good Health Practices

A mother's ability to nourish her fetus is established in her own fetal life and by her adult nutritional experience. Therefore, to prevent illness in the next generation, there must be a focus on the health practices of this generation.

A healthy mother can produce a healthy child who is less prone to develop illness. Part of the goal of *Healthy People 2020* is to enable all people to develop a healthy lifestyle so that, as parents, they can nourish and parent healthy children for the next generation (U.S. Department of Health and Human Services, 2010).

At the fourteenth week, fetal movement in response to stimuli cannot be felt by the mother, and, by the

20 weeks' gestation, the fetus may survive outside of the uterus. (This is called the age of viability.) However, special care in the neonatal intensive care unit (NICU) is required, and many preterm infants born at this stage do not survive for long. Surfactant, which helps keep the alveoli in the lungs open during respiration, is minimal even at 28 weeks' gestation (see Chapter 15). At 40 weeks' gestation, the fetus is considered full-term and ready to be born. Table 3-3 describes and illustrates the growth and development that occurs during fetal life.

The fetus that is born past 42 weeks' gestation is termed **postterm** or **postmature.** The postterm infant typically has long nails, an abundance of hair on the head, a diminished amount of vernix caseosa, diminished adipose tissue, and dry, peeling skin. A major concern in postmaturity is the decreased efficiency of the aging placenta. As the placenta ages, the fetus often is deprived of essential support, such as adequate oxygenation and waste removal. Therefore, the postterm infant is at risk for having life-threatening problems. Care of the postterm newborn is discussed in Chapter 15.

MULTIFETAL PREGNANCY

A multifetal pregnancy is one in which more than one fetus develops in the uterine cavity at the same time. Twins can be classified as monozygotic (identical twins) or dizygotic (fraternal twins).

MONOZYGOTIC TWINS

When twins result from the splitting of one fertilized egg (monozygotic), they are called identical twins. They are produced from the fertilization of a single ovum by one sperm. The ovum splits into two identical monozygotes sometime before the fifteenth day of gestation (Figure 3-9). If this division is incomplete, conjoined (formerly called Siamese) twins will result. The amniotic sacs and placentas may be shared or separate. These twins are always the same sex and are mirror images of each other.

DIZYGOTIC TWINS

If two ova are fertilized by two sperm, fraternal, or nonidentical (dizygotic), twins will result. Each fetus has its own amniotic sac and placenta. The twins can be the same sex or opposite sexes. The resemblance to each other is no closer than to other siblings. The use of fertility drugs and in vitro fertilization has increased the incidence of multifetal pregnancy (twins, triplets, quadruplets, etc.). The incidence is also increased in women who are older and have a higher parity (see Chapter 14).

Many twin or higher multiples are born prematurely because the uterus becomes overdistended. The placenta may not be able to supply sufficient nutrition to both fetuses, resulting in one or both twins being smaller than expected.

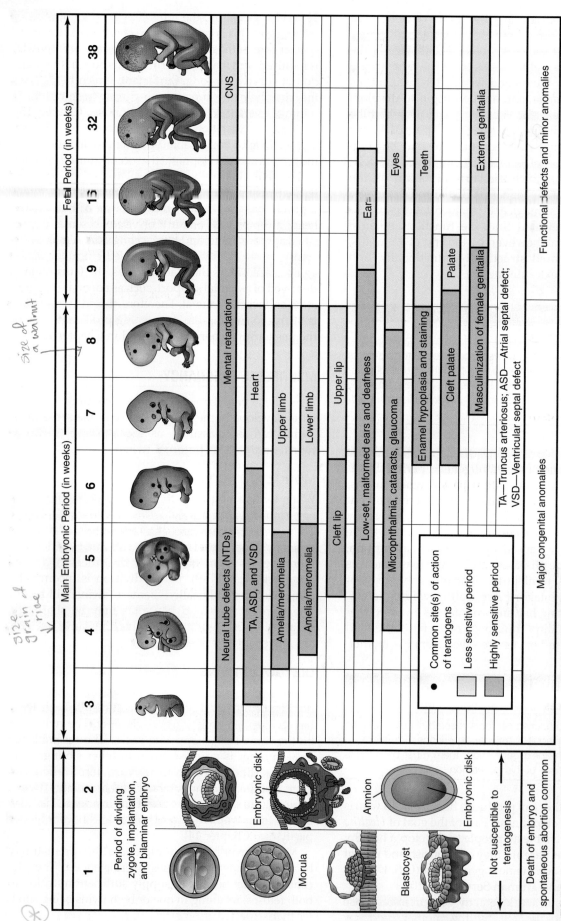

FIGURE 3-8 The sensitive or critical periods in human prenatal development. During the first 2 weeks of development, the embryo is affected by maternal influences such as nutrition status; a teratogen either damages all or most of the cells, resulting in death of the embryo, or damages only a few cells, allowing the conceptus to recover and the embryo to develop. Darker color denotes highly sensitive periods when major defects may be produced (e.g., amelia, or absence of limbs). Lighter color indicates stages that are less sensitive to teratogens when minor defects may be induced (e.g., hypoplastic thumbs). *CNS,* central nervous system.

Table 3-3 Fetal Development

AGE	LENGTH AND WEIGHT	DEVELOPMENT
Week 4 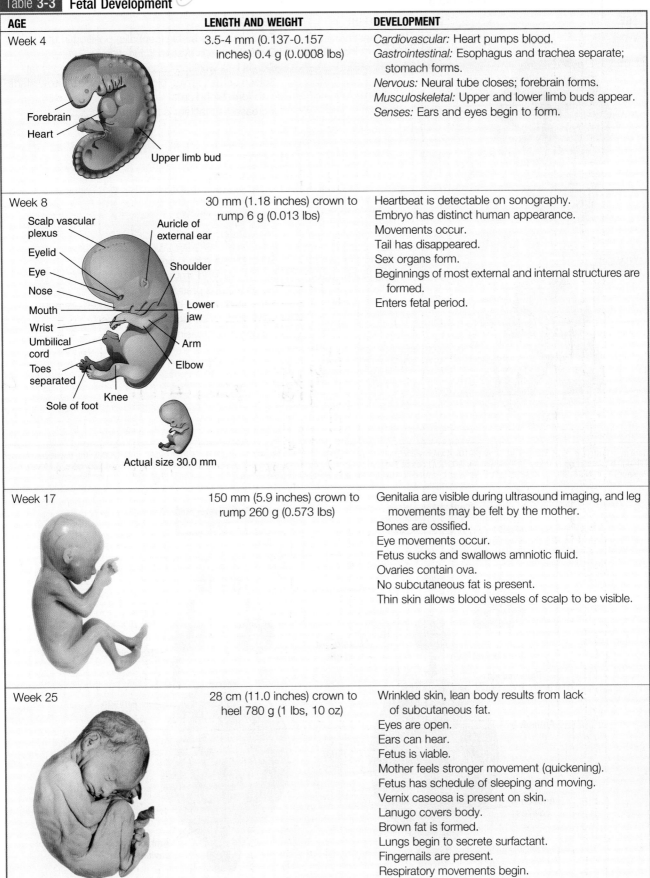 Forebrain / Heart / Upper limb bud	3.5-4 mm (0.137-0.157 inches) 0.4 g (0.0008 lbs)	*Cardiovascular:* Heart pumps blood. *Gastrointestinal:* Esophagus and trachea separate; stomach forms. *Nervous:* Neural tube closes; forebrain forms. *Musculoskeletal:* Upper and lower limb buds appear. *Senses:* Ears and eyes begin to form.
Week 8 Scalp vascular plexus / Eyelid / Eye / Nose / Mouth / Wrist / Umbilical cord / Toes separated / Sole of foot / Knee / Auricle of external ear / Shoulder / Lower jaw / Arm / Elbow. Actual size 30.0 mm	30 mm (1.18 inches) crown to rump 6 g (0.013 lbs)	Heartbeat is detectable on sonography. Embryo has distinct human appearance. Movements occur. Tail has disappeared. Sex organs form. Beginnings of most external and internal structures are formed. Enters fetal period.
Week 17	150 mm (5.9 inches) crown to rump 260 g (0.573 lbs)	Genitalia are visible during ultrasound imaging, and leg movements may be felt by the mother. Bones are ossified. Eye movements occur. Fetus sucks and swallows amniotic fluid. Ovaries contain ova. No subcutaneous fat is present. Thin skin allows blood vessels of scalp to be visible.
Week 25	28 cm (11.0 inches) crown to heel 780 g (1 lbs, 10 oz)	Wrinkled skin, lean body results from lack of subcutaneous fat. Eyes are open. Ears can hear. Fetus is viable. Mother feels stronger movement (quickening). Fetus has schedule of sleeping and moving. Vernix caseosa is present on skin. Lanugo covers body. Brown fat is formed. Lungs begin to secrete surfactant. Fingernails are present. Respiratory movements begin.

Continued

Table 3-3 Fetal Development—cont'd

AGE	LENGTH AND WEIGHT	DEVELOPMENT
Week 29	38 cm (15 inches) crown to heel 1260 g (2 lbs, 10 oz)	Fetus assumes stable (cephalic) position in utero. Central nervous system is functioning. Skin is less wrinkled because of subcutaneous fat. Spleen stops forming blood cells; bone marrow starts to form blood cells. Increased surfactant is present in lungs.
Week 36	48 cm (19 inches) crown to heel 2500 g (5 lbs, 12 oz)	Subcutaneous fat is present. Skin is pink and smooth. Grasp reflex is present. Circumferences of head and abdomen are equal. Surge of lung surfactant is produced. Lanugo is decreasing.

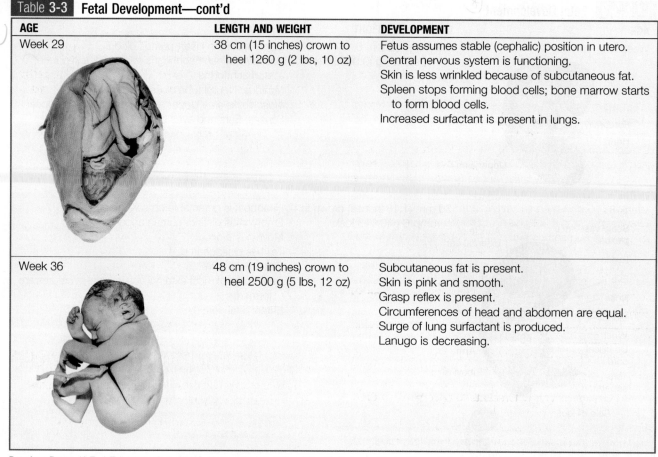

Data from Patton, K. T., & Thibodeau, G. A. (2010). *Anatomy and physiology* (7th ed.). St. Louis: Mosby; Moore, K. L., & Persaud, T. V. N. (2008). *The developing human* (8th ed.). Philadelphia: Saunders; Blackburn, S. (2007). *Maternal, fetal, and neonatal physiology: A clinical perspective* (3rd ed.). Philadelphia: Saunders; & Moore, K. L., Persaud, T. V. N., & Shiota, K. (2000). *Color atlas of clinical embryology* (2nd ed.). Philadelphia: Saunders.

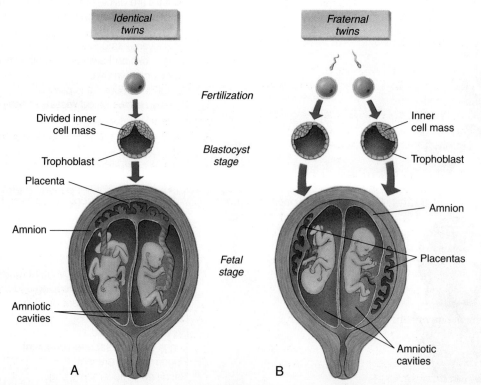

FIGURE 3-9 **Multiple births. A,** Identical (monozygotic) twins develop when the embryonic tissue from a single egg splits to form two individuals. The placenta is shared by the twins. **B,** Fraternal twins (dizygotic) develop when two different ova are fertilized by two separate sperm producing separate zygotes. Each twin has its own placenta, amnion, and chorion.

Get Ready for the NCLEX® Examination!

Key Points

- A new human life begins with the fusion of a sperm and ovum.
- What we inherit from our parents is determined by genes contained in chromosomes, which are located within the nucleus of each body cell.
- Chromosomes are located in the cell nucleus and are made up of long chains of building blocks of DNA. Genes, a segment of the DNA chain, are coded for inherited traits. In the tiny gene, four-protein molecules (A, T, C, and G) carry dominant and recessive traits.
- Every soma (body) cell has 46 chromosomes arranged in 22 pairs of autosomes and one pair of sex chromosomes (one from each parent) within the nucleus.
- The determination of fetal sex depends on whether the female X chromosome unites with the X or Y chromosome from the male. An XY match produces a male, and an XX match produces a female.
- Fertilization (fusion of the nuclei of the sperm and ovum) normally takes place in the outer third of the fallopian tube (uterine tube) 6 to 24 hours after ovulation.
- Approximately 2 to 3 weeks after fertilization, three cell layers form the ectoderm, mesoderm, and endoderm. These cell layers later differentiate to become all of the tissues and organs of the embryo.
- Embryonic membranes are the amnion (inner layer, which contains amniotic fluid and the embryo) and chorion (outer layer that encloses the amnion).
- The preembryonic period begins with conception and ends at 3 weeks' gestation. Early organ formation occurs.
- The embryonic period lasts through 8 weeks' gestation, with continued development of organs with limited function. Teratogenic agents are most likely to disturb development and cause damage to the embryo during the first 8 weeks of gestation.
- The fetal period (9 weeks until birth) is when the organs continue to develop, and the body systems get ready for extrauterine life.
- The placenta is an organ that provides for fetal respiration, nutrition, and excretion. It is also a temporary endocrine gland, producing progesterone, estrogen, hCG, and hPL.
- The umbilical cord contains two arteries that carry deoxygenated blood away from the fetus and one vein that carries oxygenated blood to the fetus. The cord is embedded in Wharton's jelly, which prevents kinking.
- The placenta, umbilical cord, and fetal circulation support fetal growth and development.
- Changes in fetal circulation at birth include closing of the ductus arteriosus, ductus venosus, and foramen ovale, which occurs as the umbilical cord is cut and blood flows to the lungs for oxygenation.
- Multifetal pregnancy means that more than one fetus develops in the uterus at the same time.
- Identical twins develop from a single fertilized ovum, and nonidentical (or fraternal) twins occur when two ova are fertilized by two separate sperm.

Additional Learning Resources

Review Questions for the NCLEX® Examination

1. Spiral structures found within the nucleus of each cell made up of building blocks of DNA are:
   1. Genes
   2. Chromosomes
   3. Gametes
   4. Molecules

2. The amount of amniotic fluid normally present at term is approximately:
   1. Less than 300 milliliters
   2. 1000 milliliters   *800 – 1,000ml*
   3. 2 liters
   4. 4 liters

3. The umbilical vein:
   1. Prevents kinking of the umbilical cord
   2. Carries deoxygenated blood
   3. Carries oxygen and nutrients from the placenta to the fetus
   4. Releases carbon dioxide and other waste products

4. The nurse tells a pregnant patient that the fetus is first capable of surviving outside of the uterus at:
   1. 8 weeks' gestation
   2. 10 weeks' gestation
   3. 16 weeks' gestation
   4. 20 weeks' gestation

5. The fetal heartbeat is first detectable on sonography at week:
   1. 4
   2. 8
   3. 17
   4. 25

6. The placenta's function(s) include: *(Select all that apply.)*

(1.) Protection
(2.) Nutrition
(3.) Respiration
4. Excretion
(5.) Hormone production

7. Amniotic fluid has which function(s)? *(Select all that apply.)*

1. Fetal oxygenation and exchange of waste products
2. Formation of tissues and organs of the embryo
(3.) Prevention of umbilical cord compression
(4.) Maintenance of a constant temperature
5. Provision of immunologic function for the fetus

8. Put the following stages of embryonic development in sequential order by numbering 1 *(first)* to 5 *(last).*

_2_ Formation of zygote
_1_ Fertilization
_4_ Blastocyst formation
_5_ Implantation
_3_ Morula formation

Critical Thinking Questions

1. The embryonic period presents the greatest risk of cell injury (by teratogens) to the embryo. What would you include in a preconception health teaching plan?

2. A prenatal patient at 18 weeks' gestation asks you how and when the sex of the baby is decided. What would you tell her? Remember to formulate your response in terms that she can understand.

chapter

Physiologic and Psychological Changes During Pregnancy

4

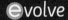

Objectives

1. Define key terms listed.
2. Calculate the expected date of delivery and duration of pregnancy.
3. Relate the difference between probable, presumptive, and positive signs of pregnancy.
4. Outline the physiologic changes in pregnancy.
5. Explain how pregnancy affects blood volume and blood plasma.
6. Describe aortocaval compression or supine hypotension during pregnancy.
7. Explain why frequency of urination occurs early and late in pregnancy.
8. Recognize the changes in skin pigmentation during pregnancy.
9. Discuss the influence of pregnancy on the skeletal system.
10. Differentiate the risk categories assigned to drugs as they relate to use during pregnancy.
11. Summarize the psychological changes that occur during pregnancy.
12. Describe the developmental tasks of pregnancy.
13. Discuss the impact and special needs of pregnancy on the adolescent, single parent, and extended family.

Key Terms

Braxton Hicks contractions (p. 50)
chloasma (klō-ĂZ-mă, p. 53)
colostrum (kŏ-LŎS-trŭm, p. 50)
diastasis recti abdominis (dī-ĂS-tă-sĭs RĔK-tīăb-DŎM-ĭnĭs, p. 53)
effacement (ĕFĀS-mĕnt, p. 50)
lightening (p. 50)
lordosis (lŏr-DŌ-sĭs, p. 53)

Nägele's rule (nah'gĕ-le, p. 44)
orthostatic hypotension (ŏr-thō-STĂT-ĭc hī-pō-TĔN-shŭn, p. 50)
striae gravidarum (STRĪ-ā grăv-ĭDĂrŭm, p. 54)
supine hypotensive syndrome (SOO-pīn hī-pō-TĔN-sĭv, p. 51)
trimesters (trī-MĔS-tĕrz, p. 44)

The nurse and other caregivers need to understand the physiologic and psychological changes that occur during pregnancy to promote health and prevent complications. Also, the nurse should know appropriate nursing and medical interventions for the uneventful (normal) pregnancy. Because culture often determines health beliefs, values, and family expectations, the assessment of cultural beliefs is important to include in patient care. With this knowledge, the nurse can develop adequate nursing care plans that include nursing diagnoses, nursing interventions related to body changes, and appropriate outcomes. Patient self-care should be a part of the care plan.

TERMINOLOGY

Understanding terms used to describe the pregnant woman is important in studying maternity care. Commonly used terms include:

Ante: before
Antepartum: time before delivery
Gravida: any pregnancy, regardless of duration, including the present one
Prenatal: time before birth
Nulligravida: a woman who has never been pregnant
Para: number of births after 20 weeks' gestation, regardless of whether the infants were born alive or dead (multifetal pregnancies are considered a single birth)
Preterm: a pregnancy that ends after 20 weeks' and before 37 weeks' gestation
Postterm: a pregnancy that goes beyond 40 weeks' gestation
Primigravida: a woman pregnant for the first time
Multigravida: a woman who is in her second or a subsequent pregnancy
Nullipara: a woman who has not given birth at more than 20 weeks' gestation

Primipara: a woman who has given birth to a fetus (dead or alive) that had reached at least 20 weeks' gestation

Multipara: a woman who has given birth two or more times to fetuses that had reached at least 20 weeks' gestation

Stillbirth: a fetus born dead after 20 weeks' gestation
EDD: estimated date of delivery

PROFILE OF PREVIOUS OBSTETRIC HISTORY

GTPALM is a mnemonic (an aid to memory) that is commonly used for recording, with the use of shorthand symbols, a woman's pregnancy history (Box 4-1). It provides a systematic, quick way to indicate the number of pregnancies the woman has had, as well as the outcomes. The letters indicate the following: *G*, gravida; *T*, term pregnancies; *P*, preterm births; *A*, abortions; *L*, number of living children; and *M*, multiple gestations and births. For example, a pregnant woman who has four living children, all single births, and who has had no preterm births and no abortions would be a gravida 5-4-0-0-4-0.

Some institutions use only two letters, *P* and *G*, to indicate **para** and **gravida.** A woman pregnant for the first time would be P0, G1.

DETERMINING DATE OF BIRTH

After the diagnosis of pregnancy, the woman's question usually is, "When is the baby due?" In the past, the term *estimated date of confinement* (EDC) was used to describe the time of birth as a period of confinement. Currently, the term *estimated date of delivery* (EDD) is considered the more accurate term. Some texts, however, also use the term *estimated date of birth* (EDB). Therefore, EDC, EDD, and EDB are interchangeable terms that refer to the expected time of labor and birth. This text uses EDD.

Nägele's rule is a method for obtaining an EDD (Box 4-2). To calculate the EDD, identify the first day of the last normal menstrual period (LNMP), count

---

Box 4-1 Two Methods of Documenting Obstetric History

GTPALM
G: gravida (total number of pregnancies, including current pregnancy)
T: number of term pregnancies
P: number of preterm deliveries
A: number of abortions
L: number of live births
M: number of multiple births

PG
P: para (number of births after 20 weeks' gestation)
G: gravida (total number of pregnancies, including current pregnancy)

Box 4-2 Nägele's Rule to Determine Estimated Date of Delivery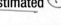

1. Determine first day of last normal menstrual period.
2. Count back 3 months.
3. Add 7 days.
4. Correct year if needed.

---

backward 3 months, and then add 7 days. An example is as follows:

1. First day of LNMP: November 18
2. Minus 3 months: August 18
3. Add 7 days: August 25

The average duration of pregnancy is approximately 280 days. This period is calculated in 28-day months, called **lunar months.** There are 10 lunar months (40 weeks, 280 days) in a full-term pregnancy, which is approximately the same as 9 calendar months. For convenience, the 9 months of pregnancy are divided into three trimesters, each generally representing a 3-month period. Although most women refer to their pregnancy in terms of months, the medical community refers to pregnancy in terms of weeks. The first trimester is considered the first 14 weeks, the second trimester is 15 to 28 weeks, and the third trimester is 29 weeks to delivery (Gabbe, Niebyl, & Simpson, 2007).

Not all pregnancies continue to term (40 weeks). A pregnancy that terminates before the fetus reaches 20 weeks' gestation is called an **abortion** (laypersons use the term **miscarriage**). A pregnancy that terminates after the age of 20 weeks but before full-term is called a **preterm** (premature) **birth.** A pregnancy that terminates 2 weeks after the EDD, or 42 weeks' gestation, is called a **postterm birth.**

SIGNS OF PREGNANCY

It is important to establish the diagnosis of pregnancy or to confirm that the woman is pregnant. Many signs of pregnancy assist in the confirmation. These signs are divided into the following three categories: (1) **presumptive** signs, which suggest pregnancy; (2) **probable** signs, which indicate that the woman is probably pregnant; and (3) **positive** signs, which give definite evidence that the woman is pregnant (Table 4-1). The three positive signs are the only signs that clearly establish a diagnosis of pregnancy. They are hearing fetal heart sounds (Figure 4-1), which are audible by a Doppler device by 10 to 12 weeks' gestation; palpating active fetal movements; and visualizing the fetus via ultrasound. The gestational sac can be detected as early as 10 days after implantation. Many of the signs and symptoms that are present in pregnancy also may be present in other conditions.

In recent years, the accuracy of pregnancy tests has improved. These tests are based on the presence of the

(handwritten in left margin: each month = 5wks)

Table **4-1**   Signs of Pregnancy: Presumptive, Probable, and Positive

SIGNS	DESCRIPTION	POSSIBLE ALTERNATIVE CAUSES
Presumptive (May Suggest Pregnancy)		
Amenorrhea	Cessation of menses; often the first sign of pregnancy	Emotional stress, chronic disease, or metabolic factors such as menopause
Nausea and vomiting	Occurs during first trimester in 50% of pregnancies; called "morning sickness" because it is usually present in morning	Gastrointestinal disorders or acute infections
Urinary frequency	Related to pressure on bladder	Urinary tract infection
Fatigue	Noticed during early pregnancy by many women	Response to increased hormones or depression
Quickening	Feeling of slight, fluttery movements of fetus at about 18-20 weeks of pregnancy	Gas movements within bowel or increased peristalsis
Breast tenderness	Tenderness and tingling caused by hormonal changes	Premenstrual status or oral contraceptives
Probable (Strongly Indicate Pregnancy)		
Uterine enlargement	Enlarged abdomen occurring as a result of growth of uterus from fetal growth	Obesity or pelvic tumors
Pigmentation changes	Darkening of skin such as linea nigra on abdomen and of nipples and areolae because of hormonal increase	Hormone stimulation related to a medical condition
Goodell's sign	Softening of cervix	Estrogen related to oral contraceptives
Hegar's sign	Softening of lower portion of uterus	Abnormal hormonal activity
Chadwick's sign	Bluish purple discoloration of vaginal mucous membrane caused by increased vascularity or pelvic congestion	Pelvic congestion due to inflammation
Ballottement	Rebounding of fetus in amniotic fluid felt by examiner during pelvic examination	Uterine polyps or ascites
Braxton Hicks contractions	Painless, irregular uterine contractions; may be felt by the woman as a tightening across the abdomen → *Pregnant women still need to be monitored.*	Medical condition such as fibroids
Positive pregnancy tests	Presence of human chorionic gonadotropin indicative of pregnancy	False results because of timing or technique or use of recreational drugs
Positive (Confirm Pregnancy)		
Ultrasound visualization	One of three signs that clearly establish a pregnancy: fetal heart sounds heard, fetal movements palpated by the examiner, and fetal outline visualized by ultrasound	Ultrasound visualization of fetus is a positive sign of pregnancy

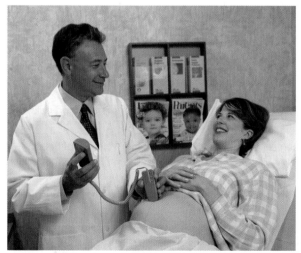

FIGURE 4-1 The fetal heart is audible by Doppler ultrasound by 10 to 12 weeks' gestation and is checked at each prenatal visit. Hearing the fetal heartbeat helps the mother accept the reality of her pregnancy.

hormone human chorionic gonadotropin (hCG), which is produced by the chorionic villi of the placenta. It is present in a pregnant woman's urine or blood as early as 1 week after conception. Home pregnancy test kits are uncomplicated and convenient and are capable of greater than 97% accuracy; however, the instructions must be followed precisely to obtain this accuracy. Pregnancy test kits are probable indicators because several factors may interfere with their accuracy, including medications such as antianxiety drugs or anticonvulsant drugs, blood in the urine, malignant tumors, and menopause.

PHYSIOLOGIC CHANGES IN BODY SYSTEMS

Many physiologic changes occur during pregnancy. Because of these changes, a number of minor symptoms or discomforts result. Most of these discomforts do not require medical treatment. However, they do require evaluation, explanation, and re-assurance to allay fears and anxieties. Many discomforts during pregnancy can be alleviated by relatively simple nursing care, including patient self-care instruction.

The two major sources of the physiologic changes during pregnancy are changes in the endocrine system and the physical changes in the body. The hormonal changes and mechanical pressures that occur from an enlarging uterus account for many of the physiologic changes and psychological adaptations that occur during pregnancy (Table 4-2).

CHANGES IN THE ENDOCRINE SYSTEM

The dramatic increase in hormones during pregnancy affects all body systems. Hormones are essential to maintain pregnancy. Most are produced initially by the corpus luteum and later by the placenta. The most striking change in the endocrine system during pregnancy is the addition of the placenta as a temporary

Table 4-2   Physiologic and Psychological Changes in Pregnancy, Nursing Interventions, and Teaching

MATERNAL CHANGES	SIGNS AND SYMPTOMS	NURSING INTERVENTIONS AND TEACHING
First Trimester		
Fertilization occurs. Increased progesterone results in amenorrhea. Sodium (Na) retention increases. Nitrogen (N) store decreases.	Pregnancy test is positive. Amenorrhea occurs.	Guide patient regarding nutritional needs and folic acid requirements. Encourage patient to seek early prenatal care. Assess attitude toward this pregnancy and how it affects family.
Blood volume increases. Levels of relaxin hormone increase. Levels of human chorionic gonadotropin (hCG) hormone increase.	Fainting is possible. Morning nausea can occur. Relaxation of gastrointestinal muscles can cause "heartburn." Sensitivity to odors increases.	Teach patient how to rise slowly from prone position. Teach patient how to cope with nausea without medication: *⊖ Skipping meals* • Eat dry crackers before arising. • Use acupressure.
Pituitary gland releases melanocyte-stimulating hormone.	Pigmentation deepens on face (chloasma) and on abdomen (linea nigra).	Discuss body changes and reassure patient that most pigmentation will fade after puerperium.
Fetus grows.	Abdomen enlarges at end of first trimester when uterus rises out of pelvis. Small weight gain occurs.	Teach methods to minimize fetal problems: • Avoid high temperatures around abdomen (baths and spas). • Discuss the effect of medications and herbs on fetal development. • Discuss nutritional and folic acid needs, control of caffeine intake in second and third trimesters, and omega-3 fatty acid intake. Facilitate communication with partner concerning relationships during pregnancy.
Uterus begins to enlarge.	Enlarged uterus presses on bladder.	Discuss effect of frequency of urination on lifestyle and activities.
For fathers, the announcement phase begins when pregnancy is confirmed, followed by an adjustment phase, and, finally, the focus phase in third trimester and during labor, when "feeling like a father" develops.	Parents adjust to the reality of pregnancy.	Review father's or partner's role and mother's responses. Refer to community agencies as needed. Assess for misinformation and knowledge deficit. Help parents identify concerns. Answer questions. Discuss care of siblings, role of grandparents, etc.
Second Trimester		
Corpus luteum is absorbed and placenta takes over fetal support (between third and fourth months).	Blood volume increases in placental bed.	Teach patient how to minimize risk of habitual abortion between third and fourth months when placenta begins to take over.
Broad ligament stretches as uterus enlarges.	Occasional pain in groin area occurs.	Teach patient Kegel exercises to strengthen pelvic muscles.
Vascularity of pelvis increases.	Sexual pleasure and desire increase. White discharge may occur.	Discuss modifications of positions for sexual comfort and pleasure. Teach patient to avoid routine douches. Teach patient perineal skin hygiene.

Table 4-2   Physiologic and Psychological Changes in Pregnancy, Nursing Interventions, and Teaching—cont'd

MATERNAL CHANGES	SIGNS AND SYMPTOMS	NURSING INTERVENTIONS AND TEACHING
Second Trimester—cont'd		
Blood volume and vasomotor lability increases.	Orthostatic hypotension can occur.	Teach patient to change positions slowly and to avoid warm, crowded areas.
Cardiac output increases.	Physiologic anemia may occur.	Iron supplements may be prescribed for anemia. Teach patient how to prevent constipation, and teach change in stool color during iron therapy.
Renal threshold decreases.	Perineal itching may occur.	Test for sugar in urine and require glucose tolerance test in second trimester to rule out gestational diabetes. Teach patient hygienic measures when high glucose is present (front to back wiping; wearing cotton panties).
Uterus rises out of pelvis.	Center of gravity of body changes.	Teach patient proper shoe heel height to avoid falling. Teach placement of automobile restraints across hips rather than across abdomen. Teach patient to avoid lying supine in bed after the fourth month of pregnancy to prevent supine hypotensive syndrome. Teach posture and pelvic rocking exercises. Instruct patient that clothes should hang from shoulders.
Estrogen relaxes sacroiliac joint.	Pressure on bladder and rectum increases.	Anticipate urinary frequency during long trips. Teach patient Kegel exercises to strengthen pelvic floor.
Enlarging uterus compresses nerves supplying lower extremities.	Leg muscle spasms occur, especially when reclining.	Check for Homans' sign. Teach patient how to dorsiflex the foot to help relieve spasms. Massage foot.
Decreased calcium levels and increased phosphorus levels are possible.	Abnormal laboratory results.	Use oral aluminum hydroxide gel to reduce phosphorus levels if elevated (when recommended by health care provider).
Decreasing cardiac reserve and increasing respiratory effort start late in the second trimester.	Physiologic stress is possible if exercise levels are not decreased.	Teach patient to monitor pulse (maximum 90 beats/minute), and teach patient that inability to converse without taking frequent breaths is a sign of physiologic stress. Teach patient to stop exercising if numbness, pain, or dizziness occurs.
Hormonal influence causes "id" to come to the surface.	Mood swings occur.	Prepare spouse or significant other and family for mood swings, outspoken behavior, and labile emotions ("speaks before she thinks").
Levels of relaxin hormone increase.	Sphincter of stomach relaxes, and gastrointestinal motility is slowed.	Teach patient how to prevent constipation. Instruct patient to increase fluid intake and avoid gas-forming foods.
Increase in estrogen causes increased excretory function of the skin.	Skin itches.	Teach patient to wear loose clothing, shower frequently, and use mild soaps and oils for comfort.
Anterior pituitary secretes melanocyte-stimulating hormone.	Skin pigmentation deepens.	Prepare patient to anticipate development of spider nevi and skin pigmentation. Reassure patient that most fade after the puerperium.
Estrogen levels increase.	Increased estrogen develops increased vascularity of oral tissues, resulting in gingivitis and stuffy nose.	Teach proper oral hygiene techniques.
	Estrogen levels develop network of increased arterioles.	Edema can occur. Assess blood pressure and report proteinuria.

Continued

Table 4-2 Physiologic and Psychological Changes in Pregnancy, Nursing Interventions, and Teaching—cont'd

MATERNAL CHANGES	SIGNS AND SYMPTOMS	NURSING INTERVENTIONS AND TEACHING
Second Trimester—cont'd		
Pituitary gland secretes prolactin.	Colostrum leaks from nipples and sometimes cakes. Breasts enlarge.	Teach patient to cleanse nipples to keep ducts from being blocked by colostrum. She should avoid soaps, ointments, and alcohol that dry skin. Teach patient not to stimulate nipples by massage or exercise because doing so may increase the risk for preterm labor.
Traction on brachial plexus is caused by drooping of shoulders as breast size increases.	Fingers tingle.	Teach patient proper posture. Encourage the use of a supportive maternity bra.
Placental barrier allows certain elements and organisms to pass through to the fetus.	Some medications can pass through the placental barrier and cause fetal defects.	Advise patient not to smoke and not to self-treat with medications. Teach patients to avoid certain jobs (e.g., working as a parking attendant, in a dry cleaning plant, or in a chemistry laboratory).
Travel during pregnancy Lowered oxygen levels can cause fetal hypoxia.	Traveling to countries that have endemic diseases can have negative effect on fetus; certain active immunizations should be avoided.	Advise patient regarding travel. Most commercial airlines have cabin pressure controlled at or below 5000-ft level and therefore do not pose a risk to the fetus.
Platelet levels increase.	Women are prone to thrombophlebitis if they are inactive for long periods.	Encourage patient to keep hydrated because of low cabin humidity in airplanes and to move around to help prevent thrombophlebitis.
Fetal growth continues.	Mother feels signs of life; fetus moves and kicks.	
Third Trimester		
Maternal weight gain of 9-22 kg (20-25 lbs) occurs.		Teach proper nutrition to foster fetal growth without adding extra "empty" calories. Encourage patient to attend childbirth or parenting classes.
Colostrum forms.	Colostrum may leak from breasts.	Teach patient the need for rest periods and organization of work. Teach patient care of nipples. Introduce nipple pads. Teach patient to avoid nipple stimulation to prevent preterm labor.
Increased estrogen levels causes edema of larynx.	Voice changes. Patient tires easily.	Professional singers may lose voice quality. Teach patient the need for rest periods.
Maximum increase in cardiac output (increase in stroke volume) occurs.	Maximize cardiac output when woman lies on her side.	Teach patient signs of gestational hypertension, and assess water retention.
Edema of hands and wrists is possible.	Risk for carpal tunnel syndrome increases.	Elevate hands; decrease repetitive motion activities.
Uterus increases in size.	Pressure on stomach occurs. Pressure on diaphragm occurs. Venous congestion increases.	Discuss how to cope with decrease in appetite and shortness of breath. Teach "talk test" for self-evaluation of exercise tolerance to prevent fetal hypoxia (must be able to finish a sentence before taking a breath). Teach patient how to avoid constipation and leg varicosities.
Sensitivity to Braxton Hicks contractions increases.	Fetal head may engage (uterus drops) (lightening).	Teach patient the signs of labor and when to come to hospital. Offer tour of labor and delivery unit.
Hormone levels increase.	"Id" is at the surface. Woman becomes self-centered and worries how she will manage labor.	Review labor management learned in prenatal classes. Discuss sibling care and support system.

endocrine organ whose role is to produce large amounts of estrogen and progesterone to maintain the pregnancy (as well as hCG and hPL [human placental lactogen]).

Table 4-3 highlights the major hormones and their influence during pregnancy. The hPL increases maternal insulin resistance during pregnancy, providing the fetus with glucose needed for growth.

CHANGES IN THE REPRODUCTIVE SYSTEM

Uterus

The uterus changes dramatically during pregnancy. Before pregnancy, the uterus is a small, semisolid, pear-shaped organ weighing approximately 60 g (2 oz). At the end of pregnancy, it is a thin-walled, muscular container housing the fetus, placenta, and amniotic fluid that weighs approximately 1000 g (2 lbs, 3 oz).

This enlargement is primarily the result of an increase in size of preexisting muscle cells (hypertrophy) and the formation of new cells (hyperplasia). The ease with which the fetus can be palpated through the abdominal wall indicates its thin structure.

The circulatory requirements of the uterus greatly increase as it enlarges and the fetus and placenta develop. The growth of the uterus is stimulated by hormones (estrogen and progesterone) and by pressure of the growing fetus against the uterine wall.

The growth and position of the uterus provide useful information about fetal growth. The position of the uterus helps confirm the EDD. For example, by 12 weeks' gestation, the uterus can be felt above the symphysis pubis, and at 20 weeks, the fundus is near the umbilicus. By 36 weeks, the fundus is at its highest,

Table **4-3**   Hormones Essential in Pregnancy

HORMONE	SIGNIFICANCE
Estrogen	Produced by ovaries and placenta Responsible for enlargement of uterus, breasts, and genitalia Promotes fat deposit changes Stimulates melanocyte-stimulating hormone in hyperpigmentation of skin Promotes vascular changes Promotes development of striae gravidarum Alters sodium and water retention
Progesterone	Produced by corpus luteum and ovary and later by placenta Maintains endometrium for implantation Inhibits uterine contractibility, preventing abortion Promotes development of secretory ducts of breasts for lactation Stimulates sodium secretion Reduces smooth muscle tone (causing constipation, heartburn, varicosities)
Thyroxine (T_4)	Influences thyroid gland's size and activity and increases heart rate Increases basal metabolic rate 23% during pregnancy
Human chorionic gonadotropin (hCG)	Produced early in pregnancy by trophoblastic tissue Stimulates progesterone and estrogen production by corpus luteum to maintain pregnancy until placenta takes over Used in pregnancy tests to determine pregnancy state
Human placental lactogen (hPL); also called chorionic somatomammotropin	Produced by placenta Affects glucose and protein metabolism Has a diabetogenic effect—allows increased glucose to stimulate pancreas and increase insulin level
Melanocyte-stimulating hormone	Produced by anterior pituitary gland Causes pigmentation of skin to darken, resulting in brown patches on face (chloasma [melasma gravidarum]), dark line on abdomen (linea nigra), darkening of moles and freckles, and darkening of nipples and areolae
Relaxin	Produced by corpus luteum and placenta Remodels collagen, causing connective tissue of symphysis pubis to be more movable and cervix to soften Inhibits uterine activity
Prolactin	Prepares breasts for lactation
Oxytocin	Produced by posterior pituitary gland Stimulates uterine contraction → can cause miscarriages if there is an ↑ of prolactin ↓ Testrogen/progesteron Is inhibited by progesterone during pregnancy After birth, helps keep uterus contracted Stimulates milk ejection reflex during breastfeeding

at the xiphoid process of the rib cage (see Figure 5-3). By 40 weeks, the fetus descends, with the fetal head entering into the pelvis (**lightening** occurs; see Chapter 6).

Early in pregnancy, irregular, painless uterine contractions (**Braxton Hicks contractions**) occur. As pregnancy progresses, these contractions help move the blood through the placenta to the fetus. They can be mistaken for labor contractions, especially near term.

Cervix

The cervix of the uterus becomes shorter and softer during pregnancy. These adjustments prepare the cervix for thinning (**effacement**) and enlargement (**dilation**) of the opening, which are necessary to permit the fetus to pass from the uterus at birth. The softening of the cervix is caused by (1) a hormonal influence that causes an increased blood supply and (2) an increase in secretions from the cervical glands. The secretions from the cervical glands form a mucous plug in the cervical canal that acts as a barrier to prevent organisms from entering the uterus. The mucous plug is usually expelled from the vagina during labor.

Ovaries

During pregnancy, follicles in the ovaries cease to develop to maturity. Ovulation does not occur. The corpus luteum persists and produces estrogen and progesterone for the first 7 to 10 weeks' gestation to maintain the pregnancy until the placenta develops and can take over hormone production. The corpus luteum of pregnancy also secretes the hormone **relaxin**. The role of relaxin, along with placental progesterone, is thought to be relaxing the symphysis pubis and other pelvic joints and ripening (or softening) the cervix in preparation for labor.

(handwritten margin note, left side: vaginal pH is acidic)

(handwritten margin note, left side near figure: darkens that way so baby can see where the nipple is located.)

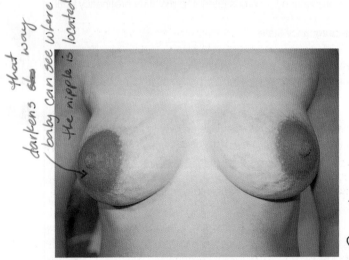

FIGURE 4-2 Striae and pigmentation of breasts. Note the darkened pigmentation of areolae and the pink-white lines at the base of the breasts that are caused by a stretching of the elastic tissue as the breasts enlarge. Pigmentation will disappear after pregnancy, and striae will fade into silvery strands.

Vagina

The changes that occur in the vagina prepare it for the tremendous stretching necessary for the birth of the baby. The proliferation of cells and hyperemia of the vaginal connective tissue cause the vaginal walls to become thickened, pliable, and expandable. As the mucosa thickens, the vaginal rugae (folds) become prominent. The vaginal discharge increases, bringing on greater amounts of glycogen. This presents an increased risk for a vaginal infection and favors the growth of the yeast *Candida albicans*. However, as the pH of the vagina decreases, the acidic conditions work to prevent growth of harmful microbes typically found in the vagina.

Breasts

Several hormones, including estrogen, progesterone, prolactin, and hPL, interact during pregnancy to prepare the breasts for **lactation** (milk production). Estrogen and progesterone seem to be the most important. The breasts rapidly enlarge in the first 8 weeks, mostly from vascular engorgement. Thereafter, the breasts enlarge progressively throughout pregnancy as a result of ductal growth stimulated by estrogen and alveolar hypertrophy stimulated by progesterone.

The breast changes during pregnancy can be summarized as follows: size increases; breasts become full, sensitive, and tender; the pigmentation of the areola and nipple darkens; and Montgomery's glands become more prominent and lubricate and protect the nipple in preparation for breastfeeding. Striae may occur (pinkish-white lines caused by stretching of the elastic tissue as the breasts enlarge). Striae will fade into silvery strands after pregnancy (Figure 4-2).

Colostrum—a thin, yellowish fluid (premilk fluid)—begins to be excreted by the breasts as early as the tenth week of gestation and continues until approximately the third postpartum day, when it is replaced by milk. Lactation is initiated by the profound drop in estrogen and progesterone levels after delivery of the placenta, allowing an increase in **prolactin** levels. Prolactin is responsible for milk production.

CHANGES IN THE CARDIOVASCULAR SYSTEM

The cardiovascular system exhibits profound changes during pregnancy (Table 4-4). These changes are essential to deliver oxygen and nutrients to the growing fetus and the enlarging uterus. Blood must be delivered into uterine vessels at pressures sufficient to meet the requirements of the placental circulation, which is necessary for an adequate exchange of oxygen between mother and fetus.

Orthostatic hypotension (a decrease in blood pressure occurring when moving from a recumbent to an upright position) may cause faintness due to a temporary decrease in cardiac output. As pregnancy progresses, the vena cava can be compressed to some degree if the pregnant woman lies on her back, which

(handwritten margin note, right side: lay on L side)

Table 4-4   Changes in the Cardiovascular System During Pregnancy

PHYSIOLOGIC CHANGE	CLINICAL SIGNIFICANCE
Heart is displaced by elevation of diaphragm.	Palpitations, benign arrhythmias, and systolic murmurs result from change in position of heart.
Cardiac output increases.	Cardiac output, or volume of blood injected into the system, is increased 30% to 50% to meet demands of enlarging uterus and fetal oxygenation.
Blood flow increases in skin.	Warmth, moist skin, and nasal congestion are experienced.
Blood flow increases to kidneys.	Removal of waste products improves for mother and fetus.
Pulse rate and stroke volume increase.	Pulse rate increases approximately 10-20 beats/minute, and the amount of blood ejected into the circulation with each heart beat increases.
Blood volume increases 30% to 45%.	Blood volume increases early in pregnancy; begins at roughly 10 weeks and peaks at 34 weeks. Blood volume increase meets circulatory and nutritional needs of maternal and fetal tissues.
Plasma and red blood volumes increase.	Plasma volume increases more than red cell mass, causing hemoglobin and hematocrit levels to fall; oral supplementation of 60-80 mg/day of elemental iron is routine. If hemoglobin level drops below 11 g/dL or hematocrit level below 35%, the patient should be evaluated for anemia.
White blood cell count increases (average >15,000/mm³).	A protective mechanism against infection, the increased white blood cell count during pregnancy makes it difficult to detect infection; the level returns to normal approximately 1 week after delivery.
Blood clotting factors increase.	This provides rapid blood clotting mechanism of placental site when expelled, increasing risk of postpartum embolism; therefore women are asked to ambulate early after delivery.
Femoral venous pressure increases.	Enlarged uterus places pressure on veins of lower extremities, and stagnation of blood in lower extremities may occur.
Compression of the inferior vena cava in the third trimester by gravid uterus can decrease cardiac output.	Supine hypotensive syndrome may occur; women are instructed to lie on the left side and to not lie flat on their backs.
Decrease in cardiac output may occur when a woman moves rapidly from a recumbent to an upright position.	Orthostatic hypotension may occur.
Blood pressure does not increase.	An arbitrary upper limit of normal is 140/90 mm Hg; an increase of ≥30 mm Hg systolic or ≥15 mm Hg diastolic above baseline may indicate a potential hypertensive disorder.
Pressure from enlarged uterus causes obstructed venous return, and progesterone causes relaxation of muscles.	Varicose veins develop in the vulva, anus (hemorrhoids), and legs. Sitting or standing for long periods should be avoided; crossing legs decreases blood flow.

[handwritten annotation: which dilutes RBC]

can decrease cardiac output. This is called supine hypotensive syndrome or *aortocaval compression* (Figure 4-3). Cardiac output doubles, and there is a 30% to 45% increase in blood volume (Blackburn, 2007). Ten percent of the maternal cardiac output is channeled to uterine blood flow in the third trimester. Cardiac output is best when the woman lies on her side. The greatest increase in cardiac output occurs during labor and delivery. An increase in various clotting factors and fibrinogen protects the woman from excess bleeding during and after birth but makes the woman more vulnerable to blood clotting events (thrombus formation). Other changes in blood values are listed in Table 4-5.

CHANGES IN THE RESPIRATORY SYSTEM

Thoracic circumference increases during pregnancy because of the relaxation of the ligaments (primarily from progesterone) and the flaring of the lower ribs. Therefore, despite the elevation of the diaphragm (as much as 4 cm [1.6 inches]) in the latter part of pregnancy, the lung capacity remains the same.

Inspiration increases during pregnancy, allowing greater intake of oxygen. Increased expiration facilitates carbon dioxide removal. In other words, the exchange of carbon dioxide and oxygen that takes place at the alveolar cell level is improved. The pregnant woman breathes more deeply (but not more frequently) to maintain oxygen for herself and her

[handwritten annotation at bottom: after neonate is born listen to the stump of umbilicus to count heart beat add a zero to the number you get.]

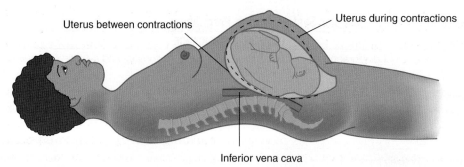

Uterus between contractions

Uterus during contractions

Inferior vena cava

FIGURE 4-3 **Supine hypotensive syndrome.** When a pregnant patient lies on her back (supine), the weight of the uterus and its fetal contents presses on the vena cava and abdominal aorta, decreasing blood flow to the heart. Maternal hypotension and fetal hypoxia may result.

Table 4-5	Normal Blood Values in Nonpregnant and Pregnant Women	
VALUE	NONPREGNANT	PREGNANT
Hemoglobin (g/dL)	12-16	11-12
Hematocrit (%)	37-48	33-46
Red blood cells (million/mm^3)	3.8-5.1	4.5-6.5
White blood cells (thousand/mm^3)	5-10	5-15; rises during labor and postpartum up to 25
Fibrinogen (mg/dL)	200-400	300-600

make flash cards

fetus. Breathing changes from abdominal to thoracic as pregnancy progresses. Oxygen consumption increases by 15% to 40% during pregnancy (Gordon, 2007).

Dyspnea

Shortness of breath (dyspnea) is a common complaint of pregnancy. The sensation of dyspnea appears to be related to a greater sensitivity of the respiratory system caused by increased progesterone. Dyspnea is also related to the pressure of the uterus on the diaphragm. Dyspnea normally does not interfere with activities of daily living and does not occur at rest.

Epistaxis

Nosebleeds (epistaxis) and nasal stuffiness are common during pregnancy. These discomforts are thought to be caused by the increased vascularity that results from increased estrogen. Another change that can occur is a change in the woman's voice. A pregnant woman's voice may become deeper because of an increase in the size of the vocal cords, which is caused by increased progesterone.

CHANGES IN THE GASTROINTESTINAL SYSTEM

Changes in the mouth often occur during pregnancy. Gum hypertrophy may occur; sensitivity and bleeding can be reduced by use of a soft toothbrush and good oral hygiene. Saliva production is often increased (ptyalism), and nausea, with or without vomiting, is common during the first trimester of pregnancy and is thought to be caused by the rising level of estrogen in the blood. During pregnancy, the peristaltic action of the gastrointestinal tract decreases, mainly because of the increase in progesterone and relaxin. With the relaxation of the cardiac sphincter, gastric contents can reach the esophagus and cause heartburn (pyrosis), a common discomfort of pregnancy. Pregnant women should be encouraged to sit up for 30 minutes after eating, rather than immediately lying down, to reduce the risk of heartburn. Common interventions to decrease nausea and vomiting are discussed in Chapter 5.

With the loss in muscle tone, there is a delayed emptying of the intestines, which allows more water to be absorbed from the bowel. This change causes constipation, another common discomfort.

Progesterone and estrogen relax the muscle tone of the gallbladder, resulting in the retention of bile salts, and this can lead to pruritus (itching of the skin) during pregnancy. Pregnancy also produces metabolic changes. Carbohydrate metabolism is altered, with increased resistance to insulin, allowing the fetus to have a source of high energy in the form of glycogen. Fat metabolism also changes, which facilitates growth and provides maternal stores for lactation. Periodic hyperglycemia can result during pregnancy, a condition called **gestational diabetes.**

CHANGES IN THE RENAL (URINARY) SYSTEM

Early in pregnancy, the growing uterus puts pressure on the bladder, causing frequent urination. Later in pregnancy, as the fetus settles down in the pelvic cavity, the woman again has pressure on the bladder, and frequency of urination returns. Stasis of urine in the bladder increases the risk of a urinary tract infection (Figure 4-4).

The ureters dilate from smooth muscle relaxation caused by an increase in progesterone and pressure from engorged circulation and an enlarging uterus. Renal plasma flow may increase by 75% to remove

↑ UTI ∵ frequent urination

metabolic wastes of the mother and fetus (Gordon, 2007). Pregnant women with asymptomatic bacteriuria (bacteria in the urine) are more prone to develop pyelonephritis (infection of the upper urinary tract).

Fluid and Electrolyte Balance

The increased glomerular filtration rate in the kidneys increases sodium filtration by 50%, but the increase in the tubular reabsorption rate results in 99% reabsorption of the sodium. Sodium retention is influenced by many factors, including elevated levels of the hormones of pregnancy. Although much of the sodium is used by the fetus, the remainder is in the maternal circulation and can cause a maternal accumulation of water (edema). This fluid retention may cause a problem if the woman in labor is given intravenous fluids containing oxytocin (Pitocin), which has an antidiuretic effect and can result in water intoxication. Agitation and delirium, possible signs of water intoxication, should be recorded and reported, and an accurate intake and output record should be kept during labor and in the immediate postpartum phase.

In pregnancy, blood is slightly more alkaline than in the nonpregnant state, and this mild alkalemia is enhanced by hyperventilation that often occurs during pregnancy. This status does not influence a normal pregnancy.

CHANGES IN THE INTEGUMENTARY AND SKELETAL SYSTEMS

The relaxation and softening of the pelvic joints and widening of the symphysis pubis are primarily caused by relaxin and placental progesterone. In the last trimester, when the fetal presenting part settles into the brim of the pelvis and a slight separation of the

symphysis pubis occurs, the woman develops a "waddling" gait. This widening facilitates passage of the fetus through the pelvis in preparation for a vaginal delivery. As the uterus enlarges, the woman's center of gravity shifts forward. To compensate for this change, women develop a progressive lordosis (curvature of the lower spine). The woman may experience low backaches, and, in the last months of pregnancy, rounding of the shoulders may occur, with aching in the cervical and upper thoracic spines (Figure 4-5). A change in the center of gravity and joint instability resulting from relaxation of the ligaments predispose the pregnant woman to problems with balance. Interventions concerning safety should be part of prenatal education.

Enlargement of the uterus stretches the round ligaments that support the uterus, and this can cause an abrupt, sharp pain when the woman moves quickly, such as getting up from a chair. In addition, as the abdominal muscles are gradually stretched during pregnancy, the rectus abdominis muscles may separate, causing a condition called diastasis recti abdominis. The muscles return to their normal position after delivery. This process is facilitated by exercise.

During pregnancy, weight gain and edema can produce a compression of the medial nerve, particularly around the wrist. This is referred to as **carpal tunnel syndrome.** This syndrome commonly consists of pain, numbness, or tingling in the hand and wrist; weakness and decreased motor function can also occur.

During pregnancy, the skin undergoes hyperpigmentation (primarily as a result of melanocyte-stimulating hormone and estrogen).

Chloasma (also known as *melasma*) is a blotchy, brownish "mask of pregnancy" that typically fades

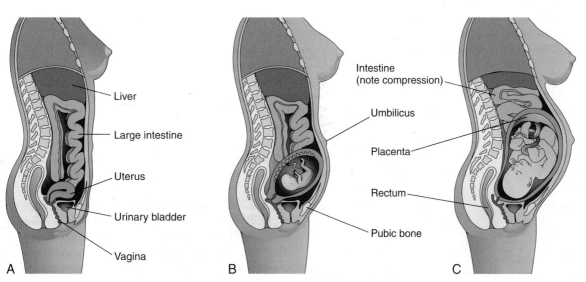

FIGURE 4-4 **Compression of abdominal contents as the uterus enlarges. A,** Nonpregnant. **B,** Twenty weeks' gestation. **C,** Thirty weeks' gestation. The bladder is compressed, causing urinary frequency.

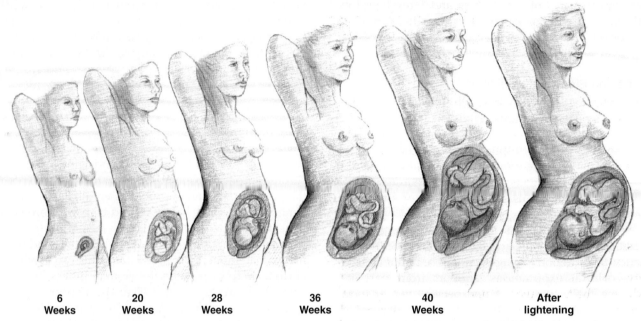

6 Weeks   **20 Weeks**   **28 Weeks**   **36 Weeks**   **40 Weeks**   **After lightening**

FIGURE 4-5 As pregnancy progresses, obvious posture changes occur and lordosis increases.

after delivery. The linea alba darkens and becomes a darkened line on the abdomen, called the **linea nigra.**

Striae gravidarum, or stretch marks, are pinkish or purplish lines caused by a weakening of the elastic tissues (Figure 4-6). Striae are often found on the abdomen, breasts, thighs, and buttocks. After delivery, these streaks turn to a fine pinkish or silver tone on fair-skinned women and a brownish color on darker skinned women. Nipples, areolae, vulva, and perineum all darken. Moles, freckles, and recent scars may also darken. In some women, hair growth may increase. In addition, blood vessels have increased permeability, causing palmar erythema and small red elevations on the skin with red lines radiating from the center, called *spider nevi.*

THE EFFECT OF PREGNANCY AND LACTATION ON MEDICATION INGESTION

The physiologic changes in pregnancy affect the metabolism of ingested medications. Subtherapeutic drug levels may occur due to the increased plasma volume, cardiac output, and glomerular filtration that occur during pregnancy. A decreased gastric emptying time during pregnancy changes absorption of drugs and can delay onset of action. Parenteral medication may be absorbed more rapidly because of increased blood flow and have a faster onset of action than in the nonpregnant state. The increased levels of estrogen and progesterone may alter hepatic (liver) function, resulting in drug accumulation in the body.

Drugs can cross the placenta and have an impact on fetal development, especially in the first trimester, and have increased absorption levels in the developing fetus in the third trimester. The mother should be taught to check with her health care provider before taking over-the-counter medications. Taking ibuprofen in the third trimester can cause early closure of the ductus arteriosus, resulting in fetal distress. Certain drugs can pass into breast milk by diffusion and be ingested by the neonate during breastfeeding. If the lactating mother must take medication, it should be administered immediately after the infant breastfeeds to minimize passage to the infant.

The U.S. Food and Drug Administration (FDA) has established a category of risk for medication use during pregnancy. All women of childbearing age should be counseled about the risk of ingesting drugs during

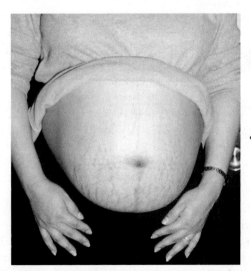

FIGURE 4-6 A pregnant woman's abdomen showing striae gravidarum (stretch marks) and linea nigra (the darkened line from the umbilicus to the pubis).

pregnancy and lactation. Pregnancy category risk allows for some assessment of risk to the fetus when a drug is prescribed to a pregnant woman (Box 4-3).

PSYCHOLOGICAL CHANGES DURING PREGNANCY

Pregnancy is a profound event in the life of a woman and her family. It is a time when she and her partner are faced with the challenges of redefining their present roles, working through previous conflicts, and taking on the parental role. The emotional and physical adjustments of pregnancy plus those required to become parents can cause varying levels of stress and anxiety.

Some specific factors that contribute to either a positive or a negative psychological response to pregnancy include body image changes, emotional security, cultural expectations, support from partners, whether the pregnancy is unexpected, and financial situations. Major factors that influence the psychological impact of pregnancy are a woman's level of maturity and readiness for childbearing. Hormonal changes that occur during pregnancy contribute to mood swings. Many women have ambivalent feelings, being both happy at the thought of parenthood and sad at the thought of lost freedom. Both the mother and father or partner identify tasks and responsibilities and begin the process of establishing a relationship with the fetus (Figure 4-7).

BODY IMAGE

Body image is a person's perception of his or her own body. Body image can be considered from four aspects: appearance, function, sensation, and mobility.

Appearance is very meaningful to some women. During pregnancy, changes in a woman's body shape and function are so noticeable that she may become anxious. Also, the speed with which the changes occur makes it difficult for some women to integrate them

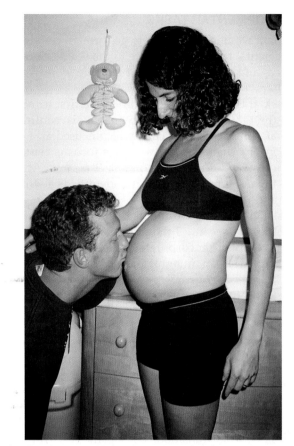

FIGURE 4-7 The father begins to develop a relationship with the fetus as he hears the fetal heart and feels movement.

into their self-perception. They may begin to feel ugly or fat, which can cause them to feel negatively about their pregnancy. These women need reassurance and must recognize that their feelings are common and normal. Other women feel beautiful during their pregnancy and will say things such as "I feel good when I am pregnant."

Function may be difficult when the pregnant woman feels that she is losing control. If she has urinary incontinence, she may feel out of control and negatively about the pregnancy. If her experience is explained as normal, she may be able to accept it with less difficulty.

Sensation may become more acute. Pregnant women may be more sensitive to touch. The change in sexuality and libido varies from woman to woman. The apparent physiologic basis of heightened sexuality is the greater vasocongestion in the pelvic area during pregnancy.

Mobility may be a problem when the woman feels restricted in her usual routine physical activities. She may be discouraged and need encouragement to participate in many of the same activities (including sports) during pregnancy that she participated in before pregnancy. Moderation is the key instruction to determining physical activity.

Box **4-3**	FDA Pregnancy Risk Category for Drugs

A: Evidence of fetal harm is remote. Controlled studies show no risk.

B: Animal studies have not shown a risk in the second or third trimesters. No available data on effect in the first trimester.

C: Studies in animals have shown negative effects on fetal development, but no controlled studies are available to know the effect on pregnant women. Risk cannot be ruled out.

D: There is positive evidence of fetal damage when the drug is used during pregnancy. The need for the drug should be carefully evaluated.

X: Studies in animals and human beings indicate definite fetal risk, and it should not be used during pregnancy.

From Meadows, M. (2001). Pregnancy and the drug dilemma. *FDA Consumer,* 35(3),16-20.

DEVELOPMENTAL TASKS

Pregnant women are known to go through certain developmental tasks. Tasks relate to the sequence of trimesters and are more apparent in some women than in others.

   Task 1: Pregnancy validation. In the first trimester (first 3 months), the pregnancy is confirmed and introversion occurs, which is used as a coping mechanism. The woman's focus is centered on nurturing and protecting the fetus. At this time, she may question her identity as a woman and mother.

   Task 2: Fetal embodiment. During the second trimester (second 3 months), the woman usually attempts to incorporate the fetus into her body image as an integral part of self. She begins to readjust her roles, and she reviews her relationships with others. At this time, repressed thoughts are dealt with, and maturation with a greater inner strength occurs.

   Task 3: Fetal distinction. When the woman feels fetal movements (quickening), the fetus starts to become distinct and separate from herself. At this time, she often daydreams about the baby, speaks of having a boy or girl, and envisions a perfect, beautiful baby (Figure 4-8).

   Task 4: Role transition. During the last trimester (last 3 months), the pregnant woman usually psychologically separates the fetus from herself and makes concrete plans for the baby. For example, she may purchase the crib and layette. At this

time, she may show greater irritability, may complain about her physical discomforts, and wants the pregnancy to end. Her normal coping mechanisms frequently do not work as well for her, and she may need additional emotional support and anticipatory guidance.

Ambivalence, acceptance, mood swings, introversion, and passivity are common and normal during pregnancy. Women commonly experience emotional lability; heightened sensitivity; increased need for affection; and greater irritability, fear, and anxiety. The pregnant woman needs to receive, rather than give, emotional support. Guidance and instruction are an important part of nursing care and can help make pregnancy a more positive and gratifying experience.

Table 4-6 shows the tasks of the parent in relation to Erikson's stages of child development. The table also includes some suggested nursing interventions that can assist in the development of effective parenting attitudes and behaviors. The growth and development of a parent begin in the first trimester of pregnancy.

RESPONSES TO PREGNANCY

Impact on the Father   Adjust & adapt.

The partner also travels through stages of adjustment to fatherhood. The *announcement* phase begins when the pregnancy is confirmed. The *adjustment* phase occurs in the second trimester, when the partner faces the reality of the pregnancy, asks questions, and participates in prenatal classes. In the *focus* phase, the partner begins to feel like a father, participates in the labor process, and discusses care of siblings and household modifications. Cultural values influence the role of the father. The nurse should not assume that a father is uninterested if he takes a less active role during the pregnancy and the birth process.

Impact on the Adolescent

Pregnant adolescents often have to struggle with feelings they find difficult to express. They are fraught with conflict about how to handle an unplanned pregnancy. Initially, they must face the anxiety of breaking the news to their parents and the father of the child. Denial of the pregnancy until late in gestation is not uncommon. There may be financial problems, shame, guilt, relationship problems with the infant's father, and feelings of low self-esteem. Alcoholism and substance abuse may be a part of the complex picture.

The nurse must assess the girl's developmental and educational level and her support system to provide the best care for her. A critical variable is the girl's age. Young adolescents have difficulty considering the needs of others, such as the fetus. The nurse helps the adolescent girl complete the developmental tasks of adolescence while assuming the new role of motherhood. Ideally, separate prenatal classes

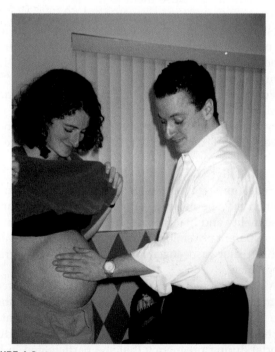

FIGURE 4-8 When the body changes of pregnancy are evident, the woman may welcome them as a sign to the world that her pregnancy is real and her fetus is thriving.

Table **4-6**   The Growth and Development of Parents

CHILD'S TASKS (ERIKSON'S STAGES)	PARENTS' TASK	NURSING INTERVENTIONS
First Trimester		
Growth	Develop attitude toward newborn: • Happy about child? • Parents of one disabled child? • Unwed mother? These factors and others will affect the parents' developing attitude.	Develop positive attitude in both parents concerning expected birth of child. Use referrals and agencies as needed.
Second Trimester		
Growth	Mother focuses on infant because of fetal movements felt. Parents picture what infant will look like, what future he or she will have, and other ideas.	Parents' focus is on child care and needs and providing physical environment for expected infant. Therefore, information concerning care of the newborn should be given at this time.
Third Trimester		
Growth	Mother feels large. Attention focuses on how fetus is going to get out.	Detailed information should be presented at this time concerning the birth processes, preparation for birth, breastfeeding, and care of sibling at home.
Birth		
Adjust to external environment	Elicit positive responses from child and respond by meeting child's need for food and closeness. If parents receive only negative responses (e.g., sleepy infant, crying infant, difficult feeder, congenital anomaly), parents' development will be inhibited.	Encourage early touch, feeding, and other practices. Explain behavior and appearance of newborn to allay fears. Help parents identify positive responses (e.g., use infant's reflexes, such as grasp reflex, to identify a positive response by placing mother's finger into infant's hand).
Infant		
Develop trust	Learn "cues" presented by infant to determine his or her individual needs.	Help parents assess and interpret needs of infant (avoid feelings of helplessness or incompetence). Do not let grandparents take over parental tasks. Help parents cope with problems such as colic.
Toddler		
Autonomy	Try to accept the pattern of growth and development. Accept some loss of control but maintain some limits for safety.	Help parents cope with transient independence of child (e.g., allow child to go on tricycle but do not yell "Don't fall" or anxiety will be radiated).
Preschool		
Initiative	Learn to separate from child.	Help parents show structure but "let go" so child can develop some independence. A preschool experience may be helpful.
School-Age		
Industry	Accept importance of child's peers. Parents must learn to accept some rejection from child at times. Patience is needed to allow children to do for themselves, even if it takes longer. Do not *do* the school project *for* the child. Provide chores for child appropriate to age level.	Help parents understand that child is developing his or her own limits and self-discipline. They should be there to guide child, but not constantly intrude. They need to help child get results from his or her own efforts at performance.
Adolescent		
Establishing identity Accepting pubertal changes Developing abstract reasoning Deciding on career Investigating lifestyles Controlling feeling	Parents must learn to let child live his or her own life and not expect total control over the child. Expect, at times, to be rejected by teenager. Expect differences in opinion and respect them. Guide but do not push.	Help parents adjust to changing role and relationship with adolescent (e.g., as child develops his or her own identify, he may become a Democrat if parents are Republican). Expose child to varied career fields and life experiences. Help child understand emerging emotions and feelings brought about by puberty.

tailored to their needs help adolescent girls learn to care for themselves and assume the role of mother (see Chapter 18).

Impact on the Older Couple

Mothers who become pregnant for the first time after age 35 years are called "elderly primips" because they are at a later stage in their childbearing cycle, and they may face special problems during pregnancy and labor. Many factors contribute to the trend of postponing pregnancy until after age 35 years:

- Effective birth control alternatives
- Increasing career options for women
- High cost of living (delays childbearing until financial status is secure)
- Development of fertilization techniques to enable later pregnancy

The "older couple" usually adjusts readily to pregnancy because they are often well educated, have achieved life experiences that enable them to cope with the realities of parenthood, and are ready for the lifestyle change. Advances in maternal care and delivery practices have decreased the risk of negative pregnancy outcomes, although special problems continue. Women over age 35 years may have a decreased ability to adjust their uterine blood flow to meet the needs of the fetus (Stables & Rankin, 2005). There may be an increase in multiple pregnancies if fertility drugs were used, which increases fetal risk. The increased risk of a congenital anomaly usually results in the offering of special tests during pregnancy (chorionic villi sampling, amniocentesis), which increases the cost of prenatal care. Although the older couple may adjust to the process of pregnancy and parenthood, they may find themselves "different" from their peers, and this can result in impaired social interaction. Concerns of the older parent relate to age and energy level as the child grows, confronting the issues of their own mortality, and child care requirements. Meeting financial needs of a college-age child at retirement is a special issue that may require discussion and planning. Many older parents are placed in a high risk prenatal group that may limit their options for selecting a birthing center. However, the pregnancy should be treated as normal unless problems are identified.

Impact on the Single Mother

The single mother may still be an adolescent, or she may be a mature woman. She has special emotional needs, especially if the father has left her, if he does not acknowledge the pregnancy, or if she does not care to have a relationship with the father. Some single mothers can turn to their parents, siblings, or close friends for support. Other single women are homosexual and have the support of their female partner. Women who do not have emotional support from significant others may have more difficulty completing the tasks of pregnancy. Their uncertainty in day-to-day living competes with the need to master the emotional tasks of pregnancy.

Some single mothers may have conceived by in vitro fertilization because of a strong desire to have a child even in the absence of a stable heterosexual relationship. These women often are nearing the end of their childbearing years and hold a "now or never" view of motherhood. Single women who plan pregnancies often prepare for the financial and lifestyle changes. Achieving social acceptance is not as difficult today as it was many years ago when single motherhood was taboo and considered a disgrace to the maternal family. The nurse should maintain a nonjudgmental attitude and assist the single mother in successfully achieving the psychological tasks of pregnancy.

Impact on the Single Father

The single father may take an active interest in and financial responsibility for the child. The couple may plan marriage eventually, but it is often delayed. A single father may provide emotional support for the mother during the pregnancy and birth. He often has strong feelings of surprise and accomplishment when he becomes aware of his partner's pregnancy. He may want to participate in plans for the child and take part in infant care after birth. However, his participation is sometimes rejected by the woman.

Impact on the Grandparents

Prospective grandparents have different reactions as well to a woman's pregnancy. They may eagerly anticipate the announcement that a grandchild is on the way, or they may feel that they are not ready for the role of grandparent, which they equate with being old. The first grandchild often causes the most excitement for grandparents. Their reaction may be more subdued if they have several grandchildren, which may hurt the excited pregnant couple.

Grandparents have different ideas of how they will be involved with their grandchildren. Distance from the younger family dictates the degree of involvement for some. They may want to be fully involved in the plans for the infant and help with child care, often traveling a great distance to be there for the big event. Other grandparents want less involvement because they welcome the freedom of a childless life again. Many grandparents are in their forties and fifties, a time when their own career demands and care of their aging parents compete with their ability to be involved with grandchildren.

If grandparents and the expectant couple have similar views of their roles, little conflict is likely. However, disappointment and conflict may occur if the pregnant couple and the grandparents have significantly different expectations of their role and involvement. The nurse can help the young couple understand their parents' reactions and help them negotiate solutions to conflicts that are satisfactory to both generations.

Get Ready for the NCLEX® Examination!

Key Points

- EDD can be calculated with Nägele's rule: subtract 3 months and add 7 days to the first day of the LNMP. However, only a small number of births occur on that exact date.
- Signs of pregnancy often resemble signs of other conditions and are therefore categorized as presumptive, probable, and positive signs of pregnancy.
- Physiologic and anatomic adaptations that occur during pregnancy are profound, but the body systems generally return to the nonpregnant state after birth.
- Being aware of the maternal adaptations that occur during pregnancy is essential to understanding the discomforts and disorders of pregnancy.
- An increase in clotting factors and fibrinogen in the blood during pregnancy makes the woman vulnerable to thrombus formation.
- Cardiac output doubles during pregnancy, and there is a 40% increase in blood volume.
- When a pregnant woman lies flat on her back, the weight of the uterus and fetal contents presses on the vena cava, abdominal aorta, decreasing blood flow and causing maternal hypotension and fetal hypoxia.
- Oxygen consumption increases 15% during pregnancy.
- Maternal insulin resistance increases during pregnancy.
- Many metabolic functions increase during pregnancy.
- Frequency of urination often occurs early in pregnancy because of the pressure on the growing uterus or the bladder, and late in pregnancy because of the pressure of the fetus on the bladder as it settles in the pelvic cavity.
- During pregnancy, hyperpigmentation of the skin occurs due to the melanocyte-stimulating hormone and estrogen. The pigmentation fades following pregnancy.
- Stretch marks (striae) occur as the elastic tissue of the skin stretches, resulting in pinkish or purplish lines on the abdomen, breasts, or buttocks. Striae fade to silver lines after pregnancy.
- Categories of drug safety during pregnancy include A, B, C, D, and X. Only drugs in the A or B category may be considered safe during pregnancy.
- Psychological changes during pregnancy are influenced by appearance, function, sensation, and mobility.
- Developmental tasks are related to the trimesters of pregnancy.
- Pregnancy has an impact on all family members.

Additional Learning Resources

SG Go to your Study Guide on pages 479–480 for additional Review Questions for the NCLEX® Examination, Critical Thinking Clinical Situations, and other learning activities to help you master this chapter content.

evolve Go to your Evolve website (http://evolve.elsevier.com/Leifer/maternity) for the following FREE learning resources:
- Animations
- Answer Guidelines for Critical Thinking Questions
- Answers and Rationales for Review Questions for the NCLEX® Examination
- Concept Map Creator
- Glossary with pronunciations in English and Spanish
- Patient Teaching Plans
- Skills Performance Checklists and more!

Online Resources
- www.alexandertechnique.com/articles/pregnancy
- www.allaboutparenting.org/parenting-skills.htm
- www.lamaze.org
- www.nursingcenter.com
- www.mypyramid.gov
- www.makewayforbaby.com/prenatalcare.htm

Review Questions for the NCLEX® Examination

1. A pregnant woman arrives at her first obstetric appointment and asks, "When is the baby due?" The woman's last normal menstrual period started on June 11. Using Nägele's rule, the nurse determines that the estimated date of delivery is:

    -3month + 7days

   1. March 4
   2. March 18
   3. September 4
   4. September 18

2. The nurse can expect to palpate the uterine fundus at its highest, at the xiphoid process of the rib cage, by:

   1. 12 weeks' gestation
   2. 20 weeks' gestation
   3. 36 weeks' gestation
   4. 40 weeks' gestation

3. The hormone responsible for the production of breast milk is:
   1. Estrogen
   2. Oxytocin
   3. Progesterone
   4. Prolactin

4. A pregnant woman reports pain and a tingling sensation in her hand and wrist. The nurse is aware that these symptoms are most likely related to:
   1. Carpal tunnel syndrome
   2. Striae gravidarum
   3. Chloasma
   4. Diastasis recti abdominis

5. Which woman would be considered an "elderly primip?"
   1. 30-year-old pregnant for the first time
   2. 35-year-old pregnant for the third time
   3. 37-year-old pregnant for the first time
   4. 40-year-old pregnant for the second time

6. Which FDA risk category for drugs indicates the least risk if taken during pregnancy?
   1. A
   2. B
   3. C
   4. X

7. What would be considered positive sign(s) of pregnancy? *(Select all that apply.)*
   1. Positive home pregnancy test
   2. Doppler auscultation fetal heart sounds
   3. Palpation of active fetal movements by examiner
   4. Ultrasound visualization of the fetus

8. Put the following developmental tasks of pregnancy in sequential order by numbering 1 *(first)* to 4 *(last)*.
   3 Fetal distinction
   1 Pregnancy validation
   4 Role transition
   2 Fetal embodiment

Critical Thinking Questions

1. A woman in her first trimester of pregnancy asks, "What procedures will the nurse-midwife do to determine that I am pregnant?" What explanation would you give her?

2. A woman in the first trimester of pregnancy would like information about her pregnancy. Her first question is, "Why do I have brown patches on my face, a brown line down my abdomen, and darker nipples?" She also asks, "Why do I urinate so often?" Why do you think these are concerns?

Health Care and Fetal Assessment During Pregnancy

Objectives

1. Define key terms listed.
2. Discuss the concept of preconception care.
3. Explain the significance of prenatal care.
4. Outline the care given during the initial prenatal visit.
5. Review care given on subsequent prenatal visits.
6. Explain five factors that place the fetus at risk.
7. Describe four methods of assessing the fetal condition during the antepartum period.
8. Explain the uses of ultrasonography during pregnancy.
9. Explain the uses of amniocentesis as a diagnostic tool.
10. Compare chorionic villi sampling with amniocentesis.
11. Explain the biophysical profile.
12. Describe the purpose of the nonstress test.
13. Determine the causes of common discomforts during pregnancy and the appropriate measures to alleviate them.
14. Demonstrate three exercises to strengthen and stretch muscles in preparation for childbirth.
15. Outline four safety precautions for exercising during pregnancy.
16. Discuss the benefits and limitations of immunizations during pregnancy.
17. Individualize various optimum weight gain patterns during pregnancy.
18. Identify the suggested dietary alterations during pregnancy.
19. Describe a common pica substance ingested by a pregnant woman.
20. Identify the basic philosophy of preparation for childbirth.
21. Illustrate three different breathing patterns used during labor and birth.

- 8wk into pregnancy most people realize they are pregnant.

Key Terms

cleansing breath (p. 86)
doulas (DOO-lăz, p. 87)
effleurage (ĕf-loo-RĂZH, p. 85)
Kegel exercises (KĒ-gŭl, p. 69)
Lamaze technique (p. 84)
Leopold's maneuvers (p. 64)

MyPlate (p. 81)
paced breathing (p. 86)
pelvic tilt exercise (p. 69)
pica (PĪ-kă, p. 84)
preconception care (p. 61)
Valsalva's maneuver (văl-SĂL-văz, p. 87)

PRECONCEPTION CARE

Preconception care is health care and screening conducted before pregnancy occurs so that medical risk factors or lifestyle behaviors can be identified, managed, or changed before conception. The normalcy of pregnancy is greatly influenced by prepregnancy health. Most women who seek medical care as soon as they realize they may be pregnant are already at or past 8 weeks' gestation, which may be too late for some interventions to be effective. Most birth defects occur between 2 and 8 weeks' gestation. These missed opportunities include ensuring an adequate daily intake of folic acid, updating immunization status, ceasing smoking, treating current infections, and obtaining genetic counseling or testing. Prenatal data collection includes physical, psychological, and psychosocial factors that will affect the health of the mother and fetus. This includes exposure to hazardous materials in the workplace. Ideally, prenatal care starts before pregnancy occurs. Preconception care is best achieved when a pregnancy is planned.

PRENATAL CARE

Early and regular prenatal care dramatically reduces infant and maternal morbidity and mortality and offers a unique opportunity for nurses to influence the family's health. Early detection of potential problems leads to prompt assessment and treatment, which greatly improves the pregnancy outcome. Pregnancy is a normal process, and the primary focus is education for self-care. Pregnancy affects the mother's body and the family's integrity; therefore, the entire family is included in the care plan (Figure 5-1). The major goals of prenatal care are listed in Box 5-1.

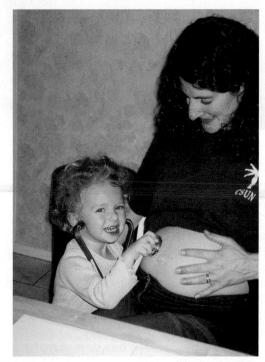

FIGURE 5-1 A sibling begins to anticipate the birth of her brother.

Box **5-1**	Major Goals of Prenatal Care

- Ensuring a safe birth for mother and child by promoting good health habits and reducing risk factors
- Teaching health habits that may be continued after pregnancy
- Educating about self-care during pregnancy
- Providing physical assessment and care
- Preparing parents for adaptation to parenthood

COLLABORATIVE CARE

To collaborate is to work together with others. Collaborative care involves the patient and the nurse with other members of the health care team contributing to the care plan for the woman. The nurse, along with other multidisciplinary health team members, can tailor interventions to meet specific needs of the patient and family.

CULTURAL COMPETENCE

The woman's lifestyle may include culturally unique beliefs and behaviors that must be considered in a care plan. The focus of education should stand out as a key part of prenatal care and patient-nurse communication. Cultural considerations are important in caring for a woman during her pregnancy. Some cultures view pregnancy and childbirth as normal conditions that do not require any special health care.

Cultural Considerations

Providing Culturally Effective Prenatal Care

- Non–English-speaking parents should be offered interpreters who are familiar with their culture and their language in the labor room, the clinic, or the home setting.
- Parenting classes should have culturally appropriate content related to the minority groups they serve.
- Documentation should include the interpreters used in patient teaching plans.
- Illustrative material or handouts should be provided in the native language of the patient at the appropriate reading level and clearly provide information concerning informed choices.
- In-service educational classes should be offered to staff on a regular basis and emphasize how to communicate with patients from different cultures (relative to patients served).

Cultural competence is the awareness of, acceptance of, and respect for beliefs, values, traditions, and practices that are different from one's own. The ability to adapt health care so that it does not violate the culture or religion of the patient is the core of cultural competence. Achieving cultural competence is aided by knowledge, skills, and encounters with others of different cultures. The assumption that all people of one culture believe and behave the same way is cultural stereotyping and should be avoided. Individual differences should be identified and respected (Figure 5-2). For example, in some cultures, such as Orthodox Judaism, the husband may not view the newborn as it is delivered; only verbal encouragement is allowed. Many non-Western cultures expect the woman to have 40 days of rest after delivery. Chinese, African American, Hispanic, and Southeast Asian cultures usually avoid full washing of the body and hair until lochia has ceased. The "hot and cold" theory is observed by many cultures, and, because labor and delivery are considered a "cold" experience, it is balanced by "hot" conditions; therefore, ice water and air-conditioning are avoided. Cambodian women often discard colostrum. In the traditional Japanese culture, newborns are bathed twice a day, and the bathing is accompanied by loud noises to ward off evil spirits.

PRENATAL VISITS

The initial assessment interview can establish a trusting relationship between the nurse and the pregnant woman. It is a planned, purposeful communication that focuses on specific assessments. Observations include the woman's subjective interpretations of her health status and the nurse's objective examination. During the initial communication, the nurse observes the woman's body language, such as her posture and facial expressions, as well as other physical and emotional signs.

Cultural Assessment Data Collection Tool to Assist in Developing an Individualized Plan of Care
(This tool can be translated into multiple languages and allows the nurse to compare the client's answers to those on an identical tool written in the nurse's dominant language. This data collection will enable the nurse to provide care to clients in a way that is culturally satisfying to them.)

Birth Plan
Providing answers to the following questions will give us information that will enable us to make your birthing experience a more positive experience.

Whom do you plan on having present to support you while you are in labor?
- ❏ Husband
- ❏ Female family member
- ❏ Friend
- ❏ No one

Have you attended a childbirth class?
- ❏ Yes
- ❏ No

If yes, what method of childbirth preparation?
- ❏ Lamaze
- ❏ Bradley
- ❏ Other

Gender of health care provider preferred?
- ❏ Male
- ❏ Female
- ❏ No preference

During pelvic examinations does your husband wish to be present if done by a male physician?
- ❏ Yes
- ❏ No

During labor will you:
- ❏ Prefer to be involved in decision making
- ❏ Prefer to have someone tell you what to do

When you are in pain do you:
- ❏ Become quiet
- ❏ Verbally express your pain
- ❏ Yell and/or cry

Regarding pain medicine do you:
- ❏ Prefer to ask for it when you want it
- ❏ Have the nurse offer it to you

Do you feel comfortable in freely making requests to MD/CNM/nurse?
- ❏ Yes
- ❏ No

Do you prefer to be addressed by:
- ❏ Your first name
- ❏ Your last name

What type of infant feeding are you planning?
- ❏ Breastfeeding
- ❏ Bottle feeding
- ❏ Both
- ❏ Breastfeeding after colostrum changes to milk

Do you prefer to drink water:
- ❏ At room temperature
- ❏ With ice

After delivery do you prefer:
- ❏ Hot beverages
- ❏ Cold beverages

Do you want to know the sex of the baby:
- ❏ When an ultrasound is done
- ❏ Immediately after birth
- ❏ After the placenta is delivered

While in the hospital after having your baby, do you prefer:
- ❏ Showers
- ❏ Baths
- ❏ Sponge baths
- ❏ None

Do you believe it is okay to wash your hair in the first few days after delivery?
- ❏ Yes
- ❏ No

According to your cultural practices, when do women who have had a baby usually get up to walk around?
- ❏ Within the first few hours after delivery
- ❏ The day after delivery
- ❏ Prefer to stay in bed

According to your cultural practices, who usually provides most of the infant care in the first few days of life?
- ❏ Mother of infant
- ❏ Both parents of infant
- ❏ Nurse and/or family members

If infant is male, do you plan to have him circumcised?
- ❏ Yes
- ❏ No

If yes, when do you prefer it should be done?
- ❏ During hospitalization
- ❏ Day eight
- ❏ After discharge

According to your cultural practices when is it acceptable for others to praise your baby?
- ❏ Any time
- ❏ Only if they are touching infant
- ❏ Never

After delivery how long will it be before you resume normal activities outside the home?
- ❏ At least 1 week
- ❏ Two weeks
- ❏ One month
- ❏ 45 days
- ❏ Over 45 days
- ❏ No specific amount of time

FIGURE 5-2 **Cultural assessment data collection tool to assist in developing an individualized plan of care.** This tool can be translated into multiple languages and allows the nurse to compare the patient's answers to those on an identical tool written in the facility's dominant language. This data collection will enable the nurse to provide care to patients in a way that is culturally satisfying to them.

INITIAL HEALTH AND SOCIAL HISTORY

A health history summary, including a thorough medical and obstetric history, is taken during the first prenatal visit to determine the present status of the woman's health. First, the nurse obtains personal information, including age, marital status, education, and occupation. Second, the nurse takes the medical history of the woman and her family. The family history and partner's history are important to identify certain health problems, such as heart disease and genetic disorders that could affect the outcome of pregnancy. The woman's personal history, including her nutritional history, is important in assessing her present and past health. A cultural history that includes the use of self-medication, complementary or alternative medicine (CAM), alcohol use, or the use of recreational drugs is part of every pregnant woman's initial health history because it may have an impact on fetal development. Third, the nurse obtains information about the woman's obstetric history, including any previous pregnancies, birth weight of previous infants, length of previous labors, present attitude toward this pregnancy, date of last normal menstrual period (LNMP), and any problems that arose during a previous pregnancy, labor, birth, and postpartum period. This information can provide clues of what to expect during the present pregnancy.

Social history provides information about the woman's and partner's occupations, education, marital status, ethnic or cultural background, and socioeconomic status. Perception of this pregnancy, coping mechanisms, and family support are explored.

PHYSICAL EXAMINATION

In the physical examination, the physician or nurse-midwife examines all body systems. This includes a head-to-toe assessment. The patient's weight and blood pressure are recorded, and microscopic urine examination is performed in the first visit. Baseline weight and blood pressure are important because a sudden change in either is significant. A sudden elevation in blood pressure or sudden excessive weight gain may be a symptom of gestational hypertension (see Chapter 13). The pregnancy examination includes a pelvic examination, which is performed to determine the status of the reproductive organs and the birth canal. Pelvic measurements may be taken to determine whether the pelvis will allow the passage of a fetus at delivery (see Chapter 2). Before the pelvic examination is conducted, the nurse should advise the woman to empty her bladder and to take deep breaths during the examination to lessen her discomfort. Routine laboratory tests are performed throughout the pregnancy (Table 5-1).

SUBSEQUENT VISITS

Prenatal visits are scheduled every month for 7 months, every 2 weeks during the eighth month, and every week during the last month if the pregnancy is uneventful (normal). The woman's weight and blood pressure are recorded, and the urine is checked for protein, acetone, and glucose. These three assessments enable the early detection of hypertension and gestational diabetes mellitus. In addition, the physician or midwife measures the height of the fundus to see whether the pregnancy is progressing at the expected rate (Figure 5-3).

The woman's abdomen is palpated with Leopold's maneuvers to assess the presentation and position of the fetus (see Chapter 7). These consist of four basic maneuvers: (1) determining what is in the fundus,

either breech or head (the head is firm and round, whereas the breech feels softer); (2) determining the location of the fetal back (opposite from the extremities); (3) noting what part of the fetus is above the symphysis pubis, either head or breech; and (4) noting the position of the cephalic prominence.

Having determined the presentation and position of the fetus, the nurse then listens to the fetal heart rate. The fetal heart rate can be detected with a Doppler device or with a fetal stethoscope. Tenderness over the woman's kidney area (costovertebral angle [CVA]) or tenderness in the calf of her leg (Homans' sign) is assessed because, during pregnancy, a woman is at greater risk for renal infection and thrombophlebitis.

The woman is asked whether she has any discomforts. Sometimes, vague symptoms or subtle clues are the first indication of an impending complication. If the woman has complaints, nursing or medical measures are suggested to relieve them. Early in the subsequent visits, the type of delivery anticipated and how she intends to feed her baby should be discussed. Reassurance of the woman's capacity to be a good mother is important.

PRENATAL FETAL ASSESSMENT

High-risk pregnancies are those in which maternal and fetal outcomes are potentially not as good as in a normal pregnancy. The improved understanding of fetal disorders and extraordinary technical advances are changing the management of high-risk pregnancies. Newer diagnostic and therapeutic approaches are being used in the management of complex problems. High-risk pregnancy presents one of the most critical challenges in medical and nursing care. Emphasis must be placed on the safe birth of infants who can develop to their maximum potential (Box 5-2).

This section discusses a range of technologies and procedures designed to reduce risks to the woman and the fetus. These procedures include nursing responsibilities that must be carried out to provide safe care, reduce risks, and meet emotional needs. See Chapter 13 for detailed information concerning complications of pregnancy.

DIAGNOSTIC TECHNIQUES AND NURSING CONSIDERATIONS

A variety of tests can be used to assess fetal well-being during pregnancy and are indicated when maternal high-risk factors are present (Table 5-2). These tests include diagnostic ultrasound, Doppler ultrasound blood flow, chorionic villi sampling, amniocentesis, percutaneous cord blood sampling, nonstress test (NST), contraction stress test (CST), biophysical profile (BPP), vibroacoustic stimulation test, and maternal assessment of fetal movements (Figures 5-4 to 5-6 on p. 69).

Septic baby's will have low temp.
not an ↑ temp.

Table 5-1   Prenatal Laboratory Tests

TEST	PURPOSE
First Trimester (Routine)	
Blood type, Rh factor, and antibody screen	Determines risk for maternal-fetal blood incompatibility
Complete blood count (CBC)	Detects anemia, infection, or cell abnormalities
Hemoglobin or hematocrit	Detects anemia
Venereal Disease Research Laboratory (VDRL) test or rapid plasma reagin (RPR)	Syphilis screen mandated by law
Rubella titer	Determines immunity to rubella
Tuberculosis test	Screening test for exposure to tuberculosis
Hepatitis B screen	Identifies carriers for hepatitis B (recommended by American College of Obstetricians and Gynecologists)
Human immunodeficiency virus (HIV) screen	Detects HIV infection; required by some states (counseling concerning prevention and risks should be provided to all prenatal patients)
Urinalysis and culture	Detects infection, renal disease, or diabetes (recommended by U.S. Preventive Services Task Force to screen for asymptomatic bacteriuria)
Papanicolaou (Pap) test	Screens for cervical cancer (recommended if not done within 6 months before conception)
Vaginal or cervical culture	Detects group B streptococci, bacterial vaginosis, or sexually transmitted infections (STIs) such as gonorrhea, chlamydia
First Trimester (If Indicated)	
Hemoglobin electrophoresis	Identifies presence of sickle cell trait or disease in women of African or Mediterranean descent
Endovaginal ultrasound	Performed when high risk of fetal loss is suspected
Second Trimester (Routine)	
Blood glucose screen: 1 hr after ingesting 50 g of glucose liquid	Routine test done at 24-28 weeks' gestation to identify gestational diabetes mellitus; results >135 mg/dL require medical follow-up
Serum alpha-fetoprotein	Optional routine test to identify neural tube or chromosomal defect in fetus
Ultrasonography	Optional noninvasive routine test to identify some anomalies and confirm estimated date of delivery
Second Trimester (If Indicated)	
Amniocentesis	Performed at a 16-20 weeks' gestation when high-risk problem is suspected or if the mother is over 35 years of age
Third Trimester (If Indicated)	
Real-time ultrasonography	Performed when problem is suspected Identifies reduced amniotic fluid, which can result in fetal problem Identifies excess amniotic fluid, which would indicate fetal anomaly or maternal problem Confirms gestational age or cephalopelvic disproportion Determines fetal lung maturity (lecithin/sphingomyelin ratio) with amniocentesis Confirms presence of anomaly that may require fetal or neonatal surgery
Cervical fibronectin assay	Determines risk of preterm labor when problem is suspected

Modified from Leifer, G. (2011). *Introduction to maternity and pediatric nursing* (6th ed.). Philadelphia: Saunders.

Nursing care during assessments of fetal health, especially with all of the new tests being performed, is important; the woman must understand the reason that specific tests are being performed. The nurse can provide an opportunity for the woman to ask questions regarding the procedure. Clarifying and interpreting test results should be carried out collaboratively by all health care providers involved in the procedures. However, the nurse is often the person who spends the most time with the woman (Nursing Care Plan 5-1 on p. 70).

 Communication

Antepartum Fetal Test

Before any antepartum fetal test, parents should know the answer to each of these questions:

- What information will the test provide that is not already known?
- How will the information be used in the management of the mother and the baby?
- What is the risk for the mother and the baby?
- If an abnormal condition is detected, is treatment available?

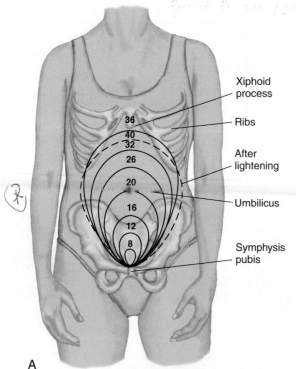

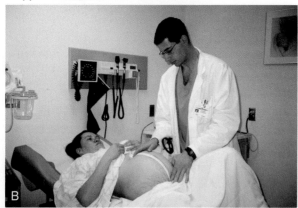

FIGURE 5-3 **Height of the fundus of the uterus during pregnancy.** **A,** The numbers represent the weeks of gestation, and the circles represent the height of the fundus expected at that stage of gestation. The dotted line at the fortieth week indicates lightening has occurred. **B,** A health care provider measures the height of the fundus at a clinic visit.

Box 5-2	Prenatal High-Risk Factors Indicating Need for Special Prenatal Testing

- Maternal condition that increases risk for uteroplacental insufficiency such as diabetes mellitus or hypertension
- History of previous stillbirth
- Mother's age less than 16 or more than 35 years
- Multifetal pregnancy
- Postterm pregnancy
- Decreased fetal movement
- Oligohydramnios
- Intrauterine growth restriction (IUGR)
- History of congenital abnormalities

PSYCHOLOGICAL REACTIONS TO DIAGNOSTIC TESTING

Few psychological studies have been performed regarding the impact of antepartum diagnostic testing and monitoring of the fetal heart rate during labor on women's anxiety levels. However, health care providers have subjectively noticed that the need for testing produces fear. Ultrasound use during pregnancy has become almost routine, and many women expect it to be a part of prenatal care. Some women look forward to the ultrasound because it confirms the pregnancy with visualization of the fetus and the fetal heartbeat. They often learn the sex of the fetus at this time. These factors can have a positive effect on the woman and even promote psychological preparation for attachment to the fetus. Because other prenatal diagnostic testing can provoke anxiety and fear, it is important to allow time for the woman to ask questions and discuss her feelings. The nurse must be particularly sensitive to and respond to the emotional, informational, and comfort needs of the woman and her family. Fetal assessment during labor is discussed in Chapter 7.

PATIENT TEACHING FOR SELF-CARE AND COMMON DISCOMFORTS OF PREGNANCY

During the 9 months of pregnancy, women experience various types of discomforts, many of which are a result of normal physiologic changes that take place during pregnancy (discussed in Chapter 4). Nurses and other health care professionals often refer to these discomforts as minor, but the pregnant woman does not consider them minor. If discomforts are not anticipated or expected, they can make her feel anxious and worried. These discomforts can usually be relieved or prevented by simple measures (Table 5-3 on pp. 71–72). Teaching women about self-care is important (Figure 5-7 on p. 72).

The nurse should provide anticipatory guidance of changes to expect during pregnancy, labor, and birth and after childbirth. The nurse reviews positive health practices and discusses their adaptation during pregnancy (Nursing Care Plan 5-2 on pp. 73–75).

Patient Teaching

Assessing Communication Barriers

Assess the reading level and native language of the woman before giving written information concerning instructions or care during pregnancy.

BATHING

Women typically perspire profusely during pregnancy. Frequent baths or showers are needed. Bathing in the tub may become a problem later in pregnancy because of awkwardness; therefore, she should consider safety measures such as rubber mats and handrails. Bathing in

Table 5-2 Tests to Assess Fetal Well-Being

TEST AND DESCRIPTION	MAJOR USES DURING PREGNANCY
Ultrasound imaging: High-frequency waves are used to visualize internal organs or tissues within the body (e.g., fetus, placenta, or moving object such as a beating fetal heart); also called ultrasonography; a transvaginal probe or abdominal transducer is used. Abdominal ultrasound requires a full bladder for better visualization (have the woman drink 1-2 qt of water before the examination). Procedure is noninvasive, is painless, and lasts approximately 20 minutes.	Confirms the pregnancy Confirms gestational age Identifies site of implantation (uterine or ectopic) Verifies fetal viability or death Identifies multifetal pregnancy (e.g., twins) Rules out specific fetal abnormalities Evaluates vaginal bleeding and location of placenta Determines amniotic fluid volume Observes fetal movements (fetal heartbeat, breathing, activity, and body movements) Used to guide procedures such as amniocentesis and chorionic villus sampling
Doppler ultrasound blood flow: Method of noninvasively studying blood flow in maternal and fetal circulations; a hand-held ultrasound device is used. Echo Doppler scan detects fetal heart activity at 6-10 weeks' gestation.	Assesses maternal-fetal blood flow Detects fetal anemia in Rh isoimmunization May identify intrauterine growth restriction (IUGR) and placental insufficiency Color Doppler imaging views heart and blood vessel structure and can detect anomalies in vessels within the umbilical cord
Chorionic villus sampling: A first-trimester alternative to amniocentesis for prenatal diagnosis of some conditions; small amount of the developing placenta (chorionic villi) is aspirated by syringe under the guidance of ultrasound and analyzed. Performed at 10-12 weeks' gestation.	Recommended only for women at risk for giving birth to baby with a genetic chromosomal or metabolic abnormality (cannot be used to determine spina bifida or anencephaly) Results of chromosome studies available in 24-48 hours Risk of abortion higher than in amniocentesis; potential limb reduction defect in fetus Rh$_0$(D) immune globulin (RhoGAM) is given to Rh-negative women Can be done earlier in gestation
Amniocentesis: Performed to obtain amniotic fluid–containing fetal cells; under direct visualization of ultrasound, a thin needle is inserted through the abdominal and uterine walls to withdraw amniotic fluid into a syringe (with cast-off cells). Sufficient fluid must be present for the test to be done (15-17 weeks' gestation and 12-14 weeks' gestation for some disorders).	*Early pregnancy* Used to assess genetic disorders (e.g., Tay-Sachs disease) Tests for level of alpha-fetoprotein (AFP), which is also present in maternal blood High AFP levels found in neural tube defects such as spina bifida (open spine) or anencephaly (incomplete development of skull and brain) Low levels of AFP associated with chromosomal disorders or gestational trophoblastic disease *Late pregnancy* Assesses for severity of maternal-fetal blood incompatibility and fetal lung maturity; RhoGAM given to Rh-negative women Minimal risk for abortion in late pregnancy but higher in early pregnancy *Safety concerns:* risk of infection, pregnancy loss (although slight), and needle injuries to fetus or placenta
Tests for fetal lung maturity: Amniotic fluid obtained by amniocentesis is tested to indicate if fetal lungs are mature enough to adapt to extrauterine life. Lecithin/sphingomyelin (L/S) ratio: a 2:1 ratio indicates fetal lung maturity (3:1 ratio is desirable for diabetic mother) Presence of phosphatidylglycerol (PG) Foam stability index (FSI, or "shake test"): if ring of bubbles persists for 15 minutes after shaking solution, test is termed positive and indicates surfactant is present and fetal lungs are mature.	Determines whether the fetus is likely to have respiratory distress in adapting to extrauterine life Sometimes used to determine whether the fetal lungs are mature enough before cesarean birth Also evaluates whether the fetus should be removed immediately or whether the lungs should be allowed to develop more in utero after the membranes have ruptured and gestation is <37 weeks (or date is questionable) Absence of PG associated with respiratory distress Blood or meconium in the amniotic fluid alters accuracy of results
Percutaneous umbilical blood sampling (cordocentesis): Obtaining fetal blood sample from placental vessel or from the umbilical cord by guidance with ultrasound (see Figure 5-6).	Evaluates whether the fetus is anemic and needs a blood transfusion Identifies Rh isoimmunization in the blood and chromosomal disorders and acid-base status of fetus
Nonstress test (NST): Assessment of fetal well-being by evaluating the fetal heart's ability to accelerate (speed up) in association with fetal movement by using an electronic fetal monitor; accelerations occur either spontaneously or in association with fetal movement. An external electronic	With adequate accelerations of the FHR, confirms that the placenta is functioning properly and that the fetus is well oxygenated with autonomic functions Blurred response indicative of hypoxia, acidosis, drugs, or fetal sleep

Table 5-2 Tests to Assess Fetal Well-Being—cont'd

TEST AND DESCRIPTION	MAJOR USES DURING PREGNANCY
monitor is applied while the woman is in a semi-Fowler's or left-lateral position; conduction gel is put on the abdomen; two belts are applied on the woman's abdomen; one belt and a device to detect fetal heart rate (FHR) and the other belt detects fetal movement; the woman is given a button to press, which records the time she feels movement on the strip on which the FHR is recorded. The test is continued for up to 40 minutes, or until the criteria for reactivity are met; because almost all accelerations are accompanied by fetal movement, the movement need not be recorded for the test to be reactive.	Nonreactive NST indicates the fetal heartbeat does not accelerate adequately and further assessment may be required A reactive NST indicates the fetal heartbeat accelerated adequately with fetal movement
Contraction stress test (CST): Evaluation of the FHR response to mild uterine contractions by using an electronic fetal monitor. Contractions are induced by intravenous oxytocin (Pitocin) infusion or by self-stimulation of the nipples, which causes the woman's pituitary gland to release oxytocin; the woman must have at least three contractions of at least 40-seconds duration in a 10-minute period for interpretation of the CST test.	Same purposes as for the NST Negative CST indicates there were no late decelerations of the FHR with three uterine contractions in a 10-minute period Variable accelerations that occur with CST may indicate cord compression
Nipple stimulation: Done if inadequate contractions occur. Woman brushes her palm across nipple for 2-3 minutes, stopping when contraction begins; after 5-minute rest period, same process is repeated. To avoid hyperstimulation (uterine contractions lasting 90 seconds or more often than every 2 minutes), bilateral stimulation should not be done unless unilateral stimulation fails.	Stimulate contractions to result in FHR accelerations Intermittent nipple stimulation preferred to prevent hyperstimulation of the uterus
Biophysical profile (BPP): Method to evaluate the condition of the fetus that uses five observations: fetal breathing movements, gross fetal movements (movements of body), FHR variability and reactivity (the NST), and the volume of amniotic fluid (amniotic fluid index [AFI]). Some facilities omit the NST, and others assess only the NST or ultrasound and AFI.	Used after 26 weeks' gestation to assess fetal oxygenation; as fetal hypoxia increases, FHR changes occur first, then decreased breathing movement (<1 breath in 30 minutes), gross body movements (<3 in 20 minutes), and finally loss of muscle tone (failure to open and close the hand) Results immediately available and allow for delay of induction if fetal well-being is confirmed
Vibroacoustic stimulation test (vibration and sound): Stimulation of fetus by artificial larynx device; used as an adjunct to the NST. The artificial larynx is applied to the woman's abdomen over the fetal head, then is activated with a 2- to 3-second stimulus.	Used to clarify whether fetus was sleeping (or inactive) during previous NST Has reduced number of nonreactive NSTs as well as time and cost Fetal accelerations in response to stimulus indicate fetal health
Maternal assessment of fetal movement (kick counts): Simple but valuable method for monitoring fetus. It should be encouraged after 28 weeks' gestation, with women setting aside a consistent time to do the "kick counts." Mother should count the number of fetal movements for 30-60 minutes 2-3 times a day; other protocols may be used.	Recognizes that the presence of fetal movements is a reassuring sign of fetal health. Decreased fetal movements possibly caused by sleep Cessation of movements correlated with hypoxia and fetal death In the third trimester, woman counts and documents fetal movement for 30-60 minutes twice a day; <4 movements in 30 minutes on 2 consecutive days or <10 movements in 12-hour period should be reported to the health care provider NOTE: Maternal use of drugs may affect fetal activity.
Amniotic fluid index (AFI): This ultrasound scan measures the amniotic fluid pockets in all 4 quadrants surrounding the mother's umbilical area and produces an AFI. A reading of 15-19 cm is considered normal; <5 cm is known as oligohydramnios (decreased amniotic fluid); >30 cm is hydramnios (excess amniotic fluid).	Identifies oligohydramnios, which is associated with growth restriction and fetal distress during labor because of kinking of the umbilical cord Identifies hydramnios, which is associated with fetal anomalies such as gastrointestinal obstruction or fetal hydrops
Alpha-fetoprotein test (AFP): Determines the level of this protein in the pregnant woman's blood serum (MSAFP) or in a sample of amniotic fluid (AFAFP). Correct interpretation requires accurate gestational age. The test is usually performed at 16-18 weeks' gestation.	High levels associated with open defects such as spina bifida Low levels associated with chromosomal anomalies or hydatidiform mole
Triple marker screening: Detects levels of human chorionic gonadotropin (hCG) and unconjugated estriol. This is often done with AFP test.	May indicate trisomy 18 or 21 if estriol is low and hCG is high. May indicate trisomy 21 if Inhibin A is elevated

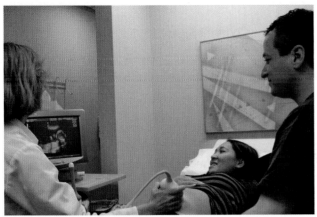

FIGURE 5-4 Ultrasonography is a noninvasive, painless method of scanning a pregnant woman's abdomen with high-frequency waves to determine fetal growth and development. The ultrasound transducer is moved over the mother's abdomen to obtain an image.

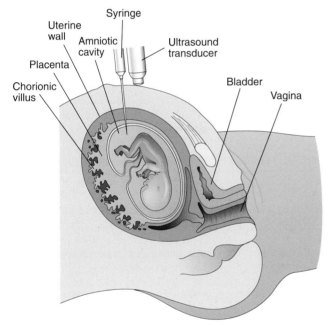

FIGURE 5-5 **Amniocentesis.** The woman is scanned by ultrasound to locate the placenta and determine the position of the fetus. A needle is inserted through the skin, fascia, and uterine wall, away from the placenta and body of the fetus. When the needle is within the uterine cavity, amniotic fluid is withdrawn.

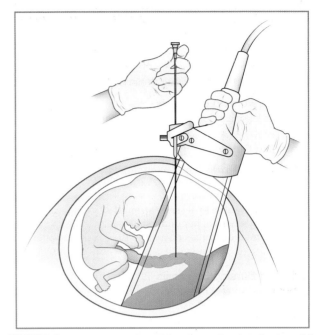

FIGURE 5-6 **Fetoscopy and cord blood sampling (cordocentesis).** A fine-gauge fiberoptic scope is passed into the amniotic sac under ultrasound direction, and cord blood is aspirated from umbilical vessels.

strengthen muscles while minimizing the risk of joint and ligament injuries. Fatigue and elevated temperatures should be avoided.

Mild to moderate exercise is known to be beneficial during normal pregnancy. The nurse should provide guidance, based on the understanding that the maternal circulatory system is the lifeline to the fetus and that any alteration can affect growth and survival of the fetus. The maternal cardiac status and fetoplacental reserve should determine the exercise levels during all trimesters of pregnancy. Current health and fitness lifestyles mandate the inclusion of information concerning exercise during pregnancy in prenatal education programs.

A history of the exercise practices of the woman is important, and gathering such information is the first step in the nursing process. Active women may have a higher tolerance for exercise than women who have a sedentary lifestyle. The goal of exercise during pregnancy should be the maintenance of fitness, not improvement of fitness or weight loss. The type of exercise is also important. The woman should not lie supine, twist, bounce, or make jerky movements during exercise (Box 5-3 on p. 76).

Specific exercises that are helpful during pregnancy include the pelvic tilt exercise, which involves alternately arching and straightening the back while on the hands and knees or while standing against a wall (Figure 5-8 on p. 77), squatting, and Kegel exercises to strengthen pelvic muscles. Kegel exercises involve the voluntary contraction and relaxation of the

(Text continued on p. 76)

hot tubs or saunas should be avoided because they increase body temperature, which may lead to fetal compromise. Tub baths are contraindicated when the amniotic membranes have ruptured or the mucous plug has been expelled. Can cause the fetus to become hypoxic > can affect major organs

PHYSICAL ACTIVITY AND EXERCISE DURING PREGNANCY

Pregnant women may benefit both psychologically and physically from retaining some portion of their prepregnancy fitness. The goal of exercising is to

Scenario

A multigravida (P2, G5) is 37 years old. The woman is approaching her twenty-fourth week of gestation. She has cut down on smoking. This pregnancy is unplanned, and financial status is unstable. She relates that her appetite has been poor when asked questions about her small amount of weight gain for the past 2 months. The certified nurse-midwife notes that fetal growth is delayed according to her estimated date of birth.

Selected Nursing Diagnosis

Deficient knowledge of conditions and equipment used

Expected Outcomes	Nursing Interventions	Rationales
Patient will verbalize understanding of procedure.	Explain nature of test being performed, whether invasive or noninvasive, and what she may experience.	Informing woman helps relieve anxiety and concern for fetal well being.
Patient will be able to describe strengths and weaknesses of her understanding of potential outcomes of tests.	Review data to be obtained. This may be information about fetal growth, placental location, or number of fetuses.	Honest and open discussion promotes better understanding and trust. It satisfies need for recognition of value of data to be obtained.

Selected Nursing Diagnosis

Fear related to the unknown

Expected Outcomes	Nursing Interventions	Rationales
Patient will respond that all questions have been satisfactorily answered and will be able to discuss correctly.	Listen to woman's concerns about the test(s) that have been scheduled.	Helps woman develop realistic view of situation.
Patient will state her understanding of what she is to do and will cooperate throughout the procedure.	Instruct the woman in specific terms regarding what she will be required to do if she must participate in obtaining any data.	Avoids fear of the unknown.
Patient will demonstrate bonding with nurse and confidence by responding positively to instructions.	Encourage verbalization; offer appropriate reassurance.	May reveal other concerns not yet addressed.

Selected Nursing Diagnosis

Pain related to invasive procedures

Expected Outcomes	Nursing Interventions	Rationales
Patient will maintain and verbalize comfort throughout the procedure(s).	Offer clear, simple, short explanations.	Provides opportunity for open communication at all times.
	Give her directions on slow, deep breathing in a calm, soothing manner.	Maintains a calm and confident, caring environment.
	Attempt to keep woman as comfortable and dry as possible.	Comfort increases compliance.

Selected Nursing Diagnosis

Anxiety related to external monitor used for nonstress test or contraction stress test of fetal heart rate

Expected Outcomes	Nursing Interventions	Rationales
Patient will state her understanding of what she is to do and will cooperate throughout the procedure.	Explain how and why electronic monitoring is used and what to expect.	Women and families sometimes express dissatisfaction with noise, beeps, and sounds of monitor and even concern that the monitor is a substitute for nursing care.
	Assure woman that someone will be with her or nearby continuously.	Reassures help is at hand.

Additional Nursing Diagnosis

Anxiety related to pregnancy and its outcome; *ineffective health maintenance* related to lack of material resources

Critical Thinking Questions

1. A woman in her twenty-fourth week of pregnancy states she is feeling fine and asks whether an ultrasound needs to be done. She states she does not want any invasive procedures done to her. How would you respond?
2. What are some nursing responsibilities in the care of a woman receiving an amnioinfusion after labor starts?

Table 5-3   Self-Care for Common Discomforts of Pregnancy

DISCOMFORT	INFLUENCING FACTORS	SELF-CARE MEASURES
First Trimester		
Nausea with or without vomiting	Elevation in hormones, decrease in gastric motility, fatigue, emotional factors; usually does not last beyond 16 weeks if vomiting persists, may lead to hyperemesis gravidarum	Avoid an empty stomach. Eat dry crackers or toast ½ to 1 hour before rising in the morning. Eat small, frequent meals. Drink fluids between meals. Avoid greasy, odorous, spicy, or gas-forming foods. Increase vitamin B_6.
Breast tenderness	Increased vascular supply and hypertrophy of breast tissue caused by estrogen and progesterone Results in tingling, fullness, and tenderness	Wear a supportive bra (to alleviate tingling and tenderness). Avoid soap to the nipples (to prevent cracking).
Urinary frequency	Pressure of growing uterus on bladder in both first and third trimesters Progesterone relaxes smooth muscles of bladder	Void when urge is felt (to prevent urinary stasis); increase fluid intake during day. Decrease fluid in late evening to lessen nocturia; limit caffeine. Practice Kegel exercises.
Vaginal discharge (leukorrhea)	Increased production of mucus by endocervical glands in response to elevated estrogen levels and increased blood supply to the pelvic area, causing white, viscid vaginal discharge	Bathe or shower daily. Wear cotton underwear. Avoid tight undergarments and pantyhose. Keep the perineal area clean and dry. Avoid douching and using tampons. Wipe the perineal area from front to back after toileting. Contact health care provider if there is a change in color, odor, or character of discharge.
Second and Third Trimesters		
Heartburn (pyrosis)	Increased production of progesterone causing relaxation of esophageal sphincter Regurgitation or backflow of gastric contents into the esophagus causing burning sensation behind the sternum, burping, and sour tastes in mouth	Sit up for 30 minutes after eating a meal. Avoid gas-forming and greasy foods. Avoid overeating. Use low-sodium liquid antacids such as Gelusil or Maalox (liquid will coat lining better than tablets); avoid sodium bicarbonate and Alka Seltzer.
Constipation and flatulence (gas)	Increased levels of progesterone causing bowel sluggishness, with increased water absorption (results in hardened stool) Pressure of enlarging uterus on intestine Diet, lack of exercise, and decreased fluids Iron supplements contributing to hardening of stools	Increase fluid intake (a minimum of 8 glasses per day, not including carbonated or caffeinated beverages because of their diuretic effect), roughage in diet, and exercise. Exercise to stimulate peristalsis. Establish regular schedule for bowel movement. Do not take mineral oil or enemas. Consult health care provider about taking a stool softener (docusate).
Hemorrhoids	Varicosities (distended veins) of rectum caused by vascular enlargement of pelvis, straining from constipation, and descent of fetal head into pelvis May disappear after birth, when pressure is relieved	Use anesthetic ointment, cool witch hazel pads, or rectal suppositories. May disappear after birth, when pressure is relieved Take sitz baths, increase fiber in diet, and have regular bowel habits to avoid constipation.
Backaches	Result of the spine's adaptation to posture changes as the uterus enlarges Enlarging uterus altering center of gravity, resulting in lordosis (exaggeration of lumbosacral curve) and muscle strain	Maintain correct posture with head up and shoulders back; use good body mechanics. Avoid exaggerating lumbar curve. Squat rather than bending over when picking up objects (bend at knees, not waist). Wear low-heeled shoes to help maintain better posture. Do exercises such as tailor sitting (cross-legged), shoulder circling, and pelvic rocking. Rest; applying localized heat may help.

Continued

Table 5-3	Self-Care for Common Discomforts of Pregnancy—cont'd	
DISCOMFORT	**INFLUENCING FACTORS**	**SELF-CARE MEASURES**
Round ligament pain	Abdominal ligaments stretched by enlarging uterus, causing pain in lower abdomen after sudden movements	Avoid jerky or quick movements. Use pillow support for abdomen. Use good body mechanics.
Leg cramps	Pressure of uterus on blood vessels that impairs circulation to legs, causing muscle strain and fatigue Imbalance in the calcium/phosphorus ratio	Dorsiflex foot and straighten leg with downward pressure on knee or stand with feet flat on floor when cramps occur (see Figure 5-7). Evaluate diet and calcium intake.
Headache	Emotional tension and fatigue Increased circulatory blood volume and heart rate causing dilation and distention of cerebral vessels	Obtain emotional support. Practice relaxation exercises. Eat regular meals. If headaches continue, report to caregiver (potential gestational hypertension).
Varicose veins	Relaxation of smooth muscle in walls of veins caused by elevated progesterone Pressure of enlarging uterus causing pressure on veins, resulting in development of varicosities in vulva, rectum, and legs	Avoid lengthy standing or sitting, constrictive clothing, and bearing down during bowel movements. Walk frequently. Rest with legs elevated. Wear support stockings; avoid tight knee-highs. Exercise (to stimulate venous return). Relieve hemorrhoid swelling with warm sitz baths, local application of astringent compresses, or analgesic ointment.
Edema of feet and ankles	Circulatory congestion of lower extremities	Elevate legs when sitting. Increase rest periods. Avoid constrictive clothing and prolonged standing or sitting.
Faintness and dizziness	Vasomotor instability or postural hypotension Standing for long periods with venous stasis in lower extremities	Avoid sudden changes in position, prolonged standing, and warm crowded areas. Move slowly from rest position. Avoid hypoglycemia by eating 4-5 small meals daily. Lie on left side when resting to avoid supine hypotensive syndrome (pressure of uterus on vena cava). If symptoms do not lessen, report to caregiver.
Fatigue	Hormonal changes in early pregnancy and periodic hypoglycemia as glucose is used by embryo for rapid growth More prominent in early months of pregnancy	Try to get 8-10 hours of sleep. Take naps during the day if possible. Use relaxation techniques, meditation, or change of scenery.
Dyspnea	Later in pregnancy, caused by uterus rising into abdomen and pressing on diaphragm	Sleep with several pillows under head. Use deep chest breathing before going to sleep. Use proper posture while sitting or standing. Avoid exertion.

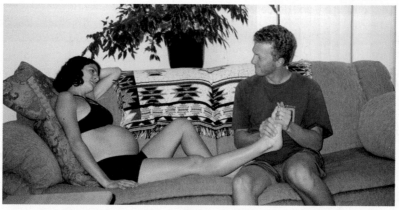

FIGURE 5-7 Relieving a leg cramp in pregnancy. Extend the affected leg, keeping knee straight, and dorsiflex the foot (point toes toward head). Foot massage also aids in relaxation and is an effective technique for pain relief during labor.

Nursing Care Plan 5-2   Prenatal Care Plan

Scenario

A 21-year-old woman comes to the clinic for her first prenatal visit. She is pregnant for the first time and states she is very tired and feels it may be caused by her poor dietary habits. She wants to know "all there is to know" about having a healthy pregnancy. She asks the nurse for advice.

Selected Nursing Diagnosis

Deficient knowledge related to lack of education or experience

Expected Outcomes	Nursing Interventions	Rationales
Patient will be able to describe activities she can engage in that will promote wellness of self and fetus.	Assess current level of understanding, questions, and concerns.	Provides baseline information needed to assist in forming an individualized teaching plan Provides insight regarding any misconceptions the patient may have that need correcting
	Develop rapport with patient, and create pleasant learning environment.	To decrease patient anxiety level; high anxiety impedes learning. When adequate rapport has been established between nurse and patient, the patient usually feels more at ease to ask questions or share concerns.
	Teach support person along with patient.	The support person can reinforce information learned during the teaching sessions and can encourage patient to consistently put into practice what is learned. In some cultures, it is essential to include the father in teaching sessions; he may dictate decisions of what will or will not be done.
	Explain the importance of prenatal care and keeping all appointments.	Increased knowledge is often correlated with an increased level of compliance. Some cultures do not view prenatal care as important, so patients need to understand why they should attend prenatal visits.
	Teach about normal physiologic changes that occur during pregnancy (fatigue, average weight gain expected, gastrointestinal changes, urinary frequency, onset of quickening, etc.).	Anticipatory guidance of what to expect alleviates anxieties and fears from misconceptions that changes are abnormal.
	Explain how to alleviate common discomforts of pregnancy associated with normal physiologic changes.	Improves comfort level
Patient's actions will indicate an understanding of what is needed to promote wellness of self and fetus.	Explain self-care needs (exercise, nutrition, rest, etc.) and ways to best meet these needs.	Provides information needed regarding health-promoting behaviors that will help optimize pregnancy outcomes
	Explain activities that are contraindicated during pregnancy (smoking, hot tubs, alcohol consumption, use of street drugs or over-the-counter medications, x-ray examinations, changing litter boxes, eating raw meat, etc.).	These activities can compromise fetal development and well-being.
Patient will be able to state at least five danger signs to report to health care provider.	Teach danger signs of pregnancy to report immediately to health care provider (decreased fetal movement, vaginal bleeding, dysuria, edema of face and hands, blurred vision, frequent headaches, bag of waters rupture, etc.).	Ensures prompt interventions when complications occur.
	Provide patient with handouts, videos, and diagrams in a language the woman can read and understand.	To reinforce verbal teaching and to provide information that the patient can refer to at a later time

Continued

Expected Outcomes	Nursing Interventions	Rationales
	Inform patient of pregnancy-related classes that are available.	A variety of childbirth classes may be available to enhance the patient's learning (prenatal classes, sibling classes, childbirth classes, etc.). Classes also provide the opportunity for patients to interact with other pregnant women who can validate each other's experiences and support one another.
Patient will state that her questions have been answered satisfactorily.	Encourage patient to call whenever she has questions or concerns.	Providing permission to call will increase likelihood that patient will use this opportunity for increased learning and to have her concerns addressed.

Selected Nursing Diagnosis

Imbalanced nutrition, less than body requirements related to nausea, vomiting; knowledge deficit related to nutritional needs during pregnancy

Expected Outcomes	Nursing Interventions	Rationales
Intake of nutrition will be adequate to meet maternal metabolic needs and to support normal fetal growth and development as evidenced by:	Determine weight at each prenatal visit.	Maternal weight gain during pregnancy should average 1.4-1.6 kg during the first trimester and 0.44 kg/weeks during the last two trimesters.
Maternal weight gain of 1.6 kg (3½ lbs) during first trimester and 0.44 kg (1 lb) per week until delivery. A lack of excessive nausea and vomiting	Determine degree of nausea and vomiting.	Nausea and vomiting, which commonly occur during the first trimester as a result of hormonal changes that decrease gastric mobility, can, if excessive, interfere with adequate nutritional intake.
Ensures adequate intake of essential nutrients	If patient is experiencing nausea and vomiting, instruct her to eat dry crackers or toast ½ hour before getting out of bed in the mornings, eat small frequent meals, drink noncaffeinated carbonated beverages, and increase intake of vitamin B$_6$.	These practices decrease nausea and vomiting because they prevent the stomach from becoming empty or distended and decrease gastric acidity.
	If patient has nausea and vomiting, instruct her to avoid beverages with meals; vitamins containing iron in the first trimester; and foods that are spicy, greasy, or have noxious odors.	Food that are spicy, greasy, or have noxious odors can increase episodes of nausea and vomiting. Iron supplements taken during the first trimester and ingestion of beverages with meals have both been associated with a higher incidence of nausea and vomiting.
	Teach patient to report excessive nausea and vomiting to health care provider.	Allows for early intervention of alternative forms of nutritional delivery if an oral diet cannot be tolerated.
24-hour dietary recall reflecting a balanced nutritional diet	Review 24-hour dietary intake and ask if this is typical of the normal diet.	Provide baseline information of patient's nutritional habits and provides insight regarding areas of deficiencies that need to be addressed.
	Determine current knowledge of nutritional needs during pregnancy.	Provides information needed to develop an individualized teaching plan. During pregnancy increased nutrients are required to meet the increased maternal metabolic rate and the needs of the developing fetus.
	Use a food guide to teach patient to eat a nutritional diet; provide her with a copy of the guide or the Internet address.	Food guides are easy-to-use visual references for what a healthy diet should consist of that can be adapted to accommodate cultural preferences.

Nursing Care Plan 5-2   Prenatal Care Plan—cont'd

Expected Outcomes	Nursing Interventions	Rationales
	Refer to dietitian as needed.	Patients with specific chronic illnesses or special nutritional needs may require additional nutritional counseling and support.
Hemoglobin ≥12 g/dL and hematocrit ≥37%	Review hemoglobin and hematocrit laboratory values.	Hemoglobin <12 g/dL or hematocrit <37% is indicative of iron deficiency anemia.
	Teach patient the importance of taking prenatal vitamins, iron supplements during the last two trimesters, and folic acid supplements as prescribed.	Prevents vitamin deficiencies, iron deficiency anemia, and neurotubular defects that have been associated with folic acid deficiencies
Fundal height reaching 28 cm by 28 weeks and then increasing 1 cm/week until delivery	Determine fundal height at each prenatal visit.	Measures fetal growth pattern. Fundal height averages 28 cm at 28 weeks and then increases approximately 1 cm/week.
Access to adequate nutrition	Discuss socioeconomic factors that can interfere with adequate nutrition.	If finances prohibit the purchase of foods necessary for a nutritional diet, referrals to community agencies may be required.
	Refer to community agencies and WIC program as needed.	Local organizations may be available to supply food to low-income families. WIC is a federally funded food program that supplies low-income women with both food vouchers and nutritional education.

Selected Nursing Diagnosis
Fatigue related to effects of physiologic changes of pregnancy

Expected Outcomes	Nursing Interventions	Rationales
Patient will state she has sufficient energy to carry out required activities of daily living.	Explain to patient physiologic changes responsible for increased feelings of fatigue during pregnancy.	Information provides knowledge that can motivate an individual to make lifestyle changes that will enhance energy level by promoting adequate rest.
	Assist patient in developing a plan to increase amount of rest and sleep (napping when children nap or during work lunch break, going to bed earlier, adjusting work schedules, etc.).	Mutually deciding on a plan increases the likelihood that the patient will follow through with the actions needed to successfully implement the plan.
	Instruct patient on ways to decrease insomnia (avoid drinking beverages with caffeine or exercising during the evening; promote relaxation with music, a warm bath, imagery, reading, etc.).	Caffeine and exercise late at night can act as stimulants to the body. Relaxation techniques before bed can eliminate stress that is inhibiting sleep.
	Instruct patient to limit fluid intake during the evening.	Prevents frequent awakenings from nocturia
	Instruct patient to position self in bed for maximum comfort (using pillows for support while side-lying or in a semi-Fowler's position).	Comfort promotes rest. As pregnancy progresses, it is important to avoid lying supine to prevent supine hypotensive syndrome. As the uterus enlarges upward, pressure is exerted against the diaphragm, which can make breathing more difficult; an upright position can alleviate dyspnea.
	Assist patient in eliminating nonessential tasks from her schedule.	Prevents fatigue from excessive demands and allows time for additional rest periods.

Critical Thinking Questions
1. A patient discovers she is pregnant for the first time. She is determined to give her baby the best environment possible in which to develop and asks you what she should avoid. What should you discuss with her?
2. A patient complains of feeling nauseated in the mornings with occasional episodes of vomiting. What teaching can you provide?

WIC, Women, Infants, and Children program.

@ Risk for falls r/t to unbalance

fetus can become hypoxic →

pubococcygeal muscles, as if starting and stopping urine flow (Box 5-4). Exercise can elevate the maternal temperature and result in decreased fetal circulation and cardiac function. Maternal body temperature should not exceed 38° C (100.4° F), thereby ruling out hot tub and sauna use during pregnancy.

When the supine position is assumed and the uterus presses on the vena cava, the increasing uterine weight and size can cause poor venous return and result in **supine hypotensive syndrome**. Orthostatic hypotension can occur and reduce the blood flow to the fetus. Certain positions need to be modified during pregnancy to avoid these problems, which can cause fetal hypoxia.

Pregnancy increases the workload of the heart. The increase in peripheral venous pooling during pregnancy results in a decrease in cardiac output reserves for exercise. When exercise is allowed to exceed the ability of the cardiovascular system to respond, blood may be diverted from the uterus, causing fetal hypoxia. Exercise increases catecholamine levels, which the placenta may not be able to filter, resulting in fetal bradycardia and hypoxia. Strenuous and prolonged exercise will cause blood flow to be distributed to the skeletal muscles and skin and away from the viscera and uterus. If the reduction in uterine blood flow exceeds 50%, serious adverse effects to the fetus may

occur. For this reason, moderate exercise is preferred for pregnant women over strenuous or prolonged exercise. Exercise does increase maternal hematocrit levels, and uterine oxygen uptake increases during exercise, so moderate exercise will not cause decreased supplies to the fetus.

Joint instability related to hormonal changes can result in injury if the woman engages in deep flexion or extension of joints. Range of motion (ROM) should not be extended beyond prepregnancy abilities.

Safety measures should be used because of the changes in the body's center of gravity as the uterus enlarges. Liquid and caloric intake should be adjusted to meet the needs of pregnancy and the demands of exercise. Women who have complications or conditions, such as hypertension or multiple gestations, should consult a health care provider before engaging in any exercise program during pregnancy.

Prenatal Yoga

Yoga is an exercise that includes mental centering (meditation), physical stretching (posing), and breath awareness and control. It is a popular labor preparation experience for women with minimal obstetric and medical complications. Bikram (hot) yoga is not recommended for pregnant women and Ashtanga yoga (vigorous) may be too strenuous for the novice (Kinser, 2008). The American College of Obstetricians and Gynecologists (ACOG) provides guidelines for exercise during pregnancy that can be beneficial to most pregnant women as preparation for labor as well as psychological well-being (ACOG, 2003).

SEXUAL ACTIVITY DURING PREGNANCY

In a healthy pregnancy, there is no valid reason to limit sexual activity. The woman should be advised that pregnancy may cause changes in comfort and desire. Some women experience heightened sexual tension during pregnancy, which is partly caused by greater blood congestion of the pelvis. Sexual intercourse should not be engaged in after the "bag of waters" (the membranes containing the amniotic fluid that surrounds the fetus) ruptures or after labor begins.

The couple may consider alternative positions, such as side-by-side or female-superior positions, if this increases the woman's comfort. The woman should communicate with her partner about physical changes, including discomfort, decreased mobility, increased urinary frequency, leg cramps, fatigue, and sexual desire. Increased uterine activity is often noted after sexual intercourse; this may be from breast stimulation, female orgasm, and prostaglandin in male ejaculate.

— women should not lie on her back

Eats up the mucous plug

Box 5-3	Exercise During Pregnancy

- Consult the health care provider before starting an exercise program.
- The goal of the exercise program should be maintenance of fitness rather than improvement of fitness.
- Concentrate on non-weight-bearing exercise, such as swimming or cycling.
- Decrease high-impact activities as the third trimester approaches.
- Avoid activities that require balance and coordination.
- Avoid activities that involve holding the breath (Valsalva's maneuver).
- Avoid excessive intensity and sweating during exercise. Inability to complete a sentence in one breath indicates shortness of breath.
- Do not exercise in the supine position after the first trimester.
- Do not use hot tubs or saunas that raise the body temperature above 38° C (100.4° F).
- Prepare joints by warming up before exercise.
- Wear a supportive bra and appropriate shoes. Be aware of changes in the center of gravity.
- Heart rate should not exceed 140 beats/minute.
- Prevent dehydration by drinking fluids liberally before, during, and after exercise.
- Avoid becoming overly warm.
- Recognize warning signs that indicate the need to stop exercise.
- Avoid scuba diving or exercising above 5000 feet in altitude.

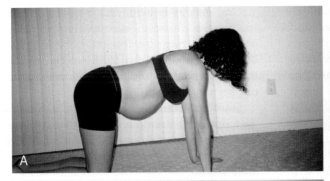
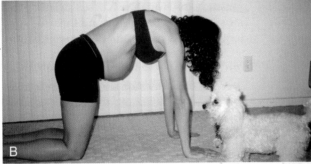
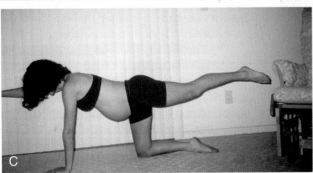
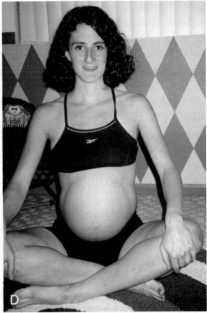
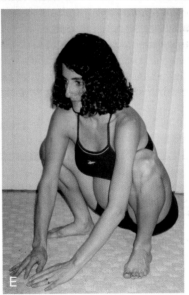

FIGURE 5-8 **Exercises during pregnancy. A** and **B,** The pelvic tilt. **C,** Proper stretch position. **D,** Tailor sitting. **E,** Proper squat position.

DOUCHING → alters normal flora

Although normal vaginal secretions are intensified during pregnancy, the pregnant woman should not douche unless prescribed by a health care provider. Douching changes the vaginal pH and alters the normal vaginal flora, which has a protective effect against pathogenic organisms. If a douche is ordered by the health care provider, specific instructions will be given to keep the douche bag no more than 15 cm (6 inches) above the level of the vagina while douching so that the water pressure is kept low.

CLOTHING

Clothing in pregnancy is generally an important factor influencing the woman's feelings about herself and her appearance in public. Clothing should be adjustable,

Box 5-4	Exercises for Muscle Strengthening and Relaxation

Pelvic tilt: Seated with knees bent and arms in back for support, the woman arches the lower back then relaxes to the neutral position. This exercise strengthens back and abdominal muscles. The exercise can also be done on hands and knees as shown.

Tailor sitting: The woman sits cross-legged on the floor to strengthen thigh and pelvic muscles.

Kegel exercises (perineal muscle tightening): The woman contracts the pubococcygeal muscles, which surround the vagina and urinary meatus. This perineal exercise strengthens muscle tone and increases elasticity.

Relaxation: The woman relaxes body muscle groups, starting from head to toe. She relaxes all parts of the body, including face and hands.

loose, washable, and lightweight. For greatest comfort, maternity dresses should hang from the shoulders and allow for the enlargement of the abdomen.

The woman should avoid wearing such articles as knee-high or thigh-high stockings, tight garters, or panty girdles because they can interfere with the blood circulation of the legs. When constriction of the blood vessels in the legs occurs, edema and varicose veins may develop.

As pregnancy progresses, the woman's center of gravity moves forward, and she will have a greater tendency to fall. Thus, it is best for her not to wear high-heeled shoes. Also, high-heeled shoes aggravate back discomfort by increasing the curvature of the lower back. Low-heeled shoes improve balance and alleviate back pain.

BREAST AND NIPPLE CARE No soap!

During pregnancy, the breasts increase one or two cup sizes. The pregnant woman should wear a supportive bra to prevent the breakdown of elastic tissue within the breasts. If the woman plans to breastfeed her baby, the use of nursing bras should be encouraged.

During bathing, no soap should be applied to the nipple area of the breasts because it has a drying effect and removes the natural oils provided by Montgomery's glands.

Women should be advised that their breasts will secrete a substance called **colostrum**, a yellow fluid, before or during the last trimester. If colostrum secretion is profuse, she may need to place pads inside her bra to maintain dryness; otherwise, constant moisture next to the breast tissue may cause nipple excoriation. Nipple cups, designed for correcting inverted nipples, may be recommended during the last 2 months of pregnancy. The woman also needs to know that the size of her breasts has nothing to do with sufficient production of milk for the baby.

DENTAL CARE

Pregnant women can continue routine dental care, but radiologic procedures should be delayed until the completion of pregnancy. It is advisable to have cavities filled and infected teeth treated. Using a soft toothbrush will lessen bleeding from the gums, which increase in vascularity during pregnancy.

Pregnancy affects oral tissues. Estrogen levels cause gum hyperplasia and can predispose the woman to gingivitis, which is evidenced by inflamed and sensitive gums. Dry mouth (xerostomia) or excessive saliva production (ptyalism) may occur during pregnancy. Esophageal reflux or vomiting during pregnancy can erode tooth enamel. Women with periodontal disease are at increased risk for preterm or low-birth-weight newborns. Increased levels of prostaglandin (PGE_2) are associated with the inflammatory process of periodontal disease and also with the onset of labor.

Oral health is achieved by brushing with a soft toothbrush, flossing, adequately controlling plaque, obtaining regular professional check-ups, and maintaining adequate nutrition. Elective professional dental care is recommended during the second trimester of pregnancy.

Fetal tooth development begins in the sixth week of gestation for primary teeth and in the tenth week of gestation for permanent teeth. Taking prenatal vitamins and fluoride and consuming foods rich in vitamins A, C, and D and calcium, phosphorus, and protein during pregnancy is essential. Nurses should provide instructions concerning oral care and the need for professional dental prophylaxis and adequate nutrition.

IMMUNIZATIONS DURING PREGNANCY

The pregnant woman needs to know that immunizations with some attenuated live viruses should not be administered during pregnancy because of the possibility of a teratogenic effect (potential for fetal damage) of the live viruses on the developing embryo or fetus. The woman should be encouraged to notify health care providers that she may be pregnant before any immunization is administered.

The benefits of vaccination in pregnant women may outweigh the risks when the likelihood of disease exposure is high and infection would pose a risk to the mother or the fetus. Pregnant women who have not received a tetanus-diphtheria (Td) vaccination in the past 10 years can receive a booster. Women who have not received the Td vaccine series can start the process in the second trimester of pregnancy. The tetanus, diphtheria, and pertussis (Tdap) vaccine may be given after delivery (Centers for Disease Control and Prevention [CDC], 2006). During the influenza season, the influenza vaccine can be given to pregnant mothers in their second or third trimester. In high-risk situations, vaccines for yellow fever and anthrax can be given to pregnant women after the first trimester (CDC, 2007). Because a hepatitis B virus (HBV) infection in the pregnant woman can result in severe disease for both mother and newborn, women at high risk for HBV infection can be vaccinated during pregnancy; the vaccine contains noninfectious hepatitis B surface antigen (HBsAg) particles and should cause no risk to the developing fetus. A known allergy to yeast is a contraindication to the HBV vaccine in the United States (CDC, 2005).

Pregnancy is a contraindication for pneumococcal; hepatitis A; polio (oral [OPV] and inactivated [IPV]); measles, mumps, rubella (MMR); and varicella vaccines. Women should be counseled not to become pregnant for at least 28 days after an MMR or varicella vaccine has been administered. Women who are susceptible to rubella should be vaccinated immediately after delivery. No known risk exists for passive immunization of pregnant women with immune globulin preparations (CDC, 2005).

Congenital defects if mom have mmr

EMPLOYMENT DURING PREGNANCY

In 1978, Congress passed the Pregnancy Discrimination Act, and an amendment in Title VII of the Civil Rights Act of 1964 requires employers to treat pregnancy-related disabilities the same as other disabilities. A federally mandated 12-week unpaid leave of absence is available for the birth or adoption of a child under the Family Medical Leave Act (FMLA). Flexibility options for work also include telecommuting, part-time, flexible hours, or light duty.

Healthy pregnant women may work until their delivery date if the job has safeguards, such as frequent rest periods and no heavy lifting is required. Strenuous physical exercise, the need to maintain body balance or stand for a prolonged period, work on industrial machines, and other adverse environmental factors should be modified as necessary. Women in sedentary jobs should not sit or stand in one position for long periods. Movement is necessary to counter the sluggish circulation that encourages the development of varicosities and thrombophlebitis.

Some occupations are more hazardous because they bring women into contact with harmful substances. These occupations include those that involve working at refineries, research laboratories, sites where chemical fumes are present, and radiation sites. Pregnant nurses may be exposed to waste anesthetic gases in the OR or anesthetic gases expired by patients in the PACU. Exposure to radiation while assisting with portable x-rays also presents an occupational hazard to pregnant nurses (Alex, 2011).

TRAVEL DURING PREGNANCY

Many women choose to maintain a normal lifestyle and travel during pregnancy. Pregnant women should be advised against prolonged sitting during travel. Because of the increased levels of clotting factors and plasma fibrinogen that normally occurs during pregnancy, there is an increased risk of developing thromboembolism with prolonged sitting (Steffen, Dupont, & Wilder-Smith, 2007). The recommendation is a maximum of 6 hours a day driving, with stops made at least every 2 hours for 10 minutes to allow the woman to walk around. Walking will increase venous return from her legs. Although pregnant women should wear seatbelts like everyone else, they should adjust the lap belt so that it fits under the abdomen and across the pelvic bones (Figure 5-9). Traveling by plane shortens traveling time and is not contraindicated as long as the plane has a well-pressurized cabin and sitting time is not prolonged.

Late in pregnancy, the possibility of early labor should be considered when traveling. The woman should be advised to ask her health care provider for a copy of her prenatal records to have, in case of an unexpected complication. Guidance concerning hand hygiene and dietary precautions to prevent diarrhea are essential. If needed, special oral rehydration solutions may be available, or bottled drinks may provide the fluid, sugar, and electrolytes needed. An oral rehydration formula recommended by the World Health Organization (WHO) is to combine 1 L of water that contains 1 teaspoon of salt, 4 teaspoons of cream of tartar, ½ teaspoon of baking soda, and 4 tablespoons of sugar (Caroll, 2005). The woman should be advised to wear comfortable shoes and long-sleeved clothing and use mosquito nets around the bed in insect-prone areas. Insect repellants with DEET are usually safe after the first trimester. Sunblock should be applied as appropriate.

EFFECT OF PREGNANCY ON MEDICATION METABOLISM

The normal physiologic changes that occur during pregnancy affect the metabolism of medications administered to the mother. Subtherapeutic levels may occur because of the increase in plasma volume, cardiac output, and glomerular filtration rate that occurs during pregnancy. Decreased gastric emptying time during pregnancy changes the absorption time of oral drugs and can delay onset of action. The increased levels of estrogen and progesterone may alter hepatic (liver) function resulting in drug accumulation in the body. Drugs can cross the placenta and have an impact on fetal development. Taking ibuprofen during the third trimester can cause an early closure of the ductus arteriosus, resulting in fetal distress. Drugs can pass into the breast milk after delivery and be ingested by the nursing newborn. The woman must be cautioned against taking *any medication* during pregnancy and lactation without first consulting her health care provider.

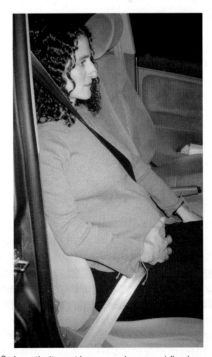

FIGURE 5-9 A seatbelt must be worn whenever riding in an automobile. The lap portion of the belt should be placed low, just below the protruding abdomen. The shoulder belt should be placed above the uterus in pregnancy.

The FDA has established risk categories for medication use during pregnancy, and it is published in all drug reference books (see Box 4-3). The nurse should carefully review the safety classification of any drug—prescription or over-the-counter (OTC)—administered to a pregnant woman. Maternal drug exposure is related to the occurrence of birth defects. More than 80% of pregnant women use OTC or prescription medication during pregnancy and may not realize the potential dangers involved. The woman should be informed about the effects of substance abuse on the developing fetus (see Chapter 16).

! Medication Safety Alert

OTC Medications

The pregnant woman should be advised not to take any OTC medication without first consulting her health care provider.

DANGER SIGNS

The pregnant woman should be taught the danger signs that must be reported to the nurse-midwife or physician. Each woman should be given written information listing the important signs, written at a level and in a language that she can read. She should have specific directions and telephone numbers so that she can obtain assistance immediately.

! Safety Alert

Danger Signs During Pregnancy

- Headaches, visual disturbance, or dizziness
- Increase in systolic blood pressure of 30 mm Hg or greater
- Increase in diastolic blood pressure of 15 mm Hg or greater or blood pressure greater than 140/80 mm Hg
- Epigastric, abdominal, or severe flank pain → Pilo
- Burning during urination or severe backache
- Abnormal fatigue and nervousness
- Anginal pain and shortness of breath noted with activity
- Muscular irritability, confusion, or seizures   eclampsia
- Vaginal bleeding or fluid leaking from the vagina
- Decrease in fetal movement (decreased kick count)
- Fever greater than 38° C (100.4° F)

WEIGHT GAIN AND FETAL GROWTH

Adequate weight gain during pregnancy is required for maternal health and normal fetal growth and development (Table 5-4 and Figure 5-10). Mothers who are underweight or who have a small weight gain during pregnancy place their infants at a higher risk for low birth weight, prematurity, low Apgar scores, and morbidity. The accepted weight gain in pregnancy for a healthy outcome in women of normal weight is 11.5 to 16 kg (25 to 35 lbs). The recommended weight gain during the first trimester is approximately 1.3 kg (3 lbs), and after the first trimester, 0.45 kg (1 lb) per week. The weight gain during the first trimester is almost entirely growth of

maternal tissues. In the second trimester, growth is primarily maternal tissue with some fetal tissue. Growth is mainly fetal in the third trimester. Obese women face a greater risk of certain medical complications. Emphasis must be placed on the quality of food intake.

NUTRITION

The mother's nutritional status can affect the outcome of her pregnancy. Pregnancy is a time when the well-being of one (fetus) directly depends on another (mother). With this knowledge, nursing strategies to determine the nutritional health of a pregnant woman include obtaining a complete nutritional history of food habits and preferences, monitoring nutritional status, and promoting nutritional education (see Evolve for more information). Studies have shown that poor fetal growth resulting from an inadequate maternal intake of nutrients can have long-term consequences for the fetus and be the cause of certain diseases in adulthood. Allergies and cultural factors

Table 5-4	Recommended Weight Gain During Pregnancy	
Underweight women (BMI* less than 18.5)	12.5-18 kg (28-40 lbs)
Normal weight women (BMI 18.5-24.9)	11.5-16 kg (25-35 lbs)
Overweight women (BMI 25-29.9)	7-11.5 kg (15-25 lbs)
Obese women (BMI over 30)	5-9 kg (11-20 lbs)

Data from Institute of Medicine. (2009). *Weight gain during pregnancy: Re-examining the guidelines.* National Academy Press. Washington, D.C.: Author. BMI, body mass index.
*BMI is calculated by dividing weight in kilograms by height in meters squared or by dividing weight in pounds by height in inches squared multiplied by 703 (CDC, 2007a). A calculator for measuring BMI is available on Evolve.

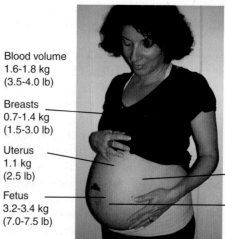

FIGURE 5-10 Weight gain in an average pregnancy.

Blood volume 1.6-1.8 kg (3.5-4.0 lb)
Breasts 0.7-1.4 kg (1.5-3.0 lb)
Uterus 1.1 kg (2.5 lb)
Fetus 3.2-3.4 kg (7.0-7.5 lb)
Maternal reserves 1.8-4.3 kg (4.0-9.5 lb)
Extravascular fluids 1.6-2.3 kg (3.5-5.0 lb)
Amniotic fluid 0.9 kg (2.0 lb)
Placenta 0.5-0.7 kg (1.0-1.5 lb)

may alter the dietary practices of some women. For example, in some cultures, milk is not a part of the traditional diet. Intake of some dark green, leafy vegetables, and tofu can provide calcium and iron.

🌐 Cultural Considerations

Common Foods Considered "Hot" or "Cold" in Some Cultures*

SOUTHEAST ASIA
Hot Foods (Yang)
Pepper
Onion
Meat, poultry, fish
Eggs
Sweets
Cold Foods (Yin)
Flour
Fruits
Cold or sour foods
HISPANIC
Hot Foods
Onions

Chili peppers
Potatoes
Cheese
Evaporated milk
Chicken, lamb
Flour tortilla
Kidney beans
Cold Foods
Fruits and vegetables
Milk
Fish
Corn tortilla
Red beans

*Some cultures classify illnesses or conditions as *hot* or *cold*. A balance is sought so that "hot" foods are preferred in conditions considered "cold," and "cold" foods are preferred for conditions considered "hot." Special care is required when counseling the woman to increase needed nutrients without deviating from the culturally required diet.

FOOD GUIDES

MyPlate (Figure 5-11) provides a quick reference for recommendations needed for a healthy diet. These guidelines were updated by the combined efforts of the U.S. Department of Health and Human Services and the U.S. Department of Agriculture (USDA) in 2011. A well-balanced, nutrient-dense diet combined with adequate physical activity is the core of the revised guidelines. Dietary guidelines, sample menus, recipes, and many other resources for consumers are available online (see Online Resources). Women who follow this guide during pregnancy can be well nourished at the time of delivery.

Different countries and cultures have their own food guides based on cultural food preferences and food availability (Figure 5-12). Universal guidelines are not effective for all populations. They should be used as guides in providing a well-balanced diet and avoiding empty calories. The guidelines can be designed to meet the individual needs of the pregnant woman.

NUTRITIONAL REQUIREMENTS DURING PREGNANCY

Good nutrition influences the outcome of pregnancy, and a determination of nutritional needs is an important part of prenatal care. Research has shown that a daily supplement of 0.4 mg folic acid *in the first weeks of pregnancy* significantly reduces neural tube defects in newborns, such as spina bifida (CDC, 2010). Foods high in folate include beans, leafy green vegetables, and whole grains.

🍎 Nutrition Considerations

Nutritional Risk Factors During Pregnancy

- Adolescence (demands of normal growth spurt added to needs of the pregnancy)
- Short interval between pregnancies because depleted nutrient stores are not replenished
- Unusual eating patterns (pica, or eating inedible and nonnutritive substances)
- Vegetarian diets with incomplete intake of the eight essential proteins
- Previous iron deficiency anemia
- Inadequate nutritional intake
- Low income
- Inadequate weight gain
- Sudden weight gain
- Weight loss
- Substance abuse (alcohol, tobacco, illicit drugs)
- Medical conditions such as diabetes or kidney dysfunction

In 2000, the FDA mandated folic acid fortification of cereal grain (but not corn mesa grain) because folic acid supplements do not help those women with unplanned pregnancies. Folic acid is needed in the first few weeks of pregnancy before many women are aware they are pregnant. In 2004, the CDC and Emory University formed the Flour Fortification Initiative (FFI) with the goal of having 80% of the world's wheat flour fortified with folic acid by the year 2015 (Berry, 2010). This will significantly reduce the occurrence of neural tube defects around the world. (The upper limit of RDI folic acid intake is 1000 μg.) The recommended calorie increase from prepregnancy needs is approximately 340 calories in the second trimester and 450 to 500 calories in the third trimester. Breastfeeding requires an increase of 500 calories from prepregnancy needs.

A fluid intake of six to eight glasses (1500 to 2000 mL) per day is recommended to maintain body temperature and prevent constipation. Although an excessive intake of caffeine-containing fluids may cause constriction of blood vessels and has been associated with fetal growth restriction, a moderate intake of caffeine (limit to 2 cups of coffee or tea) may protect against gestational diabetes (Cox, 2009).

Most women do not have iron stores to meet the demands of pregnancy (Gabbe, Niebyl, & Simpson, 2007). Because iron needs of pregnancy cannot be met by diet alone, supplementation of one 325-mg tablet of ferrous gluconate per day starting at 14 to 20 weeks' gestation is recommended. Taking iron on an empty stomach between meals increases its absorption (Gabbe et al., 2007), and eating citrus or foods high in vitamin C also aids in the absorption of iron. The ferrous form of iron is the only type readily absorbed by the intestine, and the nausea common to the first trimester usually subsides between 14 and 20 weeks' gestation. A stool softener, such as docusate sodium, may

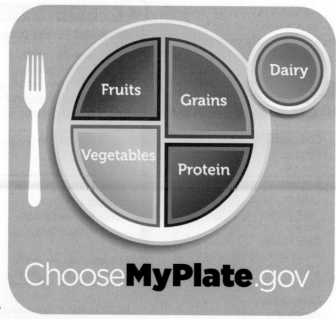

A

Food Group	1st Trimester	2nd and 3rd Trimesters	What counts as 1 cup or 1 ounce?	Remember to...
	Eat this amount from each group daily.*			
Fruits	2 cups	2 cups	1 cup fruit or juice ½ cup dried fruit	*Focus on fruits—* Eat a variety of fruits.
Vegetables	2½ cups	3 cups	1 cup raw or cooked vegetables or juice 2 cups raw leafy vegetables	*Vary your veggies—* Eat more dark-green and orange vegetables and cooked dry beans.
Grains	6 ounces	8 ounces	1 slice bread 1 ounce ready-to-eat cereal ½ cup cooked pasta, rice, or cereal	*Make half your grains whole—*Choose whole instead of refined grains.
Meat & Beans	5½ ounces	6½ ounces	1 ounce lean meat, poultry, or fish ¼ cup cooked dry beans ½ ounce nuts or 1 egg 1 tablespoon peanut butter	*Go lean with protein—* Choose low-fat or lean meats and poultry.
Milk	3 cups	3 cups	1 cup milk 8 ounces yogurt 1½ ounces cheese 2 ounces processed cheese	*Get your calcium-rich foods—*Go low-fat or fat-free when you choose milk, yogurt, and cheese.

*These amounts are for an average pregnant woman. You may need more or less than the average. Check with your doctor to make sure you are gaining weight as you should.

In each food group, choose foods that are low in "extras"—solid fats and added sugars.

Pregnant women and women who may become pregnant should not drink alcohol. Any amount of alcohol during pregnancy could cause problems for your baby.

Most doctors recommend that pregnant women take a prenatal vitamin and mineral supplement every day **in addition to** eating a healthy diet. This is so you and your baby get enough folic acid, iron, and other nutrients. But don't overdo it. Taking too much can be harmful.

B

FIGURE 5-11 A, MyPlate is a guide to healthful eating for all people. The colors represent the basic food groups in the diet, with approximate recommended amounts to consume in relation to the total diet plan. Portion size can be individualized for the consumer by accessing the site, www.choosemyplate.gov, and entering the individual's weight, gender, and activity level. The orange color represents whole grains; green represents vegetables; red represents fruit; blue represents a calcium source such as milk; and purple represents meat, poultry, eggs, and beans. **B,** The USDA provides specific recommendations for pregnant women.

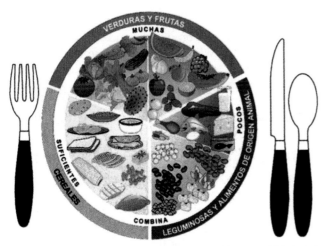

FIGURE 5-12 **Food guide plate from Mexico.** The use of foods that respect dietary limitations or restrictions may increase compliance when teaching parents and children concerning a balanced diet that promotes optimum health.

be taken to avoid constipation. Large amounts of iron and folic acid may reduce zinc absorption, and sources of zinc, such as shellfish and whole grains, should be part of the diet.

⚠ Medication Safety Alert

Iron Supplements

Iron supplements should be taken between meals or at bedtime. Milk, tea, coffee, antacids, calcium and oxalic acids in some vegetables such as spinach, and EDTA additives present in some foods can decrease the absorption of iron.

Nondairy sources of calcium, such as collard or turnip greens, juices with added calcium, and nonanimal protein sources, are available for lactose-intolerant or vegetarian women.

🍎 Nutrition Considerations

Proteins for Vegetarians

- Dry peas and beans
- Soybeans and lentils
→ Peanut butter
- Nuts and sesame seeds
- Sunflower seeds
→ Cottage cheese
- Cheese
→ Eggs

Use complementary proteins to supply all essential proteins (amino acids).

A calcium supplement may be prescribed when the imbalance of the calcium/phosphorus ratio causes leg cramps. Vitamin D supplementation may be recommended for dark-skinned women, for women who cover most of their bodies when outdoors, or for those who use sunscreen with an SPF rating of 15 or above because sunlight on the skin aids in vitamin D production. The FDA and the USDA have developed uniform food labels to inform consumers of contents of packages and

canned food. The woman should be educated to carefully read food labels, especially sodium content, to promote the intake of nutrient-dense foods.

🍎 Nutrition Considerations

Reading Labels Concerning Sodium Content

Salt free, sodium free: <5 mg
Low sodium: <35 mg
Unsalted or no added salt: No salt added during processing (but the food itself may not be salt-free)

During pregnancy and lactation, the maternal intake of docosahexaenoic acid (DHA), an omega-3 fatty acid, is essential for optimum brain development of the fetus and infant. The WHO recommends that a term infant receive 20 mg DHA per kilogram per day. Maternal sources of DHA include fatty fish, such as Atlantic and sockeye salmon, halibut, tuna, and flounder; egg yolk; red meat and poultry; canola oil; and soybean oil. Frying foods negatively alters DHA content (Colombo, Carlson, & Levine, 2004). Choline is an essential nutrient that is best obtained via foods such as chicken liver, eggs, soybeans, salmon, chicken, and cauliflower. Malabsorption syndromes and medications such as Phenytoin and barbiturates can interrupt absorption of choline and folates (Zeisel & da Costa, 2009).

Because the need for additional calories during pregnancy and lactation is less than the increased need for specific nutrients, nutrient-dense foods (foods that are high in nutrients related to the calories provided) are recommended. Nutrient-dense foods include whole grain breads, fresh fruits and vegetables, and dried peas and beans. Low-nutrient foods should be limited. Low-nutrient foods, also known as foods with "empty calories," include sweets and fats. The health care provider should be consulted before adding nutritional supplements during pregnancy because excessive amounts of some supplements can be toxic to the fetus (Box 5-5).

👥 Patient Teaching

Diet and Fetal Health

A correlation exists between maternal diet and fetal health. The nurse should guide women of childbearing age concerning the value of a well-balanced diet so that they can be in a good nutritional condition at conception and birth.

Box **5-5**   Complementary and Alternative Therapies
Supplements to avoid during pregnancy include licorice, papain, and black cohosh. Large amounts of green tea can have an antifolate action. Dietary supplements containing herbs are not recommended during pregnancy because concentrations are not monitored, and interactions can be detrimental.

FOODS TO AVOID DURING PREGNANCY

Women who are pregnant should avoid eating shark, swordfish, and king mackerel because these fish contain high levels of mercury that could be toxic to the fetus's developing nervous system. The mercury binds to the amino acids rather than to the fats and is retained after cooking. Other fish that should be limited include grouper, red snapper, trout, halibut, white albacore tuna, and marlin; they also have high levels of methyl mercury. The Environmental Protection Agency (EPA) advises pregnant women to limit fish intake to 170 g (6 oz) freshwater fish per week. Tuna, sushi, and all raw fish should be avoided during pregnancy. Eating limited amounts of salmon, trout, sardines, anchovies, and herring can provide needed DHA with minimal risk (Taylor, 2010).

Guidance from a dietitian should be sought if the woman is a strict vegetarian, is lactose intolerant, experiences pica, or has a high-risk medical condition. Large amounts of liver should be avoided, especially in the first trimester, because of high levels of preformed vitamin A (Cox, 2009). Saccharine-containing sweeteners should be avoided because it may accumulate in fetal tissue; however, other non-nutritive sweeteners are safe in moderation. Foods high in nitrites can cause fetal methemoglobinemia. Although nitrates are not harmful, some foods high in nitrates convert to nitrites and can be toxic, especially around 30 weeks' gestation (Cox, 2009).

RECOMMENDED DIETARY ALLOWANCES AND DIETARY REFERENCE INTAKES

In the United States, the Food and Nutrition Board of the Institute of Medicine (IOM) and the National Academy of Science, in cooperation with the USDA and the U.S. Department of Health and Human Services, developed recommended dietary allowances (RDA) of dietary nutrient intake required to maintain optimal health. Research has shown an increase in the use of dietary supplements, resulting in the need to describe the upper limits of intake levels to prevent toxicity. Consuming dietary supplements containing trace elements can result in toxicity if upper limits of intake are consistently exceeded. In response, a committee of the USDA Human Nutrition and Research Center published recommended dietary intakes (RDI) focusing on specific nutrients. *Dietary reference intakes (DRIs)* are an umbrella term that includes RDA and RDI.

⚠ Safety Alert

Exceeding Recommended Doses

Avoid exceeding recommended doses of vitamin and minerals because a balance is needed. For example, excess intake of vitamin C can inhibit the utilization of vitamin B_{12}.

PICA

Pica is the consumption of substances usually considered inedible and with no nutrient value, such as cornstarch, laundry starch, red clay, or ice cubes. Iron deficiency anemia is a common concern with pica. There is no evidence-based research that shows pica or food cravings reflect the body's need for the nutrient.

NUTRITION AND THE PREGNANT ADOLESCENT

The pregnant adolescent may be nutritionally at risk because of social and economic factors. The pregnant teenager has the dual demands of pregnancy and adolescence. She must consume enough nutrients for her growing fetus and for her own continued growth.

Many adolescents eat frequently during the day. They often indulge in soft drinks, tortilla chips, French fries, or fad diets. Counseling adolescents may be difficult because they often are not in charge of buying or cooking their food. Therefore, the person responsible for buying and cooking their food should be included in the counseling sessions. The adolescent should gain in the upper limit of the range recommended for normal adult women.

EDUCATION FOR CHILDBIRTH

The goals of education for childbirth are to help the expectant parents and family become knowledgeable consumers, to be active participants in maintaining health during pregnancy and birth, and to learn applicable coping strategies that empower women and their partners to decide how to best manage their pregnancy and discomforts within the limits of medical safety. Parents are informed about the numerous comfort and pain-relief strategies available to them, as well as the benefits and risks. Throughout the decision-making process, they need support for their choices. The various childbirth education programs, such as Lamaze technique (psychoprophylactic method) and Bradley technique, share these common goals. Many hospital-based childbirth education programs cover a variety of options and techniques. Several nonpharmacologic forms of pain relief can be used alone or as complements to pharmacologic interventions (see also Chapters 8 and 21).

Relaxation is one form that is taught in most childbirth preparation classes. Relaxation can keep the abdominal wall from becoming tense and allow the uterus to rise with contractions. It also can serve as a distraction technique. **Focusing** and **imagery** are another method for distraction and for keeping the sensory input of pain from reaching the cortex of the brain. **Breathing techniques** help relax the abdomen and also have a distraction value. Touch and massage provide comfort and may release endorphins.

Effleurage is a technique of gentle abdominal massage often taught in childbirth classes (see Chapter 8). Women can perform effleurage of their abdomens during contractions by using fingertip circular motions with both hands (Figure 5-13, *A*). Applying **sacral pressure** (firm pressure against the sacrum) is helpful when the woman experiences pain in her back during contractions (Figure 5-13, *B*). Other methods, discussed in Chapter 21, include hydrotherapy, biofeedback, acupuncture, transcutaneous electrical nerve stimulation, and hypnosis.

Preparing for coached childbirth emphasizes working in harmony with the body by using breath control, abdominal breathing, and general body relaxation. Breathing techniques are encouraged and are the basis for most prepared childbirth classes in the United States. Controlled breathing patterns are used to avoid losing control. Coping strategies include concentrating on a focal point, such as a favorite picture, to keep nerve pathways occupied so that they cannot respond to painful stimuli. Specific relaxation strategies (e.g., touch, imagery, music, and hydrotherapy) are used to deal with pain. The woman is taught to contract specific muscle groups while relaxing the remainder of her body. Instead of tensing during uterine contractions, the woman responds with conditioned relaxation and breathing patterns.

The basic underlying principles of most childbirth education include partner participation and support, relaxation and breathing strategies, muscle conditioning, and knowledge of choices and alternatives that can empower a laboring woman and her support person.

Early prenatal classes focus on the first and second trimesters and discuss early gestational changes, self-care during pregnancy, fetal development, nutrition, rest, posture, exercises, and relief measures for common discomforts of pregnancy (Box 5-6). Emphasis is placed on how to have a healthy pregnancy and avoid injury to the fetus. Later prenatal classes focus on changes that occur during middle pregnancy, danger signs to report, and preparation for labor and birth and include anticipatory guidance, birth choices, postpartum care, infant care and feeding, and newborn safety issues.

Patient Teaching

Packing the Labor Bag

Items the woman can take to the hospital for personal use during labor and after delivery may include:
- Lotion for massage
- Warm socks
- Personal washcloths
- Portable mini-fan
- Tennis balls for back massage
- Sugarless lollipops for dry mouth
- Lip balm
- Simple games for early labor
- CDs and CD player, iPod, or headphones
- Robe or nightgown
- Nursing bra
- Toiletries
- Clothes for mother and baby for hospital discharge

Childbirth preparation classes are available for grandparents and siblings, and most hospitals have

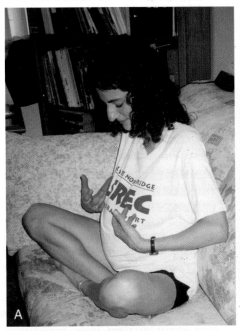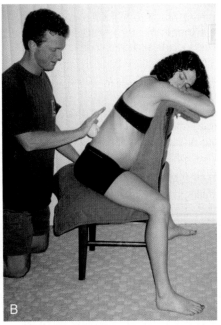

FIGURE 5-13 A, Effleurage. Slow massage of the abdomen in a circular motion using the fingertips stimulates large-diameter nerve fibers, thus interfering with transmission of pain sensations. Pressure should be firm enough to prevent a tickling sensation. **B,** Firm sacral pressure helps relieve back pain. The partner can use the palm of the hand, the knuckles, or a tennis ball to apply controlled sacral pressure. Practicing the technique during pregnancy enables effective application during labor.

Box 5-6   Types of Prenatal Classes

CHILDBIRTH PREPARATION CLASSES
- Changes of pregnancy
- Fetal development
- Prenatal care
- Hazardous substances to avoid
- Good nutrition for pregnancy
- Relieving common pregnancy discomforts
- Working during pregnancy and parenthood
- Coping with labor and delivery
- Care of the infant, such as feeding methods, choosing a pediatrician, and selecting clothing and equipment
- Early growth and development

GRANDPARENT CLASSES
- Trends in childbirth and parenting styles
- Importance of grandparents to a child's development
- Reducing conflict between the generations

EXERCISE CLASSES
- Maintaining the woman's fitness during pregnancy
- Postpartum classes for toning and fitness
- Positions and environments to avoid

BREASTFEEDING CLASSES
- Processes of breastfeeding
- Feeding techniques
- Solving common problems
- Continuation of some classes after birth with lactation specialists

GESTATIONAL DIABETES MELLITUS
- Monitoring blood glucose levels
- Diet modifications
- Need for frequent prenatal visits
- Preventing infection and complications

INFANT CARE CLASSES
- Growth, development, and care of the newborn
- Needed clothing and equipment
- Adolescent classes for birth and parenthood preparation

SIBLING CLASSES
- Helping children prepare realistically for their new brother or sister
- Helping children understand that feelings of jealousy and anger are normal
- Giving parents tips about helping older children adjust to the new baby after birth

VAGINAL BIRTH AFTER CESAREAN (VBAC) CLASSES
- What to expect during labor when previous childbirth was a cesarean section

Box 5-7   Breathing Techniques

- Breathing techniques are used during a contraction.
- Inspiration and expiration should be equal in length.
- Hyperventilation (a decrease in carbon dioxide) can occur as a result of rapid breathing. Carbon dioxide depletion can cause tingling of fingers and mouth. Dizziness may also occur. The woman should be instructed to rebreathe some carbon dioxide from cupped hands. If hyperventilation is allowed to continue, the infant can be deprived of oxygen.
- A cleansing breath, or deep breath, before each contraction helps the woman relax. If the woman inhales through her nose (rather than her mouth), she will lessen dryness of her mouth.
- "Pant-blow" breathing is rapid, shallow, or light chest breathing used in late labor.
- Expulsive breathing is modified pant-blow breathing. The woman can set a pattern by using a random number of pant breaths followed by a blow (exhalation).

Paced breathing is a method in which the woman paces herself by breathing rhythmically and, by self-regulation, is able to conserve energy. A cleansing breath should be as effortless and as deep as is comfortable. It helps the woman relax and may play a role in enhancing oxygenation. Simple measures to overcome hyperventilation include rebreathing some exhaled carbon dioxide from cupped hands or breathing normally while compressing one nostril with the index finger. Another technique is to have the woman breathe in a paper surgical mask to rebreathe some carbon dioxide. The key is to change the rapid shallow breathing to slow, deep breathing. This may be accomplished by having the woman count aloud and pace herself.

Relaxation is the foundation of all breathing patterns. The breathing rate should be comfortable for the woman. If the woman chooses to inhale through her mouth instead of her nose, she should be taught ways to protect her mucous membranes from drying out, such as sucking on crushed ice or sipping clear liquids. The overall goals of teaching breathing techniques (or paced breathing) are to (1) maintain adequate oxygenation of the mother and fetus, (2) increase physical and psychological relaxation and possibly decrease discomfort and anxiety, and (3) provide a means of focusing attention.

There is no "correct" breathing technique to prepare the woman for childbirth. The woman should be allowed to do what is most comfortable for her. If the woman has not attended childbirth classes, she can be taught as needed. It is important that each breathing pattern begin and end with a cleansing breath, which is a deep inspiration and expiration similar to a deep sigh. The cleansing breath helps the woman focus on relaxing.

separate classes for adolescents and women with high-risk pregnancies.

BREATHING PATTERNS USED DURING LABOR

Breathing techniques are used to help the woman relax and override the pain of the uterine contractions (Box 5-7).

First-Stage Breathing

Slow Paced Breathing. In the early stages of labor, the woman uses a slow, deep breathing technique that increases relaxation. She starts with a cleansing breath and then breathes slowly, as during sleep. At the end of a contraction, a cleansing breath is taken.

Modified Paced Breathing. Modified paced breathing begins and ends with a cleansing breath. During the contraction, the woman's breaths are more rapid and shallow. The rate should be no more than twice her usual rate. Some women combine both slow and modified paced breathing during the contraction. The primary considerations are adequate oxygenation and the woman's comfort.

Patterned Paced Breathing. Patterned paced breathing is used during the later part of cervical dilation. It begins with a cleansing breath, which is followed by more rapid breaths, with an interspersed soft blow, which is often called "pant-blow" or "hee-hoo" breathing. If the woman feels an urge to push before her cervix is fully dilated, she should be encouraged to use a series of soft blows to counteract the desire to push (Figure 5-14).

Second-Stage Breathing (Expulsion Breathing)

When the woman has the urge and it is time for her to push, she should take a cleansing breath, then take another deep breath, and push down while exhaling (open-glottis technique). There is controversy about whether pushing over an extended period is a safe and effective method. The question is: Can it decrease the cardiac output and reduce placental blood flow? Traditional pushing with sustained breath holding against a closed glottis (Valsalva's maneuver) results in an increase in intrathoracic pressure, possibly resulting in fetal hypoxia. Proponents of open-glottis pushing assert that pushing while exhaling, as if blowing out a candle, does not inhibit venous return to the heart or impair blood flow to the fetus. If the woman does hold her breath, it is important that it be for a maximum of 6 seconds, followed by a deep cleansing breath.

The nurse may position the woman with her head and shoulders bent forward, leaning on the diaphragm, to encourage the pushing sensation. Also, the woman may prefer a 45-degree recumbent position.

NATURAL CHILDBIRTH

Today, natural childbirth is the process of giving birth with minimum medical and pharmacologic interventions. The woman who requires or accepts assistance with pain relief should not be made to feel she has failed in her efforts. Prenatal classes also review the

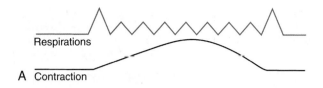

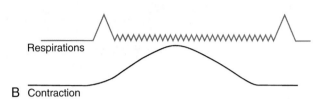

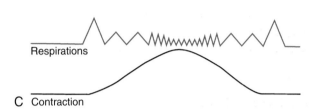

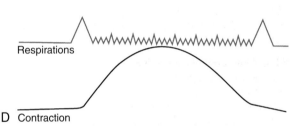

FIGURE 5-14 **A,** Slow paced breathing. The pattern starts with a cleansing breath as the contraction begins. The woman breathes slowly, at about half her usual rate, and ends with a second cleansing breath at the end of the contraction. **B,** As labor intensifies, the woman may need to use modified paced breathing. The pattern begins and ends with a cleansing breath. The woman breathes rapidly, no faster than twice her usual respiratory rate, during the peak of the contraction. **C,** In this variation of modified paced breathing the woman begins with slow paced breathing at the beginning of the contraction, switching to faster breathing during its peak. A cleansing breath also begins and ends this pattern. **D,** Patterned paced breathing begins and ends with a cleansing breath. During the contraction, the woman emphasizes the exhalation of some breaths. She may use a specific pattern or may randomly emphasize the blow.

birth process (Figure 5-15), pain management choices, and care provider choices. Obstetricians and nurse-midwives usually staff labor and delivery rooms in hospitals. Doulas are professionally trained to provide support during labor to the woman and her partner. The care of the newborn, breastfeeding, family adaptation at home, and telephone advice lines to call for help after discharge are all important components of a childbirth education program.

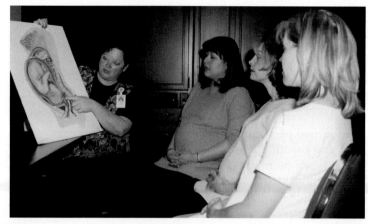

FIGURE 5-15 The nurse teaching a prenatal class discusses the movement of the fetus through the pelvis.

Get Ready for the NCLEX® Examination!

Key Points

- Adequate prenatal care improves the maternal and infant outcome. Emphasis is placed on health maintenance.
- Preconception care enables screening for medical or lifestyle risk factors that can be managed before pregnancy. It is best achieved when pregnancy is planned.
- Culturally sensitive childbirth education should be available to all pregnant women.
- The initial prenatal visit involved data collection concerning the woman's health history, lifestyle, cultural practices, and current health status.
- The pregnant woman should have approximately 13 prenatal visits to the health care provider to monitor weight, vital signs, height of the fundus, FHR, and other assessments as needed.
- Ultrasound is a noninvasive, painless, and safe method of assessing fetal and placental conditions. It offers a valuable means of confirming pregnancy, assessing fetal growth, determining placental and fetal position, and ruling out fetal and placental abnormalities.
- Doppler ultrasound blood flow analysis is a noninvasive study of blood flow changes that occur in fetal and uteroplacental circulations.
- Chorionic villus sampling is a first-trimester alternative to amniocentesis for prenatal diagnosis of some genetic conditions.
- Amniocentesis is performed to obtain amniotic fluid cells, under the visualization of an ultrasound, through the abdominal and uterine walls into the amniotic sac. Sufficient amniotic fluid must be present for the test to be done. It is used in high-risk pregnancies to assess conditions such as genetic disorders, alpha-fetoprotein levels, and maternal-fetal blood incompatibility.
- BPP is used to evaluate the condition of the fetus by observing five variables: fetal breathing movements, gross fetal movements, fetal heart rate (FHR) variability and reactivity, fetal muscle tone, and the volume of amniotic fluid index (AFI).
- The NST is used to assess fetal well-being by evaluating the ability of the fetal heart to accelerate with fetal movement. The CST evaluates the response of fetal heart rate to uterine contractions.
- The common discomforts of pregnancy occur as a result of hormonal, physiologic, and anatomic changes. The nurse provides the pregnant woman with facts about self-care actions aimed at relieving discomforts and anxiety.
- The nurse provides education and encouragement concerning ways to promote a healthy lifestyle, including exercises, body mechanics, and travel precautions.
- The pelvic tilt, Kegel exercises, and tailor sitting are exercises taught in prenatal classes.
- Exercises should not increase body temperature above 38° C (100.4° F); should not be performed while lying flat on the back; should not cause the heartbeat to exceed 140 beats/min; and should focus on maintenance of fitness instead of improving fitness or weight loss during pregnancy.
- Passive immunization with immune globulin is safe during pregnancy. Live virus vaccines such as MMR, varicella, or rubella can cause fetal damage and should not be administered during pregnancy.
- The nurse reviews hazards that can occur, such as supine hypotension syndrome.
- The optimum weight gain during pregnancy is 11.5 to 16 kg (25 to 35 lbs) for normal weight women.
- There is a high correlation between an adequate diet during pregnancy and fetal health.
- Folic acid supplementation is advised to prevent neural tube defects.

- Iron supplementation is recommended after 20 weeks' gestation. An adequate intake of iron is difficult to obtain from dietary sources alone.
- An adequate DHA intake by the pregnant woman is essential for optimum brain development in the fetus.
- Pica is the consumption of inedible items such as laundry starch, ice chips, or clay that has no nutrient value.
- Education for childbirth helps couples become more knowledgeable, active participants in pregnancy, labor, and birth.
- Several types of classes are available for pregnant women and their partners. In addition, classes are available for siblings and grandparents.
- Relaxation and conditioning exercises during prenatal classes are used to lessen discomfort during labor and birth.
- Commonly used breathing techniques, such as slow, modified, and patterned paced breathing, and conscious relaxation are beneficial to the woman in labor.

Additional Learning Resources

SG Go to your Study Guide on pages 481–482 for additional Review Questions for the NCLEX® Examination, Critical Thinking Clinical Situations, and other learning activities to help you master this chapter content.

evolve Go to your Evolve website (http://evolve.elsevier.com/Leifer/maternity) for the following FREE learning resources:
- Animations
- Answer Guidelines for Critical Thinking Questions
- Answers and Rationales for Review Questions for the NCLEX® Examination
- Concept Map Creator
- Glossary with pronunciations in English and Spanish
- Patient Teaching Plans
- Skills Performance Checklists and more!

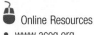 Online Resources
- www.acog.org
- www.cdc.gov/niosh/docs/2007-151/pdfs/2007-151.pdf
- www.cdc.gov/nip
- www.cdc.gov/travel/spec_needs.htm
- www.choosemyplate.gov
- www.epa.gov/waterscience/fish/states.htm
- http://fnic.nal.usda.gov
- www.lamaze.org
- www.marchofdimes.com
- www.preconception.com

Review Questions for the NCLEX® Examination

1. Pregnancy is a contraindication for all of the following vaccines except:
   1. Inactivated polio (IPV) vaccine
   2. Hepatitis B vaccine
   3. Varicella vaccine
   4. Measles, mumps, and rubella (MMR) vaccine

   Hep. A
   Pneumococcal

2. According to the Family Medical Leave Act (FMLA), how long is the Federally mandated leave of absence available for a parent following the birth or adoption of a child?
   1. 6 weeks
   2. 8 weeks
   3. 10 weeks
   4. 12 weeks

3. Which medication would be contraindicated for a woman in the 3rd trimester of pregnancy?
   1. Acetaminophen
   2. Ibuprofen
   3. Ferrous sulfate
   4. Docusate sodium

4. At her first prenatal visit, a woman asks the nurse how much weight is acceptable to gain during pregnancy. The nurse correctly responds that a woman of normal weight prior to pregnancy should gain:
   1. 10 to 15 pounds
   2. 25 to 35 pounds
   3. 30 to 40 pounds
   4. 40 to 50 pounds

5. When counseling a woman on nutritional requirements during pregnancy, the health care provider should provide which instruction(s)? *(Select all that apply.)*
   1. A daily supplement of 0.4 mg folic acid in the first weeks of pregnancy significantly reduces neural tube defects in newborns.
   2. The recommended calorie increase in the second trimester is approximately 500 calories greater than pre-pregnancy needs.
   3. Moderate caffeine intake is acceptable.
   4. Breastfeeding requires a decrease of 500 calories.
   5. Fluid intake of six to eight glasses per day is recommended.

6. Women who are pregnant should limit their intake of:
   1. Calcium
   2. Liver
   3. Poultry
   4. Tuna

7. A couple attending an early prenatal class would most likely learn about:
   1. Postpartum care
   2. Birth choices
   3. Fetal development
   4. Newborn safety

8. A woman in labor is 8 cm dilated and feels the urge to push. The nurse should encourage this woman to use:
   1. Patterned-paced breathing
   2. Slow-paced breathing
   3. Modified-paced breathing
   4. Expulsion breathing

Critical Thinking Questions

A 28-year-old patient is GTPALM 100000. She came to the clinic because her home pregnancy test was positive, and she states she has been trying to get pregnant. Her only complaint is nausea in the mornings. She states her husband is a fisherman, and she loves to eat all kinds of fish. She asks whether it is OK to continue eating fish during her pregnancy. Her physical exam reveals an enlarged uterus and a positive Chadwick's sign.

1. What does GTPALM stand for?

2. If today is April 10 and her last menstrual period was March 1, what is her due date?

3. What is Chadwick's sign? Is it normal? Is it a positive sign of pregnancy?

4. What advice would you give to the patient to relieve her nausea and vomiting in the mornings?

5. What advice will you give concerning her diet?

Process of Normal Labor

*e*volve

Objectives

1. Define key terms listed.
2. Explain *labor, lightening, vaginal show, effacement,* and *cervical dilation.*
3. Recognize spontaneous rupture of membranes.
4. Interpret the events that signal approaching labor.
5. List the four main variables in the birth process.
6. Describe the ability of the uterine muscles to contract and relax.
7. Differentiate three distinctive characteristics of labor contractions.
8. Differentiate between false and true labor.
9. Illustrate how frequency, duration, and intensity of contractions are monitored.
10. Describe fetal attitude, fetal lie, and fetal presentation.
11. List the six positions that the occiput of the fetal head may occupy in relation to the maternal pelvis.
12. Describe the term *station* as it relates to the maternal pelvis.
13. Distinguish six factors that influence the course of labor.
14. Interpret what is accomplished in each of the four stages of labor.
15. Summarize the response of each body system to the labor process.

Key Terms

acme (p. 96)
Braxton Hicks contractions (p. 98)
crowning (p. 95)
decrement (DĔK-rē-mĕnt, p. 96)
dilation (dī-LĀ-shŭn, p. 96)
duration of contraction (p. 98)
effacement (ĕ-FĀS-mĕnt, p. 96)
engagement (p. 95)
episiotomy (p. 102)
extension (p. 100)
external rotation (p. 100)
false labor (p. 99)
fetal attitude (p. 92)

fetal lie (p. 92)
fetal position (p. 93)
fetal presentation (p. 92)
floating (p. 95)
frequency of contraction (p. 96)
increment (ĬN-krĕ-mĕnt, p. 96)
intensity of contraction (p. 98)
internal rotation (p. 99)
labor (p. 91)
lightening (p. 98)
molding (p. 92)
show (p. 98)
station (p. 93)

The time of labor and birth, though short compared with the length of pregnancy, is perhaps the most dramatic and significant period of pregnancy for the expectant mother, newborn, and family. The process of labor and birth is a fairly predictable sequence of events that usually occurs in a manner that results in a healthy mother and baby.

THE PROCESS OF LABOR - can be predictable

The process by which the fetus, placenta, and amniotic membranes are expelled from the uterus is called labor. What initially causes labor to begin is not known, but it is thought to be a cascade of events. Changes in maternal hormone levels; stretching of the uterus by the growing fetus; and an interaction between the placenta and the fetal pituitary, hypothalamus, and adrenal glands all contribute to the onset of labor. Although many people focus on the uterine contractions when they define labor, the process of labor is actually an interaction of four important variables, known as the "four *P*s": the *P*assageway, *P*assenger, *P*owers, and *P*syche. These variables are discussed in this chapter. Other factors can influence the process of labor, including (Vande Vusse, 1999):

Preparation: Attendance at prenatal classes reduces fear of the unknown.

Position: Maternal preferences for horizontal, vertical, sitting, squatting, or side-lying positions may influence the progress of labor.

closes within 12-18 months

Professional help: A supportive nurse or doula (specially trained labor coach) can coach the woman through the labor process.

Procedures: The number of vaginal examinations and other invasive procedures can interrupt concentration and rapport during the labor process.

People: The presence of supportive partners or family members can influence the smooth progress of labor.

MAJOR VARIABLES IN THE BIRTH PROCESS

The four factors most significant in the process of labor include (1) **passageway** or pelvis (its size and shape), (2) **passenger** (fetus) size and position, (3) **powers** (effectiveness of contractions), and (4) **psyche** (preparation and previous experience). An ideal labor is one in which the woman's bony pelvis is adequate, the fetus is of average size, and the strength of the uterine contractions increases sufficiently to cause the cervix to fully efface and dilate. The woman's psyche—her ability to relax and concentrate on muscle groups and to maintain a low level of anxiety—also plays a role in the normal progress of her labor.

PELVIS

ideal pelvis gynecoid

The anatomy of the pelvis and uterus is discussed in Chapter 2. The angles of the birth canal are downward, forward, and upward, somewhat similar to the letter *J*. The pelvic curve must be negotiated by the fetus during the birth process. If the pelvic anteroposterior (AP) diameter is shortened by the sacral promontory or narrowed by the transverse diameter from the protrusion of the ischial spines or by the presence of a narrow pubic arch, the fetus will have difficulty coming through the birth canal. A clinical estimation of the pelvic measurements is an important part of prenatal care to determine adequacy for the birth process. An x-ray pelvimetry (measurement of the pelvis) is rarely performed. Other methods of estimating pelvic size such as a vaginal examination are discussed in Chapter 2 (Gabbe, Niebyl, & Simpson, 2007).

PASSENGER

The passenger includes the fetus along with the placenta, membranes, and amniotic fluid.

Fetal Head

The fetal head is engineered to withstand the pressure of uterine contractions and descent through the birth canal. Great pressure is exerted on the fetal head during labor, and even stronger pressure is applied to the head after the rupture of membranes because the amniotic fluid no longer serves as a cushion between the fetal head and the bony pelvis.

Bony Skull of the Fetal Head

The fetal head is composed of several bones separated by strong connective tissue, called *sutures*. A wider area, called a *fontanelle,* is formed where the sutures meet. The following two fontanelles are important in obstetrics:

- The *anterior fontanelle*, a diamond-shaped area formed by the intersection of four sutures (frontal, sagittal, and two coronal)
- The *posterior fontanelle*, a tiny triangular depression formed by the intersection of three sutures (one sagittal and two lambdoid)

The sutures and fontanelles of the fetal head allow it to change shape as it passes through the pelvis (molding). The fontanelles are important landmarks in determining how the fetus is oriented within the mother's pelvis during birth.

The main transverse diameter of the fetal head is the *biparietal diameter*, which is measured between the points of the two parietal bones on each side of the head. The AP diameter of the fetal head can vary, depending on how much the head is flexed or extended (Figure 6-1).

Fetopelvic Relationship: Terminology

Some common terms are used in a special way to describe the fetopelvic relationship. It is important to know each term to understand the course of labor and birth.

Fetal Attitude. Fetal attitude is the relation of the fetal parts to one another. The normal attitude of the fetus is one of flexion. The fetus is flexed with head on chest, arms and legs folded, and legs drawn up onto the abdomen. Changes in fetal attitude, particularly in the extension of the head, cause the fetus to present a larger diameter of the fetal head to the maternal pelvis. Extension of the fetal head, especially full extension in which the chin or face presents, makes vaginal birth difficult and sometimes impossible (Figure 6-2).

Fetal Lie. Fetal lie is the relation of the longitudinal axis of the fetus to the longitudinal axis of the mother. The ideal is a parallel relation in which the long axes of the fetus and mother are the same. In rare instances the fetus lies crosswise in the uterus (transverse lie), which necessitates a cesarean birth.

Fetal Presentation. Fetal presentation is determined by the body part of the fetus that is lowest in the mother's pelvis (Figure 6-3). A cephalic, breech, or shoulder presentation may occur. Cephalic (head first) presentation is the most common, occurring in approximately 95% of all births, and labor most often proceeds normally. If the head is flexed, the position is referred to as a *vertex presentation*. Breech presentation occurs in approximately 3% of all births. In the breech

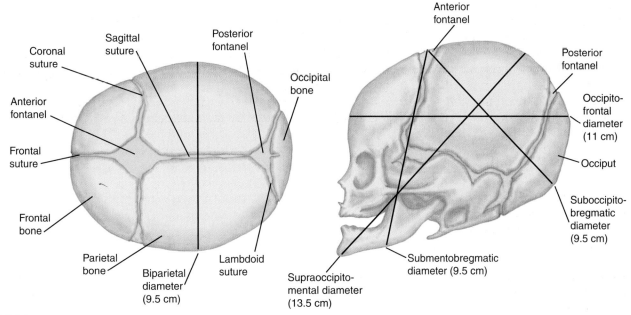

FIGURE 6-1 **The fetal head with bones, sutures, and fontanelles.** Note that the anterior fontanelle is diamond-shaped, whereas the posterior fontanelle is triangular.

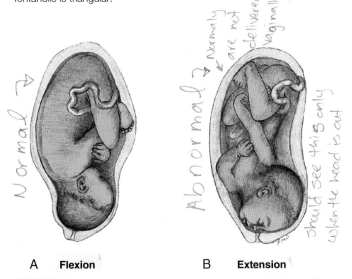

Normally are not delivered vaginally

Should see this only when the head is out

A   **Flexion**   B   **Extension**

FIGURE 6-2 **Attitude. A,** Fetus is in the normal attitude of flexion, with the arms and legs flexed tightly against the trunk. **B,** Fetus is in an attitude of extension, which is abnormal. Face presentation is illustrated.

presentation, the presenting parts may be either the buttocks (complete or frank breech) or one or both feet (footling breech) (see Chapter 14). The rarest type of presentation is the transverse (or oblique), which occurs in approximately 1% of births. These are referred to as *malpresentations* and do not proceed normally.

Fetal Position. Fetal position, a more specific indication of the fetopelvic relationship, is the relation of some designated point on the presenting part to the four quadrants of the maternal pelvis: anterior, posterior, left side, and right side. If the reference point is directed toward the transverse diameter of the maternal

pelvis, it is referred to as a *transverse position*. The notations used to describe the fetal position are:

R or L: Right (R) or left (L) side of the maternal pelvis; correlates with the right or left side of the woman's body

O, S, or M: Designated point (landmark) of fetal presenting part: occiput (O), sacrum (S), or mentum (face) (M)

A or P: Location of the designated point to the anterior (A) (front toward symphysis pubis) or posterior (P) (back toward the sacrum) of the maternal pelvis or to the transverse diameter of the maternal pelvis (midway between symphysis and sacrum)

Anterior is recorded as *A*, posterior is recorded as *P*, and transverse is recorded as *T*. The abbreviations (notations) help the caregivers communicate the fetal position. If the back of the fetal head (occiput) is directed to the left of the woman's body and anteriorly toward the pubis, it is described as **LOA** (left occiput anterior). When the occiput is directed to the left of the woman's body and to the back toward the sacrum, it is **LOP,** and the labor is often longer with the woman experiencing more backache, which is often referred to as *back labor*. The left occiput anterior and right occiput anterior positions are the most common and facilitate a normal progression of labor. Abbreviations for fetal presentations are shown in Box 6-1.

Station. Station is the relation of the presenting part of the fetus to an imaginary line drawn between the ischial spines of the maternal pelvis (Figure 6-4). To

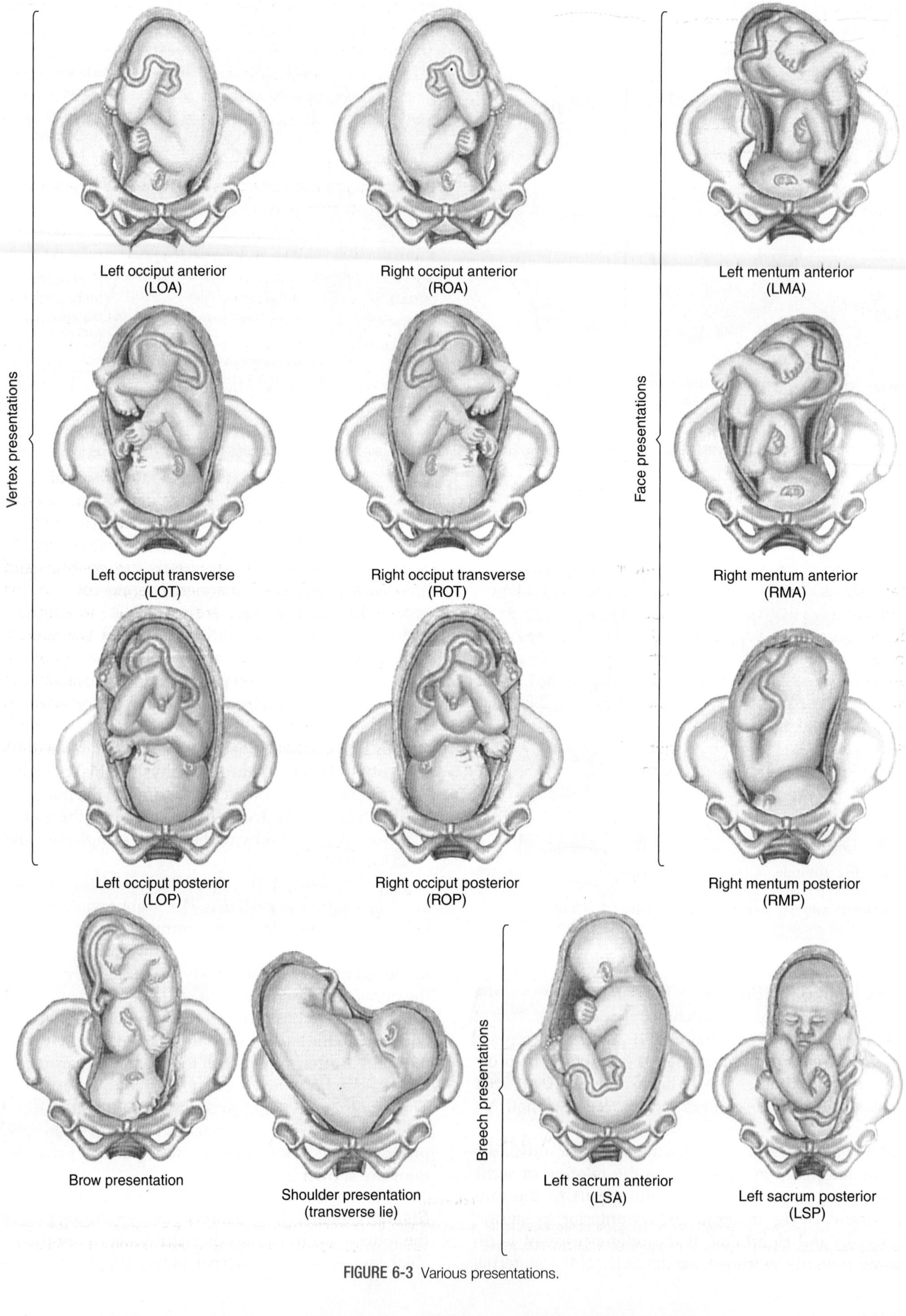

Vertex presentations

Left occiput anterior
(LOA)

Right occiput anterior
(ROA)

Left occiput transverse
(LOT)

Right occiput transverse
(ROT)

Left occiput posterior
(LOP)

Right occiput posterior
(ROP)

Face presentations

Left mentum anterior
(LMA)

Right mentum anterior
(RMA)

Right mentum posterior
(RMP)

Brow presentation

Shoulder presentation
(transverse lie)

Breech presentations

Left sacrum anterior
(LSA)

Left sacrum posterior
(LSP)

FIGURE 6-3 Various presentations.

Box 6-1 Classification of Fetal Presentations and Positions*

CEPHALIC PRESENTATIONS
Vertex
LOA	Left occiput anterior
ROA	Right occiput anterior
ROT	Right occiput transverse
LOT	Left occiput transverse
OA	Occiput anterior
OP	Occiput posterior

Face (Mentum)
LMA	Left mentum anterior
RMA	Right mentum anterior
LMP	Left mentum posterior
RMP	Right mentum posterior

BREECH PRESENTATIONS
LSA	Left sacrum anterior
RSA	Right sacrum anterior
LSP	Left sacrum posterior
RSP	Right sacrum posterior

*Abbreviations that designate brow (or military) and shoulder presentations are not included here because they occur infrequently.

put it simply, the station is how far the fetal presenting part has descended into the mother's pelvis. Station defines the progression of (usually) the fetal head down toward the pelvic floor. It is measured in centimeters above or below the ischial spines. When the presenting part is above the ischial spines, it is at minus station, with −5 at the inlet. When the presenting part is 1 or 2 cm below the spines, it is at the +1 or +2 station. Station +5 is at the outlet. When the presenting part is level with the spines, it is said to be at the 0 (zero)

station, and the head is referred to as *engaged*. This progress is significant because when engagement occurs, the widest biparietal diameter of the baby's head has entered the inlet (middle of pelvis). Before the head becomes engaged, it is said to be floating. When the station is +2 or +3, the mother's perineum begins to bulge.

Crowning takes place when the fetal head is forced against the pelvic floor and can be seen at the vaginal opening during contractions. During labor, the presenting part moves from the negative into the positive stations. Failure of the presenting part to descend in the presence of strong contractions may be caused by a disproportion between the maternal pelvis and the fetal presenting part. The movement of the presenting part downward toward the outlet of the pelvis occurs in the ninth month and is known as *lightening*. Engagement takes place when lightening occurs.

POWERS: UTERINE CONTRACTIONS

Understanding labor requires an understanding of the dramatic and unique physiology of the uterus. The uterine muscle (myometrium) is a smooth muscle that possesses the same properties as other smooth muscles in the body. Each muscle can contract and relax in a coordinated manner. Uterine contractions occur when uterine cells are stimulated to contract, and the stimulation spreads throughout the uterus. During labor, the contractions begin in the top of the uterus (fundus) and spread throughout the uterus in approximately 15 seconds. Because each contraction starts at the top, the nurse is able to ascertain the beginning of the contraction by placing her or his hands on the fundus.

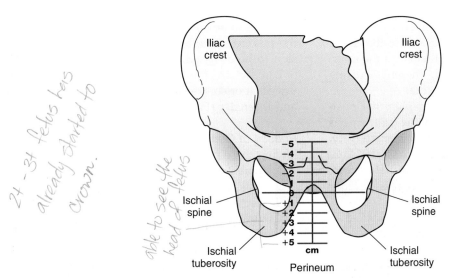

FIGURE 6-4 **Stations of presenting part (degree of engagement).** In this diagram, the presenting part has reached the +1 station. The lower pelvis, from the ischial spines to the pelvic floor, represents positive stations (+1, +2, +3), and the upper pelvis, from the inlet or pelvic brim to the ischial spines, represents negative stations (−3, −2, −1).

A unique property of the uterine muscle is its ability to retain some of the shortening achieved during the contraction. This ability is called *retraction* or **brachystasis**. When the myometrium cells contract, the fibers of both the fundus and the body of the uterus shorten. When the contraction ends and the muscles relax, the fibers do not return to their original size but remain shorter than before the contraction. This continued shortening of the muscle fibers in the upper portion of the uterus results in a progressive decrease in the size of the uterine cavity and a thickening of the muscle tissue of the upper portion. These changes supply the force needed to advance the fetus. With less room at the top of the uterus, the fetus is forced to descend.

Uterine contractions are referred to as the *source of power* that brings about the birth of the fetus. Because these contractions cause discomfort, they are commonly called *labor pains*. The amount of discomfort produced by the contractions varies with the intensity of the contraction and the woman's tolerance of discomfort (her psyche). During labor, the woman may first perceive the contractions as back discomfort. The discomfort then radiates to the front of the abdomen.

The Uterine (Labor) Contraction

Each contraction is followed by a period of **relaxation**, the interval between contractions. This period is significant to the mother and fetus. During the contraction, there is decreased blood flow through the uterine arteries and intervillous spaces. This decline in blood flow lowers the fetal heart rate. If the mother is being observed by electronic fetal monitor, the decrease in fetal heart rate during contractions is carefully assessed (see Chapter 7). If the contractions become more frequent and prolonged, the decrease in blood flow can be cumulative and compromise the fetus. In other words, the fetus receives a decreased oxygen supply and experiences stress during contractions. For this reason, it is important that the caregiver report to the physician if labor contractions are so close that there are no relaxation periods between them or if the intervals are progressively shortened, thereby causing significant patterns of fetal bradycardia.

Labor contractions are affected by maternal position. When a woman lies on her back, the contractions are likely to be more frequent but of lower intensity. When she lies on her side, the contractions are likely to be less frequent but of greater intensity. Therefore, a side-lying position improves the progress of labor and improves oxygenation to the fetus.

Effect of Contractions on the Cervix

Cervical changes include cervical effacement and dilation. Cervical **effacement** is the shortening and thinning of the cervix. Normally, the cervix is 2 cm (0.8 inches) in length. When effacement is complete (100%), the cervix has almost disappeared (Figure 6-5).

Cervical **dilation** is the enlargement of the cervical opening (os) from 0 to 10 cm (complete dilation). Both cervical effacement and dilation are measured by a vaginal examination. If the cervix is beginning to dilate or is thinned, the onset of labor is near. Dilation of 4 cm is significant because, at this point, the woman's active labor usually progresses to completion.

Contractions cause the cervix to efface (thin) and dilate (open) to allow the fetus to descend in the birth canal. Before labor begins, the cervix is a tubular structure about 2 cm (0.8 inch) long. Contractions simultaneously push the fetus downward as they pull the cervix upward (an action similar to pushing a ball out of the cuff of a sock). This causes the cervix to become thinner and shorter. Effacement is determined by a vaginal examination and is described as a percentage of the original cervical length. When the cervix is 100% effaced, it feels like a thin, slick membrane over the fetus.

Dilation of the cervix is also determined during a vaginal examination. Dilation is described in centimeters, with full dilation being 10 cm. Both the dilation and effacement are estimated by touch rather than being precisely measured.

When the cervix is fully dilated (second stage of labor), the woman often uses her abdominal muscles to superimpose intraabdominal pressure on the contraction pressure. The bearing-down effort with the abdominal muscles is consciously controlled and is of great assistance in the final push to expel the fetus. It is important that someone (the nurse or significant other) coach the woman in her bearing-down effort during labor contractions.

Characteristics of Uterine (Labor) Contractions

Uterine contractions are the important source of power that (1) produces cervical effacement and dilation, (2) causes the fetus to engage and rotate, (3) causes the fetus to be delivered, and (4) detaches and expels the placenta (afterbirth). Therefore, for labor progression to be assessed, it is important to know the type of contractions the woman is having. The characteristics of labor contractions include **frequency, duration,** and **intensity** (Figure 6-6).

Phases of Contractions. Each contraction has the following three phases:
1. Increment, the period of increasing strength
2. Peak, or acme, the period of greatest strength
3. Decrement, the period of decreasing strength

Contractions are also described by their average frequency, duration, intensity, and interval.

Frequency of Contraction. Frequency of contraction is the elapsed time from the beginning of one contraction until the beginning of the next contraction. Frequency is described in minutes and fractions of minutes,

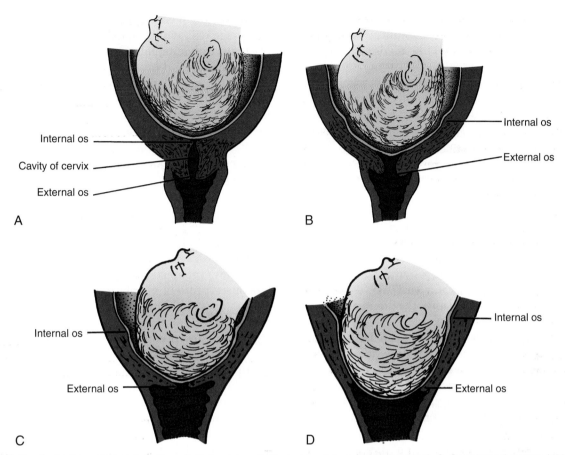

FIGURE 6-5 **Cervical effacement and dilation. A,** Before labor. **B,** Beginning effacement (dilation 2 cm). **C,** Complete effacement (100%). **D,** Complete dilation (10 cm).

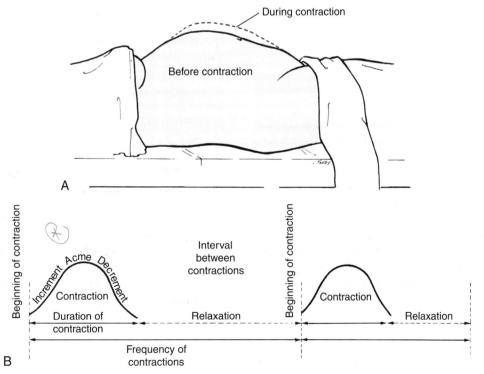

FIGURE 6-6 **A,** Changes in abdominal contour before and during uterine contraction. **B,** Assessment of frequency, duration, and intensity of uterine contractions during labor.

such as "contractions every 4½ minutes." Contractions occurring more often than every 2 minutes may reduce fetal oxygen supply and should be reported.

Duration of Contraction. Duration of contraction is the elapsed time from the beginning of a contraction until the end of the same contraction. Duration is described as the average number of seconds for which contractions last, such as "duration of 45 to 50 seconds." Persistent contraction durations longer than 90 seconds may reduce fetal oxygen supply and should be reported immediately.

Intensity of Contraction. Intensity of contraction is the approximate strength of the contraction. In most cases, intensity is described in words such as *mild, moderate,* or *strong,* which are defined as follows:

  Mild contractions: Fundus is easily indented with the fingertips; the fundus of the uterus feels similar to the tip of the nose.

  Moderate contractions: Fundus can be indented with the fingertips but with more difficulty; the fundus of the uterus feels similar to the chin.

  Firm contractions: Fundus cannot be readily indented with the fingertips; the fundus of the uterus feels similar to the forehead.

Interval. The interval is the amount of time the uterus relaxes between contractions. Blood flow from the mother into the placenta gradually decreases during contractions and resumes during each interval. The placenta refills with freshly oxygenated blood for the fetus and removes fetal waste products. Persistent contraction intervals shorter than 60 seconds may reduce fetal oxygen supply.

⚠ Safety Alert

When to Report Contractions

Report to the registered nurse any contractions that occur more frequently than every 2 minutes, last longer than 90 seconds, or have intervals shorter than 60 seconds.

PSYCHE

The psyche is recognized as part of the labor process. For example, anxiety and fear can decrease a pregnant woman's ability to cope with pain in labor. Maternal catecholamines (stress hormones secreted when the woman is anxious or fearful) are known to inhibit uterine contractility and placental blood flow. However, relaxation augments the natural process of labor.

Prenatal care and childbirth classes prepare the mother to cope with the labor process. The nursing responsibilities during labor include the use of strategies to reduce anxiety and promote relaxation.

Conservation of energy until it is needed in the expulsion stage will avoid exhaustion and the development of an electrolyte imbalance, which can occur with hyperventilation and profuse perspiration.

Culture, expectations, past experiences, language barriers, and availability of a support person are factors that influence a woman's ability to cope with the experience of labor and delivery. Traditional and nontraditional forms of therapy used to deal with the discomforts of labor and delivery are discussed in Chapters 8 and 21.

EVENTS BEFORE THE ONSET OF LABOR

Any of the following signs noticed by the expectant woman indicates that labor usually is not far away: lightening, vaginal discharge (show), false labor, spontaneous rupture of membranes, and cervical changes.

LIGHTENING

Lightening describes what happens when the fetus begins to settle in the maternal pelvis and move downward toward the pelvic outlet. In referring to lightening, some women say, "The baby has dropped down" because the fundus no longer presses on the diaphragm. However, there is more pressure from the fetal head on the maternal blood vessels, nerves, and bladder. The physical changes that occur in the mother as a result of lightening include (1) easier breathing, (2) more frequent urination, (3) leg cramps, and (4) edema of the lower extremities.

VAGINAL DISCHARGE (BLOODY SHOW)

With cervical changes caused by increased pressure in the pelvic region, a blood-tinged mucous plug becomes dislodged from the cervical os. The blood is from the rupture of superficial blood vessels. Bloody show appears as pink-stained mucus and is different from the bleeding that occurs during menstruation or from a cut finger.

ENERGY SPURT

Some women have a sudden burst of energy 1 or 2 days before labor. The cause of this energy spurt is unknown. Some call it a "nesting time" when the woman prepares the nursery or cleans house. The woman should be warned not to overexert herself during this high-energy phase. Rather, she should conserve this energy so that she will not be exhausted when labor begins.

FALSE LABOR

Later in pregnancy, the expectant mother becomes aware of Braxton Hicks contractions that are painless but may be felt when she places her hand on her abdomen.

Braxton Hicks contractions are irregular contractions that begin during early pregnancy and are rarely perceived by the pregnant woman. They may intensify as term approaches. When the woman becomes more aware of and sensitive to the Braxton Hicks contractions, she may believe that labor has started (see the discussion of true and false labor later in the chapter). Although Braxton Hicks contractions are often called *false labor*, they do play a part in preparing the cervix to dilate and in adjusting the fetal position within the uterus.

Uterine activity increases during the last 2 to 3 weeks of pregnancy, but the contractions remain uncoordinated and irregular. These contractions help demarcate the uterus into the upper segment (the muscular, contractile portion) and the lower segment, which is relaxed.

If the woman is near term and the contractions are uncomfortable, the woman may come to the hospital. If the cervix has not dilated and the contractions remain irregular or stop, the condition is called false labor, or prodromal labor. The conclusive difference between true labor and false labor is **cervical change** such as dilation, which occurs with true labor (Table 6-1). False labor has no clinical significance except that it causes maternal anxiety and premature admission to the hospital. The experience may be disappointing and embarrassing to the woman and her family.

SPONTANEOUS RUPTURE OF MEMBRANES

Spontaneous rupture of the amniotic membranes (SROM) occasionally occurs before labor begins. SROM is what women mean when they say, "My water broke." At term, it is not unusual for women to go into labor within 24 hours after SROM. If labor does not begin within 24 hours, it is often induced because of the risk of infection because of the open passageway into the uterus. The induction of labor by artificially rupturing the membranes is not done until the pregnancy is near term. When the membranes rupture, there is a danger of a prolapsed cord if the fetal head has not settled in the pelvis (the umbilical cord can descend along with the discharge of amniotic fluid). Initially, there can be either a trickle or a rush of fluid. For SROM to be differentiated from urine or vaginal fluid, a Nitrazine paper test is used to determine the pH of the fluid. Amniotic fluid is slightly alkaline (which turns the paper blue), whereas urine is generally acidic. When the amniotic membranes are artificially ruptured, it is referred to as AROM; PROM refers to **premature** rupture of the membranes.

LABOR

MECHANISMS OF LABOR

The mechanisms (cardinal movements) of labor are a series of movements that reflect changes in the fetus's posture as it adapts to the birth canal. Most of the changes in posture take place during the second stage of labor; however, descent and some flexion may take place earlier.

The posture changes (mechanisms of labor) are dictated by the pelvic diameters, maternal soft tissues, the size of the fetus, and the strength of contractions. The fetus must turn and twist to locate the easiest path. In essence, labor proceeds along the path of least resistance through the adaptation of the smallest achievable fetal dimensions to the contour of the maternal pelvis. The mechanisms of labor are the series of adaptive movements of the fetal head and shoulders and include (1) engagement and descent, (2) flexion, (3) internal rotation, (4) extension, (5) external rotation, and (6) expulsion (Figure 6-7).

Descent cannot be isolated from the other adaptive movements because it occurs throughout the labor process. As the head moves toward the pelvic inlet, it is described as floating.

Engagement occurs when the biparietal diameter of the fetal head reaches the level of the ischial spine of the mother's pelvis (presenting part is at a 0 station or lower). This descent may occur before or after labor begins and is caused by the pressure of contractions and of the amniotic fluid.

Flexion occurs as the fetal head descends. The head flexes so that the chin rests on the chest. Flexion enables the smallest fetal diameter to enter the maternal birth canal. It normally occurs when the fetal head meets resistance from the pelvis and soft tissues of the pelvic floor.

Internal rotation occurs as the fetal head rotates from the transverse position to the anterior position,

Table 6-1 Comparison of True Labor and False Labor

CHARACTERISTIC	TRUE LABOR	FALSE LABOR
Show (pinkish mucus)	Usually present; increases as the cervix changes	None present
Contractions	Regular with increases in intensity and duration	Irregular; no change in frequency and intensity
Discomfort	Often begins in lumbar region and then is felt in abdomen	Often located in abdomen
Activity	Contractions often intensified by activity (walking)	Contractions often lessened by walking
Cervical changes*	Effacement and progressive dilation of cervix	No cervical changes

*The most distinguishing characteristics between true and false labors are the cervical changes that occur in true labor.

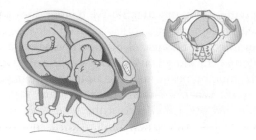

1. Head floating, before engagement

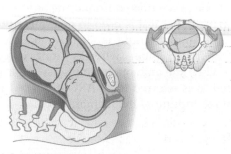

2. Engagement, flexion, descent

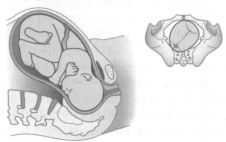

3. Further descent, internal rotation

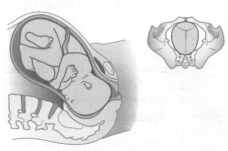

4. Complete rotation, beginning extension

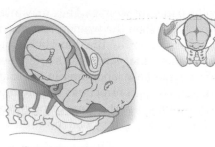

5. Complete extension

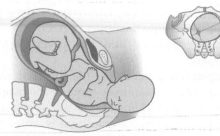

6. Restitution, external rotation

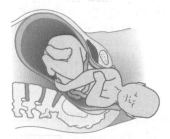

7. Delivery of anterior shoulder

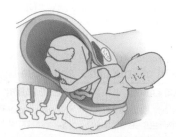

8. Delivery of posterior shoulder

FIGURE 6-7 Mechanisms of normal labor in a left occipitoanterior vertex position. 1, Head floating before engagement; 2, engagement, flexion, and descent occur as the head moves toward the pelvic inlet; descent continues; 3, descent and internal rotation to occiput anterior (OA) position; 4, complete rotation and beginning extension as the head reaches the pelvic floor; 5, the head is born by complete extension; 6, restitution and external rotation, returning to left OA (LOA) position and alignment with the shoulders; 7, delivery of the anterior shoulder; 8, with delivery of the posterior shoulder, expulsion occurs as the body of the baby is rapidly born.

aligning itself with the AP diameter of the maternal pelvis. Pressure from the pelvic floor encourages the fetal head to rotate anteriorly and rest beneath the symphysis pubis.

Extension begins as the fetal head reaches the pelvic floor, at which point it pivots under the symphysis pubis and advances upward. This results from a combination of pressure from the uterine contractions, abdominal pressure exerted by the mother's pushing, and resistance from the pelvic floor. As extension occurs, the occiput appears at the vaginal opening (crowning), followed by the forehead, nose, mouth, and chin. Extension is complete when the entire head is born.

External rotation, often called restitution, occurs after the head is delivered. The head immediately rotates back to the transverse position to be in alignment with the shoulders, and then the shoulders align themselves to the AP diameter of the pelvic outlet.

Expulsion usually proceeds as follows. First, the anterior shoulder rotates forward under the symphysis pubis and is delivered, followed by delivery of the posterior shoulder; then the delivery of the rest of the baby's body is rapid. The expulsion, or birth of the fetus, ends the second stage of labor.

Placental expulsion, or delivery of the afterbirth, is not one of the mechanisms of labor but normally occurs between 5 and 30 minutes after the birth of the baby. The uterus begins to contract, reducing its size, immediately after the birth of the baby, and the placenta is sheared off from the endometrium (lining of the uterus). Signs of placental separation are (1) lengthening of the cord, (2) change in the shape of the uterus, and (3) a trickle or gush of blood from the vagina. If the dull (maternal) side of the placenta appears first, it is referred to as a **Duncan mechanism;** if the shiny (fetal) side appears first, it is referred to as a **Schultze mechanism** (see Figure 7-15). Periodic studies have not shown any significant differences between the two mechanisms. Placentas implanted low in the uterus are usually delivered by the Duncan mechanism. Placentas implanted near the fundus of the uterus are usually delivered by the Schultze mechanism. The delivery of the placenta ends the third stage of labor.

THE FOUR STAGES OF LABOR

Labor is divided into four stages. Each stage has its own changes that set it apart from the others. The powers of labor and variables mentioned earlier that influence the course of labor should be considered in the assessment of each stage.

First Stage

The first stage of labor is the longest and most variable stage. The first stage begins with the onset of regular contractions and is complete when the cervix is fully dilated and effaced. The first stage is referred to as the **stage of dilation and effacement.** The contractions bring about two important changes in the cervix: (1) complete effacement of the cervical canal (100%) and (2) complete dilation of the cervix (10 cm).

The first stage of labor is divided into **latent, active,** and **transition** phases, each characterized by certain physical and psychological changes. The first stage of labor may last from 8 to 20 hours in the primipara and 5 to 14 hours in the multipara.

Latent Phase. The latent phase is the early, slow part of labor, which begins with the onset of regular contractions and lasts until the cervix has dilated to at least 4 cm. During this phase, the contractions become stabilized and are usually mild. They occur every 10 to 15 minutes and last approximately 15 to 20 seconds. At this point, the woman feels that she is able to cope with discomfort. She is often talkative and smiling and relieved that labor has finally started. She is encouraged to be out of bed, watching TV, or talking with her partner. This is a good time to ask the woman whether she has any questions about what to expect and, if she is anxious, to teach her some of the relaxation techniques. At this time, she is able to focus clearly on what is being taught.

Active Phase. The active phase causes the woman different degrees of discomfort. The contractions are stronger and last longer, with the result that cervical dilation progresses from 4 to 7 cm. Fetal descent proceeds. The duration of contractions increases to 30 to 45 seconds. They occur approximately 5 minutes apart and are of moderate to strong intensity. During this phase, the woman can be assisted in her breathing techniques and relaxation. She may continue to walk until she is uncomfortable or until her amniotic membranes rupture. As her contractions increase, her anxiety and discomfort increase. She may begin to doubt her ability to cope with the labor contractions.

Transition Phase. The transition phase is the last part of the first stage. Cervical dilation continues at a slower rate but becomes complete (8 to 10 cm). The contractions are now more frequent, last longer (60 to 90 seconds), and are stronger. During this phase, the woman may exhibit the decreased ability to cope with her contractions and pain. The woman often becomes very restless, frequently changing positions and feeling as if she has been abandoned. It is crucial that the nurse stay with the woman at this time as a backup or relief for the support person. The woman often needs to be reminded of how to relax and focus or refocus with each contraction. She may also become irritable and not want to be touched during her contractions (Box 6-2). The woman often fears losing control and is completely self-focused.

Box 6-2 Characteristics of the Transition Phase

- Restlessness
- Sense of bewilderment and sometimes anger
- Statements that she "cannot continue" or "can't take it"
- Difficulty in following directions; need for instruction with each contraction
- Requests for medication to ease the pain
- Hyperventilation caused by increased breathing rate
- Perspiration on face
- Belching or hiccupping
- Nausea and vomiting
- Increasing rectal pressure; statements that she has to have a bowel movement
- Feelings of warmth; throwing off covers (exposure may embarrass partner)
- Irritability
- Contractions often only 1 to 2 minutes apart and last up to 90 seconds

The woman may feel a splitting sensation by the force of the contractions and pressure of the fetal head near the opening of the cervix. As the fetal head descends, she likely will feel the urge to push because of the pressure from the fetal head on the sacral nerves. As she pushes, her abdominal muscles exert additional pressure, which helps the fetal head descend. As the fetal head continues its descent, the perineum begins to bulge and flatten, and soon the fetal head can be seen at the vaginal opening. The first stage of labor ends when the cervix is completely dilated and effaced.

Second Stage

The second stage of labor **(stage of expulsion)** begins when the cervix is completely dilated (10 cm) and ends with the birth of the baby. At this time, the woman usually feels the urge to bear down (as if she has to have a bowel movement). She may now use her abdominal muscles to assist the involuntary uterine contractions as a force to cause the descent of the baby. She should be coached not to hold her breath more than 5 seconds at a time when she pushes. Prolonged breath holding may trigger Valsalva's maneuver, which results from the closing of the glottis, thereby increasing intrathoracic and cardiovascular pressure. This can diminish the perfusion of oxygen across the placenta and result in fetal hypoxia and abnormalities in the fetal heart rate. An open-glottis method should be used in which air is released through the mouth during pushing. This method avoids the intrathoracic buildup of pressure.

The second stage generally lasts from a few minutes to 2 hours. Descent of the fetal head causes bulging of the perineum. Crowning occurs when the fetal head is seen in the external opening of the vagina. Between contractions, the fetal head appears to recede. With succeeding contractions and the woman pushing, the birth is imminent. The uterine contractions are forceful but now are usually only every 2 to 3 minutes in frequency and last 60 to 90 seconds. There usually is an increase in bloody show.

As the fetal head reaches the perineal floor, it appears at the vaginal opening. To prevent laceration, the physician or midwife may perform an episiotomy (a midline or mediolateral incision in the perineum). An episiotomy may also be done to shorten the second stage. An episiotomy is not routine but is used when indicated. The physician or midwife supports the fetal head as it delivers and rotates, either to the left or to the right; the mouth and then nose of the baby are suctioned as they appear. When the head is delivered, a quick check is made to ensure that the umbilical cord is not around the baby's neck (nuchal cord). After the head rotates to align the occiput with the baby's back, the shoulders and the rest of the baby's body is delivered. After the second stage of labor ends with the birth of the baby, the woman usually is relieved.

Third Stage

The third stage of labor is referred to as the **placental separation stage**. It begins with the birth of the baby and ends with the expulsion of the placenta. This process can last up to 30 minutes, with an average length of 5 to 10 minutes. After the birth of the fetus, the umbilical cord is clamped in two places and cut between the two clamps. The mouth and nose of the baby may be suctioned again to clear them of mucus (see Chapter 7). An oxytocin drug (commonly Pitocin) may be given to the woman to keep the uterus firm and lessen the maternal blood loss immediately after the placenta has been delivered.

Fourth Stage

The fourth stage of labor **(stage of recovery)** begins with the delivery of the placenta and lasts through the first 1 to 4 hours or until the mother's vital signs are stable. Major readjustments of the mother's body occur. Blood loss can range from 250 to 500 mL, which can cause the blood pressure to drop and the pulse rate to increase. The uterine muscles must stay contracted to compress the open blood vessels at the placental site and minimize blood loss. The uterus is palpable as a firm rounded mass at or below the level of the umbilicus. For the first hour after delivery, it is critical to observe the mother for excessive bleeding and assess the firmness of the contracting uterus.

The mother may feel thirsty and hungry, and she may experience a shaking chill. Nursing care is discussed in Chapter 7. The mother is interested in touching and holding her baby, and she should be encouraged to begin the mother-infant attachment process. Family bonding and the initiation of breastfeeding are an important part of the fourth stage of labor.

PHYSIOLOGIC CHANGES IN LABOR

Labor can affect all systems in the body. The major changes that occur in the various body systems in response to labor are shown in Table 6-2.

Table **6-2**   Physiologic Changes in Labor and Nursing Interventions

PHYSIOLOGY	CLINICAL SYMPTOMS	NURSING INTERVENTIONS
Cardiovascular System		
Uterine contractions release 400 mL of blood into vascular system, causing increase in cardiac output.	BP increases by 10 mm Hg; pulse rate slows.	Assess BP between contractions. Assess level of consciousness.
Ascending vena cava and descending aorta are compressed by weight of uterus.	Supine hypotension can occur.	Have woman avoid lying on back; encourage left side-lying position.
Holding the breath and forceful pushing increase intrathoracic pressure and reduce venous return and can cause fetal hypoxia.	Forceful rather than spontaneous pushing (Valsalva's maneuver) causes redness of face, increase in BP, slowing of pulse rate.	Encourage open-glottis pushing and discourage forceful pushing during second stage.
WBC count increases to 25,000/mm^3.	Increase in WBC count is not related to infection.	Correct interpretation of laboratory results intrapartum and postpartum is important.
Alterations in the fetal heart rate and rhythm may occur in response to contraction patterns.	The normal fetal heart rate is 110-160 beats/minute.	Monitor fetal heart rate frequently. Time the frequency and duration of contractions.
Respiratory System		
Increased physical activity of labor increases oxygen consumption. Anxiety can also increase oxygen consumption.	Respiratory rate increases.	Encourage relaxation between contractions.
Paced breathing techniques can prevent the development of respiratory alkalosis. *using paper bag/cupped hands.*	Tingling of the hands and feet, dizziness, or numbness may indicate hyperventilation, which can cause respiratory alkalosis.	Coach the laboring woman in breathing techniques.
Renal System (Kidneys)		
Breakdown in muscle tissue resulting from work of labor can cause proteinuria.	A full bladder may be palpable above the symphysis pubis.	Palpate above symphysis to detect a full bladder. Encourage voiding every 2 hours; catheterize if bladder is distended and if the woman is unable to void.
Full bladder can be obstructed by full uterus and fetal head.	Spontaneous voiding may occur during contractions.	Do not confuse spontaneous urination with rupture of bag of waters. Nitrazine paper can detect whether fluid discharge is urine or amniotic fluid.
Musculoskeletal System		
Muscle activity increases during labor. Increased joint laxity can cause backaches.	Diaphoresis, fatigue, and increased temperature may occur.	Observe for diaphoresis, fatigue, and increased temperature. Encourage rest between contractions. Use comfort measures for diaphoresis and positioning for back and joint pain.
Neurologic System		
Euphoria changes to self-centeredness as labor progresses. Amnesia during second stage is common, and fatigue and elation occur in third and fourth stages. Endorphins produce natural, general sedation, whereas ischemia of perineal tissues by pressure of presenting part causes decrease in perception of perineal pain.	Behavior of patient may change during each stage of labor.	Provide support and acceptance of behavior. Allow sleep whenever possible. Provide for safety and privacy.

Continued

Table 6-2   Physiologic Changes in Labor and Nursing Interventions—cont'd

PHYSIOLOGY	CLINICAL SYMPTOMS	NURSING INTERVENTIONS
Gastrointestinal (GI) System		
Mouth breathing during labor dries the lips and tongue.	Dry lips and mouth may be noted.	Assess for signs of dehydration. Use ice chips to moisten lips and tongue during active labor.
GI motility is decreased during labor.	Nausea and vomiting of undigested food may occur.	Do not allow food or drink during active labor. Rectal pressure and urge to defecate may indicate imminent delivery.
Endocrine System		
Estrogen increases and progesterone decreases. Metabolism increases during labor; work of labor may decrease glucose levels.	Increased metabolism may influence blood glucose level.	Encourage rest whenever possible between contractions and during fourth stage. Close monitoring of mother with diabetes (including blood glucose levels) during labor is essential.
Blood		
The increased blood volume during pregnancy enables a 500-mL blood loss during delivery without problem unless woman is anemic.	Blood pressure may decline; pulse rate may increase.	Monitor vital signs during labor and delivery. Report decrease in blood pressure and increase in pulse rate, which may indicate hypovolemia.
Increased levels of fibrinogen and other clotting factors during pregnancy prevent hemorrhage during delivery but increase risk for thrombosis.		If possible, avoid prolonged use of stirrups to support legs during delivery.
The increased fetal hemoglobin level enables fetus to carry increased level of oxygen during labor. Placental exchange of oxygen and waste occurs between contractions.	Contractions that exceed 90 seconds may impact fetal oxygenation.	Monitor contraction patterns and fetal heart rate closely during labor. Contractions that exceed 90 seconds should be reported to the health care provider.

BP, Blood pressure; *WBC*, white blood cell.

Get Ready for the NCLEX® Examination!

Key Points

- The four *Ps*—pelvis, passenger, powers, and psyche—are essential components of labor and birth. Each of these components involves both the maternal and fetal adjustments.
- It is necessary for the maternal passage (pelvis) to be adequate in shape and size to accommodate the descent and birth of the fetus.
- The passenger (fetus) negotiates through the maternal pelvis and usually passes head first through the various diameters of the pelvis. As the fetus descends, bony structures and soft tissues exert pressure, which forces the fetus to negotiate the birth canal by a series of passive movements (mechanisms of labor or cardinal movements).
- The powers (uterine contractions) are coordinated and of ample quality and strength to efface and dilate the cervix. With the aid of maternal expulsive efforts, contractions help expel the fetus, and birth occurs.

- The maternal psyche allows the woman to cope with the physical demands and pain of labor to push the fetus out of the birth canal.
- The conclusive difference between true and false labor is that progressive dilation and effacement of the cervix occur in true labor.
- Labor contractions increase in intensity, duration, and frequency. They are involuntary and intermittent during the first stage and are augmented by maternal bearing-down efforts during the second stage.
- The time between contractions is necessary to allow resumption of the placental blood flow and exchange of oxygen and waste products between the maternal and fetal circulations.
- The systemic response to labor guides both nursing assessments and nursing interventions during labor.
- The woman's cultural attitudes and beliefs about labor and birth influence whether labor is a stressful or positive experience.

Additional Learning Resources

SG Go to your Study Guide on pages 483–484 for additional Review Questions for the NCLEX® Examination, Critical Thinking Clinical Situations, and other learning activities to help you master this chapter content.

 evolve Go to your Evolve website (http://evolve.elsevier.com/Leifer/maternity) for the following FREE learning resources:

- Animations
- Answer Guidelines for Critical Thinking Questions
- Answers and Rationales for Review Questions for the NCLEX® Examination
- Concept Map Creator
- Glossary with pronunciations in English and Spanish
- Patient Teaching Plans
- Skills Performance Checklists and more!

Online Resources
- www.awhonn.org
- www.gowingo.com/health

Review Questions for the NCLEX® Examination

1. The relation of the presenting part of the fetus to an imaginary line drawn between the ischial spines of the maternal pelvis is referred to as:

   1. Engagement
   2. Lie
   3. Presentation
   4. Station

2. The best position to promote progress for a woman in labor is:

   1. Supine
   2. Semi-Fowler's
   3. Side-lying
   4. Prone

3. A woman in labor reports that her "contractions are occurring every 3 minutes." The characteristic of labor the woman is most likely describing is:

   1. Duration
   2. Increment
   3. Frequency
   4. Intensity

4. When assessing the intensity of contractions of a laboring woman, the nurse finds that the fundus is easily indented with the fingertips. The nurse will document the intensity of contractions for this woman as:

   1. Mild
   2. Moderate
   3. Firm
   4. Severe

5. Expected physical changes that occur in the mother as a result of lightening include: *(Select all that apply.)*

   1. Hypotension
   2. Easier breathing
   3. More frequent urination
   4. Leg cramps

6. A woman has just entered the fourth stage of labor. The most important nursing assessment during this stage of labor is:

   1. Fetal heart rate
   2. Cervical dilation
   3. Uterine firmness
   4. Pain

7. The anterior fontanelle of the fetal head is formed by the intersection of which suture(s)? *(Select all that apply.)*

   1. Sagittal
   2. Frontal
   3. Coronal
   4. Lambdoid

8. Put the following mechanisms of labor in sequential order by numbering 1 *(first)* to 6 *(last).*

   __2__ Flexion
   __1__ Engagement and descent
   __6__ Expulsion
   __5__ External rotation
   __3__ Internal rotation
   __4__ Extension

Critical Thinking Questions

1. Why are the mechanisms of labor outlined in the chapter necessary for the fetus to negotiate through the maternal pelvis? How will labor be affected if one part of these mechanisms is altered?

2. How does a full bladder influence the progress of labor?

Nursing Care During Labor

Objectives

1. Define key terms listed.
2. Describe three variations in cultural practices.
3. Compare alternative birth settings.
4. Outline three nursing assessments and interventions during each stage of labor.
5. Discuss the significance of psychological support during labor.
6. Review ways to protect the woman from infection.
7. Compare external and internal fetal monitoring during labor.
8. Compare the advantages and disadvantages of electronic fetal monitoring during labor.
9. Describe the cleansing of the woman's perineum in preparation for birth.
10. Compare reassuring and nonreassuring fetal heart rates.
11. Relate the nurse's role in fetal monitoring.
12. Describe the purpose of amnioinfusion.
10. Discuss the role of a doula in the delivery room.
14. Explain the common nursing responsibilities during birth.
15. Identify nursing priorities when assisting in an emergency (precip) delivery.
16. List four items that are important to record about the infant's birth.
17. Discuss the immediate care of the newborn.
18. Explain the reason the neonate requires administration of vitamin K at birth.
19. Describe the nursing assessments that are important in the woman's recovery period after birth.
20. Illustrate two ways to encourage maternal-newborn bonding after birth.
21. Discuss fetal pulse oximetry.

Key Terms

accelerations (ăk-sĕl-ĕr-Ā-shŭnz, p. 123)
amnioinfusion (ăm-nē-ō-ĭn-FŪ-zhăn, p. 127)
Apgar score (p. 140)
decelerations (dē-sĕl-ĕr-Ā-shŭnz, p. 123)
doula (DOO-lă, p. 132)
Duncan mechanism (p. 136)
early decelerations (p. 125)
external fetal monitoring (p. 121)
ferning (p. 127)
fetal pulse oximetry (ŏk-SĬM-ĕ-trē, p. 125)

internal fetal monitoring (p. 122)
late decelerations (p. 125)
Leopold's maneuvers (p. 127)
Nitrazine paper test (NĪ-tră-zēn, p. 127)
nonreassuring heart rate pattern (p. 120)
precipitate delivery (p. 143)
reassuring heart rate pattern (p. 120)
Schultze mechanism (p. 136)
variable decelerations (p. 125)

The labor and birth process is an exciting, anxiety-provoking, but rewarding time for the woman and her family. They are about to undergo one of the most meaningful and stressful events in life. The adequacy of their preparation for childbirth will now be tested. Labor begins with regular uterine contractions, continues with hours of hard work, and ends as the woman and her family begin the attachment process with their newborn.

The primary goal of nursing care is to ensure the best possible outcome for the mother and the newborn. Nursing care focuses on establishing a meaningful, open relationship; determining the fetal status; encouraging the woman's self-direction and ability to cope; and supporting the woman and her family throughout the labor and birth process. Research-based goals for normal labor and delivery include allowing labor to start on its own, allowing freedom of movement during labor, providing continuous labor support without routine interventions, allowing spontaneous pushing in a non-supine position, and keeping mother and infant together in skin-to-skin contact immediately after birth (AWHONN, 2007).

BIRTH SETTINGS

Birth settings can include traditional hospital birth settings, independent birthing centers, or home birth services. They often are designed, in principle, to emphasize the naturalness of childbirth. The nurse-midwife, in collaboration with the physician, assumes the overall management of the birth and prenatal and postpartum care. However, some alternative birth settings are managed by a nurse-midwife without a physician present. In these settings, the nurse assumes a variety of responsibilities, including childbirth education and assistance with the birth itself.

An important advantage of alternative birth settings to the woman and family is that they have more control over the events surrounding the birth experience. The woman has an opportunity to decide on her activities during labor. She is usually allowed to modify her eating and drinking patterns and can select different positions for comfort during labor and birth. In addition, her companions and family are given the opportunity to participate more in the birth process. Some common obstetric practices, such as artificial rupture of the membranes, intravenous administration of fluids, and administration of drugs, are minimized in alternative birth settings. If complications occur, the woman is transferred to a labor and delivery unit in a hospital.

IN-HOSPITAL BIRTHING ROOMS

An in-hospital birthing room is a hospital room or suite furnished to provide a homelike atmosphere conducive to the parents' participation in the birth (Figure 7-1). The woman stays in the same room for labor, delivery, and recovery; thus, the setting is called an *LDR room*. In some hospitals, the woman also remains in the same room during the postpartum stay, and that setting is known as an *LDRP room*. Siblings can visit and become acquainted with the newborn shortly after birth.

FREESTANDING CENTERS (OUT-OF-HOSPITAL BIRTHING CENTERS)

Some families choose the out-of-hospital birthing center for maternity care. These centers combine a home environment with a short-stay, ambulatory health facility with access to in-hospital obstetric and newborn care. Their advantage over home birth is quick access to the hospital facility if needed. The program usually provides comprehensive prenatal, birth, and postpartum care.

HOME BIRTH

A community-based nurse-midwife usually manages a home birth. The advantage of a home birth is that the woman is in familiar, comfortable surroundings during the labor and birth process with her family present. If hospitalization is not required, some couples decide on home birth because it is less expensive. However, the couple should know the risks involved in a home birth before making their decision. For example, there usually is a lack of emergency equipment and additional staff to handle emergencies, and their home may be too far from a hospital and medical care if any unforeseen complications arise.

CULTURAL CONSIDERATIONS

Knowledge about the beliefs, customs, and practices of different cultures should be incorporated in labor care (Table 7-1). **Modesty** is an important consideration for all women, but women in some cultures are particularly uncomfortable about exposure of their bodies. Exposure of as little of the woman's body as possible is recommended.

Pain expression varies with the cultural background. In some cultures, it is important for individuals to act in a manner that will not bring shame on the family; women, therefore, may not express pain outwardly. In other cultures, women may be vocally expressive during labor and cry out or moan with contractions and request pain relief.

Position preference varies with cultures, and there are differences within cultures. In many non-European societies uninfluenced by westernization, women assume an upright position in childbirth. In some cultures, kneeling or squatting during childbirth is common.

A **female care provider** is preferred in some cultures. Regardless of cultural background, the woman feels more comfortable and less stressed when her wishes are respected.

The **support person** with whom the woman feels comfortable varies according to her beliefs and

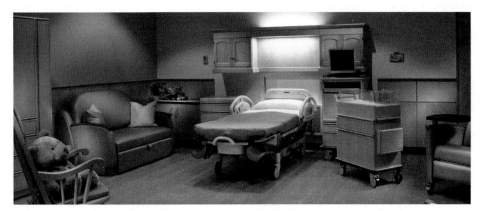

FIGURE 7-1 **A room used for labor, delivery, recovery, and postpartum (LDRP) care.** All of the furniture opens up to reveal the monitors and equipment needed.

Table 7-1   **Birth Practices of Selected Cultural Groups**

ROLE OF WOMAN IN LABOR AND DELIVERY	ROLE OF FATHER OR PARTNER IN LABOR AND DELIVERY
African American	
Participates actively Is vocal in labor Wants sponge bath postpartum only Avoids hair washing until lochia ceases	Female attendants are usually preferred.
American Indian	
Is stoic May have indigenous plants in room May wear special necklaces May use meditation chants Prefers water at room temperature to drink Prefers chicken soup and rice postpartum	Husband avoids eating meat during perinatal phase. Husband may provide support during labor.
Arabic	
Is passive but expressive Views keeping body covered as important May wear protective amulets May have low pain tolerance Values male newborn more than female Expects 20 days of bed rest after birth	Husband is not expected to participate but remains in control. Female family member is preferred as coach. Husband must be present if male health care provider examines woman. Husband may whisper praises in newborn's ear.
Brazilian	
May not participate in coping techniques during delivery Needs to be offered pain relief options Stays at home for 40 days postpartum except for medical appointments	Presence of husband in delivery room is discouraged.
Cambodian (Khmer)	
Is stoic in labor If walking during labor, must not pause in doorway (thought to delay birth) Does not want the infant's head touched without permission Colostrum discarded Will not nurse after delivery or eat vegetables in first week	Individual family preference decides whether father is present during delivery.
Central American (Guatemala, Nicaragua, El Salvador)	
Is vocal and active during labor May prefer to wear red (a protective color) If more affluent, prefers bottle feeding Prefers chicken soup, bananas, meat, and herbal tea Showers postpartum Avoids "cold foods"	Husband is expected to be present for support, but female family members participate more.
Chinese	
May be vocal during labor Must not pause in doorway if walking during labor (thought to delay birth) All doors and windows to be unlocked (thought to ease passage of infant) Do not use first name of woman May not shower for 30 days postpartum Covers ears to prevent air from entering body Prefers breastfeeding Needs to be encouraged to ask questions	Husband usually does not play an active role in labor and delivery, but oldest male makes decisions. Woman's mother may participate.
Cuban	
Is vocal but passive during labor and delivery Uses formal name at introduction Must stay at home 41 days postpartum and be sheltered from stress	Mother of woman is preferred as coach. Husbands are not usually involved in labor but must be informed first of problems and progress.

Table 7-1   Birth Practices of Selected Cultural Groups—cont'd

ROLE OF WOMAN IN LABOR AND DELIVERY	ROLE OF FATHER OR PARTNER IN LABOR AND DELIVERY
Eritrean, Ethiopian	
Is stoic but takes active role Modesty very important; must remain covered Prefers breastfeeding for 2 years Remains in seclusion 40 days postpartum Consumes warm food and drinks during puerperium	Traditionally, husbands are not allowed to be present during labor and delivery.
Falkland Islands Native	
Places keys (unlock) and combs (untangle) under pillow of labor bed	
Filipino	
Prefers slippery foods (such as eggs) so infant will "slip through birth canal" Prefers midwife support Assumes active role in labor Prefers sponge baths postpartum	Husband is not usually with woman during labor.
Hindu, Sikh, Muslim, Nepalese, Fijian, Pakistani	
Assumes passive role and follows directions of trained professionals May keep head covered during labor Prenatal care started on 120th day of gestation Should not reveal sex of newborn until after placenta is delivered (to avoid upsetting the mother if the sex is not of her preference) Takes sponge baths postpartum Remains in seclusion 40 days postpartum	Female coach is preferred, although father waits near labor room for consultation. Husband must be present if male physician examines woman. Ceremony of *A quqah* involves father shaving head of newborn and whispering praises into ear of newborn. Coach may chant scriptures during birth.
Hmong (Laos, Myanmar [Burma], Thailand)	
Is usually quiet and passive Avoids multiple caregivers Avoids internal examinations Views full genital exposure as unacceptable Prefers squat position Do not remove amulets on wrists and ankles Do not use first name initially Prefers chicken, white rice, and warm fluids postpartum Bottle feeding popular	Husband is usually present and makes all decisions.
Israeli (Orthodox Jewish)	
Prefers nurse-midwife Maintains modesty Must not be intimate with husband until 7 days after lochia stops Males circumcised on the eighth day Females named on first Saturday after birth	Husband may not participate in prenatal classes. Husband may not touch wife during labor, view perineum, or view baby being born. Husband may participate from afar with verbal encouragement during labor. Woman's mother participates in birth process.
Japanese	
Prefers north part of room May cut hair and take special vows Is assertive during labor but may not ask for pain relief Values modesty Will bathe and shower postpartum May expose infant to loud noises and music twice a day for a week to ward off evil spirits	Husband chants and throws rice to ward off evil spirits. Modern-day husbands are present and participate during labor and delivery. In modern Japan, husbands are compliant with health education.
Korean	
Is compliant with health care provider Avoids ice water Is an active participant in labor Do not address by first name initially Prefers sponge bath postpartum May not wish to ambulate early	Husband participates in labor and delivery. Husband prefers not to be told in advance of fetal prognosis. Family makes medical decisions.

Continued

Table **7-1**   Birth Practices of Selected Cultural Groups—cont'd

ROLE OF WOMAN IN LABOR AND DELIVERY	ROLE OF FATHER OR PARTNER IN LABOR AND DELIVERY
Mexican American	

Believes supine position is best for fetus
Selects her preferred coach
Prefers privacy
Accepts pain but is active in labor
Will not shower postpartum and walks to bathroom only
Avoids beans postpartum
Uses alternative therapies for mother and newborn
  (see Chapter 21)
	Husband is in control of decisions but is not present
	  during labor.
	Female relatives provide support.
	Husband prefers not to be told in advance of serious
	  fetal prognosis.

Puerto Rican	

Is active in labor
Prefers hospital care
Keeps body covered
Does not eat beans, starch, or eggs if breastfeeding
Will not wash hair for 40 days postpartum
Prefers sponge bath and lotions
	Husband assumes supportive role during labor and
	  delivery.
	If not present during delivery, husband expects to be
	  kept informed.

Vietnamese	
Woman expected to "suffer in silence" Needs to be offered options for pain relief Prefers upright position for labor and delivery Prefers warm fluids to drink Sponge bathes only for 2 weeks postpartum Newborn not praised to protect from jealousy	Female family member is preferred. Husband is expected to remain nearby. Sexual intercourse is prohibited during pregnancy and puerperium.
West Indian (Trinidad and Tobago, Jamaica, Barbados)	
Prefers midwife Maintains passive role and follows instructions Prefers bed rest for 1 week postpartum Do not address by first name initially	Female relative or friend as coach is preferred. Husband is not present in area.

Data from Leifer, G. (2010). *Introduction to maternity and pediatric nursing* (6th ed.). Philadelphia: Saunders; Lowdermilk, D. I., Perry, S., & Hockenberry, D. (2010). *Maternal child nursing care,* St. Louis: Mosby; Wong, D.I., Perry, S.E., & Hockenberry-Eaton, M. (2009). *Maternal and child nursing care.* (2nd ed.). St. Louis: Mosby; Nichols, F. H., & Zwelling, E. (1997). *Maternal-newborn nursing: Theory and practice.* Philadelphia: Saunders; Minark, P. A., Lipson, J. G., & Dibble, S. I. (1996). *Culture and nursing care.* San Francisco: University of California; Lipson, J.F., & Steiger, N.J. (1996). *Self-care nursing in a multicultural context.* Thousand Oaks, CA: Sage publications; Murasaki, S. (1996). *Diary of Lady Murasaki.* New York: Penguin Books.
Note: Use professional translators whenever possible. Family members may not accurately convey cultural preferences.

customs. The woman's mother or a female relative (rather than her husband or male partner) may give support during labor. Women from a strong matriarchal family structure may prefer their mothers or female extended family members to be with them during the labor process. Cultural sensitivity will assist nurses in being nonjudgmental, and they will be less likely to impose their own values and beliefs on women they care for (Nursing Care Plan 7-1).

CARE MANAGEMENT

WHEN TO GO TO THE HOSPITAL OR BIRTH CENTER

During late pregnancy, the woman should be instructed about when to go to the hospital or birth center. This is *not* an exact time, but the general guidelines are:

→ *Contractions:* The woman should go to the hospital or birth center when the contractions have a pattern of increasing frequency, duration, and intensity. The woman having her first child is usually

advised to enter the facility when contractions have been regular (every 5 minutes) for 1 hour. Women having second or later children should go sooner, when regular contractions are 10 minutes apart for a period of 1 hour.

→ *Ruptured membranes:* The woman should go to the birth facility if her membranes rupture or if she thinks they may have ruptured.

→ *Bleeding other than bloody show:* Bloody show is a mixture of blood and thick mucus. Active bleeding is free flowing, bright red, and not mixed with thick mucus.

→ *Decreased fetal movement:* The woman should be evaluated if the fetus is moving less than usual. Many fetuses become quiet shortly before labor, but decreased fetal activity can also be a sign of fetal compromise or fetal demise (death).

→ *Any other concern:* Because these guidelines cannot cover every situation, the woman should contact her health care provider or go to the birth facility for evaluation if she has any other concerns.

Nursing Care Plan 7-1 **Culturally Sensitive Care**

Scenario
Mrs. G. is a 24-year-old para 1, gravida 2, patient who recently immigrated to the United States. She is in active labor and appears frightened. You are responsible for admitting Mrs. G. to the labor and delivery unit. Mrs. G. speaks no English, and her husband's English is extremely limited.

Selected Nursing Diagnosis
Decisional conflict related to the desire to please health care workers and desire to engage in cultural rituals and practices

Expected Outcomes	Nursing Interventions	Rationales
Patient will participate with nurse in developing a culturally acceptable plan for obstetric care.	Assess cultural rituals and practices that are important to the patient by interview, with an interpreter if necessary or with a birth plan questionnaire.	Information obtained aids in the development of a culturally congruent individualized care plan.
	Approach patient and support person in an unhurried manner, allowing sufficient time for discussions with them.	Relieves anxiety and conveys a message of acceptance.
	Explain to patient that she has the right to help develop the care plan and request that the care include specific cultural rituals and practices.	Patients and support persons are more likely to make requests when they are informed it is acceptable to participate in the care plan.
Patient will freely verbalize her desires when asked to participate in practices that do not agree with her cultural preferences.	Allow patient to engage in cultural rituals and practices whenever it is medically safe to do so.	Allows patient to engage in activities that can be comforting and can enhance her coping abilities.
Patient will express satisfaction with the care received during her hospitalization.	Whenever possible, provide choices to patients (e.g., "Would you like to take a shower now or would you prefer to wait?").	Allows patient to choose culturally acceptable ways of doing things without feeling as if she is being disrespectful to health care provider.

Selected Nursing Diagnosis
Impaired verbal communication related to the effects of a language barrier

Expected Outcomes	Nursing Interventions	Rationales
Patient and support persons will have all essential information communicated to them in a manner that they can understand.	Whenever possible, assign a nurse who speaks the same language as the patient.	Allows for direct communication between nurse and patient and lessens risks of misinterpretation.
Patient and support persons will have their questions answered.	Provide a hospital interpreter of the same sex whenever possible, and inform patient that all information will be kept confidential.	Knowing that the information they reveal will be kept confidential may encourage verbalization.
Health care providers will become aware of needs of patient and support persons as they arise.	Face the patient and support person when speaking, and direct conversation to them rather than to the interpreter.	Enhances communication between nurse and the patient and support person, and allows observation of nonverbal communication.
	In the absence of an interpreter, provide a questionnaire in the patient's native language to be given on admission that includes assessment information that can be answered with numbers, yes/no answers, or multiple choice answers.	Can be compared with an identical questionnaire written in English or the dominant language of health care workers to provide important assessment data.
	Assess for patient's and support person's nonverbal signs of needs or concerns.	Facial expressions or tone of voice used as the patient and support person interact can be clues that they have questions or concerns.
	Write down short yes/no questions and simple commands you can use to communicate with the patient and support person.	Allows for quick assessments to be made in the absence of an interpreter. It is important to remember that some patients may respond "yes" even when they do not understand the question; therefore, it is important to look for agreement between the verbal and nonverbal responses or behaviors.

Continued

Nursing Care Plan 7-1   **Culturally Sensitive Care—cont'd**

Expected Outcomes	Nursing Interventions	Rationales
	Communicate with support person by using simple words and short sentences.	When English is limited, the ability to understand what is said decreases as the complexity of the words and sentence structure increases.
	Assess ability to read, and provide literature to patients in their native language if appropriate.	If patient can read written information, it can be an effective way of communicating when verbal communication is impaired.
	Use pictures, diagrams, flash cards, or body signals to communicate.	Can be an effective way to convey information or directions in the absence of an interpreter.
	As much as possible, avoid unnecessary communication with others in the presence of the patient or support person.	Carrying on long conversations with others in a language the patient and support person cannot understand can be construed as being disrespectful and elicit unnecessary fears and anxieties.

Selected Nursing Diagnosis

Fear related to unfamiliarity with the dominant culture's environment or childbirth practices

Expected Outcomes	Nursing Interventions	Rationales
Patient will freely express her feelings and concerns.	Orient patient to the environment, equipment, procedures, routines, and anticipatory guidance of what she can expect. Use interpreter as needed.	Knowledge can reduce fears and anxieties by clearing up misconceptions.
Patient will verbalize and use coping strategies to alleviate fear.	Use events to identify or estimate when things will occur (e.g., before sunset, after lunch).	Many cultures rely on events rather than a clock to determine time. When patients can anticipate approximate time frames, fear and anxiety can be reduced.
Patient will state she is less afraid.	Encourage family members to visit or stay with patient.	Provides support to the patient.
Patient will have relaxed facial expressions.	Encourage patient to express fears and concerns.	Provides the opportunity to correct misconceptions or misunderstandings.
	Assess childbirth and newborn cultural practices and rituals that are important to patient. Unless contraindicated or unsafe, allow patient to participate in those practices.	Provides insight into cultural belief system that can be used to individualize a care plan. Participating in cultural practices can provide feelings of security, which help alleviate fear.
	Maintain a nonjudgmental attitude toward cultural practices that are safe to implement.	Conveys feelings of acceptance and decreases patient's fears of not acting in expected manner.
	Provide scientific rationale for practices that are contraindicated or unsafe and develop mutually acceptable compromises for these practices.	Knowledge allows patients to make informed decisions about adopting safer practices.
	Provide frequent encouragement to the patient and support person.	Increases patient's and support person's feelings of well-being and self-worth.

Critical Thinking Question

1. In the absence of an interpreter or a questionnaire in the woman's native language, what other methods can you use to obtain necessary data?

The woman's knowledge of her own body complements professional knowledge. Thus, when the woman feels "something is different," she should be given positive encouragement for her self-monitoring of symptoms rather than her focusing on the exact symptoms of true or false labor (Palmer & Carty, 2006).

Data collection begins at the first contact with the woman, whether by telephone or in person. Women are encouraged to call the hospital labor and delivery unit or birthing center if they have questions about when to come to the hospital to be evaluated. The manner and expression or tone of voice in which the nurse communicates with the woman during their first contact can influence how the woman will feel about her birth experience.

PREADMISSION FORMS

The nurse should review the available preadmission forms because they may have been completed a few weeks before admission. The prenatal record has information, including nursing and medical parameters, laboratory results, and nutritional guidance, that has been provided. Expressed psychosocial and cultural factors, including the woman's birth plan and her special requests or needs, may also be documented.

CARE PLAN

A major challenge for the nurse is the formulation of a care plan for labor and birth. An individualized plan should include the woman's coping mechanisms and support systems (see Chapter 5). The plan also includes whether the woman will labor, give birth, and recover in the same room or be transferred to a delivery room to give birth. Also, the care plan reflects the degree to which the partner will participate in the labor process.

The teaching aspect of the plan should incorporate what the woman can expect in labor care. The nursing care plan provides an important means of communication between the woman and the nurse (Nursing Care Plan 7-2).

DATA COLLECTION AND ADMISSION PROCEDURES

The nurse is responsible for collecting data concerning the woman being admitted. Components of the admission information can be obtained from the prenatal record and then verified or updated. Women who have not had prenatal care will need to give more information to the nurse. The nurse's data collection during admission focuses on three priorities: to determine (1) the condition of the mother and the fetus, (2) whether birth is imminent, and (3) whether the woman's labor appears uneventful. Most facilities have a preprinted form to guide admission data collection. Women who have had prenatal care should have a prenatal record on file for the retrieval of information. Women who have not had prenatal care will have additional laboratory tests, which may include a complete blood count,

---

⭐ Nursing Care Plan 7-2   Uncomplicated Labor and Delivery

Scenario
A woman, Para 0, Gravida 1, is admitted to the labor unit in active labor and placed on an external electronic fetal monitor. She appears anxious and fearful and states she is worried about the welfare of her baby.

Selected Nursing Diagnosis
Ineffective coping related to fear, anxiety, and feelings of powerlessness

Expected Outcomes	Nursing Interventions	Rationales
Patient will exhibit appropriate coping mechanisms and will be able to cooperate with support person and nursing staff.	Introduce yourself to the patient and support person.	Establishing rapport with patient and her support person decreases their anxiety.
	Orient patient to the unit. Explain equipment, procedures, and what to expect before each intervention.	Instruction enhances understanding of anticipated events. Knowledge decreases anxiety.
	Assess for signs and symptoms of ineffective coping (e.g., verbalization of feelings of powerlessness or inability to cope, crying spells, rapid speech, inability to follow directions or make decisions, muscle and facial tension).	Allows for early interventions to enhance coping abilities. Ineffective coping can increase the perception of pain, decrease ability to tolerate pain, and decrease comprehension of verbal instruction. Fear and anxiety cause the adrenal glands to release catecholamines, which can inhibit uterine contractions and divert blood flow from the placenta.
	Explain all procedures before initiating them; use simple, concise terms; and repeat explanations as needed.	Anticipatory guidance helps alleviate fears and anxieties. When anxiety level is high, patients may be able to comprehend only small amounts of information at one time and often require repeat instructions.
	Encourage patient and support person to ask questions. Also, encourage verbalization of fears and concerns, and use active listening techniques.	Allows for the opportunity to correct misconceptions and misunderstandings that might be contributing to fears and anxieties. Active listening techniques encourage the woman and support person to share information, acknowledge their feelings, and convey to them feelings of acceptance.
	Explain pain control options that are available.	Reassures patient that pain control measures are available and that she has a choice of whether to use them.

Continued

Nursing Care Plan 7-2 | Uncomplicated Labor and Delivery—cont'd

Expected Outcomes	Nursing Interventions	Rationales
	Approach patient in a calm, confident manner (do not appear rushed). Remain with patient as much as possible; when you leave, reassure her you will be nearby and will respond to call light. If central monitoring is used, reassure patient that fetal well-being is being continuously monitored.	Promotes feelings of security. Patient often perceives the nurse as "expert" and experiences less fear and anxiety when the nurse is perceived as being competent and readily available. Knowing that fetal well-being is continuously being monitored relieves concerns that prompt intervention will be delayed if required.
	Keep patient informed of labor progress and fetal well-being.	Reassurance that labor is progressing normally and the fetus is doing well decreases fears and anxieties.
Patient will be able to make informed decisions regarding treatment options.	Provide patient with choices as much as possible. Whenever possible, offer suggestions rather than give commands.	Decreases feelings of powerlessness and may be helpful in gaining inner control.
Patient will express increased feelings of control.	Help patient identify situations that she does have control over (e.g., positioning, pain control methods, relaxation techniques).	Decreases feelings of powerlessness and may be helpful in gaining inner control.
	Encourage use of cultural or religious rituals and practices unless contraindicated.	Can provide strength, comfort, and enhanced ability to cope; may help alleviate feelings of powerlessness.
	Help patient identify coping mechanisms that have been helpful in the past, review those taught in childbirth classes, and teach new coping mechanisms as needed.	Use of coping mechanisms that have been helpful in the past may be successful in the current situation. Helping the patient with relaxation techniques and diversional activities can increase coping abilities and sense of control.
	Accept verbal expressions of anger.	Verbalizing feelings of frustration and anger can be an effective coping mechanism for some patients.
	When patient is out of control or during transition, provide firm, short, concise directions.	Preventing destructive behaviors (such as physically hitting others or pushing before completely dilated) can help preserve self-esteem and prevent injury to self and others.
	Provide positive feedback for use of coping mechanisms and childbirth methods used.	Encouragement enhances self-confidence and provides the strength to continue.

Selected Nursing Diagnosis

Ineffective tissue perfusion (fetal) related to impaired gas exchange during labor and delivery process

Expected Outcomes	Nursing Interventions	Rationales
Fetal heart rate (FHR) variability will be present, with an FHR baseline of 110-160 beats/minute and FHR accelerations.	Obtain an initial 20-minute electronic fetal monitoring tracing.	Provides baseline status of fetal well-being. FHR baseline should be 110-160 beats/minute, with baseline variability of 6-10 beats/minute. Accelerations of 15 beats/minute for 15 seconds are a reassuring sign of fetal well-being. Nonreassuring findings would allow for immediate intervention.
	Continue monitoring fetus by continuous electronic fetal monitoring; intermittent electronic monitoring for 15 minutes every hour, by Doppler every hour during latent phase of labor, every 30 minutes during active phase of labor, and every 15 minutes during second stage of labor; or per hospital protocols or provider orders.	Allows for prompt intervention when nonreassuring FHR patterns are observed.
	Monitor FHR immediately after rupture of bag of waters.	When membranes rupture and the fetal head is not engaged, cord prolapse (an obstetric emergency) can occur.

Nursing Care Plan 7-2   Uncomplicated Labor and Delivery—cont'd

Expected Outcomes	Nursing Interventions	Rationales
	When bag of waters ruptures, note color and odor of amniotic fluid.	Foul odor is indicative of infection. Green tinge to the amniotic fluid indicates that the fetus has defecated in utero, which occurs during hypoxic episodes.
	Monitor maternal heart rate and blood pressure every hour and as needed or per hospital protocols or provider orders.	Decreased cardiac output or maternal hypotension can result in decreased blood flow to the placenta.
Absence of nonreassuring FHR patterns (late decelerations, severe variable, absent variability, etc.) will indicate adequate tissue perfusion to uterus.	If nonreassuring patterns occur, reposition the patient.	Changing positions to the side or knee-chest can relieve pressure on the umbilical cord, allowing more blood to flow through it. Repositioning also prevents supine hypotension, which decreases blood flow to the placenta.
	If nonreassuring patterns occur, provide oxygen at 8-10 L/minute by mask.	Hyperoxygenation of the mother's blood increases the delivery of oxygen to the fetus.
	If nonreassuring patterns occur, stop oxytocin (Pitocin) infusion.	Oxytocin intensifies uterine contractions, which decrease placental blood flow.
	Notify the health care provider of nonreassuring FHR patterns.	Allows additional interventions that require an order or health care provider interventions.
	Administer tocolytics as ordered.	Tocolytics decrease the number and intensity of uterine contractions, which allow for increased blood flow to the placenta.
	Assist with placement of internal fetal monitors as indicated.	Internal fetal monitoring allows for accurate monitoring of FHR variability and gives true intensity of uterine contractions.
	Assist with amnioinfusion as indicated.	Provides a fluid cushion around the umbilical cord, which aids in decreasing cord compression and allows more oxygen to reach the fetus.
	Increase nonadditive intravenous fluids as ordered.	Corrects maternal hypotension.
	Assist with obtaining fetal scalp blood sample for pH testing and fetal pulse oximetry.	Provides acid and base levels of fetus and allows for prompt intervention if indicated.
Normal Apgar score will be ≥7 at 5 minutes	Prepare for cesarean birth or vacuum extraction per hospital protocol when ordered.	When nonreassuring FHR patterns, scalp pH, or fetal pulse oximetry indicates fetal hypoxia, immediate delivery often becomes the only safe option to protect the fetus from injury.

Critical Thinking Question
1. What is a priority nursing action when a nonreassuring FHR appears on the monitor during active labor?

---

hematocrit, drug screen, tests for sexually transmitted infections, and others as indicated. Box 7-1 outlines nursing responsibilities during patient admissions.

NURSING CARE OF PATIENT IN FALSE LABOR

True labor is characterized by changes in the cervix (effacement and dilation), which is the key distinction between true and false labors. See Table 6-1 for other characteristics of true and false labors.

A better term for false labor might be *prodromal labor* because these contractions help prepare the woman's body and the fetus for true labor. Many women are observed for a short while (1 to 2 hours) if their initial assessment suggests that they are not in true labor and their membranes are intact. The mother and fetus are assessed during observation as if labor were occurring.

Most facilities run an external electronic fetal monitor (EFM) strip for at least 20 minutes to document fetal well-being. The woman can usually walk about when not being monitored. If she is in true labor, walking often helps intensify the contractions and causes cervical effacement and dilation.

After the observation period, the woman's labor status is reevaluated by the health care provider, and another vaginal examination is performed. If there is no change in the cervical effacement or dilation, the woman is usually sent home to await true labor. Sometimes, if it is her first child and she lives nearby, the woman in very early labor is sent home because the latent phase of most first labors is quite long.

Each woman in false labor (or early latent-phase labor) is evaluated individually. Factors to be

Box 7-1   Admission Data Collection

1. Place identification bracelet on woman.
2. Obtain necessary information for labor record.
3. Document vital signs. Report blood pressure greater than 140/80 mm Hg.
4. Record fetal heart rate. Report rates less than 110 or more than 160 beats/minute.
5. Determine whether amniotic membranes have ruptured. Describe any vaginal discharge.
6. Assess uterine contractions.
7. Monitor intravenous fluids if ordered.
8. Document allergy history.
9. Document time of last food intake. Explain NPO (nothing by mouth), ice chips, or clear liquid only status during labor.
10. Determine recent illness or medication use.
11. Obtain required consent signatures with appropriate witness signatures.
12. Review results of laboratory tests from prenatal chart. Document blood Rh status and vital signs.
13. Orient woman and partner to unit.
14. Discuss care preferences (see Figure 5-2).
15. Secure the woman's personal items.

considered include the number and duration of previous labors, distance from the facility, and availability of transportation.

Legal and Ethical Considerations

The Woman in False Labor

Encourage the woman in false labor to return to the hospital or birthing center when she thinks she should. It is better to have another "trial run" than for her to stay home until she is in advanced labor.

The woman in false labor is often frustrated and needs generous reassurance that her symptoms will eventually change to true labor. No one stays pregnant forever, although it sometimes feels that way to a woman who has had several false alarms and is tired of being pregnant. Guidelines for coming to the facility should be reinforced before she leaves. If her membranes are ruptured, she is usually admitted even if labor has not begun because of the risk for infection or a prolapsed umbilical cord (see Chapter 14).

FOCUSED DATA COLLECTION FOR FIRST AND SECOND STAGES OF LABOR

In addition to creating an environment of trust and security, meeting informational needs, promoting relaxation, and providing a support system, the nurse must address specific physical concerns throughout the labor process. These nursing assessments and interventions begin during the first stage and continue through the labor process.

Priority activities are performed to assess the condition of the mother and fetus and to determine when the birth is imminent. Several assessments relate to the safety of both the mother and the fetus and therefore need to be carried out in a consistent time frame. In addition, any departure from the normal progress of labor should be promptly documented and reported.

⚠ Safety Alert

Warning Signs of Potential Complications

- Maternal fever greater than 38° C (100.4° F)
- Contractions lasting more than 90 seconds
- Contractions less than 2 minutes apart
- Fetal bradycardia or tachycardia
- Loss of baseline variability on fetal monitor
- Meconium-stained amniotic fluid
- Foul-smelling vaginal discharge = infection
- Excessive bleeding and hypotension
- Fetal heart rate less than 110 or greater than 160 beats/minute

[handwritten annotations: "Report to doctor immediately." and "indicates fetal distress."]

MONITORING FETAL HEART RATE

The fetal heart rate (FHR) should be assessed by auscultation with a Doppler transducer or fetoscope if the woman is not on an EFM. The location of the strongest fetal heart tone depends on the fetal position because the heart tone is best heard over the fetal back (Figure 7-2). If the woman and fetus are determined to be at low risk, the FHR is monitored and documented per routine (Skill 7-1). A sudden change in FHR or a measurement outside of the range of 110 to 160 beats/minute should be immediately reported. FHR should be taken immediately after the rupture of membranes because any prolapse of the umbilical cord is most likely to occur at this time. In addition, the FHR should be taken after a vaginal examination, administration of medications, and notation of abnormal fetal activity.

A Doppler transducer or a fetoscope is used to auscultate the FHR between, during, and immediately after uterine contractions. Advantages of continuously monitoring FHR with an EFM include the ability to evaluate FHR variability and to identify abnormalities in FHR patterns.

When a woman is on an EFM, the nurse should closely observe the FHR tracing. The nurse should report signs of fetal distress to the physician or nurse-midwife immediately. These signs include (1) a loss of baseline variability, (2) variable or late decelerations that persist after maternal position change, and (3) persistent fetal tachycardia. Meconium in the amniotic fluid when the fetus is in a vertex position, a sign of fetal distress, should also be reported.

Intermittent Fetal Heart Monitoring During Labor

Fetal monitoring during labor is an integral part of nursing care. Intrapartum fetal monitoring is surveillance used to identify the healthy fetus or the

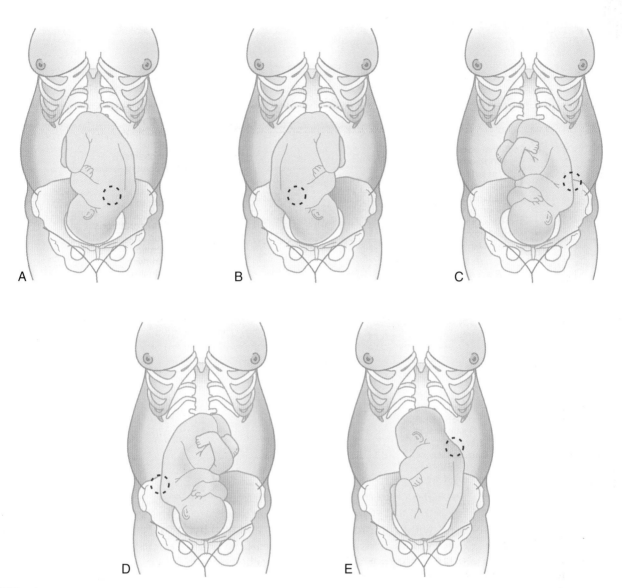

FIGURE 7-2 **Best location for hearing fetal heart tone on woman's abdomen corresponding to fetal positions. A,** Left occiput anterior. **B,** Right occiput anterior. **C,** Left occiput posterior. **D,** Right occiput posterior. **E,** Left sacral anterior.

Skill 7-1   Auscultating Fetal Heart Rate*

PURPOSE

To assess and document fetal heart rate.

Steps

1. Use Leopold's maneuvers to identify fetal back (see Skill 7-3). (FHR is best heard through the fetal back.)*
2. Assess FHR with a fetoscope, Doppler transducer, or external fetal heart monitor.
3. Using the fetoscope, place the bell over the fetal back with the head plate pressed against your forehead. Move the fetoscope until you locate where the sounds are the loudest.
4. Using the Doppler transducer, review instructions.
5. Place water-soluble conducting gel over the transducer, and turn the instrument on.
6. Place the transducer on the abdomen over the fetal back, and move it until you clearly hear the sounds.
7. Palpate the mother's radial pulse to see whether it is synchronized with the sounds of the fetoscope. If so, try another location to get fetal heart sounds that do not synchronize with the maternal pulse.
8. Assess the FHR for 30 to 60 seconds. Average rate is 110 to 160 beats/minute. Report nonreassuring signs. FHR outside of the normal limit (less than 110 or more than 160 beats/minute) and slowing of FHR that persists after the contraction ends. Further evaluation may be necessary.

*See Figure 7-2 for approximate locations of the fetal heart rate (FHR) at different fetal positions.

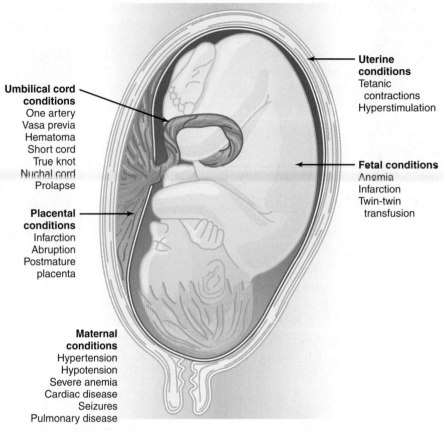

Uterine conditions
Tetanic contractions
Hyperstimulation

Umbilical cord conditions
One artery
Vasa previa
Hematoma
Short cord
True knot
Nuchal cord
Prolapse

Fetal conditions
Anemia
Infarction
Twin-twin transfusion

Placental conditions
Infarction
Abruption
Postmature placenta

Maternal conditions
Hypertension
Hypotension
Severe anemia
Cardiac disease
Seizures
Pulmonary disease

FIGURE 7-3 Clinical conditions associated with fetal distress in labor.

fetus showing signs associated with compromise (Figure 7-3). During labor, uterine contractions compress the spiral arteries, temporarily stopping maternal blood flow into intervillous spaces. Between contractions, during the period of relaxation, fresh oxygenated maternal blood reenters the intervillous spaces, and waste products drain out. A normal fetus can withstand the stress of uterine contractions without developing hypoxia because sufficient oxygenation occurs between contractions. Prolonged contractions can lead to uterine placental insufficiency (UPI) and fetal hypoxia. Fetal well-being during labor is measured by the response of the FHR to uterine contractions.

Low-risk technology is a method of fetal monitoring that uses **intermittent auscultation** of FHR by a hand-held Doppler ultrasound device or a fetoscope between, during, and immediately after uterine contractions. The FHR is assessed at 30-minute intervals during the first stage of labor and at 15-minute intervals during the second stage of labor (AAP, 2007) (Box 7-2). In addition, the FHR is assessed after the

Box **7-2**   **When to Auscultate and Document the Fetal Heart Rate**

Use these guidelines for documenting the fetal heart rate (FHR) when the woman has intermittent auscultation or continuous electronic fetal monitoring.

ROUTINE AUSCULTATION
- Every hour in the latent phase
- Every 30 minutes in the active phase of first stage (after a contraction)
- Every 15 minutes in the second stage

WOMEN WITH HIGH-RISK FACTORS
- Every 15 minutes in the first stage
- Every 5 minutes in the second stage

SPECIAL AUSCULTATIONS
- When the membranes rupture (spontaneously or artificially)
- Before and after ambulation
- Before and after medication or anesthesia administration or a change in medication
- At the time of peak action of analgesic drugs
- After a vaginal examination
- After the expulsion of enema
- After urinary catheterization
- If uterine contractions are abnormal or excessive
- When the IV rate of oxytocin is changed
- Every 15 minutes for 1 hour after start of epidural
- Upon recognition of abnormal uterine activity

Data from Hacker, N. F., Moore, J. G., & Gambone, J. (2009). *Hacker and Moore's essentials of obstetrics and gynecology* (5th ed.). Philadelphia: Saunders; Leifer, G. (2010). *Introduction to maternity and pediatric nursing* (6th ed.). Philadelphia: Saunders; and Miller, D. (2010). Intrapartum fetal monitoring. *Contemporary OB/GYN,* 55(2), 26-36.

contraction, and an increase or decrease in FHR is documented. This type of fetal assessment is more commonly done in home births and birthing centers (Skill 7-2). In hospitals, most women have EFM at some period during their labor. In some institutions, a 20-minute EFM strip is obtained for all patients admitted to the labor unit; intermittent FHR monitoring may then be done (Table 7-2).

The ideal method of fetal assessment during labor contractions continues to be debated. The advantage of auscultation of FHR is that it places fewer restrictions on maternal activity. Health care providers in the United States usually prefer to use continuous EFM for their labor patients because they feel legally vulnerable when prescribing intermittent auscultation. Because continuous FHR monitoring is so widely used in the United States, it has been implicated in the higher incidence of cesarean births. For a woman who is considered to be at low risk, a short recorded strip of approximately 5 minutes every 30 minutes or in accordance with the hospital's policy may be used.

Continuous Electronic Fetal Monitoring During Labor

Electronic FHR monitoring can detect changes in FHR during labor that indicate inadequate oxygenation of the fetus. Immediate interventions can safeguard the fetus against some possible complications. EFM provides a visual display of the FHR. A continuous tracing of the FHR can be obtained, allowing many characteristics to be observed and evaluated. Uterine activity is also measured and displayed. Data obtained from the fetal monitor are transcribed on a continuous strip of graph paper (Figure 7-4). EFM data can be electronically transmitted

Skill 7-2   Determining Manual Fetal Heart Rate

PURPOSE
To assess and document fetal heart rate.

Steps
Location
1. Identify where the clearest fetal heart sounds will most likely be found (over the fetal back and usually in the lower abdomen).

Fetoscope
a. Place the head attachment (if there is one) over your head and the earpieces in your ear.
b. Place the bell of the scope in the approximate area of the fetal back and press firmly while listening for the muffled fetal heart sounds. When they are heard, count the rate for 1 full minute.
c. Count the rate in 6-second increments for at least 1 minute. Multiply the low and high numbers by 10 to compute the average range of the rate (e.g., 130 to 140 beats/minute).
d. Assess rate before and after at least one full contraction cycle.
e. Check the mother's pulse at the same time if uncertain whether the fetal heart sounds are being heard; the rates and rhythms will be different.

Doppler Transducer
a. Put water-soluble gel on the head of the hand-held transducer.
b. Put the earpieces in your ear, or connect the transducer to a speaker.
c. Turn the switch on and place the transducer head over the approximate area of the fetal back.
d. Count the heart rate as instructed previously. If earpieces are used, let the parents hear the fetal heartbeat.

Chart the Rate
1. Promptly report rates less than 110 beats/minute or more than 160 beats/minute for a term fetus.
2. Report slowing of the rate that lingers after the end of a contraction.

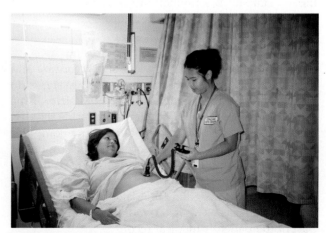

Doppler fetal heart rate (FHR) monitoring. The FHR is checked during each prenatal visit and during labor. Hearing the fetal heartbeat is reassuring to the expectant mother and helps her accept the reality of her pregnancy.

Table 7-2   Classification of Fetal Heart Rate Patterns

CLASSIFICATION	CHARACTERISTICS	NURSING INTERVENTIONS
Category 1 (Reassuring)	Baseline 110-160 BPM Moderate variability Accelerations may be present No late decelerations Early decelerations may be present	Continue monitoring Q 30 minutes first stage and Q 15 minutes second stage
Category 2 (Questionable)	Any FHR not stated in category 1 or 3 Tachycardia Bradycardia No accelerations with fetal stimulation	Continue monitoring Q 15 minutes first stage; Q 5 minutes 2nd stage Interventions to improve fetal blood flow and oxygenation: e.g., change maternal position; administer O$_2$; adjust IV fluids
Category 3 (Abnormal)	Recurrent late decelerations Bradycardia Sinusoidal pattern	Prepare for expedited delivery

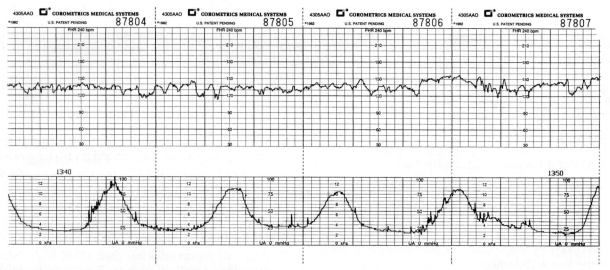

FIGURE 7-4 **Normal (reassuring) fetal heart rate (FHR) pattern.** Upper grid represents the FHR, and lower grid represents uterine contractions. The FHR is in the normal range of 110 to 160 beats/minute. Note the saw-toothed appearance of the FHR tracing, which indicates variability.

to a bank of video screens centrally located in the nurses' station for continuous assessment when health care providers are not at the bedside.

Documenting Electronic Fetal Monitoring

Recent advances also permit electronic recording and storage of EFM on disk. Some of the new systems do not use graph paper or produce the EFM strip. If the nurse wants to review FHR patterns or uterine activity, he or she retrieves the information with a computer program that displays the information on a monitor (Figure 7-5). Computers are increasingly used to help nurses manage the large amount of information generated. Computer programs may alert the nurse to abnormal patterns. The fetal monitor strip becomes part of the patient's medical record.

Because the nurse often maintains some responsibility for fetal monitoring, he or she is also responsible for acquiring and interpreting knowledge about advances in technology as they are introduced in the labor unit.

THE NURSE'S ROLE

The nurse's role is to continually assess whether the FHR pattern is a reassuring heart rate pattern, which reflects adequate fetal oxygenation (Figure 7-6). Nonreassuring heart rate patterns indicate fetal distress, and appropriate nursing interventions must be taken. Management of labor patients includes careful documentation on the patient's chart and the monitor strip. Appropriate nursing care during labor includes knowing FHR patterns and initiating interventions as necessary. Early recognition of changes in the FHR pattern serves as a warning that will enable early intervention to prevent fetal death or irreversible brain damage.

Before beginning fetal monitoring, the nurse explains the procedure to the woman and her support person. As the monitor strip continues to run and care is provided, interventions (vaginal examinations, voiding, etc.) are recorded on the strip and on the medical record. This information is significant in the assessment of the tracing and provides permanent

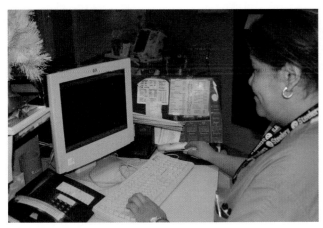

FIGURE 7-5 Nurse is checking the electronic fetal monitor on the computer at the nursing station.

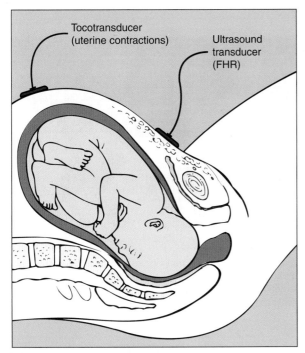

Tocotransducer
(uterine contractions)

Ultrasound
transducer
(FHR)

FIGURE 7-6 **External fetal monitoring.** Placement of external transducers. Tocotransducer (top) records the pressure of uterine contractions.

documentation of care given. It is important to record the times EFM is discontinued and restarted.

Maternal vital signs are recorded, intake and output monitored, and contraction patterns documented. The positioning of the monitors for FHR and uterine contractions should be adjusted as needed. If an internal spiral electrode is used, the connection to the leg plate should be checked and the leg plate secured to the woman's thigh. Emergency interventions when nonreassuring FHR patterns occur include administering oxygen, 8 to 10 L/minute by mask; turning the patient to the side-lying position; stopping the oxytocin infusion but keeping the intravenous line open; and notifying the health care provider.

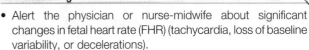

Safety Alert

Nonreassuring Fetal Heart Rate: Prioritization Guidelines

- Alert the physician or nurse-midwife about significant changes in fetal heart rate (FHR) (tachycardia, loss of baseline variability, or decelerations).
- Reposition the woman to avoid the supine position (correct hypotension by a side-lying position).
- Administer oxygen by facemask at 8 to 10 L/minute (increases oxygen saturation, making more available for the fetus).
- If oxytocin is being infused, stop administration. Keep the intravenous line open.
- Closely monitor uterine activity.
- Increase rate of nonadditive intravenous fluid to expand the woman's blood volume.
- Monitor vital signs to identify fever, hypotension, or hypertension.
- Observe perineum for bulging, crowning, or a prolapsed cord.
- If nonreassuring pattern is severe, begin the preparation for possible internal monitoring or cesarean birth, unless vaginal birth is imminent.

TYPES OF ELECTRONIC FETAL MONITORING

External Fetal Monitoring

External fetal monitoring is accomplished by securing an ultrasound transducer and a tocodynamometer to the woman's abdomen (Skill 7-3). When placed correctly, the electronic monitor picks up the sound waves of the fetal heart. Uterine contractions can also be monitored for frequency and duration; however, uterine contraction intensity *cannot* be monitored with an external monitor. External devices are secured on the mother's abdomen by elastic straps, belts, or a tube of wide stockinette. The external devices are noninvasive, and they do not require ruptured membranes or cervical dilation.

The equipment is easily applied by the nurse, but it must be repositioned as the mother or fetus changes position. The woman is asked to assume a semi-sitting or lateral position. This type of monitoring often confines the woman to the bed; therefore, the equipment is removed periodically to wash the applicator sites and to give a back massage. This method is valuable during the first stage of labor in women with intact membranes.

A beltless tocodynamometer is available. This system consists of an adhesive transducer that is applied to the woman's abdomen with a double-sided adhesive film. This method is preferred by the laboring woman because it allows her more freedom of movement. However, with the advent of epidurals and high-tech monitoring of even routine labors, the woman may not be able to ambulate freely. In early labor, intermittent external electronic monitoring is used in most hospitals to provide adequate information while allowing the woman to ambulate, shower, and interact with family until the bag of water ruptures or high-tech interventions are instituted.

Skill 7-3 Applying an External Fetal Monitor

PURPOSE

To monitor the fetal heart rate continuously.

Steps

1. Follow instruction manual for equipment (learn how to operate the equipment before using it on the patient).
2. Perform function test—print online—to see whether calibrated correctly for accurate data. Determine whether date and time are correct.
3. Explain to mother and partner that two belts will be placed around the abdomen—one for the fetal heart rate (FHR) sensor and one with a device to assess uterine contractions.
4. Slide belts under woman's back without sensors attached. Keep belts smooth (no wrinkles). If stockinette is used, slide it up from her feet to her abdomen.
5. Locate fetal back. Locate loudest sound of FHR (best heard through fetal back).
6. Apply conduction gel to the Doppler ultrasound transducer and place on woman's abdomen at location of fetus's back. Move transducer until clear FHR is heard. Unit may have a green or flashing light to indicate a good signal.
7. Place uterine activity sensor on the fundal area, where uterine contractions feel the strongest when palpated. Observe tracing line for uterine activity when the woman has a contraction. The line will be jagged because it also senses the movement of the abdomen with breathing. Fetal or maternal movement will cause a spike in the line.
8. Observe the tracing strip for baseline FHR. Palpate contractions for intensity and relaxation (external monitor does not measure intensity).
9. Document voiding, stooling, and care procedures on tracing.
10. Report any abnormal findings to the physician or nurse-midwife.

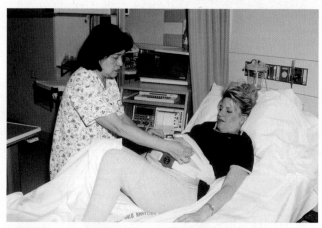

A nurse places the external transducers for fetal monitoring. The transducer placed over the fundus of the uterus records uterine contractions. The lower sensor monitors the fetal heart. Note that this patient has two fetal heart monitors because she is pregnant with twins.

Internal Fetal Monitoring. Accuracy is the main advantage of using internal fetal monitoring (Figure 7-7). However, it requires ruptured amniotic membranes and at least 2 cm of cervical dilation. The fetal presenting part must be known and down near the cervix. After the perineum is cleansed, a sterile internal spiral electrode is inserted into the vagina and placed against the presenting part, usually the head. The spiral electrode is rotated clockwise until it is attached to the presenting part (head or buttocks; never on the face, fontanelles, or genitalia). Wires that extend from the electrode are attached to a leg plate (which is placed on the woman's thigh) and then attached to the fetal monitor. A pressure transducer is introduced into the uterine cavity to monitor uterine activity.

Evidence-Based Practice

External Fetal Monitoring

Advantages
- Because it is noninvasive, it reduces the chance of infection.
- It can be conducted at any time (before amniotic membranes have ruptured and before cervix is dilated).
- Placement of transducers can be done by the nurse.
- Tracing gives a permanent record.

Disadvantages
- Uterine contraction intensity is not measurable.
- It may decrease personal contact with staff.
- Movement of woman may require frequent repositioning of transducers.
- Obesity and fetal position affect the quality of recording.

Best ♡ rate of the fetus is found on their back!

As the uterus contracts, it compresses the pressure transducer. The pressure is sensed and then converted into a pressure reading, and the intensity of the contraction is recorded. FHR is evaluated by assessing the tracing for baseline FHR, baseline variability, and periodic changes. The characteristics of fetal heart patterns, their causes, and nursing interventions required are discussed in Table 7-3.

Reassuring and Nonreassuring Patterns

The Normal Pattern. The normal FHR pattern is accepted as a heart rate of 110 to 160 beats/minute measured over 2 minutes in a 10-minute window of time. There are no decelerations, but there may be an acceleration. A fetus born with this normal *reassuring* heart rate pattern is virtually always normally oxygenated. Fetal problems can be predicted when abnormal FHR patterns occur. Abnormal patterns are called *nonreassuring* heart patterns.

Accelerations. Accelerations are brief, temporary increases in FHR of at least 15 beats/minute above the baseline lasting 15 seconds to under 2 minutes. They usually occur with fetal movements, just as heart rate increases in adults during exercise. They may occur with vaginal examinations, uterine contractions, fundal

pressure, and breech presentations. Accelerations are a reassuring FHR pattern and a sign of well-being.

Decelerations. Decelerations are transitory decreases in FHR from the baseline that are classified according to patterns—early, late, and variable—and according to the time of their occurrence in relation to the uterine

↰ *can put fetus in distress*

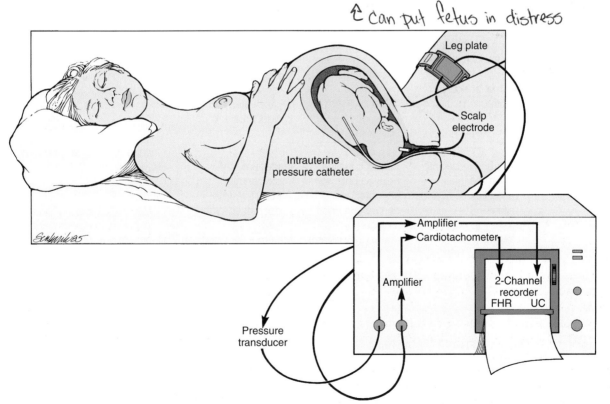

FIGURE 7-7 **Internal fetal monitoring with fetal scalp electrode.** The fetal electrocardiogram is obtained by applying the electrode directly to the fetal scalp, and then attaching the electrode to a leg plate on the mother's thigh. The signal is transmitted to the monitor, counted, and displayed. The uterine contractions are assessed with an intrauterine pressure catheter attached to a pressure transducer. The signal is then displayed on the monitor, where it is amplified, counted by the cardiotachometer, and recorded. *FHR,* fetal heart rate; *UC,* uterine contraction.

Table 7-3 Characteristics of Electronic Fetal Monitoring and Nursing Interventions

TERM	DEFINITION	CHARACTERISTIC	CAUSE	NURSING INTERVENTIONS
Baseline FHR	FHR between contractions	Normal rate 110-160 beats/minute	Good oxygenation	No intervention is necessary.
Baseline variability	Change of baseline FHR Fluctuations of FHR that result in irregular printed line on monitor strip.	Normal variability 6-25 beats/minute Moderate variability over 25 beats/minute Loss of baseline variability denoted by flat (smooth) baseline of <5 beats/minute	Decreased variability indicative of fetal sleep Loss of variability indicative of depressants or uteroplacental insufficiency (UPI) Variability is normal; loss of variability is abnormal	If variability is lost, change maternal position to side (left side, if possible) If FHR is abnormal, provide oxygen 8-10 L/minute by mask; notify physician.
Bradycardia	Abnormally slow heart rate	FHR <110 beats/minute for ≥10 minutes	Severe fetal hypoxia Drugs Heart block Maternal hypotension Oxytocin infusion	Discontinue drugs (if cause); provide oxygen by mask. Notify physician. Change maternal position.
Tachycardia	Persistent abnormally fast FHR	FHR <160 beats/minute for ≥10 minutes	Maternal fever Fetal hypoxia Fetal infection Cardiac anomalies	Change maternal position to side-lying. Check maternal vital signs. Assess emotional status (anxiety). Provide oxygen; notify appropriate personnel. Stop oxytocin but keep intravenous line open.
Periodic FHR patterns	Changes in FHR that occur with uterine activity	Transient	Normal or expected	No intervention is required.
Early deceleration	Slowing of FHR when contraction begins Return of FHR to normal at end of contraction	Mirrors contraction; return of FHR to baseline at end of contraction FHR usually within range of 110-160 beats/minute	Fetal head compression resulting from uterine contraction Vaginal examination Fundal pressure	No intervention is required.
Late deceleration	Slowing of FHR after contraction begins (when uterine blood flow is at a minimum) Recovery to normal delayed (until blood flow has resumed)	Return of FHR to normal baseline delayed until well after uterine contraction ends (Is a non-reassuring pattern)	UPI Inadequate fetal oxygenation (resulting from decreased blood flow) Maternal hypertension	Change to left side-lying position. Provide oxygen 8-10 L/minute by mask. Monitor BP. Correct hypotension if present in response to epidural analgesia. Decrease rate of maintenance infusion. Discontinue oxytocin infusion. Prepare for tocolytic drug administration. Assist with fetal blood sampling. Notify physician.
Variable deceleration Prolonged deceleration	Slowing of FHR under 15 BPM lasting between 15 seconds and 2 minutes Slowing below FHR baseline 2 minutes but under 10 minutes	Abrupt, transitory decrease in FHR that is variable in duration, intensity, and timing relative to contraction	Indicates compression of cord Short cord Prolapsed cord Cord around neck Oligohydramnios	Change maternal position. Provide oxygen if FHR does not respond. Correct hypotension if present. Notify physician if above measures do not correct FHR. Prepare for amnioinfusion or forceps delivery.

Table 7-3 Characteristics of Electronic Fetal Monitoring and Nursing Interventions—cont'd

TERM	DEFINITION	CHARACTERISTIC	CAUSE	NURSING INTERVENTIONS
Acceleration	Abrupt increase of FHR of 15 BPM above baseline lasting between 15 seconds and 2 minutes	Variable Increases with fetal movement Decreases with fetal sleep cycle	Indicates intact CNS response to fetal movement Vaginal examination Fundal pressure	Spontaneous accelerations are basis of reactive NST. No intervention is necessary. Slow oxytocin infusion if repeated accelerations occur. Prolonged fetal tachycardia may be associated with maternal infection.
Prolonged acceleration	Acceleration above baseline of 15 BPM lasting more than 2 minutes but under 10 minutes		Acceleration lasting more than 10 minutes is considered a change in baseline	
Sinusoidal pattern	A smooth wavelike undulating pattern of FHR baseline	Wavelike frequency of 3-5 per minute lasting 20 minutes Variability may be absent	Is an ominous sign of impending fetal death	Notify health care provider immediately

BP, blood pressure; *CNS*, central nervous system; *FHR*, fetal heart rate; *NST*, nonstress test; *BPM*, beats per minute.

contraction (Figure 7-8). Decelerations indicate an interruption of oxygen transfer to the fetus. Nursing interventions are required to prevent fetal compromise such as CP or death.

Early decelerations. Early decelerations typically start with the contraction, end when the contraction is over, stay within the normal range of FHR greater than 110 beats/minute, and produce a V-shaped pattern. A common cause of early decelerations is compression of the fetal head, which stimulates a vagal response of the fetal parasympathetic nervous system. No intervention is necessary.

Late decelerations. Late decelerations frequently begin at approximately the peak of the contraction and end *after* the contraction ends. They are often associated with uteroplacental insufficiency. The depth and time to return to the baseline are significant. Persistence or recurrence of late decelerations usually indicates hypoxia or lack of oxygen to the fetus. Late decelerations can be caused by maternal hypotension, excessive uterine activity (e.g., during induction of labor), and deficient placental perfusion. A drop of 30 beats/minute or a loss of the baseline variability (less than 3 to 5 beats/minute) is a significant indicator of fetal distress. Prolonged late deceleration followed by tachycardia and loss of variability may indicate fetal acidosis.

Repetitive late decelerations are problematic and require immediate intervention, including repositioning the woman, administering oxygen 8 to 10 L/minute by mask, discontinuing oxytocin infusion (if being administered), increasing intravenous fluids to correct dehydration, evaluating vital signs to identify hypotension, and promptly reporting these occurrences to the physician or nurse-midwife.

Variable decelerations. Variable decelerations involve a transient drop in the FHR before, during, or after the uterine contraction. They are related to a brief compression of the umbilical cord. The decelerations are abrupt and often associated with accelerations before or after the deceleration. They are rarely associated with hypoxia because the accelerations before and after are protective. The mother's position should be changed. If variable decelerations become prolonged and repetitive, they may indicate a tight cord around the fetus's neck, which may require an emergency cesarean birth. Variable decelerations occurring early in labor are often a result of oligohydramnios (a decrease in amniotic fluid).

FETAL PULSE OXIMETRY

Fetal pulse oximetry ($FSpO_2$) was approved by the U.S. Food and Drug Administration (FDA) in May 2000. However, the value of fetal pulse oximetry remains controversial (Oats & Abraham, 2005). A transcervical catheter positioned against the fetal cheek can measure fetal oxygen saturation. The amniotic membranes must have ruptured and the cervix must be at least 2 cm dilated and the fetus in vertex presentation at the cervix. The normal term fetus during labor has an oxygen saturation level of 40% to 70%. Levels less than 30% may indicate fetal metabolic acidosis, which would indicate hypoxia and require rapid delivery of the fetus. Fetal pulse oximetry may be indicated to enable continuing labor and avoid a cesarean birth, especially when a nonreassuring FHR is present in a term fetus.

MONITORING UTERINE CONTRACTIONS

When the woman is admitted, a 20- to 30-minute baseline electronic monitoring of uterine contractions and FHR is usually performed. This monitoring may be continued during labor. However, if the woman is at low risk for complications, palpation, a less precise method, may be used to determine the contraction

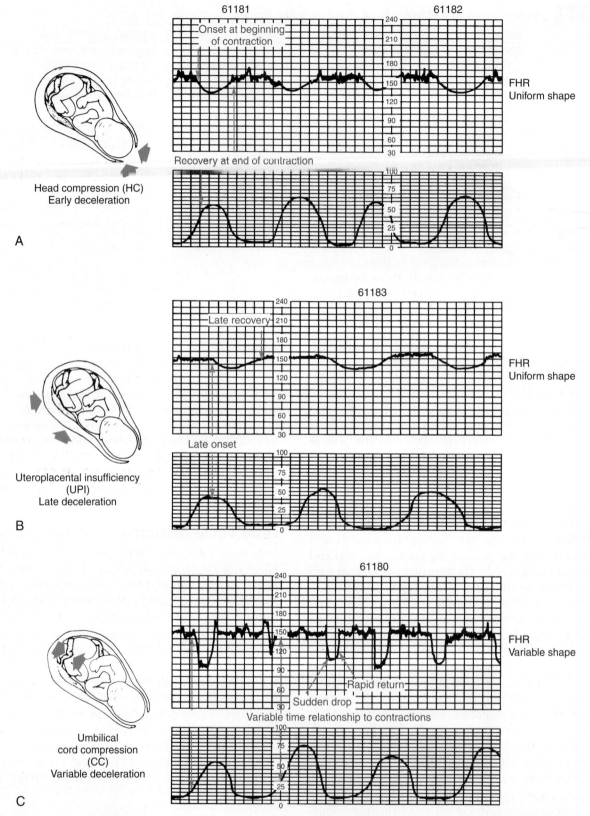

61181   61182

Onset at beginning
of contraction

FHR
Uniform shape

Recovery at end of contraction

Head compression (HC)
Early deceleration

A

61183

Late recovery

FHR
Uniform shape

Late onset

Uteroplacental insufficiency
(UPI)
Late deceleration

B

61180

FHR
Variable shape

Rapid return
Sudden drop
Variable time relationship to contractions

Umbilical
cord compression
(CC)
Variable deceleration

C

FIGURE 7-8 Fetal heart rate (FHR) stress patterns, showing early deceleration **(A),** late deceleration **(B),** and variable deceleration **(C).** *UC,* uterine contractions.

Skill 7-4 Determining Contractions by Palpation

PURPOSE

To provide intermittent assessment of uterine contractions.

Steps

1. Place the fingertips of one hand lightly on the upper uterus. Keep the fingers relatively still, but move them occasionally so that mild contractions can be felt.
2. Palpate at least three to five contractions for an accurate estimate of their average characteristics.
3. Note the time when each contraction begins and ends. Calculate the **frequency of contractions** by counting the elapsed time from the beginning of one contraction to the beginning of the next. Calculate the **duration of contractions** by determining the number of seconds from the beginning to the end of each contraction.

4. Estimate the **intensity of contractions** by trying to indent the uterus at the contraction's peak. If it is easily indented (like the tip of the nose), the contraction is mild; if it is harder to indent (like the chin), it is moderate; if nearly impossible to indent (like the forehead), it is strong.
5. Document the average frequency (in minutes and fractions), duration (in seconds), and intensity.
6. Report contractions that occur more frequently than every 2 minutes or last longer than 90 seconds or intervals of relaxation shorter than 60 seconds.
7. Guidelines for minimum interval between fetal heart rate (FHR) assessment:
   a. Hourly during latent period
   b. Every 30 minutes during active phase
   c. Every 15 minutes during second stage
   d. More frequently if abnormal pattern exists (see Box 7-2).

pattern. To palpate contractions, the nurse places his or her fingertips on the woman's abdomen over the uterine fundus. A summary of the frequency, duration, and intensity of contractions should be recorded in the woman's medical record. A guideline to the assessment of contractions by palpation is presented in Skill 7-4.

DETERMINING FETAL POSITION BY ABDOMINAL PALPATION

← the way the pelvis is positioned.

By using abdominal palpation (Leopold's maneuvers), the registered nurse or health care provider can ascertain the position, presentation, and engagement of the fetus (Skill 7-5). Abdominal palpation will sometimes reveal a multifetal pregnancy at the time of admission. Also, because FHR is best heard through the fetal back, determining the location of the fetal back is helpful. In a vertex presentation, the FHR is heard below the mother's umbilicus in either the right or left lower quadrant of the abdomen. In a breech presentation, the FHR is heard above the mother's umbilicus (see Figure 7-2).

MONITORING STATUS OF AMNIOTIC FLUID

Another important nursing responsibility is to determine whether the amniotic membranes are intact or ruptured. If the amniotic membranes have ruptured, the nurse should note the time of rupture and the color, amount, and odor of amniotic fluid. Normally, amniotic fluid is clear and pale and has little odor.

↑ should not be a foul odor.

Greenish fluid suggests fetal passage of meconium. Wine-colored amniotic fluid indicates the presence of blood and possible premature separation of the placenta. A foul or unpleasant odor of fluid suggests infection.

The nurse should perform a Nitrazine paper test, after donning gloves, to confirm whether the amniotic membranes have ruptured (Skill 7-6). The test strip is sensitive to pH and will turn deep blue if amniotic fluid is present. The blue color indicates the alkalinity of the fluid. If leakage is actually urine, the fluid will be slightly acidic, and the strip will remain yellow.

Ferning is a characteristic pattern of crystallization in amniotic fluid when it dries. Ferning may be observed by placing vaginal fluid on a glass slide, allowing it to dry, and then observing it under a microscope. Urine and other vaginal discharge will not show this pattern.

AMNIOINFUSION

Amnioinfusion is the infusion of warmed normal saline or Ringer's lactate solution into the uterine cavity after the amniotic membranes have ruptured. Amnioinfusion is performed to decrease the compression of the umbilical cord, increase fluid when oligohydramnios is present, dilute meconium in the uterine cavity, and reduce the risk of meconium aspiration. Contraindications to amnioinfusion include a prolapsed cord, vaginal bleeding, and severe fetal distress.

Skill 7-5   Performing Leopold's Maneuvers

PURPOSE
To determine fetal position and presentation.

Steps

1. Have woman empty bladder and lie on her back with knees flexed and small pillow under one hip.
   a. Presentation. Hands are placed on either side of the maternal abdomen to palpate the uterine fundus to determine whether a round, hard object is felt at the fundus (the fetal head, indicating a breech presentation) or a soft, irregular contour (the fetal buttocks, indicating a vertex presentation).
   b. Position. Hands are placed on either side of the maternal abdomen, supporting one side of the abdomen while palpating the other side. Palpating a hard, smooth contour indicates location of the fetal back, whereas feeling soft, irregular objects indicates the small parts or extremities.
   c. Confirm presentation. The suprapubic area is palpated to determine that the vertex (or head) is presenting. Feeling a hard, round area that does not move may indicate the head is engaged.
   d. Attitude. Attitude of the fetal head is determined by palpating the maternal abdomen with fingers pointing toward the maternal feet. The hand is moved downward toward the symphysis pubis. Feeling a hard, round object on the same side as the fetal back indicates the fetus is in extension. Feeling the hard, round object opposite the fetal back indicates the head is in flexion.
2. Document the findings, and report any abnormal findings.

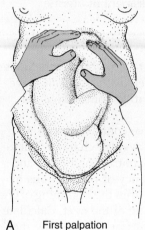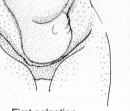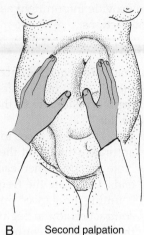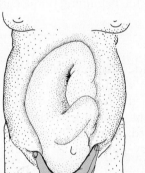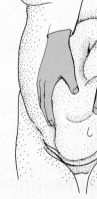

A   First palpation   B   Second palpation

C   Third palpation   D   Fourth palpation

Skill 7-6   Testing for the Presence of Amniotic Fluid (Nitrazine Paper Test)

PURPOSE
To determine the presence of amniotic fluid in vaginal secretions.

Steps

1. Explain purpose to woman.
2. Wash hands; apply clean gloves.
3. Place piece of Nitrazine paper into fluid from vagina.
4. A blue-green or deep-blue color of the Nitrazine paper indicates fluid is alkaline and most likely amniotic fluid.
5. A yellow to yellow-green color of the strip paper indicates fluid is acidic and is most likely urine.
6. Document and report results, offer and provide peri care, remove gloves, and wash hands.
7. Document the presence of bloody show, which may alter accuracy of results.

PHYSICAL CARE AND PSYCHOLOGICAL SUPPORT DURING LABOR AND BIRTH

THE NURSE'S ROLE

Because the woman's physical needs are the most apparent, it is easy to emphasize the physical aspect of care and neglect the psychological aspect of care related to the childbirth process.

The goal of psychological care is to make the labor and delivery process a more pleasant and satisfying experience and to allow more family participation. This can affect the course of labor and the woman's attitude toward the father or partner, the infant, and future pregnancies. The woman's response to each stage of labor and the nursing interventions for each stage are presented in Table 7-4.

 Health Promotion

Technology and the Nurse

The nurse's responsibility during labor is to focus on the patient. The use of technology in the labor room should not be a substitute for hands-on care. Data on a monitor cannot report the patient's feelings, which are important in providing an enriched birth experience. Establishing a therapeutic relationship with the woman and significant other upon admission is essential.

The nurse documents the progress of labor; reports abnormal findings; and provides measures of support, prevention of infection, and promotion of comfort. Position changes are effective in promoting comfort and facilitating fetal rotation and descent. Walking, standing, leaning, sitting upright, side-lying, squatting, or knee-chest positions are also effective. Periodic vaginal examinations are performed by the registered nurse or health care provider with sterile gloves and a water-soluble lubricant to determine the status of cervical dilation and effacement (Figure 7-9).

Vaginal examinations are contraindicated if vaginal bleeding is present (see Chapter 14). Maternal vital

 Evidence-Based Practice

Reassessment of Fetal Heart Rate

Reassess fetal heart rate (FHR) after:
- Rupture of membranes
- Vaginal examination
- Ambulation (before and after)
- Change in infusion rate of oxytocin
- Administration of drugs (before and after)
- Urinary catheterization
- Expulsion of enema
- Recognition of abnormal uterine activity (close, strong contractions)
- Decrease in fetal activity (as felt by mother)

 If FHR is being monitored electronically, it should be frequently observed and documented according to the institution's policy.

signs are documented every hour in the latent phase and every 30 minutes in the active phase of labor. FHR patterns are monitored closely, and frequency, intensity, and duration of contractions are documented. Any questionable FHR pattern must be reported promptly to the nurse or health care provider. A dry mouth may be relieved by ice chips or lollipops, but the laboring woman should receive nothing by mouth (NPO) in regards to solid foods because nausea and vomiting can occur during labor and delivery, and the risk for aspiration is high. Intake and output are recorded, and the bladder is checked for distention every 1 to 2 hours because the woman may not be able to sense the need to void. Palpation of a bulge above the symphysis pubis may indicate the bladder needs to be emptied. In addition to the consistent assessment of maternal and fetal conditions, the nurse helps the woman cope with labor by comforting, positioning, teaching, and encouraging her. Another aspect of intrapartal care is the attention to the woman's partner.

 Evidence-Based Practice

Using Infection Prevention and Control in Labor and Delivery

- Use barrier precautions to prevent skin and mucous membrane contact with body fluids.
- Wear eye protection or a face shield when assisting in a procedure where a splash of fluid can occur.
- Wear shoe covers and a full-length, fluid-resistant cover gown during delivery.
- Use standard precautions whenever handling sharps (e.g., suture needles and syringes with needles). Dispose of all used sharps in the appropriate container.
- Never recap needles.
- Review standard precautions on Evolve.

SUPPORTING THE PARTNER

Partners, or coaches, vary considerably in the degree of involvement with which they are comfortable. The labor partner is most often the infant's father but may be the woman's mother or friend. Some partners are truly coaches and take a leading role in helping the woman cope with labor. Others are willing to assist if they are shown how, but they will not take the initiative. Still other couples are content with the partner's encouragement and support but do not expect him or her to have an active role. The partner should be permitted to provide the type of support comfortable for the couple. The nurse does not take the partner's place but remains available as needed (Figure 7-10).

The partner should be encouraged to take a break and periodically eat a snack or meal. Many partners are reluctant to leave the woman's bedside, but they may faint during the birth if they have not eaten. A chair or stool near the bed allows the partner to sit down as much as possible.

Table 7-4   **Stages and Phases of Labor**

STAGES OF LABOR AND UTERINE CONTRACTIONS	WOMAN'S RESPONSE	NURSING INTERVENTIONS
Stage 1: Dilation		
Main Goals: Complete Dilation of Cervix, Descent of Fetus		
Latent phase: cervix 0-3 cm Contractions every 10-20 minutes, 15- to 30-second duration, mild intensity; progressing to every 5-7 minutes, 30- to 40-second duration, mild to moderate intensity	Happy, excited Talkative and eager to be in labor Exhibits need for independence Attempts to care for own bodily needs Seeks information about her care Some apprehension	Establish rapport. Monitor maternal vital signs and FHR. Assess status of amniotic fluid, whether membranes are intact or ruptured. Observe voiding time and amount. Assess coping ability, anxiety. Teach breathing techniques if needed. Encourage walking if membranes are intact. Encourage woman and support person to participate in care. Encourage relaxation if lying down (assist with techniques such as effleurage or sacral pressure). Offer fluids or ice chips. Keep woman NPO to prevent aspiration. Keep couple informed.
Active phase: cervix 4-7 cm Contractions every 2-3 minutes, 50- to 60-second duration, moderate to strong intensity	Apprehensive Ill-defined doubts and fears Exhibits increased fatigue and may feel restless As contractions become stronger, becomes anxious Becomes more dependent as she is less able to meet her needs Desires companionship Becomes uncertain whether she can cope with contractions Ritual activities or motions during contractions perhaps indicative that strong coping strategies are in place	Continue to assess and document maternal vital signs and FHR every 30 minutes. Provide support and encouragement. If on electronic fetal monitor, observe for normal or abnormal signs; explain monitor to woman and support person. Assess status of membranes. Encourage woman to void every 1-2 hours to avoid bladder distention. Observe for full bladder (woman loses urge to void with epidural block). Assess progress of labor (cervical dilation). Registered nurse may perform vaginal examination (see Figure 7-9). Provide comfort and safety measures: moisten lips, apply ointment, and provide ice chips. Apply cool cloth to woman's forehead. Provide back rubs, sacral pressure, effleurage, attention-focusing activities. Assist with oral hygiene. Keep bed linens dry and bedrails up. Provide assistance with position changes, support with pillows, or help with walking. Protect woman from infection with frequent perineal care. Inform couple about labor progress.
Transition: cervix 8-10 cm Contractions every 2-3 minutes, 60- to 90-second duration, strong intensity	Marked restlessness and irritability Amnesia between contractions Generalized discomfort, cramps in legs Sometimes hiccupping and belching Nausea and vomiting Perspiration on face Trembling legs Increased vaginal show May feel tearing open or splitting apart with contractions Desires medication May feel out of control Fear of being alone	Continue nursing interventions from active phase. Encourage woman to rest between contractions. Talk woman through the contraction by maintaining breathing pattern. Assess monitor strip for normal or abnormal signs (if on monitor); if not on monitor, assess FHR and blood pressure every 15 minutes. Recognize woman may not want to be touched during transition period; recognize this is a difficult time for woman. Do not leave woman alone. Accept behavior of throwing off covers, etc. Get blanket if woman feels cold; assist in changing positions. Apply cool cloth to head when woman feels hot. Encourage voiding; assess for full bladder. Provide support, praise, and encouragement for her efforts. Provide privacy.

Table **7-4** Stages and Phases of Labor—cont'd

STAGES OF LABOR AND UTERINE CONTRACTIONS	WOMAN'S RESPONSE	NURSING INTERVENTIONS
Stage 2: Expulsion of Fetus		
Main Goal: Descent to Birth of Baby, Complete Dilation 10 cm		
Contractions every 1½-2 minutes, 60- to 90-second duration, strong intensity	Desire to push Satisfaction if told baby is almost here Complete exhaustion Pushes with contractions May feel helpless, out of control, panicky Rectal and vaginal bulging and flattening of perineum	Encourage open-glottis grunting push technique when bearing down is spontaneous. Encourage deep breathing between contractions. Assess FHR after each contraction (if not on monitor). Assess monitor strip for normal/abnormal findings. Assess contraction for frequency, duration, and intensity. Assess progress of labor; inform woman and partner. Encourage continued support. Remain with woman at all times. Cleanse perineal area (stroke downward). Provide necessary materials and equipment for delivery. After birth, give immediate care to newborn. Assess woman for potential hemorrhage.
Stage 3: Expulsion of Placenta		
Main Goals: Expulsion of Placenta, Prevention of Hemorrhage		
Contractions temporarily ceased 2-3 contractions to expel placenta Upward rise of uterus in abdomen Visible lengthening of umbilical cord Trickle or gush of blood	Eager to get acquainted with baby Sense of relief	Assess woman's vital signs. Assess for excessive bleeding. Provide nurse-midwife or physician with necessary materials (for possible episiotomy repair). Take woman to recovery room (if in traditional facility). Encourage parent-newborn bonding.
Stage 4: Immediate Recovery Period (Minimum 1 Hour)		
Main Goals: Prevent Hemorrhage, Facilitate Maternal-Newborn Bonding		
	Exhausted but happy labor is over Eager to feed baby Hungry Thirsty Sleepy	Direct nursing assessment toward prevention of hemorrhage. Assess every 15 minutes for 1 hour minimum: fundus location (height) and consistency (if not firm, massage and report); lochia amount, color, odor; vital signs: blood pressure, pulse, temperature; perineum: episiotomy for edema, hematoma; state of hydration; bladder for distention; fatigue and exhaustion (provide atmosphere for rest). Encourage mother-newborn bonding (holding baby, breastfeeding). Provide privacy for woman, partner, and baby to get acquainted.

FHR, fetal heart rate; *NPO,* nothing by mouth.

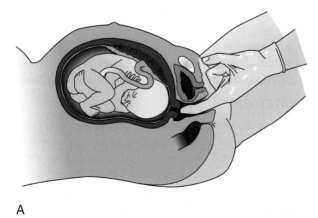
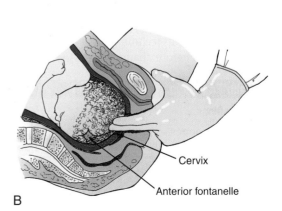

Cervix

Anterior fontanelle

A   B

FIGURE **7-9 Vaginal examination. A,** Undilated, uneffaced cervix, membranes intact. **B,** Palpation of sagittal suture line. Cervix effaced and partially dilated.

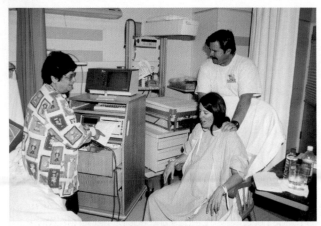

FIGURE 7-10 The nurse explains the electronic monitor that shows the acme of the contraction has passed, while the partner messages the laboring woman's back and shoulders.

 Patient Teaching

Teaching the Father or Partner

The father or partner should be taught:
- How labor pains affect the woman's behavior and attitude
- How to adapt responses to the woman's behavior
- What to expect in his or her own emotional responses as the woman becomes introverted or negative
- Effects of epidural analgesia

THE DOULA

A doula is a person other than a family member or friend who is trained to provide labor support. A doula may be certified by associations, such as the International Childbirth Education Association or the Association of Labor Assistants and Childbirth Educators, and adheres to a specific scope of practice. Doulas may be hired by the mother or couples to provide labor support, guidance, and encouragement to the mother during labor and to act as an advocate for the family (Figure 7-11).

TEACHING

Teaching the laboring woman and her partner is an ongoing task of the intrapartum nurse. Even women who attended childbirth classes often find that the measures they learned are inadequate or need to be adapted. Positions or breathing techniques that are different from those learned in class may need to be tried. A woman should usually try a change in technique or position for two or three contractions before abandoning it for another.

 Health Promotion

Changing Positions

Regular changes of position make the laboring woman more comfortable and promote the normal processes of labor.

Many women are discouraged when their cervix is about 5 cm dilated because it has taken many hours to reach that point. They think they are only halfway

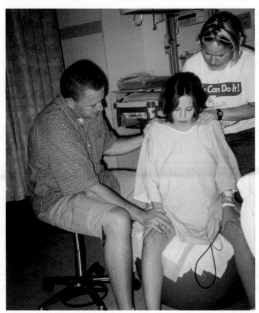

FIGURE 7-11 **The doula.** The laboring woman sits on a birthing ball as her partner provides encouragement and the doula massages her shoulders.

through labor (full dilation is 10 cm). However, a 4- to 5-cm dilation signifies that about two thirds of the labor is over because the rate of progress increases once this level has been reached. Laboring women often need support and reassurance to overcome their discouragement around this time.

The nurse often must help the woman avoid pushing before her cervix is fully dilated. She can be taught to blow out in short puffs when the urge to push is strong before the cervix is fully dilated. Pushing before full dilation can cause maternal exhaustion and fetal hypoxia, thus slowing progress rather than speeding it.

When the cervix is fully dilated, the nurse teaches or supports effective pushing techniques. If the woman is pushing effectively and the fetus is tolerating labor well, the nurse should not interfere with the woman's efforts. The nurse should encourage the woman to take a deep breath and exhale it at the beginning of a contraction. She then takes another deep breath and pushes with her abdominal muscles while exhaling. Prolonged breath holding while pushing (Valsalva's maneuver) can impair fetal blood circulation. The woman should push for about 4 to 6 seconds at a time. If she is in a semi-sitting position in bed, she should pull back on her knees, pull behind her thighs, or use the handrails on the bed.

WATER BIRTH

In May 2005, the American Academy of Pediatrics Committee on Fetus and Newborn classified water birth as an experimental procedure requiring parental informed consent (Schuman, 2006). However, a current trend in alternate delivery is delivering in a water bath (Figure 7-12). Advantages and disadvantages of a water birth are described in Table 7-5.

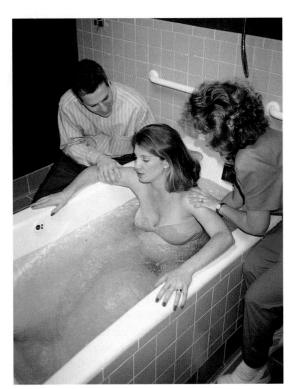

FIGURE 7-12 The use of a warm bath or a Jacuzzi during labor promotes muscle relaxation and pain relief.

Table 7-5	Advantages and Disadvantages of Water Birth	
ADVANTAGES	**DISADVANTAGES**	
To the Mother		
Pain relief from the warm water	Vasodilation	
Relaxation with the water buoyancy	Fatigue to decreased muscle tone	
	Fluid loss due to perspiration in the warm water	
	Increased hydrostatic pressure experienced during delivery	
	Difficulty in getting out of the bath if an emergency occurs	
To the Neonate		
Gentle exit during birth	Respiratory depression because of warmth of the water	
	Loss of cold stimulus that initiates respiration	
	Infection from exposure to maternal vaginal and bowel organisms	
	Aspiration	
	Difficulty with fetal monitoring	

PROVISION OF CARE DURING THE FOUR STAGES OF LABOR

BIRTH

Signs of impending birth are listed in Box 7-3. Most of the comfort measures suggested for the first stage of labor remain appropriate during the second stage (which begins with the cervix being completely effaced and

Box 7-3   Signs of Impending Birth

Specific behaviors may suggest that birth is imminent, such as:
- Sitting on one buttock (basically crowing of head)
- Making grunting sounds
- Involuntarily bearing down with contractions
- Stating "the baby is coming"
- Bulging of the perineum

If birth appears imminent, the nurse should not leave the woman alone, should prepare for the precipitate birth, and should summon help with the call bell.

dilated and ends with the birth of the baby). As the head descends, the woman has the urge to push because of pressure of the fetal head on the sacral nerves and the rectum. The woman should take a cleansing breath before each contraction to keep oxygen and carbon dioxide levels in balance. She should use the open-glottis method for pushing, in which air is released during pushing, so that intrathoracic pressure does not build up. Some women experience intense physical exertion by pushing and may feel a tearing sensation. The perineum begins to bulge and flatten, and soon the baby's head appears at the vaginal opening (crowning). The fetal head distends the perineum, and the physician or nurse-midwife applies gentle, firm support on the head in the direction of the perineum to maintain flexion. The force of the next one or two contractions and maternal effort will usually deliver the infant's head.

! Safety Alert

Impending Birth

If the mother states, "The baby is coming," believe her!

After the head is delivered, the woman is asked to stop pushing. The physician or midwife wipes the baby's face with gauze sponges and uses a bulb syringe to suction first the mouth and then the nose. The physician or nurse-midwife checks the baby's neck for the umbilical cord. If the cord is present around the neck, it is usually long enough to be slipped over the head; however, it may be necessary to clamp and cut the cord first. Meanwhile, the head realigns itself with the shoulders (*external rotation*). The woman may be asked to steadily bear down with the next contraction to deliver the shoulders. The rest of the baby's body will quickly follow. The newborn is dried (to minimize the loss of heat), and often is placed on the mother's abdomen, after which the umbilical cord is clamped. If the husband or partner is present, it is ideal to allow him or her to participate in the experience of cutting the umbilical cord. The baby may be placed on the mother's chest, with skin-to-skin contact providing warmth to the newborn and establishing mother-infant bonding.

DELIVERY

The woman most often delivers in the same room where she has labored. The maternal position for birth varies from a lithotomy position, to one in which her feet rest on a footrest while she holds a bar, to a side-lying position with the woman's upper leg held by the coach. Once the woman is positioned for birth, her vulva and perineum are cleansed (Skill 7-7). The nurse prepares the delivery table for use (Figure 7-13). The nurse (usually the same nurse as the labor nurse) continues to monitor the FHR every 5 to 15 minutes. To protect all of the care providers in the delivery room, each wears fluid-resistant gowns, gloves, and face masks that incorporate eye shields or goggles. The physician or nurse-midwife will have carried out appropriate handwashing (surgical scrub) before putting on the sterile barrier attire. The health care provider and partner coach the woman through the second stage of labor (Figure 7-14).

If the physician or nurse-midwife elects to perform an episiotomy (an incision into the perineum, performed during the second stage of labor to enlarge the perineal opening to prevent tearing as the head of the fetus is born), the circulating nurse opens the appropriate instruments and sutures for repair once the placenta has been delivered.

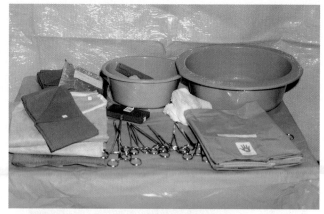

FIGURE 7-13 Sterile delivery table arranged in a convenient order.

EXPULSION OF PLACENTA

The third stage of labor begins after the birth of the baby and ends with the expulsion of the placenta. After the delivery of the baby, the uterus rapidly shrinks. The placenta, however, does not decrease in size; thus, as the placental site becomes smaller, the placenta begins to buckle and then separates; as the uterus contracts, the placenta is expelled, usually within 15 to 30 minutes after the baby is delivered. Signs of imminent delivery of the placenta include lengthening of the

---

Skill 7-7   Cleansing the Perineum Before Delivery

PURPOSE

To remove secretions and feces from perineal area.

Steps

1. Use warm water and solution per hospital policy.
2. Use a fresh sponge to cleanse each new area.
3. Using a zigzag motion, cleanse the area between the clitoris to the pubic hairline.
4. Using a zigzag motion, cleanse the area between the labia majora and inner thigh on one leg and then the other.
5. Apply a single stroke with the sponge downward from the right side of the clitoris and downward to the anus.
6. Apply a single stroke with the sponge downward on the left side of the clitoris to the anus.
7. Apply a single stroke downward in the middle over the clitoris over the vulva and perineum.

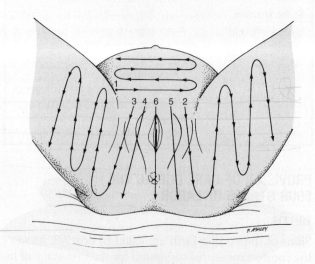

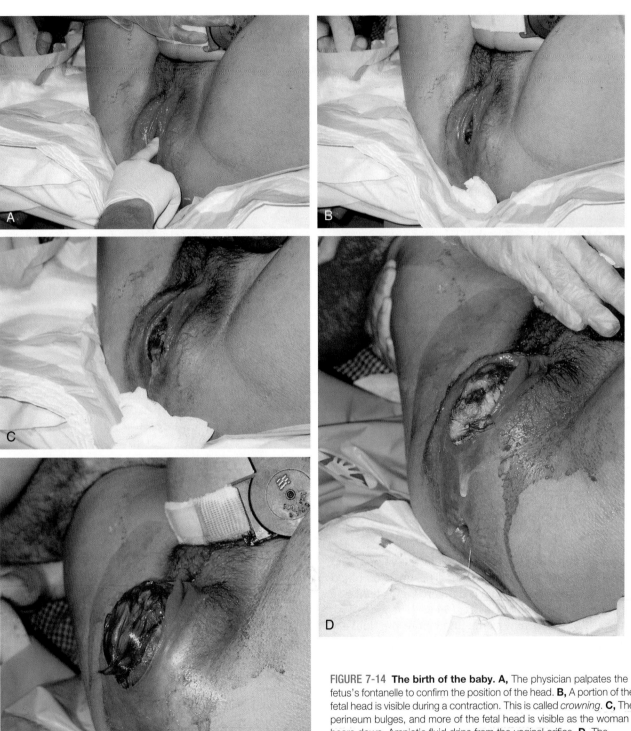

FIGURE 7-14 **The birth of the baby. A,** The physician palpates the fetus's fontanelle to confirm the position of the head. **B,** A portion of the fetal head is visible during a contraction. This is called *crowning*. **C,** The perineum bulges, and more of the fetal head is visible as the woman bears down. Amniotic fluid drips from the vaginal orifice. **D,** The perineum has been cleansed with an antibacterial solution as the fetal head begins extension. Note the distention of the perineum and anus. **E,** The head is about to be born. Note the thinning, redness, and distention of the perineal area. An episiotomy may be performed at this stage to enlarge the vaginal opening. Also, note the fetal monitor that is in place on the mother's abdomen to allow continuous monitoring of the fetal heart rate.

Continued

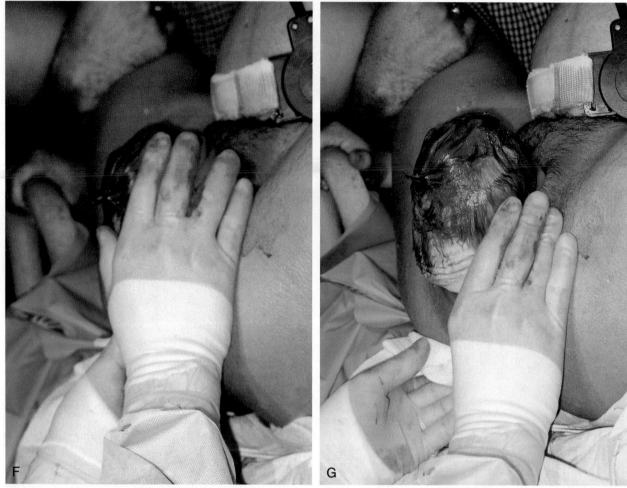

FIGURE 7-14—CONT'D **F,** The physician supports the perineum as the head emerges. **G,** The physician checks for the cord around the neck.

Continued

umbilical cord, a gush of blood from the vagina, and elevation of the uterine fundus. The gush of blood may come after the placenta is delivered if the fetal side of the placenta is expelled first (Schultze mechanism); the gush of blood may come just before the delivery of the placenta if the maternal side is expelled first (Duncan mechanism).

The third stage places the woman at risk for hemorrhage; therefore, assessment of the amount of bleeding, the woman's blood pressure, and pulse rate is very important. The nurse records the time the placenta is expelled and whether it delivered spontaneously. An oxytocin drug (e.g., Pitocin) may be given to the woman after the placenta is delivered to help the uterine muscles contract and thereby reduce the amount of blood loss. The placenta is examined by the health care provider to determine whether it is intact (Figure 7-15). The nursing responsibilities during birth are summarized in Box 7-4.

IMMEDIATE RECOVERY PERIOD

The recovery period, sometimes referred to as the *fourth stage of labor*, is the stage of physical recovery for the mother. It lasts from the delivery of the

placenta through the first 1 to 4 hours after birth. The greatest danger to the mother in the first hour after birth is hemorrhage. Vital signs are taken, and an ice bag is often applied to the perineum to reduce the amount of edema that occurs because of trauma or an episiotomy. The location and firmness of the uterine fundus are assessed and the fundus massaged as needed. The amount and color of lochia (vaginal discharge) are assessed; no more than one perineal pad per hour should be saturated. A continuous trickle of bright red blood when the fundus is firm may indicate a bleeding laceration and must be immediately reported. The bladder must be assessed for distention because the woman often does not feel the urge to urinate. A distended bladder can displace the uterus from the midline position and inhibit uterine contraction. Urinary catheterization may be required. Many women have a shaking chill after delivery, yet deny being cold. A warm blanket over the woman's body provides warmth and comfort until the shaking subsides. The return of sensation to the lower extremities is documented (see Chapter 8).

→ Rule of thumb 1 pad per hour average!

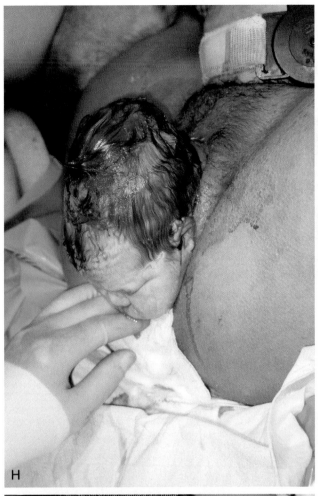

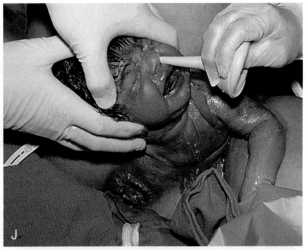

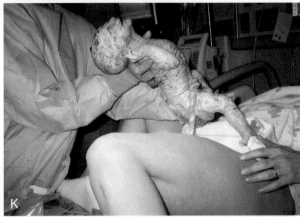

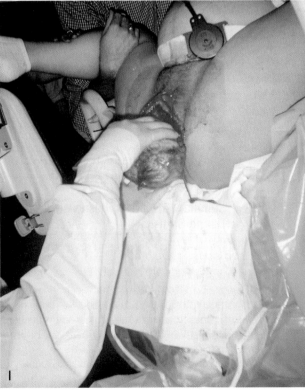

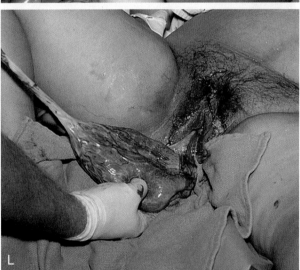

FIGURE 7-14—CONT'D H, The perineum is covered as the head is born. **I,** The physician exerts gentle pressure on the head to release the anterior shoulder from under the symphysis pubis. The posterior shoulder quickly follows, and the baby is born. **J,** The physician uses a bulb syringe to clear the infant's airway. **K,** The newborn infant, covered with thick white vernix, is lifted onto the abdomen of the mother, where the cord is cut. **L,** The placenta is delivered.

Continued

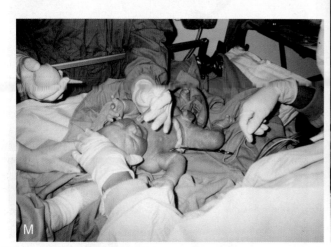
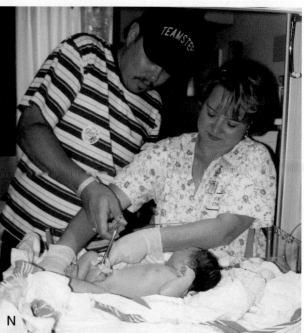

FIGURE 7-14—CONT'D **M,** The newborn is placed in the radiant warmer, where gentle resuscitative measures such as bulb syringe suctioning and whiffs of oxygen are provided. Note the metal clamp on the umbilical cord. **N,** The nurse assists the father in cutting the umbilical cord so that the disposable clamp can be applied.

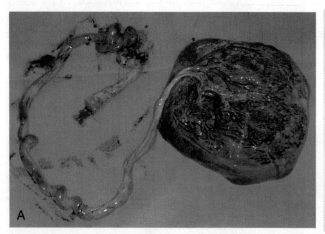
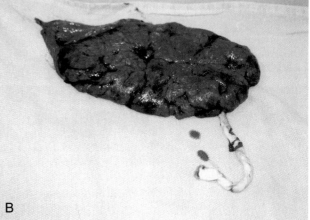

FIGURE 7-15 **Expulsion of the placenta. A,** Schultze mechanism occurs when the fetal side of the placenta, which is shiny and smooth, is delivered first. Note the knot in the umbilical cord, which was a cause of fetal distress during labor. **B,** Duncan mechanism occurs when the maternal side of the placenta, which is dull and rough, is delivered first.

The nursing assessment is performed every 15 minutes for at least 1 hour and according to hospital protocol thereafter (Table 7-6). The mother and partner should be encouraged to continue the parent-infant bonding process, and the mother should be assisted in initiating breastfeeding.

PHASE 1: IMMEDIATE CARE OF THE NEWBORN

Physiologic changes in the respiratory and circulatory systems occur as the baby is born and the umbilical cord is cut. The newborn enters a series of stages of transition from intrauterine to extrauterine life and, for the first 8 hours, may be physiologically unstable.

Box 7-4 **Summary of Nursing Responsibilities During Birth**

- Preparing delivery instruments and newborn resuscitation equipment
- Performing perineal prep
- Providing support to the woman and her partner or coach
- Administering medications as needed
- Providing phase 1 care to the newborn, such as suctioning, oxygen, drying the skin, and placing in a radiant warmer
- Performing phase 1 infant assessment
- Examining placenta to be sure it is intact and recording if it is expelled by a Duncan or Schultze mechanism
- Providing identification for mother, infant, and partner
- Assessing the fundus and perineum after delivery
- Promoting parent-infant bonding

Table 7-6	Maternal Problems That Must Be Reported in the Fourth Stage
SYMPTOM	**CAUSE**
Rising pulse rate and falling BP and decreasing urine output	Imminent hypovolemic shock
Soft, boggy uterus	Poorly contracted uterus, increasing the risk of hemorrhage
Lochia exceeding one pad per hour	Possible hemorrhage
High, displaced uterine fundus	Full bladder (can interfere with uterine contraction)

The first 30 minutes to 1 hour of life is called the *first period of reactivity* and usually takes place in the delivery room because the mother and newborn are usually kept together during the fourth (recovery) stage of labor. The physiologic changes in the newborn are discussed in Chapter 9.

NURSING CARE OF THE NEWBORN IN THE DELIVERY ROOM

Nursing care of the newborn after delivery is divided into three transitional phases: *phase 1*, the immediate care after birth, from birth to 1 hour of age; *phase 2*, from 1 to 4 hours after birth (usually when newborn is transferred to nursery or postpartum unit); and *phase 3*, from 4 hours after birth until discharge from hospital.

The goals of care of the newborn in phase 1 include:
- Maintaining thermoregulation
- Maintaining cardiorespiratory function
- Identifying mother, partner, and newborn
- Performing a brief assessment for anomalies
- Observing for and documenting passage of meconium and urine
- Facilitating parent-newborn bonding and first breastfeeding

Health care personnel always wear gloves when handling a newborn before the first bath because of the blood and amniotic fluid that is on the infant's skin.

Thermoregulation - prevent hyperthermia

Maintaining warmth of the newborn is important because hypothermia (low body temperature) forces the newborn to use glucose to warm his or her body, thereby causing hypoglycemia (low blood sugar). Hypoglycemia is associated with the development of neurologic problems. Hypothermia causes cold stress that results in an increase in the newborn's basal metabolic rate (BMR) in an effort to warm the body. An increase in the BMR results in an increased need for oxygen consumption, which can lead to hypoxia (low blood oxygen level). Therefore, once the baby is born, he or she is immediately dried with a soft towel and placed on the back or side in a heated crib or radiant warmer, with the neck slightly extended (Figure 7-16). A hat may be placed on the head after it is dried to prevent heat loss from this large body surface area. When the infant is removed from the radiant warmer, a warm blanket wrap should be applied.

Cardiorespiratory Support

The face is gently wiped to remove excess mucus and amniotic fluid. The newborn is an obligate nose breather and will not breathe through the mouth voluntarily if the nose is obstructed. Therefore, nasal suctioning with a bulb syringe contributes to a clear airway. Bulb suctioning of the mouth prevents aspiration of mucus and amniotic fluid (see Skill 10-4). As soon as the baby is placed in the radiant warmer, a heart monitor is applied because the heart rate is the most reliable indicator of need for resuscitation. A newborn with a heart rate greater than 100 beats/minute will generally need suctioning only. If the newborn is cyanotic, supplemental blow-by oxygen can be given. A cyanotic newborn with a heart rate less than 100 beats/minute requires stimulation by rubbing the back with a towel while being given blow-by oxygen. If rapid response to suction, oxygen, and tactile stimulation does not occur, bag and mask resuscitation may be initiated by the registered nurse, respiratory therapist, or other health care provider.

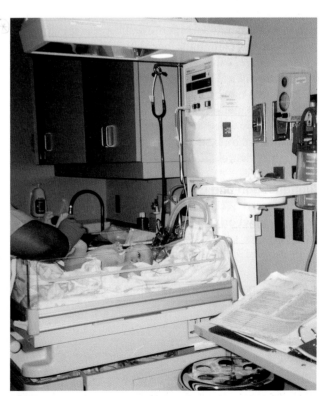

FIGURE 7-16 **Newborn in radiant warmer.** The nurse applies a thermal sensor to the newborn's abdomen and assesses the infant in the radiant warmer. Note the nurse is wearing purple nitrile (latex free) gloves when handling the newborn because newborns can be allergic to latex.

8-10 good
4-7 gentle stimulation
3-↓ active resuscitation.

Table 7-7   Apgar Scoring System

SIGN	0	1	2
Heart rate	Absent	<100 beats/minute	≥100 beats/minute
Respiratory effort	No spontaneous respirations	Slow; weak cry	Spontaneous, with a strong, lusty cry
Muscle tone	Limp	Minimal flexion of extremities; sluggish movement	Active spontaneous motion; flexed body posture
Reflex irritability	No response to suction or gentle slap on soles	Minimal response (grimace) to stimulation	Prompt response to suction, with cry or active movement with a gentle slap to sole of foot or backrub
Color	Blue or pale	Body pink, extremities blue	Completely pink (light skin) or absence of cyanosis (dark skin)

NOTE: The nurse evaluates each sign in the Apgar and totals the score at 1, 5, 10, and 15 minutes after birth to determine what interventions the infant needs. A score of 8-10 requires no action other than continued observation and support of the infant's adaptation. A score from 4-7 means the infant needs gentle stimulation such as rubbing the back; the possibility of narcotic-induced respiratory depression should also be considered. Scores ≤3 mean that the infant needs active resuscitation. If resuscitative measures are applied, the following scoring chart is added to the routine Apgar:

MINUTES	1	5	10	15
Oxygen				
PPV/NCPAP				
ETT				
Chest compression				
Epinephrine				

Data from Apgar, V. (1966). The newborn (Apgar) scoring system: Reflections and advice. *Pediatric Clinics of North America, 13,* 645; American College of Obstetricians and Gynecologists (ACOG). (2009). ACOG Practice Bulletin N. 106: Intrapartum fetal heart rate monitoring: Nomenclature, interpretation, and general management principles. *Obstetrics and Gynecology, 114*(1), 192-202; Macones, G., Hankins, G., & Spong, Y. (2008). The 2008 National Institute of Child Health and Human Development workshop report on electronic fetal monitoring: Update on definitions, interpretation, and research guidelines. *Obstetrics and Gynecology, 112*(3), 661-666.
ETT, endotracheal tube; *NCPAP,* nasal continuous positive airway pressure; *PPV,* positive pressure ventilation.

Oxygen may be given as needed until the infant cries vigorously. _Acrocyanosis (a blue color to the hands and feet of the newborn) is normal because of sluggish peripheral circulation for the first few hours after birth._

An **Apgar score** is assigned at 1 and 5 minutes after birth (Table 7-7). An Apgar score identifies the condition of the newborn and determines whether further resuscitation measures are needed. A score of 7 to 10 indicates a baby who has good cardiorespiratory function with minimal bulb suctioning assistance. Some signs of respiratory distress in the newborn are listed in Box 7-5.

Identification and Clamping of Cord
A numbered wristband and ankle band are placed on the newborn, and wristbands with matching numbers are placed on the mother and the partner (Figure 7-17). All identifying information is

documented and verified in the delivery room. The identification band numbers are verified every time the infant is separated and returned to the mother during the hospital stay. In some hospitals, a sensor is added to the newborn's wristband that will set off an alarm if the baby is removed from the unit. Footprints of the baby and fingerprints of the mother may be included in the identification process in some hospitals; some hospitals take a photograph of the newborn in the delivery room. A cord clamp is applied to the

Box 7-5   Signs of Respiratory Distress in the Newborn
- Persistent cyanosis (other than hands and feet)
- Grunting respirations (a noise heard without a stethoscope as the newborn exhales)
- Retractions on inhalation under the sternum or between the ribs
- Sustained respiration rate higher than 60 breaths/minute
- Sustained heart rate below 100 or above 160 beats/minute

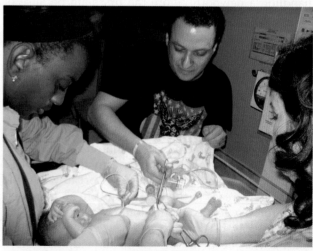

FIGURE 7-17 The nurse includes the father when clamping and cutting the umbilical cord and provides teaching care of the umbilical cord stump.

umbilical stump, and the cord is assessed to determine the presence of two arteries and one vein (a mnemonic to help remember this is *AVA*).

Documenting Urination and Passage of Meconium

The newborn cannot be discharged home before patency of the gastrointestinal and genitourinary tracts is established. If the newborn urinates or passes meconium in the delivery room, it must be recorded in the medical record.

Administering Vitamin K

The newborn should receive vitamin K (phytonadione [AquaMEPHYTON] 0.5 to 1 mg). It is given intramuscularly in the midanterior thigh (the vastus lateralis muscle), where the muscle development is adequate (Skill 7-8). Because newborns cannot synthesize vitamin K in the intestines without the presence of bacterial flora, they are deficient in clotting factors, and vitamin K must be administered as a prophylaxis to assist in clotting.

↳ usually given within 1hr of birth

Skill 7-8   Administering Intramuscular Injections to the Newborn

PURPOSE

To effectively administer an intramuscular injection to the newborn.

Steps

1. A 1-mL syringe with a 5/8-inch, 25-gauge needle is often used. A small needle reaches the muscle but potentially prevents striking the bone.
2. Locate the correct site. The middle third of the vastus lateralis muscle is the preferred site (see illustration). The middle third of the rectus femoris is an alternate site, but its proximity to major vessels and the sciatic nerve necessitates caution during injection.
3. Cleanse the area with an alcohol wipe.
4. Stabilize leg while grasping tissues (upper thigh) between thumb and fingers to prevent sudden movement by newborn and possible injury.

5. Insert needle at 90-degree angle to the thigh.
6. Aspirate; if no blood returns, slowly inject solution to distribute medication evenly and minimize discomfort. (If blood returns with aspiration, withdraw needle, discard syringe and needle, and prepare a new medication.)
7. Remove needle quickly and gently massage the site with an alcohol swab. Massage helps medication absorb.
8. Reposition infant.
9. Remove gloves, wash hands, and document in medical record.

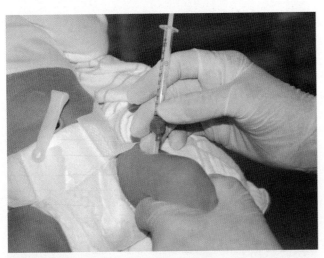

Intramuscular injection. The newborn's leg is stabilized with one hand and the needle is injected into the thigh at a 90-degree angle. Note that the nurse is wearing gloves on both hands when handling the unwashed newborn.

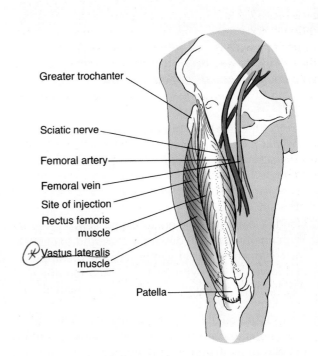

Greater trochanter

Sciatic nerve

Femoral artery

Femoral vein

Site of injection

Rectus femoris muscle

Vastus lateralis muscle

Patella

Prophylactic Eye Care

Prophylaxis against gonococcal **ophthalmia neonatorum**, an infection that can cause blindness, is required for all newborns. The newborn can acquire an eye infection, such as gonorrhea or chlamydia, when passing through an infected birth canal. Erythromycin (Ilotycin) ophthalmic ointment is commonly used for **prophylactic eye care** because it produces less eye irritation and destroys the *Chlamydia* organism. Ideally, a single unit dose (new tube) of ointment is used. The ointment is placed so that it reaches all areas of the conjunctival sac (Skill 7-9). It is recommended that eye prophylaxis be administered approximately 1 hour after birth to allow time for newborn-parent interaction without the newborn's vision being disturbed.

Promoting Parent-Newborn Bonding

As soon as the newborn is dry, warm, and stable, he or she may be wrapped in a clean blanket and placed in the mother's arms. Breastfeeding should be started if the mother desires with skin-to-skin contact and a blanket over both the baby and mother (Figure 7-18). (Breastfeeding is discussed in Chapter 11.) The alert period of the newborn in this first period of reactivity lasts for 1 hour only; the infant will then sleep for approximately 4 hours. Therefore, every effort should be made to promote bonding as soon as possible. breast-feeding should be tried to be given.

Observing for Abnormalities

The respiratory and heart rate are monitored and recorded. The newborn is observed for obvious anomalies such as symmetry of movement, cry, and the basic

startle (Moro's) reflex. A more detailed assessment is performed in phase 2 of newborn care and is discussed in Chapter 10.

The newborn is transported to the newborn nursery or couplet postpartum unit according to the facility protocol. Some hospitals transport the newborn in a radiant warmer to the nursery, where he or she is observed for 1 to 4 hours. Other hospitals wrap the newborn warmly and place him or her in the mother's arms for transport to a rooming-in unit. In an LDRP unit, the mother and newborn remain in the delivery suite until discharge.

UMBILICAL CORD BLOOD BANKING

Blood from the placenta and umbilical cord has, in the past, traditionally been treated as a waste product and discarded. It is now known that cord blood contains the same type of blood stem cells as bone marrow. Stem cells give rise to all cells found in the blood, including immune bodies. Stem cell transplants can be an invaluable aid in the treatment of many malignant and genetic diseases of children and adults.

Cord blood can be collected at birth for storage and possible future use if needed. In 2004, a bill was introduced by the U.S. Congress to establish a national network of cord blood stem cell banking under the direction of the National Health Resources and Services Administration (HRSA), and, in 2008, the American College of Obstetricians and Gynecologists (ACOG) updated the policy recognizing the use of umbilical cord blood as an accepted emerging therapy.

Skill 7-9   Administering Eye Ointment to the Newborn

PURPOSE

To protect the newborn from ophthalmia and chlamydia infection. (All newborns have this prophylactic treatment before leaving the delivery room.)

Steps

1. Gently cleanse the eye of blood and vernix.
2. With one finger, pull down the lower lid to expose the conjunctival sac, *or* gently separate the upper and lower eyelids with the thumb and forefinger.
3. Apply ointment evenly across the conjunctival sac and allow the eye to close.
4. This should be done before leaving the delivery room but after the mother and infant have had time to bond immediately after delivery.

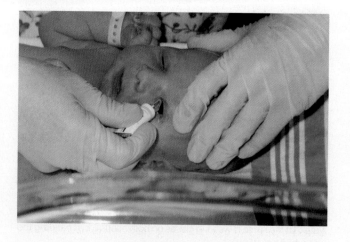

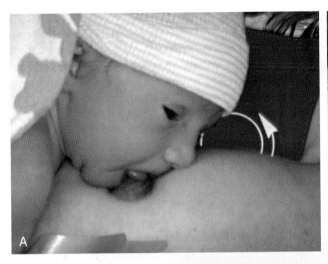
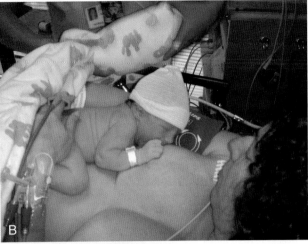
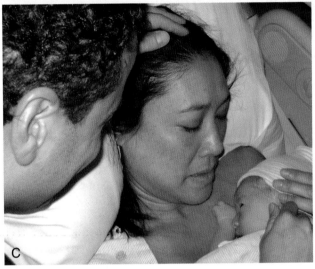

FIGURE 7-18 **Bonding. A,** This newborn infant, just a few minutes old, is placed on her mother's chest and searches for the breast nipple with her tongue to start breastfeeding. **B,** Mother and infant bond as skin-to-skin contact and breastfeeding are started just minutes after birth. Both are covered with a blanket for warmth. **C,** Mother and father bond with the newborn in the LDR room.

The collection process requires informed consent from the mother and involves using special collection kits that contain Vacutainer, screening for infectious diseases, and packaging materials required for sending the blood to the storage facility.

The Human Genome Project and development of gene therapy may further increase the value of cord blood banking. Seventy to 80 mL of cord blood is usually collected by the health care provider after delivery of the newborn and clamping of the cord but before the placenta is expelled. Cord blood must be transported to the cord blood bank storage facility within 48 hours of collection. It is then processed and cryopreserved at a temperature of −196° C (−320° F) with liquid nitrogen. No expiration date is required for undisturbed samples. All pregnant women and their partners should be counseled concerning cord blood banking. The costs of cord blood collection and banking may not be covered by health insurance.

PHASE 2 AND PHASE 3: CARE OF THE NEWBORN

Phase 2 care of the newborn occurs 1 to 4 hours after birth in the nursery or postpartum unit, and Phase 3 care of the newborn occurs from 4 hours after birth until discharge (see Chapter 10). Breastfeeding is discussed in Chapter 11.

EMERGENCY DELIVERY BY THE NURSE (WITHOUT A PHYSICIAN OR NURSE-MIDWIFE)

Labor sometimes proceeds very rapidly; a physician or nurse-midwife may not be present, and the nurse may be the most qualified health professional present to deliver the newborn. This type of delivery is called a precipitate delivery and is most likely to occur in multiparous women, although it may also occur with oxytocin stimulation and with preterm newborns.

The major nursing interventions in an emergency delivery are to:

- Remain calm and support the woman
- Provide cleanliness
- Control the birth of the baby

Reassuring the woman with a calm, confident approach lessens her fear and anxiety. This approach is helpful to the nurse as well. The nurse offers reassurance and clear instructions.

In a rapid delivery, events often happen so quickly that sterility is not the priority. However, every effort should be made to use clean linen and supplies.

Controlling the rapid birth of the baby's head is the most important thing the nurse can do in an emergency (precipitate) delivery. This is important to prevent cerebral damage to the baby and perineal lacerations to the mother. The mother should be encouraged to open her mouth and pant during the contractions to control her desire to push. Then, if possible, the nurse applies gentle pressure to the perineum and delivers the head between contractions. The rest of the baby's body usually follows with the next contraction. **The nurse should make no attempt to hold the baby's head back to prevent the birth** (Skill 7-10).

Skill 7-10   Assisting with an Emergency Birth

PURPOSE

To prioritize care and prevent injury to the mother and newborn.

Steps

1. Get the emergency delivery tray ("precip tray").
2. Do not leave the woman if she exhibits any signs of imminent birth, such as grunting, bearing down, perineal bulging, or a statement that the baby is coming. Summon the experienced nurse with the call bell and try to remain calm.
3. Put on gloves. Either clean or sterile is acceptable because no invasive procedures will be done. Gloves are used primarily to protect the nurse from secretions while supporting the infant.
4. Support the infant's head and body as it emerges. Wipe secretions from the face.
5. Use a bulb syringe to remove secretions from the mouth and nose, then clamp the cord in two places, and cut the cord between the clamps.
6. Dry the infant quickly and wrap in blankets or place in skin-to-skin contact with the mother to maintain the infant's temperature. Cover both warmly.
7. Observe the infant's color and respirations. The cry should be vigorous and the color pink (bluish hands and feet are acceptable).
8. Observe for placental detachment and bleeding. After the placenta detaches, observe for a firm fundus. If the fundus is not firm, massage it. The infant can suckle at the mother's breast to promote the release of oxytocin, which causes uterine contraction.

Get Ready for the NCLEX® Examination!

Key Points

- Nursing care focuses on establishing a healthy, open relationship between the couple and care providers. The nurse's goal should be to have the best possible outcome for the woman and her baby.
- Alternative birth settings are designed, in principle, to emphasize the naturalness of childbirth.
- The nurse is responsible for establishing an environment in which the woman and her partner are treated with kindness and respect.
- Cultural considerations in nursing care include the way pain is expressed and the significance of modesty. The nurse should be aware of various cultural traditions and integrate them with the care whenever possible.

- The data collection for an intrapartum admission includes taking a personal and obstetric history and a medical history, including a physical assessment of the woman and the fetus.
- During the first stage of labor, the nurse concentrates on the changing needs of the woman and the fetus. The support person is an important part of the team and is encouraged to participate in the woman's care.
- The nurse plays a key role in the assessment of change through the latent, active, and transition phases of labor. He or she must implement care and evaluate its effectiveness in meeting the woman's needs throughout the anticipated changes of labor and birth.

- The nurse provides continuous monitoring, support, and safety for the woman from the time she is in active labor through the recovery period.
- Fetal distress can be caused by uterine problems, fetal problems, maternal conditions, or problems with the umbilical cord. Response to medications such as epidural analgesia can also alter the FHR and cause fetal distress.
- Continuous EFM during labor can detect changes in FHR pattern that may indicate inadequate oxygenation of the fetus. This can be accomplished by an external (noninvasive) method or an internal (invasive) method.
- A nonreassuring heart rate pattern may indicate fetal distress and requires nursing interventions.
- Common nursing interventions for nonreassuring FHR patterns include lateral positioning of the mother in bed, administering oxygen by mask, monitoring the maternal hydration status, and monitoring progress of labor.
- Fetal oxygen saturation monitoring was approved by the FDA to reduce the need for cesarean birth for the term fetus with a nonreassuring FHR pattern. Its use and value remain controversial.
- An amnioinfusion is the infusion of warm normal saline or Ringer's lactate solution into the uterine cavity to decrease compression of the umbilical cord and reduce the risk of meconium aspiration.
- A doula is a specially trained person hired by the family to provide support and coaching during labor.
- The primary concern during the fourth stage of labor is the prevention of hemorrhage. Other concerns include bladder distention, comfort, and safety. During this stage (the recovery period), the nurse can facilitate parent-newborn attachment by providing skin-to-skin contact, initiating breastfeeding, and making it possible for mother and infant to get acquainted.

Additional Learning Resources

SG Go to your Study Guide on pages 485–486 for additional Review Questions for the NCLEX® Examination, Critical Thinking Clinical Situations, and other learning activities to help you master this chapter content.

 Go to your Evolve website (http://evolve.elsevier.com/Leifer/maternity) for the following FREE learning resources:
- Animations
- Answer Guidelines for Critical Thinking Questions
- Answers and Rationales for Review Questions for the NCLEX® Examination
- Concept Map Creator
- Glossary with pronunciations in English and Spanish
- Patient Teaching Plans
- Skills Performance Checklists and more!

Online Resources
- www.asia-initiative.org
- www.awhonn.org
- www.gowingo.com/health
- www.lamaze.org

Review Questions for the NCLEX® Examination

1. A woman in her last trimester of pregnancy asks, "How will I know when I am in true labor?" The nurse provides a response based on the fact that true labor is characterized primarily by:
   1. Contractions
   2. Rupture of membranes
   3. Changes in the cervix
   4. Bloody show

2. The location of the strongest fetal heart tone depends on the fetal position because the heart tone is best heard over the:
   1. Fetal back
   2. Maternal fundus
   3. Fetal occiput
   4. Placenta

3. When assessing an FHR pattern, the nurse observes early decelerations. The most appropriate nursing action for early decelerations is to:
   1. Increase rate of intravenous fluids.
   2. Assist patient into side-lying position.
   3. Administer oxygen via face mask.
   4. Continue monitoring FHR pattern.

4. The nurse is preparing a woman in labor for an amnioinfusion. Which factor would be a contraindication to amnioinfusion?
   1. Oligohydramnios
   2. Presence of meconium
   3. Vaginal bleeding
   4. Umbilical cord compression

5. A newborn will receive vitamin K:
   1. Intramuscularly in the midanterior thigh
   2. Intramuscularly in the deltoid
   3. Subcutaneously in the midanterior thigh
   4. Subcutaneously in the abdomen

6. Which of the following are signs of impending birth? *(Select all that apply.)*
   1. Increasing frequency of contractions
   2. Sitting on one buttock
   3. Bulging of the perineum
   4. Making grunting sounds

7. When nonreassuring FHR patterns occur, which emergency intervention(s) would be undertaken? *(Select all that apply.)*
   1. Stopping all intravenous fluids
   2. Administering oxygen
   3. Turning patient to side-lying position
   4. Notifying the health care provider
   5. Monitoring of intake and output

Critical Thinking Questions

A patient is G31102 at 40 weeks' gestation in active labor and handling her contractions well, sitting on a labor ball, with her husband at her side. She is 9 cm dilated, 100% effaced, and the fetus is in a −2 station. Her water suddenly breaks.

1. What is the significance of the water breaking and the −2 station?

2. What is your priority nursing action when the water breaks?

3. What stage of labor is the patient in?

4. What does G31102 mean?

5. The vaginal fluid is slightly pale yellow and watery. What is the significance of this?

6. What nursing interventions are needed at this time?

Management of Pain During Labor

Objectives

1. Define key terms listed.
2. Describe the factors that influence a woman's comfort during labor.
3. Explain the physical causes of pain during labor.
4. Explain the role of endorphins in the body.
5. Discuss three nonpharmacologic pain control strategies.

6. Review the potential effect of sedatives and narcotics on the newborn.
7. Explain the advantages and limitations of pharmacologic methods of pain management.
8. Outline the nursing responsibilities related to pharmacologic and nonpharmacologic pain management during labor.

Key Terms

anesthesia (ăn-ĕs-THĒ-zē-ă, p. 153)
blood patch (p. 155)
cognitive stimulation (KŎG-nĭ-tĭv stĭm-ū-LĀ-shŭn, p. 150)
cutaneous stimulation (kū-TĀ-nē-ŭs, p. 150)
effleurage (ef-loo-rahzh´, p.148)

endorphins (p. 148)
epidural block (ĕp-ĭ-DOO-răl, p. 153)
gate control theory (p. 148)
pudendal block (pū-DĔN-dăl, p. 153)
sacral pressure (SĂ-krăl, p. 150)

PAIN MANAGEMENT

Labor pains exist for a short time only. However, within that short time, the discomfort progresses from a slightly unpleasant experience to intense sensations. To the woman in labor, discomfort or pain may seem endless, and she may wonder whether she can tolerate it. To the nurse, the process of labor is a challenge. Armed with knowledge of the characteristics of pain in the various stages of labor, interventions for pain relief, comfort methods, and cultural responses to labor pain, the nurse is able to design a care plan to meet the specific needs of the woman in labor. Working with the woman, family, and other health professionals, the nurse can meet the challenges of making each labor and birth a safe and satisfying experience.

STANDARDS OF PAIN MANAGEMENT

The Joint Commission (TJC) recognizes the importance of pain control in all health care settings for *all* patients. Standards include:
- Patients have the right to pain management.
- Staff must competently assess and manage pain.
- Policies should be in place to support prescription of pain medication.
- Patients should be educated about pain management.
- Pain management extends past discharge.

THE UNIQUE PAIN OF LABOR

Pain is universal. How it is experienced is both personal and subjective. Childbirth pain differs from pain experienced in other conditions in the following ways:
- Labor pain is part of the **normal** process, whereas pain at other times usually indicates illness or injury.
- The sources of pain are known. The purpose of the muscle contraction helps in the birthing process.
- The woman has time for preparation. Knowledge and skills can be developed to manage the pain. The sensation is referred to as a *contraction* rather than a pain.
- The pain is known to be self-limiting. It is anticipated to last only hours, not days or weeks. Each contraction pain has a beginning, peak (or acme), and ending that can be anticipated to help the woman cope during the labor process.
- The pain ends with the birth of a baby.

Pain control during labor can be managed by nonpharmacologic (non-drug) or pharmacologic (drug) methods. General nonpharmacologic comfort measures during labor, such as adjustment of the environment, breathing techniques, or maternal positioning, are discussed in Chapter 5.

FACTORS THAT INFLUENCE LABOR PAIN

Several factors cause pain during labor and influence the amount of pain a woman experiences. Other factors influence a woman's response to and ability to tolerate or cope with labor pain.

Pain Threshold and Pain Tolerance

Two terms are often used interchangeably to describe pain, although they have different meanings. **Pain threshold,** also called *pain perception*, is the least amount of sensation that a person perceives as painful. Pain threshold is fairly constant, and it varies little under different conditions. **Pain tolerance** is the amount of pain one is willing to endure. Unlike the pain threshold, one's pain tolerance can change under different conditions. A primary nursing responsibility is to modify as many factors as possible so that the woman can safely tolerate the pain of labor and delivery.

Sources of Pain During Labor

Physical sources are the main contributors to pain during labor:

- Dilation and stretching of the cervix (stimulates nerve ganglia)
- Uterine contractions (decrease in blood supply to uterus causes ischemic uterine pain similar to ischemic heart pain)
- Pressure and pulling of pelvic structures (ligaments, fallopian tubes, and peritoneum)
- Distention and stretching of the vagina and perineum (splitting and tearing sensation)
- The intensity of labor contractions
- The length of time for cervical changes to occur
- The size and position of the fetus, which add to the length of labor

Other factors that contribute to the pain of labor include:

- The mother's fatigue and pain tolerance
- Fear and anxiety: These result in muscle tension, which exaggerates the pain sensation of the labor contraction.
- Cervical readiness: The mother's cervix normally undergoes changes that facilitate effacement and dilation in labor. If the cervix has not made these changes (ripening), more contractions are needed to cause effacement and dilation.
- Interventions of caregivers: Although they are intended to promote maternal and fetal safety, common interventions such as intravenous lines, fetal monitoring, amniotomy, or vaginal examinations can be a source of discomfort or pain in the laboring woman.
- Psychosocial factors: Culture influences how a woman reacts to pain during childbirth (see Table 7-1).

GATE CONTROL THEORY

The **gate control theory** of pain has application to labor and childbirth. According to the gate control theory, a gating mechanism occurs in the spinal cord. Pain sensations are transmitted from the periphery of the body along nerve pathways to the brain. Only a limited number of sensations can travel these pathways at one time. Distractions or focused activity can replace travel of pain sensation. When the activity fills the path, the gate is closed, and impulses are less likely to be transmitted to the brain. When the gate is open, pain impulses ascend to the brain. Similar gating mechanisms exist in the descending nerve fibers from the hypothalamus and cerebral cortex. These areas of the brain regulate a person's thoughts and emotions and can influence whether pain impulses reach the level of conscious awareness. **Effleurage**, cutaneous stimulation by a patterned massage of the abdomen, may have a direct effect on closing the gate. The gate control theory, by using descending and ascending neural pathways, helps explain the effectiveness of various types of focusing strategies taught in childbirth preparation classes, such as breathing, listening to music, verbal coaching, and effleurage. Acupuncture, external analgesics, and back massage provide relief because they help close the "gate" to the discomfort.

CHEMICAL FACTORS

Neuromodulators, also called **endorphins** or endogenous opiates, are protein chemicals found in the brain. They are produced by the anterior pituitary gland and the hypothalamus. They are natural opiate-like substances known to relieve pain. Endorphins (and **enkephalins**) are similar to morphine-like substances. They are believed to play a major role in the biologic response to pain. They may be produced by stress and increase the pain threshold, thus helping the woman tolerate the pain of labor and birth. Endorphins are believed to make the woman drowsy and sleepy. Studies have shown that the endorphin blood level in a woman during the birthing process is much higher than that of a nonpregnant woman. Women who have a positive attitude during labor and birth have more natural protection because of their body's ability to produce its own endorphin analgesia.

NONPHARMACOLOGIC PAIN CONTROL STRATEGIES

The United States is a multicultural society, and the nurse must understand the cultural traditions concerning expression of pain to provide culturally sensitive care and support. Fear, anxiety, and muscle tension increase catecholamine secretion and increase pain perception. All laboring women benefit from nursing interventions that can relieve fear, tension, and anxiety. The nurse must empower the mother to use her own method of dealing with pain.

Various nonpharmacologic measures for control of labor pain are practiced (Box 8-1). Many of these techniques are learned in childbirth education classes. These include general support, imagery or visualization, distraction, changes in temperature, touch, comfort measures, and baths (whirlpool if available). The nurse's role is to assist the woman in using the techniques she has learned during childbirth classes and

to encourage support and participation of the partner or coach (Figure 8-1).

GENERAL COMFORT MEASURES

General comfort can reduce stress and thus reduce pain. Also, comfort measures can encourage relaxation. It is important to eliminate sources of noxious (offensive) stimuli whenever possible. The nurse can try to relieve thirst, sweating, and heat through comfort measures. Providing ice chips and lollipops and

---

Box 8-1   Nonpharmacologic Pain Relief Measures

PROGRESSIVE RELAXATION
- The woman contracts and then consciously releases different muscle groups.
- Technique helps the woman to distinguish tense muscles from relaxed ones.
- The woman can assess and then release muscle tension throughout her body.
- Technique is most effective if practiced before labor.

NEUROMUSCULAR DISSOCIATION (DIFFERENTIAL RELAXATION)
- The woman strongly contracts one group of muscles and consciously relaxes all others.
- The coach checks for unrecognized tension in muscle groups other than the one contracted.
- This prepares the woman to relax the rest of her body while the uterus is contracting.
- Technique is most effective if practiced before labor.

TOUCH RELAXATION
- The woman contracts a muscle group and then relaxes it when her partner strokes or massages it.
- The woman learns to respond to touch with relaxation.
- Technique is most effective if practiced before labor.

RELAXATION AGAINST PAIN
- The woman's partner exerts pressure against a tendon or large muscle of the arm or leg, gradually increasing the pressure and gradually decreasing pressure to simulate the gradual increase, peak, and decrease in contraction strength.
- The woman consciously relaxes despite this deliberate discomfort.
- This gives the woman practice in relaxation against pain.
- Technique is most effective if practiced before labor.

EFFLEURAGE
- The abdomen or other areas are massaged during contractions.
- Massage interferes with transmission of pain impulses, but prolonged continuous use reduces effectiveness (habituation). The pattern or area massaged should be changed when it becomes less effective.
- Massaging in a specific pattern (such as circles or a figure eight) also provides distraction.

OTHER MASSAGE
- Massage of the feet, hands, or shoulders often helps relaxation.

- Habituation may occur in any type of massage. Change the area massaged if it occurs.

SACRAL PRESSURE
- Technique helps reduce the pain of back labor (see Figure 8-2).
- Obtain the woman's input about the best position. Moving the pressure point a fraction of an inch or changing the amount of pressure may significantly improve effectiveness.
- Pressure may also be applied by tennis balls in a sock, a warmed plastic container of intravenous solution, or other means.

THERMAL STIMULATION
- Technique stimulates temperature receptors that interfere with pain transmission.
- Either heat or cold applications may be beneficial. Examples are cool cloths to the face and ice in a glove to the lower back.

POSITIONING
- Any position except the supine position is acceptable if there is no need for a specific position.
- Upright positions favor fetal descent.
- Hands-and-knees position helps reduce the pain of back labor.
- Change positions about every 30 to 60 minutes to relieve pressure and muscle fatigue.

DIVERSION AND DISTRACTION
- Technique increases mental concentration on something besides the pain. It may take many forms:
  - Focal point: concentrating on a specific object or other point
  - Imagery: creating an imaginary mental picture of a pleasant environment or visualizing the cervix opening and the infant descending
  - Music: serves as a distraction or provides "white noise" to obscure environmental sounds

HYDROTHERAPY
- Water delivered by shower, tub, or whirlpool relieves tired muscles and relaxes the woman.
- Nipple stimulation by shower can increase contraction because it stimulates the pituitary to release oxytocin.

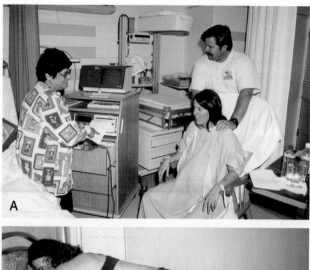

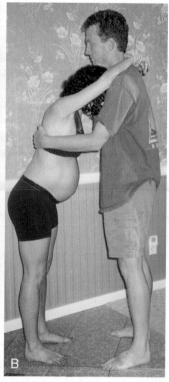

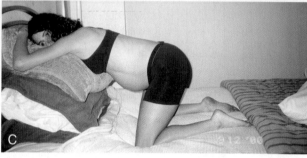

FIGURE 8-1 The nurse can best teach or support nonpharmacologic pain control during the latent phase of labor, when the woman is comfortable enough to understand the teaching. **A,** The nurse explains the electronic monitor that shows tthat the acme of the contraction has passed, while the partner massages the back and shoulders of the laboring woman. **B,** The woman walks during early labor and leans on her partner during a contraction. **C,** The woman assumes a knee-chest position to ease the pain of "back labor" caused by a fetal occiput posterior presentation.

repositioning the woman or adjusting the monitoring belts may provide relief.

COGNITIVE STIMULATION

Several cognitive stimulation methods (mental stimulation) of pain control may be tried. Imagery (imagining a pleasant experience) can help the woman by serving as a distraction from the painful stimuli. Using a focal point or focusing on breathing patterns or a spot on the wall may help the woman block out painful sensations. This behavior requires her active participation.

CUTANEOUS STIMULATION

Cutaneous stimulation, involving touching, rubbing, or massaging (back or shoulders), often decreases discomfort. Counter-pressure—a variation with the palm, closed fist, or firm object pressed at the point of back pain (sacral pressure)—is often helpful (Figure 8-2). Rhythmic stroking and massage of the abdomen (effleurage) during a contraction can also lessen discomfort (see Figure 5-13 and Chapter 21). Note that some women do not like to be touched.

THERMAL STIMULATION

During early labor, women may find a warm bath or shower relaxing. A cool, damp cloth applied to the forehead is especially comforting to some women in the later phases of labor. Hot or cold towels applied

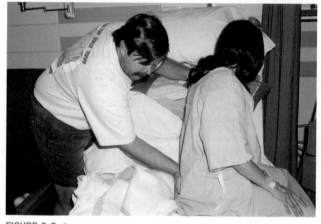

FIGURE 8-2 Sacral pressure applied by the partner during early labor.

to the back may be effective, or the use of a shower or a disposable bottle filled with warm water can be used to provide warmth and mild pressure to the back.

BREATHING TECHNIQUES

Breathing techniques change the focus during the contraction. There is no right or wrong breathing pattern, but rather the woman should use what she feels comfortable with (see Chapter 5). Breathing techniques can be taught to the unprepared woman while she is in labor (ideally during early labor). The nurse evaluates the breathing techniques used by the laboring woman.

RELAXATION

Even if the woman has attended prenatal classes, she will need continued support in achieving relaxation of her voluntary muscles. The most effective teaching time, once labor has begun, is between contractions and during the first stage of labor.

HYPNOSIS

Hypnosis can be a powerful labor intervention that appears to be safe, is without known side effects, and has positive physical and psychological outcomes. With hypnosis, the woman retains a feeling of control. The nurse can optimize the woman's hypnosis experience by understanding how his or her role in the labor room may be modified. Hypnosis is a technique that the mother may select during pregnancy; she is usually trained in self-hypnosis that can be used during labor. In the labor room, the nurse may help trigger self-hypnosis by using specific suggestions or playing specific audiotapes provided by the woman. The labor nurse must not interrupt the woman during a contraction when the woman is using self-hypnosis techniques. Characteristic signs of progression in labor may not be evident in a patient under hypnosis; therefore, careful observation and documentation concerning the progress of labor are essential.

PHARMACOLOGIC PAIN CONTROL STRATEGIES

PHYSIOLOGY OF PREGNANCY AND ITS RELATIONSHIP TO ANALGESIA AND ANESTHESIA

Specific factors in the physiology of pregnancy affect the pregnant woman's response to analgesia and anesthesia:

- The pregnant woman is at increased risk for hypoxia caused by the pressure of the enlarging uterus on the diaphragm.
- The sluggish gastrointestinal tract of the pregnant woman can result in increased risk for vomiting and aspiration.
- Aortocaval compression, also known as *vena cava syndrome* (pressure on the abdominal aorta by the heavy uterus when the woman is in a supine position), increases the risk of hypotension and the development of shock.
- The effect on the fetus must be considered.

See the effects of pregnancy on drug metabolism in Chapter 4.

ADVANTAGES OF PHARMACOLOGIC METHODS

The use of drugs for reducing pain during labor can help the woman be a more active participant in the birth process. They help her relax and work with the contractions. Drugs do not usually relieve all pain and pressure sensations.

The pain of labor may cause a "stress response" in the mother that results in an increase in autonomic activity, a release of catecholamines, and a decrease in platelet perfusion. This stress response results in fetal acidosis. The pain can also cause maternal hyperventilation and lead to respiratory alkalosis, then a compensating metabolic acidosis (Box 8-2). Metabolic acidosis in the woman results in fetal acidosis, which can compromise the fetus's health. Therefore, appropriate pain relief during labor can play an important role in the positive outcome of pregnancy for mother and infant.

LIMITATIONS OF PHARMACOLOGIC METHODS

Pharmacologic methods are effective, but they do have limits. One important limitation is that two persons are medicated: the mother and her fetus. Any drug given to the mother can affect the fetus, and the effects may be prolonged in the infant long after birth. The drug may directly or indirectly affect the fetus because of effects the drug(s) produce in the mother (such as hypotension).

Several pharmacologic methods may slow labor's progress if used early in labor. Some complications during pregnancy limit the pharmacologic methods that can be safely used during labor. For example, a method that requires the infusion of large amounts of intravenous fluids might overload the woman's circulation if she has a heart disease. If she takes other medications (legal or illicit), they may interact adversely with the drugs used to relieve labor pain.

Physical factors can influence the intensity and duration of pain that the woman experiences during labor. At times, nonpharmacologic methods of pain relief need to be combined with pharmacologic management. The nurse should provide support to the woman, who is ultimately responsible for choosing the method of pain control. The nurse can reassure the woman that pharmacologic methods are acceptable and safe when they are given and monitored as necessary. The decision to prescribe and administer

---

Box 8-2   **How to Recognize and Correct Hyperventilation**

SIGNS AND SYMPTOMS
- Dizziness
- Tingling of hands and feet
- Cramps and muscle spasms of hands
- Numbness around nose and mouth
- Blurring of vision

CORRECTIVE MEASURES
- Breathe slowly, especially in exhalation
- Breathe into cupped hands
- Place a moist washcloth over the mouth and nose while breathing
- Hold breath for a few seconds before exhaling

drugs during labor must be carefully weighed because of the effects on the newborn. Dosage and time of administration must be calculated to avoid having the baby born with respiratory depression. Because the fetus cannot metabolize the drugs as quickly as the mother, the fetal response may be intense and last much longer (Box 8-3).

Before medication is administered, baseline assessments of maternal vital signs, fetal heart rate (FHR) patterns, known allergies, and last oral intake should be documented. During the first stage of labor, administration of drugs may affect the progress of labor. If an analgesic is given too soon during the latent phase, it may slow down the labor. Labor should be well established, with a cervical dilation of 4 cm (active labor) before the woman receives pain medication. As labor progresses, some women may need medication to help them relax. It is important to record the time and amount given, the woman's vital signs, and the FHR.

Various forms of pain medication can be used in labor; herbal pain remedies may also be used in some cultures to reduce pain. When designing her birth plan, it is best for the woman to discuss the options during early labor (see Chapter 5). Analgesics during labor may reduce the hormonal and stress response to the pain of labor and be especially advantageous to the obese or hypertensive woman.

ANALGESIA

Parenteral opioids can reduce gastric emptying, thus increasing the risk of aspiration if food or fluids are in the stomach. Careful monitoring of vital signs and FHR is essential when these analgesics are used. Injections should be given at the beginning of a

---

| Box 8-3 | Factors That Influence Drug Choice for Labor |

- The woman's preference for pain relief should be considered.
- The drug should provide maximum relief to the woman, with minimum risk to the fetus.
- The drug should have minimum side effects.
- Labor should be well established.
- If the drug affects uterine contractions, the woman should be made aware of this effect.
- Adequate fetal monitoring and emergency equipment should be available.
- The drug must allow the uterus to contract during the postpartum period. (Some general anesthetics relax the uterus and increase bleeding.)
- Drugs should not be given if less than 1 hour remains before delivery because, after birth, the infant may have difficulty metabolizing them and may have respiratory depression.
- Women with a history of substance abuse have fewer safe choices for pain relief.
- Drugs cross the placenta and may cause neonatal respiratory depression.

---

contraction so that little of the drug will go to the placenta for transfer to the fetus. By the end of the contraction, much of the medication will have been transported to maternal tissues, and effect on the fetus will be minimized. Analgesics used to reduce the perception of pain in labor include the following:

- *Meperidine (Demerol)* is a common intravenous opioid that is sometimes used during labor. It has a rapid onset and a 50-minute peak of action. Ideally, birth should occur more than 2 hours after administration of opioids so that the newborn will not have central nervous system (CNS) depression that will require resuscitation. Respiratory depression in the newborn may last up to 3 days and, for this reason, this drug is not the drug of choice during labor. Maternal responses may include hypotension, sedation, nausea, and pruritus (itching). Decreased FHR and variability can occur. *[handwritten: Most common]*

- *Sublimaze (Fentanyl)* is a rapid onset, short-acting opioid agonist that lasts approximately 1 to 2 hours. Respiratory depression can occur. This drug is often used in combination with regional anesthesia.

- *Butorphanol (Stadol)* and *nalbuphine (Nubain)* are combination opioid agonist-antagonist drugs that relieve pain and nausea and have a short duration of action. These medications must not be given to women with drug dependence because a withdrawal response may be precipitated in both mother and newborn (London, Ladewig, Ball, & Bindler, 2006).

- *Naloxone (Narcan)* is used to relieve maternal itching (pruritus) that commonly occurs as a side effect to epidural anesthesia. Naloxone is also used as an adjunct to oxygenation, ventilation, and gentle stimulation in the treatment of newborn respiratory depression. Opioids may remain in the system of the newborn for several days and cause temporary alterations in neurobehavioral responses of the newborn (London, Ladewig, Ball, & Bindler, 2006). Naloxone may cause withdrawal symptoms in women with a history of illicit drug use, and symptoms may persist in the newborn.

SEDATIVES

Sedatives such as phenobarbital do not produce relief of pain. Sedatives may relieve anxiety and nausea, but they cross the placenta, affect the fetus, and usually have no antagonists (reversing agent) to assist the newborn who may have respiratory depression. Sedatives may inhibit the mother's ability to cope with the pain of labor and therefore are not usually used during active labor.

ADJUNCTIVE DRUGS

Phenothiazine medications such as *promethazine (Phenergan)* or *hydroxyzine (Vistaril)* can control nausea and anxiety and may reduce narcotic requirements during labor. These drugs do not relieve pain and are used in conjunction with opioids. Vistaril cannot be given intravenously.

Benzodiazepine drugs such as diazepam (Valium) are rarely used in obstetrics because of their depressive effects. Flumazenil is a benzodiazepine antagonist that can help reverse maternal drug-induced sedation and ventilatory depression. Adjunctive drugs such as *diphenhydramine (Benadryl)* may be given to relieve pruritus.

ANESTHESIA

Anesthesia is the partial or complete loss of sensation with or without loss of consciousness. Two types of anesthesia used in labor care are regional blocks and general anesthesia. The most commonly used regional blocks are listed in Table 8-1.

Regional Anesthesia

With regional anesthesia, the woman is able to participate in the birth and retains her protective airway reflexes, both of which are advantages. The injection sites of regional anesthetics are shown in Figure 8-3. The pudendal block is given when the woman is ready for delivery. It anesthetizes the lower vagina and part of the perineum (Figure 8-4).

In an epidural block, the anesthetic is injected into the epidural space, which is located inside the vertebral column surrounding the dural sac in the lumbar region of the spine. An epidural block can be given during the first and second stages of labor. A **spinal subarachnoid block** is commonly used for cesarean births. Frequent monitoring of maternal vital signs

Table 8-1	Regional Anesthesia Used During Labor and Birth			
TYPE OF PROCEDURE	**AREA AND EFFECT OF BLOCK**	**WHEN GIVEN**	**MAJOR DISADVANTAGES**	**NURSING INTERVENTIONS**
Pudendal Block				
Local anesthetic injected transvaginally into space in front of pudendal nerve	Perineum, vulva, rectal area; causes perineal anesthesia for repair of episiotomy or lacerations	Late second stage (10-20 minutes before birth of baby)	Broad ligament hematoma	Instruct patient about method; provide support; assess for hematoma.
Epidural Block				
Local anesthetic injected into epidural space at fifth lumbar vertebrae (caudal block is achieved at level of sacral hiatus and is rarely used today)	Affects all sensations from the level of the umbilicus to the thighs; relieves discomfort of uterine contractions and fetal descent and anesthetizes perineum	Active labor (4 cm dilated) to relieve pain	Maternal hypotension, fetal bradycardia, loss of bearing-down reflex in second stage possibly causing urinary retention	Position patient as required; instruct patient about method; assess maternal blood pressure and pulse and FHR every 5 minutes; assess maternal bladder at frequent intervals; do not let woman walk alone until all motor control has returned; assess for orthostatic hypotension.
Spinal Block				
Local anesthetic injected into subarachnoid space	Affects all sensations from the level of the nipple to the feet; given for vaginal birth and cesarean birth	May be given before cesarean birth; numbs body from nipples to feet	Limited duration of action; maternal hypotension, fetal bradycardia, loss of bearing-down reflex in second stage; potential headache during postpartum period; may cause urinary retention	Instruct patient about method; assess maternal vital signs every 5-10 minutes; assess uterine contractions, hypotension, and level of anesthesia; assess FHR tracing; provide safety and prevent injury when woman moves; recognize signs of impending birth.
Paracervical Nerve Block				
Lidocaine injected into cervical mucosa	Used early in labor to block pain of uterine contractions	Given during first stage of labor	Causes fetal bradycardia; improper technique can result in serious toxicity	Rarely used today; closely monitor labor progress because patient does not feel sensations or contractions.

FHR, fetal heart rate.

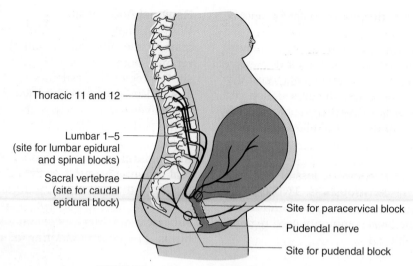

Thoracic 11 and 12

Lumbar 1–5
(site for lumbar epidural
and spinal blocks)

Sacral vertebrae
(site for caudal
epidural block)

Site for paracervical block

Pudendal nerve

Site for pudendal block

FIGURE 8-3 Injection sites of regional anesthetics.

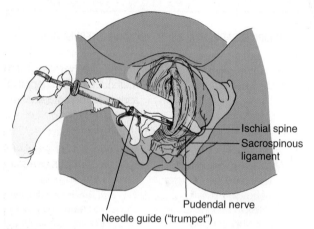

Ischial spine
Sacrospinous
ligament

Pudendal nerve
Needle guide ("trumpet")

FIGURE 8-4 Pudendal block provides local anesthesia that is adequate for an episiotomy and use of low forceps.

and FHR is important, and it is significant to observe the level of anesthesia (Figure 8-5).

The use of epidural and intrathecal opioids without an anesthetic agent allows the woman to sense the contractions without feeling pain; in addition, the ability to voluntarily bear down during the second stage of labor is not lost. This modification may also be helpful in postoperative cesarean birth pain relief because motor ability is not lost. A "walking epidural" is achieved with lower dosages of the anesthetic agent. This is known as a *spinal epidural* or *coaxial* technique. A single dose of a long-acting opioid before the epidural catheter is removed after delivery can provide the woman with long-acting pain relief for approximately 24 hours.

Contraindications to Epidural and Subarachnoid Blocks. Because hypotension is a common side effect of epidural and subarachnoid blocks, a woman who has hypovolemia (such as hemorrhage) would have difficulty maintaining blood pressure and adequate uteroplacental perfusion. Anticoagulant therapy or a blood-clotting disorder may lead to the formation of a hematoma at the injection site with serious consequences. As with other medications, allergy or infection at the injection site would also be a contraindication to epidural and spinal analgesia.

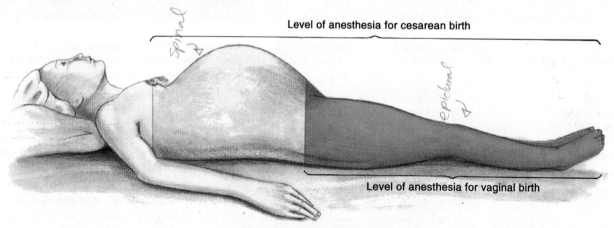

Level of anesthesia for cesarean birth

Level of anesthesia for vaginal birth

FIGURE 8-5 Levels of anesthesia for epidural and subarachnoid blocks.

Side Effects of Regional Anesthesia and the Nursing Role. The nurse should witness that informed consent was obtained for the administration of regional anesthesia and clarify information with the woman and her partner. The woman's bladder is emptied, and the nurse assists with positioning during the administration procedure. Hypotension is a common side effect of regional anesthesia, so frequent monitoring of blood pressure is required. Hypotension can decrease uteroplacental blood perfusion; therefore, close monitoring of fetal heart patterns is also essential. Intravenous fluids may be prescribed to prevent or treat dehydration. Ringer's lactate solution or normal saline is most often used because a glucose-containing solution causes the fetus to increase insulin production, which can result in hypoglycemia after birth. Glucose also causes an increase in kidney excretion of urine, and, because the woman cannot sense the urge to void, the nurse must be observant for a distended bladder and maintain an accurate intake and output. Because sensation is altered, position changes should be initiated by the nurse to preserve skin integrity. The upright position should be included in position changes. Itching is a common side effect of regional anesthesia and can be managed with a variety of comfort measures.

If an intramuscular medication is ordered for a woman receiving regional anesthesia, the upper arm (deltoid) site is preferred because of the predictable absorption rate (Bricker & Lavender, 2002). The second stage of labor may be prolonged when epidural anesthesia is used, but recent research has not shown any ill effects (Bowes & Thorp, 2004).

Toxicity with local anesthetics is a rare occurrence, but the nurse must be alert for symptoms such as disorientation, ringing in the ears, twitching, and convulsions. Hypothermia is a common side effect after birth because of vasodilation and radiant heat loss. The room should be kept warm, wet linen removed, and the woman covered with warm blankets after delivery. A headache may occur after a spinal block because of cerebrospinal fluid leakage at the site of puncture. A **blood patch** often provides dramatic relief (Figure 8-6). In a blood patch, 10 to 15 mL of the woman's blood is injected into the epidural space to seal the dural puncture. The woman should be advised to avoid straining during bowel movements or coughing for a few days after a blood patch procedure. Bed rest in a flat position and intravenous fluids relieve the postspinal headache that may occur in the postpartum period.

Headaches do not occur with epidural blocks because the dura mater of the spinal canal has not been penetrated and there is no leakage of spinal fluid. Therefore, lying flat after birth is not necessary when an epidural has been used.

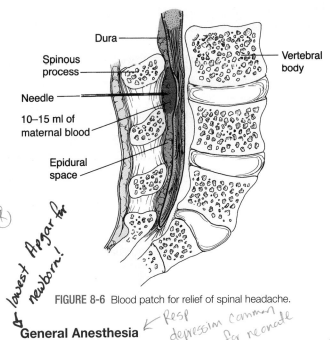

FIGURE 8-6 Blood patch for relief of spinal headache.

General Anesthesia

General anesthesia is rarely given for vaginal births. It is sometimes used in an emergency cesarean birth when the woman is not a good candidate for the spinal block. It relieves pain through the loss of consciousness. General anesthesia puts the woman at risk for regurgitation and aspiration of gastric contents. The gastric contents are highly acidic and can produce chemical pneumonitis if aspirated. Administering drugs to raise the gastric pH and make secretions less acidic reduces the risk of lung injury if aspiration occurs. General anesthesia crosses the placental barrier, and the fetus will be under its effects at birth, making resuscitation and establishment of initial respiration a challenge. In the postpartum period, the effects of general anesthesia may cause the uterus to relax. Close observation and nursing intervention are necessary to prevent postpartum hemorrhage.

THE NURSE'S ROLE IN PHARMACOLOGIC TECHNIQUES

The nurse's responsibility in pharmacologic pain management begins at admission (Nursing Care Plan 8-1). The woman should be closely questioned about allergy to foods, drugs (including dental anesthetics), or latex to identify pain relief measures that may not be advisable. She should be questioned about her preferences for pain relief. Factors that may affect the choice of pain relief should be noted, such as back surgery, infection in the area where an epidural block would be injected, or blood pressure abnormalities.

For safety reasons, the nurse keeps the side rails up on the bed if the woman is given medications for pain relief. Narcotics may cause drowsiness or dizziness. Regional anesthetics reduce sensation and movement

✦ Nursing Care Plan 8-1   Pain Relief During Labor

Scenario
A woman in the labor unit is in active labor and is 4 cm dilated. She states her contractions are very painful and asks how she can get some pain relief.

Selected Nursing Diagnosis
Acute pain related to labor and delivery process

Expected Outcomes	Nursing Interventions	Rationales
Patient will be able to make an informed decision regarding pain control options she would like to use.	Assess current knowledge of obstetric pain control measures.	Allows the nurse to develop an individualized teaching plan for the patient.
	Assess whether patient attended childbirth classes; if yes, determine the childbirth techniques taught.	Provides necessary information so the nurse can reinforce psychoprophylactic methods of coping or initiate teaching of nonpharmacologic comfort measures that can be used during stages of labor.
	Provide positive reinforcement and encouragement to patient and support persons as they apply nonpharmacologic techniques learned in childbirth classes. Assist with techniques as necessary.	Positive reinforcement and encouragement provide the patient and support person a sense of control and self-confidence.
	Assess anxiety level, and implement measures to reduce anxiety as needed.	Allows for early intervention to decrease anxiety levels. High levels of anxiety can increase the perception of pain, decrease ability to tolerate pain, and decrease comprehension of verbal instruction.
	Provide teaching between uterine contractions.	The patient is more attentive and can better internalize information when not in pain.
	Teach patient pain control options available, giving the pros and cons of each.	Providing information allows the patient to make informed decisions regarding pain control.
Patient will express relief obtained from labor pain by the use of childbirth techniques learned and/or comfort measures, analgesics, and anesthetics given.	Initiate teaching and reinforcement of nonpharmacologic comfort measures that can be used during labor if needed (e.g., use of focal point, visual imagery, breathing, and relaxation techniques). Assist with implementation of these measures as needed.	These nonpharmacologic comfort measures work by providing diversion during uterine contractions. According to the gate control theory of pain, only a limited number of sensations can travel along neural pathways at any one time, so when activities fill the pathway, pain is inhibited.
	Provide massage or counter-pressure or help patient find position of maximum comfort—standing, sitting, squatting, side-lying, on hands and knees—as needed.	Changing positions and using counter-pressure may help alleviate discomfort caused by pressure of presenting parts on bony structures, ligaments, or tissues. Massage helps relieve muscle tension and provide a diversion to inhibit pain sensations.
	If patient is considering an epidural, ensure that informed consent is obtained *before* administration of narcotics.	The patient will have to wait several hours to sign an epidural consent if narcotics are given before the request for an epidural.
Patient will have relaxed facial expressions and be able to rest between uterine contractions.	Assess for nonverbal signs of ineffective coping with pain and offer pain medications and/or epidural anesthesia.	Some patients hesitate to make requests even when they would like pharmacologic interventions. It is common for women in many cultures not to request assistance.
	Administer pain medications as ordered and assist with epidural placement.	Pharmacologic intervention may be needed to alleviate discomfort when nonpharmacologic methods of pain control are perceived to be ineffective.
	Provide comfort measures (ice chips, petroleum jelly for dry lips, dry linens, etc.).	Enhances patient's comfort level.
	Keep patient informed of progress made after each vaginal examination.	Progression of effacement, dilation, and station encourages the patient that she is making progress and that the discomfort will not last forever.
	Inform patient when uterine contractions reach peak intensity (acme).	Knowledge that a uterine contraction has reached peak intensity often promotes relaxation, which reduces muscle tension and pain sensations.

Critical Thinking Questions

1. A woman is in the early first stage of labor and states she is afraid she will not be able to tolerate the pain of labor and asks for medication to "keep the pain level low." What nonpharmacologic comfort measures can you suggest?

to varying degrees, and therefore the woman may have less control over her body.

The nurse reinforces the explanations given by the anesthesia clinician regarding the procedures and the expected effects of the selected pain management method. Women often receive these explanations when they are very uncomfortable and do not remember everything they were told. The woman is helped to assume and hold the position for the epidural or subarachnoid block. The nurse tells the anesthesia clinician when the woman has a contraction because it might prevent her from holding still. The anesthetic drug is usually injected between contractions.

The woman is observed for hypotension if an epidural or subarachnoid block is given. Hospital protocols vary, but blood pressure is measured every 5 minutes after the block begins (and with each reinjection) until her blood pressure has returned to baseline and is stable. An automatic blood pressure monitor is often used. Some facilities add a pulse oximeter to monitor oxygen saturation. At the same time, the nurse observes the fetal monitor for signs associated with fetal compromise (see Chapter 7) because maternal hypotension can reduce placental blood flow.

Evidence-Based Practice

Maternal Blood Pressure

AWHONN practice guidelines suggest assessing maternal blood pressure and FHR Q5 minutes after regional analgesia, such as epidural medication, is administered.

The epidural block is given during labor and may reduce the mother's sensation of rectal pressure. The nurse coaches her about the right time to start and stop pushing with each contraction if needed. The nurse also observes for signs of imminent birth, such as increased bloody show and perineal bulging, because the woman may not be able to feel the sensations clearly.

Nursing responsibilities related to general anesthesia include assessment and documentation of oral intake and administration of medications to reduce gastric acidity. The woman should be told that all preparations for surgery will be performed before she is put to sleep. The nurse should reassure her that she will be asleep before any incision is made. Having a familiar nurse in the operating room full of new people may be reassuring to the woman before surgery.

Safety Alert

Admission Assessments

The following are important admission assessments related to pharmacologic pain management: last oral intake (time and type), adverse or allergic reactions to drugs (especially dental anesthetics), other medications taken, any food allergies or latex allergy, medical or surgical history, and personal preferences.

The woman who has received a general anesthetic is usually awake enough to move from the operating table to her bed after surgery. Her respiratory status is observed every 15 minutes for 1 to 2 hours. A pulse oximeter provides constant information about her blood oxygen level. She is given oxygen by facemask or other means until she is fully awake. Her uterine fundus and vaginal bleeding are observed as for any other postpartum woman. Her urinary output from the indwelling catheter should be observed for quantity and color at least hourly for 4 hours.

If the woman receives narcotic drugs, the nurse observes her respiratory rate for depression. Because respiratory depression is more likely to occur in the neonate than in the mother, the neonate is closely observed after birth. Narcotic effects in the infant may persist longer than in an adult. The nurse has naloxone on hand in case it is needed to reverse respiratory depression in the mother or neonate.

The nurse observes the woman for late-appearing respiratory depression and excessive sedation if she received epidural narcotics after a cesarean birth. This may be up to 24 hours after administration, depending on the drug given. The woman's vital signs are monitored hourly, and a pulse oximeter may be applied. Facilities often use a scale to assess for sedation so that all caregivers use the same criteria for assessment and documentation. For example, landmarks can be used to measure where sensory levels begin and end. An alcohol prep pad can be used to determine sensation levels on the skin. If the woman reports numbness of the chest, tongue, or face or has difficulty taking a full breath, the anesthesia level may be too high. These symptoms should be reported immediately to the health care provider. Additional analgesics are given cautiously and strictly as ordered. If mild analgesics do not relieve the pain, the health care provider is contacted for additional orders.

Get Ready for the NCLEX® Examination!

Key Points

- Childbirth pain is unique because it is normal and anticipated. Women prepare for it by going to classes for childbirth education.
- The gate control theory is the basis for many nonpharmacologic pain relief techniques.
- Nonpharmacologic pain control strategies such as breathing techniques, effleurage, and imagery are commonly used during labor.
- Relaxation and the use of controlled breathing can reduce the amount of analgesia necessary.

- The use of opioid agonist-antagonist medications in a drug-dependent woman can cause serious withdrawal symptoms in the mother and newborn.
- Side effects of regional anesthesia include hypotension, bladder distention, postspinal headache, and pruritus.
- Aspiration of food particles can cause serious physiologic consequences; therefore, all labor patients are placed on an NPO order, except for ice chips or lollipops.
- Any drug given to the laboring woman for pain can also affect the fetus. If the mother has received narcotics during labor, the nurse should observe for respiratory depression in the newborn. A medication antagonist, such as naloxone, should be readily available for possible newborn resuscitation.
- Advantages of regional anesthesia include the woman's ability to participate in the birth and retention of protective airway reflexes.

Additional Learning Resources

SG Go to your Study Guide on page 487 for additional Review Questions for the NCLEX® Examination, Critical Thinking Clinical Situations, and other learning activities to help you master this chapter content.

evolve Go to your Evolve website (http://evolve.elsevier.com/Leifer/maternity) for the following FREE learning resources:
- Animations
- Answer Guidelines for Critical Thinking Questions
- Answers and Rationales for Review Questions for the NCLEX® Examination
- Concept Map Creator
- Glossary with pronunciations in English and Spanish
- Patient Teaching Plans
- Skills Performance Checklists and more!

 Online Resources
- www.aafp.org/afp/2003095.115.html
- www.awhonn.org
- www.childbirth.org
- www.lamaze.org
- www.parentstages.com
- www.thejointcommission.org

Review Questions for the NCLEX® Examination

1. Protein chemicals produced by the anterior pituitary gland and the hypothalamus that are similar to morphine-like substances and are believed to play a major role in the biologic response to pain are called:
   1. Catecholamines
   2. Endorphins
   3. Analgesics
   4. Narcotics

2. A woman in labor is imagining a pleasant experience to help distract her from pain. This method of distraction is considered:
   1. Cognitive stimulation
   2. Cutaneous stimulation
   3. Sacral pressure
   4. Self-hypnosis

3. Advantages of pharmacologic pain control methods include: *(Select all that apply.)*
   1. They allow more active participation by the woman in labor.
   2. They provide relief of all pain and pressure sensations.
   3. They assist with relaxation.
   4. They promote the woman to work with contractions.

4. A patient in the Labor and Birth Department received epidural anesthesia during the delivery of her son. If the patient reports pruritus of her arms, trunk, and legs, the nurse would expect the health care provider to prescribe:
   1. Naloxone (Narcan)
   2. Diphenhydramine (Benadryl)
   3. Hydroxyzine (Vistaril)
   4. Diazepam (Valium)

5. Which medical diagnosis would be a contraindication to spinal analgesia?
   1. Diabetes
   2. Hypovolemia
   3. Arthritis
   4. Mitral valve prolapse

6. The gate control theory, by using descending and ascending neural pathways, helps explain the effectiveness of various types of focusing strategies taught in childbirth preparation classes. Which of the following is an example of the application of the gate control theory of pain control? *(Select all that apply.)*
   1. Controlled breathing
   2. Listening to music
   3. Effleurage
   4. Release of endorphins
   5. Hypnosis

Critical Thinking Question

1. You are assigned to a woman who is in early labor with her first baby, and she is asking for pain medication. You discover that she did not attend childbirth preparation classes, but she is concerned about having a healthy baby. How would you help her?

Physiologic Adaptation of the Newborn and Nursing Assessment

Objectives

℞ Test!

1. Define key terms listed.
2. Describe four important neonatal adaptations to extrauterine life.
3. Explain how fluid in the lungs is replaced with air.
4. Relate how the neonate's pulmonary circulation is established.
5. Differentiate between the three fetal circulatory shunts, including their reasons for closure.
6. Recall the location of brown fat and how it is used in infant heat production.
7. Explain three reasons that the newborn should not be allowed to chill or experience cold stress.

8. Explain four ways to prevent heat loss in the newborn.
9. Recognize the normal range of neonatal vital signs.
10. Describe the assessment of the anterior and posterior fontanelles.
11. Differentiate among molding, cephalohematoma, and caput succedaneum.
12. Review key physical and behavioral assessments of the newborn.
13. Discuss normal newborn reflexes.
14. State the purpose of newborn screening tests.

Key Terms

acrocyanosis (ak′ro-si″ə-no′sis, p. 171)
brown adipose tissue (BAT) (ĂD-ĭ-pōs, p. 167)
cold stress (p. 160)
conduction (p. 165)
convection (p. 165)
cutis marmorata (ku′tis mahr″mo-ra′ta, p. 171)
desquamation (des″kwə-ma′shən, p. 171)
ductus arteriosus (p. 162)
ductus venosus (p. 162)
Epstein's pearls (p. 171)
erythema toxicum (er′ə-the′mə, p. 171)
evaporation (p. 165)
fontanelles (fon′tə-nel′, p. 170)
foramen ovale (p. 161)

forceps marks (p. 172)
functional residual capacity (FRC) (p. 161)
Harlequin color change (p. 172)
milia (mil′e-ə, p. 172)
miliaria (mil′e-ar′e-ə, p. 169)
molding (p. 170)
Mongolian spots (p. 172)
nevi (ne′vi, p. 172)
nonshivering thermogenesis (thĕr-mō-JĔN-ĕs ĭs, p. 167)
opisthotonos (o′pis-thot′ə-nəs, p. 167)
port-wine stain (p. 172)
radiation (p. 167)
surfactant (sŭr-FĂK-tănt, p. 160)
thermoregulation (thĕr-mō-RĔG-ū-LĀ-shŭn, p. 162)

[handwritten marginalia: During the 1st hour of the post-delivery skin to skin should be done so infant adjusts faster and allow baby 3 new to bond. 3. try to encourage breastfeeding]

ADJUSTMENT TO EXTRAUTERINE LIFE

In adapting to life outside of the uterus, the newborn infant must master thermoregulation, metabolic homeostasis, and respiratory gas exchange and convert from fetal to neonatal circulation pathways. These major transitions occur at a time when the infant must also respond to gestational and birth traumas. An understanding of the newborn's normal adaptation to extrauterine life will enable the nurse to prioritize assessments and nursing interventions and recognize deviations.

To live independently from the mother, the newborn must immediately establish pulmonary ventilation—that is, breathe on his or her own. The newborn must adapt to do the following:

- Quickly breathe and maintain respiration rate
- Replace fluid in the lungs with air
- Open up the pulmonary circulation and close the fetal shunts
- Allow pulmonary blood flow to increase and cardiac output (blood volume) to be redistributed
- Provide energy to maintain body temperature and support metabolic processes

- Dispose of waste products produced by food absorption and metabolic processes
- Detoxify substances entering from the external environment

RESPIRATORY AND CIRCULATORY FUNCTION

The respiratory and cardiovascular systems are required to quickly adapt to life outside of the uterus. When the cord is clamped, the placental circulation is immediately cut off. The changes that occur in the lungs are described in the following sections.

Preparatory Events to Breathing

In utero, the fetus's lungs are filled with fluid. This fluid is a combination of secretions of the alveolar cells of the lungs and some amniotic fluid. At birth, air must replace this fluid.

Surfactant, a phospholipid, is produced by the mature lungs in a term fetus. It reduces the force between the moist surfaces of the alveoli, thereby preventing them from collapsing with each expiration and thus promotes lung expansion. Also, surfactant promotes lung compliance (the lung's ability to easily fill with air). This action is important because, when the newborn begins to breathe, less effort will be required to continue and maintain breathing, reducing the chance that atelectasis (collapsed alveoli of the lung) will occur.

Onset of Breathing

For the neonate's life to be maintained outside of the uterus, the lungs must function immediately after birth. Pulmonary ventilation must be quickly established through lung expansion. The first breath of the healthy term infant occurs within seconds after birth; by 30 seconds, the neonate usually is breathing quite well on his or her own. Many powerful stimuli send messages to the respiratory center of the neonate's brain (Figure 9-1). These stimuli can be divided into four categories: sensory, chemical, thermal, and mechanical.

The **sensory stimuli** that help respirations begin as the neonate emerges from the dark warmth of the uterus to the external environment are cold, touch, movement, light, and sound. Skin sensors are stimulated by tactile drying, wrapping the neonate in warm blankets, and skin-to-skin contact. Clamping the umbilical cord is a powerful **chemical stimulus**. The newborn experiences a temporary hypoxia when the placental blood flow is stopped due to the clamping of the cord. A decreased blood oxygen level (Po_2) and an increased blood carbon dioxide level (Pco_2), along with a decreased pH, occur. Acidosis results, which activates the respiratory center in the medulla of the brain to initiate respirations.

At birth, the newborn must make an adjustment from a warm environment (in utero) to a much cooler one. This temperature change is a major **thermal stimulus** to respirations. Excessive cooling (cold stress), however, will increase the need for oxygen and can produce acidosis. A lack of oxygen (hypoxia) at the tissue level will depress respirations rather than stimulate them. Because of this, it is very important to keep the infant warm.

The important **mechanical stimuli** are chest compression and recoil, which cause air to be drawn into and out of the lungs. The chest is compressed as it passes through the birth canal and recoils or expands as it leaves the mother's body.

Changing from Fluid-Filled to Air-Filled Lungs

During a normal vaginal birth, the infant's head is delivered first, then the chest. The chest area, made up of cartilage and bones, is squeezed or compressed, promoting drainage of fluid from the lungs. Before the

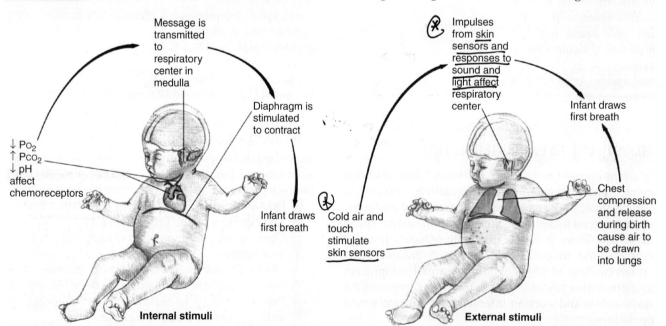

Message is transmitted to respiratory center in medulla

Diaphragm is stimulated to contract

↓ Po_2
↑ Pco_2
↓ pH
affect chemoreceptors

Infant draws first breath

Cold air and touch stimulate skin sensors

Internal stimuli

Impulses from skin sensors and responses to sound and light affect respiratory center

Infant draws first breath

Chest compression and release during birth cause air to be drawn into lungs

External stimuli

FIGURE 9-1 Internal causes of the initiation of respirations are the chemical changes that take place at birth. External causes of respirations include sensory, thermal, and mechanical factors.

chest is delivered, almost half of the fluid is forced out. As the chest returns (recoils) to its natural position, the infant sucks in air (20 to 40 mL) to replace the fluid forced out without having to make any effort of his or her own. The lung expansion creates the negative intrapleural pressure that is maintained throughout life.

The infant who is delivered by cesarean birth does not experience chest compression followed by chest recoil and thus is at greater risk for respiratory distress. However, there are other mechanisms by which the lungs are cleared besides this "vaginal squeeze." Some of the fluid is absorbed by the lymphatic vessels, and the rest of the fluid is removed by the pulmonary capillaries. If the fluid is not removed, the infant will experience labored breathing or respiratory distress.

With the first breath, functional residual capacity (FRC) is established. This means a small amount of air is left in the alveoli of the lungs, which allows them to stay partially open during expiration. Surfactant promotes lung expansion and the ability of the alveoli to fill with air. With the establishment of FRC, the second, third, and subsequent breaths do not require as much pressure; with each breath, respiration becomes easier.

⚠ Safety Alert

Emergency Equipment Needed in Case Pulmonary Circulation Does Not Adapt

- Overhead radiant warmer with warm blankets
- Heated, humidified oxygen
- Suction and sterile suction catheters (size 8 F for preterm and 10 F for term newborns)
- Wall suction set for 40 to 80 mm Hg
- Ventilation bag with pressure release valve and manometer
- Intubation equipment, including laryngoscope blades (size 0 for preterm and 1 for term newborns)
- Endotracheal tubes
- Oxygen mask with manual bag compressor
- Gloves, tape
- Drugs, intravenous fluids, or blood volume expanders
- Neonatal intravenous supplies
- Nasogastric tube

The normal newborn respiratory rate is 30 to 60 breaths/minute. The normal newborn's breathing pattern includes 5- to 15-second pauses, called *periodic breathing*, and is normal. Cessation of breathing for more than 20 seconds is called apnea and is abnormal. The newborn breathes through the nose, and any nasal obstruction can cause respiratory distress because the newborn will not typically breathe through the mouth.

Closing Down the Fetal Structures (Shunts)

During fetal life, most of the blood flow bypasses the nonfunctional lungs and liver. A small percentage of blood goes to the lungs to perfuse the tissues. After birth, the neonate's blood must begin to circulate to the lungs for oxygenation and to the liver for filtration.

In other words, the three fetal shunts—the ductus arteriosus, foramen ovale, and ductus venosus—must close. These closures occur in response to shifts in pressures in the heart, an increase in blood oxygenation level, and cord clamping (Figure 9-2).

Foramen Ovale. The foramen ovale is an opening (a flap in the septum) between the right and left atria of the heart, with blood flow and pressure being

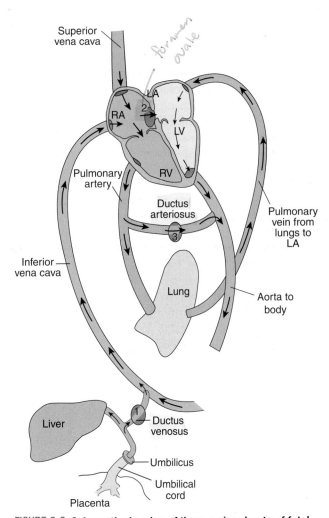

FIGURE 9-2 **Schematic drawing of three major shunts of fetal circulation.** Blood enters the fetus from the placenta; most blood bypasses the liver by the ductus venosus (1) into the inferior vena cava, which flows into the right atrium of the heart (RA). Most blood bypasses the right ventricle by way of the foramen ovale (2) and flows into the left atrium (LA) and then to left ventricle (LV) and out through the aorta to the body. Some blood does enter the right ventricle (RV) from the right atrium and flows into the pulmonary artery toward the lungs. Most blood is again diverted from the lungs by the ductus arteriosus (3) directly into the aorta, and minimum blood flows to the lungs because lung oxygenation is not needed during fetal life. The small amount of blood that flows to the lungs returns to the left atrium by the pulmonary vein and continues to the left ventricle and out to the body by the aorta. At birth, the ductus venosus (1), foramen ovale (2), and ductus arteriosus (3) will close. The right side of the heart is shaded to show that the pressure is greater on the right side during fetal life because of collapsed lungs. When the lungs inflate at birth, the pressure decreases on the right, and the increased left-sided pressure helps close the flap of the foramen ovale (2).

greater in the right atrium. It functions like a one-way valve for blood flow, from the right to the left, and shunts blood away from the lungs to the aorta. Clamping the umbilical cord causes a large stream of blood from the placenta to be cut off. As a result, the pressure on the left side of the neonate's heart becomes greater than that on the right side, placing pressure against the atrial septum, closing the flap of the foramen ovale. The foramen ovale functionally closes approximately 1 minute after birth, complete anatomic closure takes place approximately 2 hours after birth, and by 3 months the atrial septum is permanently fused together.

Ductus Arteriosus. The ductus arteriosus shunts blood from the pulmonary artery to the aorta, bypassing the lungs during fetal life. The pulmonary arterioles dilate in response to the increased aeration of the lungs at birth and the oxygen saturation of the blood increases, causing the ductus arteriosus to constrict and completely close at birth. The functional closure of the ductus arteriosus occurs approximately 15 to 24 hours after birth. The anatomic closure (fibrosis of ductus) occurs approximately 3 to 4 weeks after birth.

It is important to note that the ductus arteriosus can dilate (reopen) during the first several weeks after birth. If the neonate has a decrease in blood pressure and oxygen saturation, there may be a return to fetal-type circulation, with a reopening of the ductus arteriosus. This is referred to as **patent ductus arteriosus** and can lead to right-sided heart failure and pulmonary congestion. If the ductus arteriosus does reopen, unoxygenated blood will bypass the lungs and go through the pulmonary artery into the aorta and general circulation, and the newborn can become hypoxic and die.

Ductus Venosus. The ductus venosus is a fetal structure (shunt) that allows most oxygenated blood to bypass the liver and enter the inferior vena cava. Clamping the umbilical cord at birth cuts off the umbilical venous blood flow, causing a redistribution of blood, greatly reducing the flow of blood through the ductus venosus. The ductus venosus constricts at birth, closes anatomically approximately 1-2 weeks after birth, and eventually becomes a ligament. The closure of this bypass forces blood perfusion in the liver. The mechanisms for this closure are unknown.

It is important that the health care provider understand the basic mechanisms behind the closure of the fetal structures or shunts. Understanding the pressure changes within the heart and changes in the blood flow pattern will help the health care provider recognize problems or defects and determine appropriate management.

BODY SYSTEM ADAPTATIONS AND FUNCTIONS

Although significant events occur in the body systems before birth, the body systems of the newborn are required to adapt and function differently after birth. The major adaptations are explored in Table 9-1.

Thermoregulation

Thermoregulation, the ability to produce heat and maintain a normal body temperature, is a vital metabolic function and a continuous challenge for the newborn. Nursing responsibilities related to thermoregulation immediately after birth are discussed in Chapter 7. Cold stress effects are reviewed in Figure 9-3.

🔍 Evidence-Based Practice

Preventing Newborn Heat Loss

- Dry neonate immediately after birth.
- Dry head and cover with hat after birth.
- Place neonate in prewarmed blankets. Replace with additional prewarmed blankets if environment is less than optimal.
- Avoid newborn contact with wet linens. Change wet linens as needed.
- Encourage skin-to-skin contact with mother after newborn is dried. Mother's body heat will warm the baby.
- Maintain a warm environment by putting newborn in a radiant warmer.
- Protect infant from drafts; avoid placing infant near the air conditioner, vents, door, or window.
- Place radiant warmers, incubators, and cribs away from windows or outside walls.
- Put warm blanket between neonate's body and cool surface (e.g., examining table or scale).
- Warm hands, stethoscope, and clothing before touching neonate.
- Dress and wrap newborn quickly after any procedure.
- Maintain environmental temperature at 32° C to 34° C (89.6° F to 93.2° F) for the unclothed infant.
- Monitor abdominal skin temperature until stable at 36.5° C (97.7° F).

Temperature regulation of the newborn is maintained by balancing the amount of heat produced with the amount of heat lost. If the amount of heat lost exceeds the amount of heat produced, the body temperature will fall.

The flexed position of the extremities in a term newborn minimizes the exposure of skin surface to the air, but if the infant has poor muscle tone and the arms and legs do not remain flexed (as seen in the preterm infant), more body surface area is exposed to the air, and the risk of cold stress increases. A major responsibility in newborn care is maintaining a neutral thermal environment that prevents heat loss and cold stress. A neutral thermal environment makes minimum demands on the newborn's energy reserves, allowing a

Table 9-1 Characteristics of Body Systems Before and After Birth

BEFORE BIRTH	AFTER BIRTH
Respiratory Function	
Lungs are filled with fluid.	Fluid is removed by the chest being squeezed during vaginal delivery and is absorbed by the lymphatic system.
There is no air in lungs. Surfactant is present in mature fetuses. There is no movement of air in lungs.	Air is pulled in with first breath to open alveoli and establish FRC with the help of surfactant that keeps alveoli open. Baby begins to breathe within 30 seconds after birth. Powerful stimuli (cold, touch, clamping of cord) help initiate breathing.
Respiratory rate is slower.	Respiratory rate increases to 30-60 breaths/minute because of greater need for oxygen.
Gas is exchanged through fetoplacental unit.	Neonate must breathe on his or her own to get oxygen.
Temperature is warm and stable.	The newborn is at risk for hypothermia and hyperthermia until thermoregulation stabilizes. If the newborn becomes chilled (cold stress), oxygen needs will increase.
Circulatory Function	
Placenta provides oxygen needs.	Placental function ends; pressure changes in the heart start systemic circulation and oxygenation of blood in lungs.
Pulmonary vessels are constricted; there is minimum blood flow to lungs.	Dilation of vessels occurs with increased blood flow and oxygen to the lungs.
Umbilical cord supplies oxygen and nutrition to fetus by the placenta.	Cord is clamped; pressure increases in left side of heart, ending right-to-left shunt and sending blood to lungs for oxygenation.
Ductus arteriosus shunts blood to bypass lungs.	Ductus arteriosus closes because of increased blood oxygenation, resulting in increased blood flow to lungs; functional murmurs may be heard until closure is permanent, usually within the first weeks of life.
Ductus venosus shunts blood to bypass liver.	Ductus venosus constricts and functionally closes when the umbilical cord is clamped; the ductus venosus becomes a ligament.
Foramen ovale allows flow from right atrium to left atrium	Increased pressure in left atrium causes valve shunt to close, ending right-to-left flow of blood within the heart
Gastrointestinal (GI) Function	
GI tract is relatively inactive.	Baby is able to suck and swallow and is capable of ingesting, digesting, and eliminating breast milk or formula.
Blood glucose level is maintained via placental circulation.	The newborn's carbohydrate reserves are low and mostly in the form of glycogen. If glycogen stores are depleted, the newborn utilizes brown fat sources for energy. The newborn can be breastfed immediately after birth.
Fetus swallows amniotic fluid and demonstrates sucking and swallowing movements in utero.	Immature esophageal sphincter makes newborn prone to regurgitation.
No feeding is received by GI tract.	Baby is prone to swallowing air during feeding and crying; baby must be burped during and after each feeding because of air pocketing (retaining air in upper part of stomach); early feeding prevents hypoglycemia and promotes excretion of excess bilirubin.
No stooling occurs.	Active peristalsis in lower bowel causes baby to have frequent stools.
In hypoxia or distress, anal sphincter relaxes and meconium passes into amniotic fluid, indicating fetal distress.	Absence of stools in first 48 hours indicates bowel obstruction; first stool is sticky, dark green meconium and is passed within 24 hours of life; changes in stool color during first few days indicate healthy GI tract.
Stomach and bowel contents are sterile.	Stomach and bowel contents are no longer sterile; gastric contents become more acidic; infant is unable to manufacture vitamin K until intestinal flora (with bacteria) are established.
Basic taste sensations are present.	Baby has all basic taste sensations and reacts to strong tastes and odors.
Enzymatic and pancreatic function is immature (until gestation of 36-38 weeks).	Baby digests fat less efficiently because of inadequate amount of pancreatic enzyme lipase. Pepsinogen (the enzyme necessary for protein synthesis) is present. The newborn is deficient in pancreatic amylase for several months and has difficulty digesting starches and complex carbohydrates. The fat in breast milk may be better digested by the newborn because breast milk contains lipase and more medium-chain triglycerides.

Continued

Table 9-1 **Characteristics of Body Systems Before and After Birth—cont'd**

BEFORE BIRTH	AFTER BIRTH
Gastrointestinal (GI) Function—cont'd	
	Little saliva is produced until 3 months of age, and the stomach capacity of a newborn is approximately 50-60 mL.
	The blood glucose should stabilize at 60-70 mg/dL by the third day of life.
Endocrine Function	
Placenta functions as an endocrine gland.	Immature posterior pituitary gland limits antidiuretic hormone and vasopressin functions, placing newborn at risk for dehydration.
Renal Function	
Placenta is responsible for fetal excretion of wastes in utero.	Baby voids to excrete waste products; baby should void within the first 8 hours (document output and report if longer than 8 hours).
Fetus excretes urine into amniotic fluid.	Newborn can lose as much as 10% of body weight during the first few days of life (80% of neonate's distribution of body water is extracellular).
	Newborn voids an average volume of 15 mL, 20 times in a 24-hour period with an output of 25 mL/kg/day.
	The kidney of the newborn is limited in its ability to concentrate or dilute urine.
Immunologic Function	
Before birth, fetus is in a sterile environment.	Baby comes in contact with many pathogenic organisms and is susceptible to infections. This is attributable to the infant's delicate skin; limited phagocytosis (specialized white blood cells); and portals of entry for organisms, such as the umbilical stump.
Only immunoglobulins cross the placenta, providing maternal antibodies to the fetus that protect against bacterial and viral diseases such as diphtheria, mumps, polio, and tetanus.	The newborn acquires passive immunity from the mother; this immunity lasts for 3 to 5 months; baby does not have immunoglobulin for toxoplasmosis, rubella, cytomegalovirus, and herpes (TORCH) infections.
	Colostrum, a forerunner of breast milk, is high in IgA (thus breastfeeding provides IgA to the infant, protecting against some GI and respiratory tract infections).
Liver is immature.	Liver function is hindered by deficiency in enzymes.
Iron is stored in the liver during the last 3 months of gestation if mother's intake of iron is adequate.	A term newborn has enough iron stored to last 5 months.
Production of prothrombin is limited because of inadequate vitamin K.	Until bacterial flora in the intestine favor vitamin K production, the liver's ability to help form coagulation factors such as prothrombin is limited, predisposing infant to hemorrhage during first few days of life.
	Vitamin K (phytonadione [AquaMEPHYTON]) is administered to the newborn to bring clotting time within normal range (to prevent excessive bleeding).
	Because of a deficiency in the enzyme glucuronyl transferase, a shorter red blood cell (RBC) life span, and a higher RBC count, visible jaundice (physiologic jaundice) is seen at approximately the third day of life. Bilirubin is toxic; therefore, assessment of bilirubin levels is important.
Stressful birth hypoxia and cold stress can deplete glycogen stores in the liver.	Newborn is at risk for hypoglycemia (blood glucose levels <40 mg/dL).
	Total serum bilirubin at birth is ≤3 mg/dL, unless a hemolytic process was present in utero.
Neurologic Function	
Fetus has basic reflexes.	Baby is born with basic reflexes (grasp, sucking, rooting, Moro's, and tonic neck reflexes).
Neurologic system is immature.	Motor movements are uncoordinated.
	All neurons of the cerebral cortex are present at birth and then increase in size and complexity.
	Basic reflexes that are present at birth will disappear as myelinization occurs and voluntary control develops.
	Sensory perceptions are developed, and newborn can feel pain.
	As soon as the newborn sneezes, the amniotic fluid is forced out of the eustachian tubes.
	Hearing is well developed.
	The senses of smell, taste, and touch are well developed at birth.
Skin is thin.	The newborn skin is sensitive to touch; soft stroking, cuddling, and snug wrapping will often quiet a crying neonate.

FRC, functional residual capacity; *IgA,* immunoglobulin A.

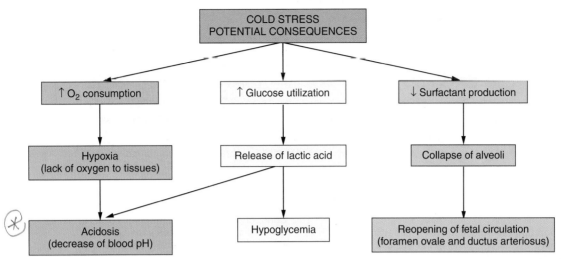

FIGURE 9-3 **Consequences of cold stress.** Cold stress increases oxygen consumption, respiratory rate, and vasoconstriction. The increase in glucose utilization in efforts to maintain warmth causes release of lactic acid, which contributes to metabolic acidosis and hypoglycemia. Metabolism of brown fat to raise the body temperature releases fatty acids into the bloodstream that can result in the interference of bilirubin transport to the liver, causing hyperbilirubinemia. Cold stress decreases surfactant production, which contributes to alveoli collapse and hypoxia. The lowered oxygen saturation caused by hypoxia may cause the reopening of the ductus arteriosus (fetal circulation), which can result in death.

basal metabolic rate (BMR) with minimum oxygen consumption needs. Maintaining an abdominal skin temperature of 36.5° C (97.7° F) will minimize oxygen consumption needs and conserve energy. A neutral thermal environment is maintenance of 32° C to 34° C (89.6° F to 93.2° F) for an *unclothed* term newborn (London, Ladewig, Ball, & Bindler, 2006). A neutral thermal environment in the nursery may be 25° C (77° F) for a newborn who is warmly wrapped in an open bassinet (Blackburn, 2007). If a neutral thermal environment is not maintained, the newborn will respond by increasing the BMR, and oxygen consumption needs will increase, resulting in cold stress, depletion of glycogen stores, and resulting acidosis. Kangaroo care (skin-to-skin contact) is the best means of thermal support (see Chapters 10 and 15). Because of this, nonvital procedures such as bathing should not be done until the newborn's body temperature and respirations have been stabilized.

Factors Contributing to Heat Loss. Newborns are prone to heat loss because they have a large body surface area in relation to their weight. Their skin is thin, blood vessels are close to the surface, and there is little subcutaneous fat for insulation. Because of these factors, newborns have a greater transfer of heat to the external environment than do adults. In addition, at birth the newborn's skin is wet with amniotic fluid, and the room temperature is cooler than the intrauterine environment.

Heat Loss to Environment. Heat loss to the environment takes place in four ways: evaporation, conduction, convection, and radiation (Figure 9-4, Table 9-2).

Evaporation. Evaporation occurs when wet surfaces are exposed to air. The loss of heat occurs as water is converted to a vapor. The newborn immediately loses heat when the amniotic fluid on the skin evaporates; therefore, drying the newborn as quickly as possible after birth is important to reduce heat loss. Drying the head, which is the largest surface area of the body, is especially important. A stockinette cap may be placed on the neonate's head to reduce heat loss. Delaying the initial bath until the neonate's temperature has stabilized is desirable to minimize heat loss by evaporation. Additional heat loss by evaporation occurs through insensible water loss from the skin and through respirations.

Conduction. Conduction is the loss of heat to a cooler surface by direct skin contact. Conduction occurs when the newborn comes in contact with cold objects. Chilled hands, cold scales, cool examining tables, and a cold stethoscope can cause heat loss by conduction. Precautions should be taken to avoid touching neonates with objects cooler than their skin. Measures to reduce heat loss by conduction include placing the infant in a prewarmed blanket or using a radiant warmer.

Convection. Convection is the loss of heat from the warm body surface to moving cooler air. Airflow from air conditioning or people moving around the room increases the loss of heat. Drafts and oxygen by mask can increase convective heat loss in the newborn. To control or prevent convective heat loss, newborns are often placed in radiant warmers or incubators (out of drafts) until their temperature is stable. Also, neonates may be transported in enclosed, warmed incubators through the hallways. Newborns should be warmly wrapped when in their bassinets.

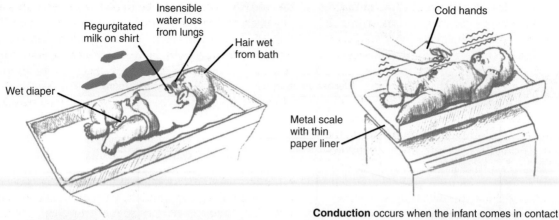

Evaporation can occur during birth or bathing from moisture on skin, as a result of wet linens or clothes, and from insensible loss.

Conduction occurs when the infant comes in contact with cold objects or surfaces such as a scale, circumcision restraint board, cold hands, or a stethoscope.

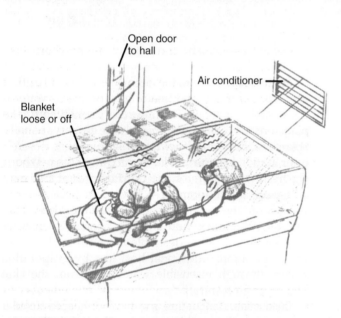

Convection occurs when drafts come from open doors, air conditioning, or even air currents created by people moving about.

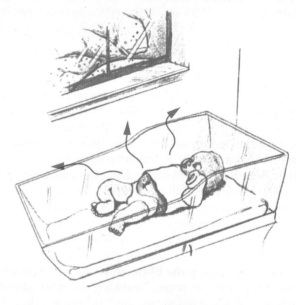

Radiation heat loss occurs when the infant is near colder surfaces. Thus, heat is lost from the infant's body to the side of the crib and to the outside walls and windows.

FIGURE 9-4 Methods of heat loss: evaporation, conduction, convection, and radiation.

Table **9-2** | Nursing Interventions to Prevent Heat Loss in Newborns

MECHANISM OF HEAT LOSS	SOURCES OF HEAT LOSS	INTERVENTIONS
Evaporation (conversion from liquid to vapor)	Evaporation of wet amniotic fluid on skin at birth	Dry infant quickly. Dry and cover head of infant.
Conduction (transfer of heat to a cooler surface)	Cool surface of bed, scale, stethoscope	Prewarm radiant warmer and stethoscope before use. Place scale paper on scale, and place warm blanket on other surfaces.
Convection (loss of heat to the surrounding cooler air)	Drafts from window, air conditioning, oxygen vents	Place crib away from windows and vents.
Radiation (loss of heat to surrounding cold environment)	Cold environment of walls, windows	Place crib away from cold walls. Wrap infant warmly.

Radiation. Radiation loss occurs from a warm object to a cooler one when the objects are not in contact with one another. For example, if the crib is near cold windows or if walls of the incubator are cold, heat is lost by radiation.

Nonshivering Thermogenesis

In the adult, response to cold involves muscle activity in the form of shivering. Compared with the adult, the newborn cannot use muscle activity (shivering) to produce heat and has difficulty conserving and dissipating heat to maintain an optimum temperature. The newborn relies on nonshivering thermogenesis, using brown fat stores, vasoconstriction in cold environments, and vasodilation in warm environments.

When exposed to a cool environment, the newborn produces heat by physiologic mechanisms, or thermogenesis. These mechanisms include increased BMR; muscular activity; and chemical thermogenesis, also called *nonshivering thermogenesis*. It is the primary method of heat production and is unique to newborns.

Nonshivering thermogenesis, a complex process that increases the metabolic rate and rate of oxygen consumption in the newborn, uses the metabolism of brown fat (brown adipose tissue [BAT]) for heat production when the newborn infant is subjected to cold stress. Brown fat (named for its dark color) develops at 28 weeks' gestation and is found around the neck; in the axillae; around the kidneys, adrenals, and sternum; between the scapula; and along the abdominal aorta (Figure 9-5).

The cells in BAT contain numerous fat vacuoles and an abundant blood and nerve supply. As brown fat is metabolized, the heat produced warms vital areas of the body. Brown fat can be depleted in newborns exposed to prolonged periods of cold stress. When this happens, thermogenesis can be impaired. Brown fat typically disappears by 3 months of age. Certain drugs such as meperidine (Demerol) given to a laboring woman before delivery can interfere with metabolism of brown fat in the newborn, resulting in neonatal hypothermia.

NURSING ASSESSMENT OF THE NEWBORN

Nursing assessment of the newborn includes observation, inspection, auscultation, palpation, and percussion. The assessment is not performed in a single examination but in a series of examinations. A complete assessment of the newborn includes detailed evaluation of all body systems. Skin color, type of respirations, temperature, activity, and feeding behavior alert the examiner to the health status of the newborn.

Phase 1 assessment and care of the newborn take place in the delivery room and were discussed in Chapter 7. At this time, the neonate is in his or her first phase of reactivity, and bonding is initiated with parents. *Phase 2* assessment and care of the newborn take place on admission to the newborn nursery, usually between 1 and 4 hours of age, where a more detailed examination is performed. *Phase 3* care of the newborn occurs from 4 hours of age until discharge and may take place in the rooming-in setting with the parents present. This allows for teaching to take place. This chapter discusses phase 2 of newborn care: general assessment.

GENERAL APPEARANCE

The resting posture and spontaneous movements can best be evaluated before the newborn is disturbed. Flexion and symmetry can be observed while the baby is resting. The term newborn rests with hips abducted and flexed and knees flexed. Arms are adducted and flexed at the elbow, with the hand in the fist position. Lack of flexion is associated with prematurity. Extension of the neck with an arched back (opisthotonos) is associated with central nervous system (CNS) problems. Spontaneous movements may provide subtle clues to potential CNS problems. Noticeable jerky or jittery movements may indicate excessive electrical discharge from the neurons or a metabolic disorder such as hypoglycemia, hypocalcemia, or hypoxia; neurologic damage; or drug withdrawal. Repetitive blinking or pedaling movements of the lower limbs may represent seizure activity caused by injury at birth. Prolonged or excessive tremors may indicate hyperactivity and should be reported to the health care provider for further evaluation. If tremors persist, a capillary blood heel stick may be done to determine the blood glucose level. Hypoglycemia in the

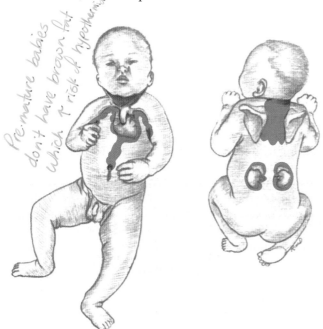

Premature babies don't have brown fat which ↑ risk of hypothermia

FIGURE 9-5 Sites of brown fat (brown adipose tissue) in the newborn.

newborn is present if the blood glucose level is 40 mg/dL or less.

The neonate's cry should be strong and lusty. A high-pitched, shrill cry is abnormal and may indicate a neurologic disorder, hypoglycemia, or drug withdrawal (neonatal abstinence syndrome). The newborn's cry is important to assess because it is the way to communicate needs, such as feeling wet, hungry, or too warm.

VITAL SIGNS

Vital signs should be taken when the newborn is quiet or resting. The heart and respiratory rates will be much faster if the baby is fussing or crying than when in the quiet state. Vital sign observation begins while the mother and infant are bonding in the delivery room. Vitals signs are measured at 15- to 30-minute intervals at first, then hourly, and every 4 to 8 hours after the infant is stable (in phase 3 care).

Heart Rate

The nurse should listen to the apical heart rate for a full minute for accuracy, noting the rate, rhythm, intensity, position of the apical pulse, and presence of abnormal sounds (Figure 9-6). The newborn's heart rate varies with activity. *Bradycardia* in the newborn refers to a heart rate less than 110 beats/minute, and *tachycardia* is a heart rate greater than 160 beats/minute. The rate should range between 110 and 160 beats/minute with normal activity. Heart rate is auscultated with a warmed stethoscope, listening to the apical beat over

the heart (precordial) region, which is slightly below the left nipple (at the fourth intercostal space and to the left of the midclavicular line). The two femoral pulses (in the groin region) should also be evaluated. A weak or slow femoral pulse suggests a coarctation stricture of the aorta. Abnormalities should be reported to the charge nurse or health care provider.

Respirations

The nurse must also count respirations for a full minute because the newborn's respiratory rate is irregular. The nurse visually watches the rise and fall of the baby's abdomen because the respirations of neonates are abdominal or diaphragmatic in character. Movement of the chest and abdomen should be synchronized. The range is typically from 30 to 60 breaths/minute. A normal finding is periodic breathing (a pause in breathing). This describes an intermittent cessation of respirations for less than 15 seconds. However, cessation of respirations for more than 20 seconds (apnea) should be further assessed. Nasal flaring, costal or substernal retractions (sucking in of the chest wall with the sternum moving inward with inspiration), and a grunting sound on expiration are abnormal and indicate respiratory distress.

🏃 **Health Promotion**

Determining Newborn's Respiratory Status

- Count respirations for 1 full minute because breathing patterns are irregular.
- Observe respiratory rate. If less than 30 breaths/minute or greater than 60 breaths/minute, report to charge nurse.
- Observe and report signs of respiratory distress, including nasal flaring, grunting, or retractions (sternal movement inward with inspiration).
- Observe mucous membranes for cyanosis.
- Observe for apnea lasting more than 20 seconds.
- Observe for need to clear airway if gagging or choking occurs.
- Suction with bulb syringe as needed.
- Report unusual findings to charge nurse.

Breath sounds should be clear over most of the area, but sounds of moisture might be heard in the lungs during the first few hours after birth. The reason is that lung fluid has not been completely absorbed. Rales, a rush of air through fluid, sound like rubbing your hair between two fingers near your ear. Rhonchi are coarse sounds resembling snoring. They represent air rushing through thick secretions. Abnormal or diminished sounds should always be verified by an experienced nurse and reported to the health care provider.

Temperature

The neonate's temperature drops immediately after birth. The internal organs are poorly insulated, and the skin is relatively thin. In addition, the newborn's

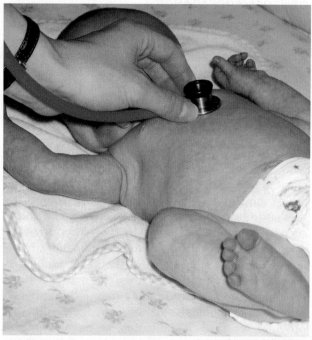

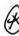 **FIGURE 9-6** **Assessing the apical pulse.** This is the most accurate technique for assessing the heart rate of a neonate.

heat-regulating center has not yet matured. The neonate's body rapidly reflects the temperature of the environment.

The newborn is unable to maintain or raise body temperature by shivering; instead, efforts to increase body temperature are aided by a special tissue, called *brown fat*. Immediately after birth, a thermal sensor is often applied to the newborn's skin on the upper abdomen (but not over bone) and secured with porous tape or a foil-covered foam pad to monitor the temperature continually. Because the skin temperature will fall before the core body temperature falls, monitoring the skin temperature enables interventions that will prevent core hypothermia.

During phases 2 and 3 care, an intermittent reading of axillary temperature is usually preferred and should be stable at 36.5° C (97.7° F) (Skill 9-1). Digital thermometers are read when the indicator sounds. The tympanic membrane sensor is used only if the tip of the sensor is small enough to fit into the newborn's ear (it registers the temperature in 2 seconds). The rectal temperature is not used as a routine method because it may cause rectal mucosal irritation and increase the chances of perforation. Temperature readings should be recorded every 30 minutes for the first hour after birth, then each hour for the first 4 hours until stable, after which the temperature is assessed a minimum of every 8 hours for healthy term newborns.

An elevated temperature can occur from dehydration, too much clothing, or infection. Subnormal temperatures (chilling or cold stress) in neonates can be the result of metabolic disturbances and infections. An environmental temperature that is too high can increase the newborn's temperature; one that is too low can decrease the temperature. The room temperature should be kept at 25° C (77° F). Because the neonate is not able to perspire effectively (the sweat glands do not fully function for the first week of life), overheating can cause the neonate to break out in a pinpoint, reddish rash that is often referred to as prickly heat or miliaria.

Blood Pressure

Blood pressure (BP) may be measured with an appropriately sized neonatal cuff and taken when the neonate is quiet. The average BP at birth is 60 to 80 mm Hg systolic and 40 to 50 mm Hg diastolic. When the newborn is crying or sucking, the BP values increase by 10 to 20 mm Hg. A Doppler BP device or electronic measurement greatly improves the accuracy of the reading. A systolic reading may be obtained by noting the pressure when palpating the return of the radial pulse if other methods are not available. If a cardiac

---

Skill 9-1   Taking the Axillary Temperature

PURPOSE
To assess body temperature.

Steps

1. Hold the infant securely.
2. Place the thermometer probe in the center of the axilla.
3. Hold the arm down against the body until the indicator sounds.
4. Record the temperature reading. Report temperature reading of under 97.0° F or over 100.4° F.

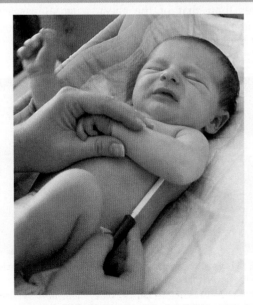

anomaly is suspected, BP is assessed in all four extremities with an appropriately sized cuff. The cuff should cover one half to three fourths of the extremity. On the neonate, two or three BP measurements should be taken and the average recorded for accuracy.

ASSESSMENT OF PHYSICAL CHARACTERISTICS

Skin

The skin provides a visible record of the newborn's health status. The skin is inspected for characteristics related to term, preterm, or postterm neonates. Some of the clinical findings are common but not significant; however, they can be of concern to parents. Other findings are potentially abnormal and should be reported to the health care provider. A greenish brown discoloration (meconium stain) of the skin, nails, and cord can result if meconium was passed before birth. Peeling or excessive cracking of the skin is associated with postterm newborns. Other skin findings include vernix caseosa (Figure 9-7), milia, lanugo, acrocyanosis, petechiae, jaundice, and birthmarks (Table 9-3).

Head

The shape of the neonate's head varies, depending on the type and length of labor. The heads of breech-born infants and those delivered by elective cesarean birth are characteristically round because pressure was not exerted on them during birth. Newborns born head first and vaginally often have an elongated head, called **molding,** which usually resolves in a few days.

The newborn's head has a large surface area compared with its body. The average head circumference is 33 to 35.5 cm (13 to 14 inches). The neonate's head circumference either equals or exceeds by about 2.5 cm (1 inch) the circumference of the chest. If the head circumference is more than 4 cm (1.6 inches) greater than that of the chest, a serial assessment for increased intracranial pressure or possible

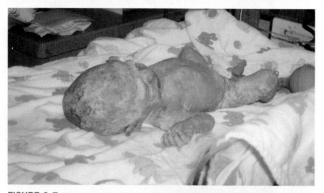

FIGURE 9-7 Vernix is the thick, white, cheesy substance covering the skin of the newborn. Preterm newborns are heavily covered in vernix, whereas postterm newborns have little vernix protection on their skin. Note the heavy covering of vernix on this newborn.

hydrocephalus is indicated. A small head, **microcephaly,** may be caused by rubella or toxoplasmosis during fetal development. The head circumference is measured at birth and at every clinic visit (see Chapter 10).

Molding and Caput Succedaneum. Molding and caput succedaneum are normal findings at birth. Molding, or overlapping of the bones of the head, occurs as a result of head compression during the birth process. The skull bones override each other for the head to fit through the vaginal canal, but this resolves within 2 or 3 days. **Caput succedaneum** is localized swelling of soft tissues of the scalp (Figure 9-8) that is caused by pressure on the head during labor. It can be palpated as a soft, fluctuant mass that may cross over the suture lines. Caput succedaneum is absorbed in a few days and requires no intervention.

Cephalhematoma. **Cephalhematoma** is a collection of blood between the periosteum and a bone of the skull that it covers (Figure 9-9). It may be unilateral or bilateral and does not cross the suture line. The area emerges as a defined hematoma between the first and second days. Its disappearance may take as long as 3 weeks. It usually results when trauma occurs to small blood vessels of the periosteum. This finding is more common when the mother has had a prolonged or difficult labor. Measurement of the head and chest is discussed in Chapter 10.

Fontanelles. The neonate's skull has anterior and posterior fontanelles, which are commonly called *soft spots.* They are covered with a sturdy membrane capable of protecting the underlying tissues. The fontanelles are openings in the bony skull (wide spaces between the cranial sutures) that allow the fetal head to mold in order to fit through the birth canal (something fused bones cannot do). The anterior fontanelle is the largest and most important for clinical evaluation. It is diamond-shaped and formed by the juncture of the cranial bones. Examination of the fontanelles is important in understanding the newborn's health status and brain development. The anterior fontanelle should be palpated to determine whether it is bulging or depressed (sunken). When the newborn cries, coughs, or vomits, the anterior fontanelle may bulge. When the newborn is quiet, it should not be elevated but should be level with the cranial bones. Growth of the head is stimulated by brain growth, which is mostly complete by 2 years of age. When the cranial sutures are fused (closed), brain growth is restricted. The size of the anterior fontanelle at birth is between 3.6 and 6 cm (1.4 and 2.4 inches) (Skill 9-2 on p. 174).

The size of the fontanelles in preterm and term newborns is the same once the preterm newborn reaches what would have been its estimated date of birth

Table 9-3   Assessment of Skin

CONDITION	APPEARANCE	NURSING INTERVENTIONS
Acrocyanosis	Cyanosis of the hands and feet in the first week of life is caused by a combination of a high hemoglobin level and vasomotor instability.	Parent education concerning this normal phenomenon is helpful.
Cutis marmorata	A lacelike red or blue pattern on the skin surface of a newborn's body.	A normal vasomotor response to low environmental temperature. Wrap infant warmly. Intense or persistent appearance should be reported.
Desquamation	Peeling of the skin at birth may indicate postmaturity. Early removal of vernix can be followed by desquamation in term newborns.	Instruct parents to avoid harsh soaps. Some hospitals do not vigorously remove vernix from the skin of newborns.
Epstein's pearls	Pearly white pinpoint papules in midline of upper palate.	Distinguish from a thrush lesion.
Erythema toxicum	Splotchy erythema with firm yellow-white papules that have a red base.	Can occur at age 2 days. No intervention is required because erythema will spontaneously clear.

Continued

Table 9-3	Assessment of Skin—cont'd	
CONDITION	**APPEARANCE**	**NURSING INTERVENTIONS**
Harlequin color change	An imbalance of autonomic vascular regulatory mechanism. Deep red color over half of body, pallor on the longitudinal half of body. Usually occurs with preterm infants who are placed on their side.	The phenomenon disappears with muscular activity. Changing position of infant is helpful. Condition is temporary and does not usually indicate a problem.
Milia	Pearly white pinpoint papules on face and nose of newborn.	No treatment. Will spontaneously disappear. Educate parents not to attempt to "squeeze out" the white material because infection can occur.
Mongolian spots	Dark blue or slate gray discolorations most commonly found in lumbosacral area. The intensity and hue of color remains until fading occurs. It is of no medical significance but can be misdiagnosed as a bruise.	These lesions are caused by melanin deposits in dark-skinned persons and gradually disappear in a few years. The nurse must distinguish these lesions from hematoma of child abuse.
Port-wine stain	Known as nevus flammeus. A collection of capillaries in the skin. It is a flat, red-purple lesion that does not blanch on pressure.	This is a permanent skin marking that darkens with age and can become elevated and vulnerable to injury. If a large area of face or neck is involved, laser surgery may be indicated to preserve the child's self-image. Can be associated with genetic disorders.
Forceps marks	A bruised area on skin in the shape of forceps or pattern of vacuum extractor.	The bruising and swelling fade within a few days and do not require intervention other than parental support and teaching.
Nevi	Known as stork bites. These are pink, easily blanched patches that can appear on eyelids, nose, lips, and nape of the neck.	These marks gradually fade and are of no clinical significance.

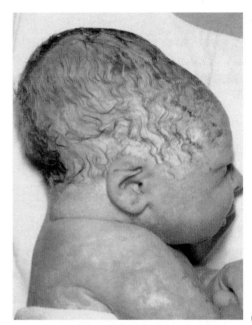

FIGURE 9-8 Caput succedaneum. Swelling on the head of the newborn is symmetric and is the result of edema under the scalp. This condition will disappear without treatment.

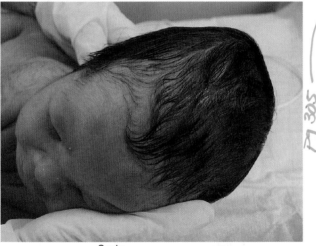

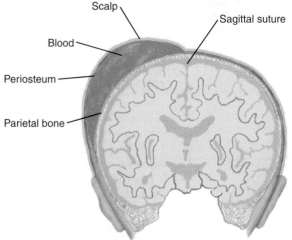

Scalp

Sagittal suture

Blood

Periosteum

Parietal bone

FIGURE 9-9 Cephalhematoma, a collection of blood between the periosteum and the cranial bone. The swelling does not cross the suture line. No treatment is indicated.

(Kiesler & Ricer, 2003). A bulging anterior fontanelle while the newborn is quiet indicates increased intracranial pressure. A depressed fontanelle is often a late sign of dehydration. A large fontanelle or delayed closure can indicate congenital hypothyroidism, Down syndrome, congenital rubella, syphilis, or increased intracranial pressure. A small anterior fontanelle or early closure is called *craniosynostosis* and is associated with abnormal brain development. It can be caused by chromosomal anomalies, fetal hypoxia, or fetal alcohol syndrome. The anterior fontanelle is usually closed by 18 months of age.

The posterior fontanelle is triangle-shaped. It is located between the occipital and parietal bones and is much smaller than the anterior fontanelle. It closes when the newborn is 2 to 3 months old. Late closure of the fontanelle may indicate hydrocephaly.

Because parents are often concerned about touching a newborn's soft spots, they should be informed that the fontanelles are covered with layers of protective tissue so that the head can be safely touched and washed. A summary of newborn observations and data collection is discussed in Table 9-4.

ESTIMATION OF GESTATIONAL AGE

Assessment of physical and neurologic findings to determine gestational age is performed by using the Ballard scoring system, in which 12 scores are totaled and a maturity rating is expressed in weeks of gestation. Gestational scoring is performed within the first few hours and repeated again at 24 hours after the newborn's neurologic system has settled (see Chapter 15). A term newborn is one who is born at 38 to 42 weeks' gestation. Preterm neonates are born at less than 38 weeks' gestation, and postterm neonates are born after 42 weeks' gestation. Fetal size is expressed as small for gestational age (SGA) if weight is less than the 10th percentile, or large for gestational age (LGA) if weight is greater than the 90th percentile for gestational age. The weight alone does not determine prematurity or maturity of the newborn. The score on the Ballard scale differentiates SGA from prematurity (see Figure 15-1). The preterm newborn is discussed in Chapter 15.

BEHAVIORAL ASSESSMENT

Assessment of the newborn's behavior provides information about behavioral alertness. Behavior changes occur in the phases of reactivity through which the newborn passes during the first 6 to 8 hours after birth. Knowledge about these reactive phases helps the parent respond appropriately to the baby's needs, thereby promoting parent-newborn attachment.

At birth, the newborn is in a state of quiet alertness during the first period of reactivity. His or her eyes are open and alert and respond to stimuli. The newborn's heart and respirations are increased. This phase is followed by a phase of active alertness. During this

Skill 9-2   Measuring the Fontanelles

PURPOSE

To determine baseline measurements of the fontanelles.

Steps

1. Obtain the size of the fontanelles by measuring the widest point of the width and the widest point of the length, adding the measurements together, and dividing by 2.

2. The normal anterior fontanelle in a newborn measures between 3.6 and 6 cm (1.4 and 2.4 inches).

3. The fontanelles should appear flat with the contour of the skull. A bulging fontanelle may indicate increased intracranial pressure. A depressed fontanelle may indicate dehydration. Both conditions should be reported.

4. Document findings.

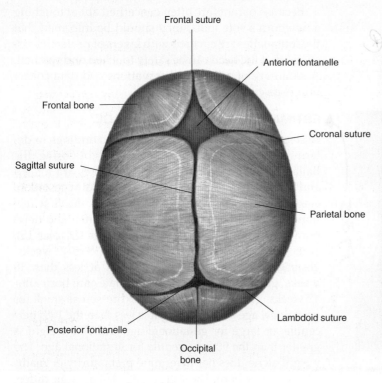

Frontal suture
Anterior fontanelle
Frontal bone
Coronal suture
Sagittal suture
Parietal bone
Lambdoid suture
Posterior fontanelle
Occipital bone

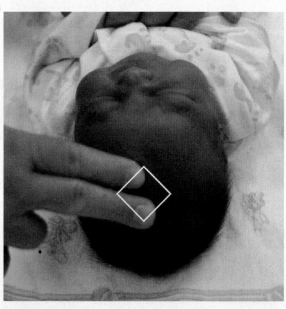

Table **9-4**   Summary of Newborn Observations and Data Collection

OBSERVATION	NORMAL	NORMAL VARIATIONS	INDICATIONS OF PATHOLOGIC CONDITION
General color	Pink (or normal for ethnic group)	Acrocyanosis	Jaundice in first 24 hours can indicate hemolytic process. Body cyanosis can indicate cardiac problem.
Muscle tone	Flexed extremities, adducted with hand in closed fist	Sharp flexion of hips from breech delivery	Extended extremities may indicate prematurity or low Apgar score. Open hand may indicate preterm neonate. Jittery movements may indicate hypoglycemia or drug withdrawal. Asymmetric movement may indicate trauma.

Table 9-4   Summary of Newborn Observations and Data Collection—cont'd

OBSERVATION	NORMAL	NORMAL VARIATIONS	INDICATIONS OF PATHOLOGIC CONDITION
Skin	Presence of lanugo, some vernix Smooth, soft, good turgor (see Table 9-3)	Heavy lanugo and vernix indicating preterm neonate Sparse lanugo and little vernix may indicate postterm infant Mongolian spots (see Table 9-3)	Peeling may indicate postmaturity. Green stain may indicate history of fetal distress. Thin, shiny skin may indicate preterm neonate. Poor turgor may indicate prematurity or dehydration.
Weight	3402-3997 g (7 lbs, 8 oz–8 lbs, 13 oz)	Loses approximately 10% of birth weight but regains it within 10 days	Variations in weight can indicate LGA, SGA, or prematurity.
Length	48-53 cm (19-21 inches)		<45 cm (17.7 inches) indicates congenital condition.
Temperature	Axillary: 36.5°-37° C (97.7°-98.6° F)	Unstable; may lead to cold stress	Hypothermia may require incubator care or proper swaddling.
Head	Circumference: 33-35.5 cm (13-14 inches)	Altered symmetry of head from molding, caput succedaneum, or cephalhematoma; will resolve in a few days without treatment	Large head may indicate hydrocephalus. Very small head may indicate microcephaly.
Sutures, fontanelles	Anterior fontanelle flat and diamond shaped; posterior fontanelle triangle shaped	Suture override; will correct in a few days	Bulging fontanelle can indicate increased intracranial pressure. Depressed fontanelle can indicate dehydration. Third fontanelle may indicate Down syndrome.
Face	Symmetric movement; sucking pads present in cheeks Face sensitive to touch.	Eyes open if newborn is tipped forward when held upright May sneeze to clear nose	Cleft in lip may indicate congenital anomaly. Asymmetric movement may indicate nerve damage.
Eyes	Symmetric movement; blue-white sclera May track moving object to midline Tearless crying. Can focus on simple, contrasting pattern that is 7-10 inches away.	Strabismus (may be temporary) Scleral hemorrhage caused by difficult delivery Permanent eye color established by 3-6 months.	Low ear-to-eye symmetry may indicate kidney problem. Yellow sclera indicates hyperbilirubinemia. Tearing before 2 months of age may indicate plugged duct or other pathology.
Ears	Cartilage firm. Assess position of ear in relation to outer canthus of eye (Figure 9-10)	Hearing established after first sneeze that clears eustachian tubes.	Lack of firm cartilage in ear pinna may indicate prematurity. Low set ears may indicate a kidney disorder.
Mouth	Gums pink and moist, no teeth Tongue sometimes extended beyond lips Sucking, rooting and extrusion reflexes present Salivary glands immature	Epstein's pearls (normal white dots) on midline of upper palate in first month (should be differentiated from white dots of thrush, which are abnormal)	Tongue that cannot extend beyond lips indicates tongue tie, which interferes with sucking and speech development. Cleft in upper palate indicates congenital anomaly. Large protruding tongue characteristic of Down syndrome. Excess oral secretions may indicate atresia.

Continued

※ the ears and Kidneys usually develop @ the same time so if there is a deformity in the ears the Kidneys might be deformed as well.

Table 9-4 Summary of Newborn Observations and Data Collection—cont'd

OBSERVATION	NORMAL	NORMAL VARIATIONS	INDICATIONS OF PATHOLOGIC CONDITION
Shoulders, clavicle	Short neck Full range of motion of arms	Long, thin neck in preterm newborn	Crepitus at clavicle may indicate fracture. Limited motion or unilateral Moro's reflex may indicate local birth trauma.
Back	Flat and straight when prone C-shaped back when in sitting position Head lag not more than 45 degrees Anus is patent. Passage of meconium must be documented before discharge.	Color of stool changes as it transitions to milk stool (Figure 9-11).	Open lesion on back may indicate spina bifida. Arching back or opisthotonos position may indicate CNS problem. Absence of stool may indicate imperforate anus
Chest	Chest circumference 30.5-33 cm (12-13 inches) Symmetric respirations 30-60 breaths/minutes Heart rate 110-160 beats/minutes Lusty cry	Breast engorgement from maternal hormones Breast tissue mass 5 mm or more. Distance between nipples 8 cm (3 inches)	Little breast tissue may indicate prematurity. Bradycardia or tachycardia may indicate distress.
Abdomen	Bowel sounds present Symmetric, protruding abdomen Umbilical cord with two arteries and one vein and is midway between symphysis pubis and xiphoid process. Abdomen moves with chest during respiration. Passes meconium within 24 hours (see Figure 9-11) Cord begins to dry within few hours and falls off within 7-9 days.	Bowel sounds absent 1-2 hours after birth Cord stump may protrude beyond skin giving appearance of hernia but will invaginate and disappear in few weeks (Figure 9-12)	Visible peristalsis may indicate pyloric stenosis. Green-stained cord may indicate history of fetal distress. Abnormal vessels may indicate congenital anomaly. Failure to pass meconium in 24 hours may indicate cystic fibrosis or nonpatent anus.
Thighs	Symmetric creases on both thighs Free range of motion	Usually flexed knees and hips in term newborn	Asymmetric creases on thighs and limited abduction may indicate congenital hip dysplasia (Figure 9-13).
External genitalia	Female labia meet at midline Male meatus at tip of penis Testes in scrotum. Deep rugae present in scrotum of full term newborn. Urination within 24 hours should be documented. Should have 6 wet diapers a day.	Rust-colored uric acid crystals in urine. White vaginal discharge may be from withdrawal of maternal hormones. Hymenal tags may protrude from vagina but will disappear in few weeks.	Meatus above or below tip of penis indicates epispadias or hypospadias. Enlarged scrotum may indicate hydrocele. Smooth scrotum with absent rugae may indicate prematurity.
Hands and feet	10 fingers and toes Nails extending to tip of finger Hands held in fisted position Strong grasp reflex Knee and foot in alignment Flat feet normal (younger than 3 years) Legs not extended at knee	Open, relaxed hand in preterm newborns	Straight simian crease in palm may indicate Down syndrome. Short fifth finger may indicate chromosomal anomaly. Nonaligned knee-foot may indicate clubfoot. Limp extremities may indicate CNS problem or Erb's palsy.

CNS, central nervous system; *LGA,* large for gestational age; *SGA,* small for gestational age. Observation of general appearance may detect external anomalies. Reflexes and behavior should also be documented.

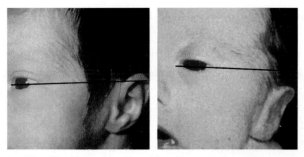

FIGURE 9-10 **Ear position.** The ears are assessed for placement; low-set ears may indicate that a congenital anomaly is present in the renal system. An imaginary line drawn from the outer canthus of the eye should be even with the upper tip of the pinna of the ear.

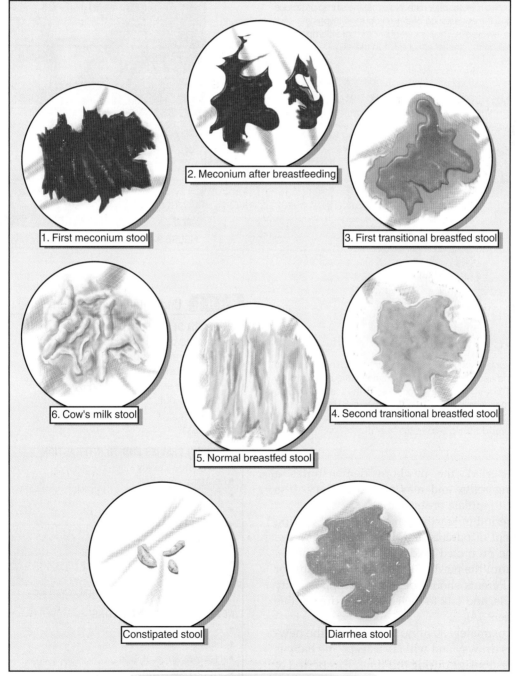

FIGURE 9-11 **Normal newborn stool cycle.** The first meconium is dark, greenish black, and tarry. It gradually changes to a greenish yellow transitional stool. The breastfed newborn's milk stool is golden yellow, and the bottle-fed newborn may have a pale yellow stool. A green, watery stool is indicative of diarrhea and should be reported to the health care provider.

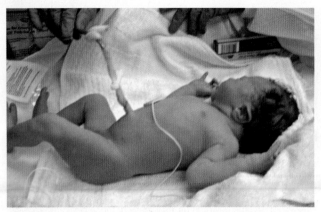

FIGURE 9-12 **The clamped umbilical cord.** The umbilical cord of this newborn was clamped minutes after birth. Note that the stump protrudes past the skin, giving the appearance of a hernia but will invaginate and disappear within a few weeks. The light weight of the cord clamp will not exert an undue pull on the area of attachment to the skin.

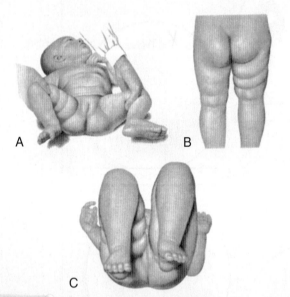

FIGURE 9-13 **A,** Ortolani maneuver to assess the hips. The newborn's legs are flexed and abducted laterally toward the mattress. A "click" sound, indicating movement of the femoral head in the acetabulum, is a positive sign of congenital hip dysplasia. **B,** The knees should be of equal length. **C,** The thigh folds should be symmetric. Asymmetry is shown in this figure.

active/alert period, the newborn demonstrates a strong sucking reflex and may appear hungry. It is an ideal time to initiate breastfeeding.

The first period of reactivity facilitates the bonding and attachment of parents and newborns. Eye-to-eye contact can be promoted by delaying insertion of eye medication until the newborn can interact with his or her parents. Parents should be given an opportunity to hold, cuddle, and talk to their newborn during this period (Figure 9-14).

After approximately 30 minutes to 1 hour, the newborn becomes drowsy and will fall asleep. The baby is typically unresponsive during this time. This period of inactivity may last from 2 to 4 hours. After the sleep

period, the newborn enters the second period of reactivity. This second period may last 4 to 6 hours. The newborn is awake, is alert, and may cry. The newborn shows activity such as rooting, sucking, and swallowing and appears hungry. The newborn may respond to eye-to-eye contact at this time, and bonding can be promoted. Feeding may be initiated if it was not started in the first period of reactivity. The nurse can help the parents understand newborn cues that will indicate newborn needs (Box 9-1).

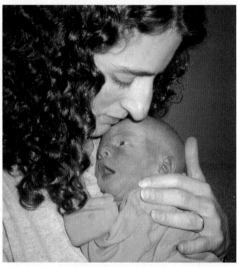

FIGURE 9-14 A mother bonds with her newborn.

Box **9-1**   Understanding Newborn Cues

NEWBORN DESIRES INTERACTION
- Focuses on face of parent
- Ceases random body movement
- Turns head to parent
- Has wide and bright, open eyes
- Reaches out
- Coos
- Babbles

NEWBORN DESIRES END TO INTERACTION
- Turns head away
- Is fussy
- Turns eyes away
- Yawns
- Squirms

NEWBORN IS HUNGRY
- Places hand at mouth
- Sucks, roots
- Flexes arm and clenches fist over body

NEWBORN IS FINISHED EATING
- Arches back
- Falls asleep
- Relaxes arms at side
- Turns head away from nipple

Behavioral States

Various states of consciousness or awareness are commonly observed in the newborn; reactions vary as the baby passes from one state to another. However, most newborns move smoothly between these states. The sleep states vary from deep sleep to irregular (light) sleep. Nurses should teach parents how to recognize and respond to the various behavior states of the newborn (Table 9-5). Newborns prefer to look at human faces and shapes in contrasting colors such as black and white. The newborn can see objects most clearly that are 7 to 10 inches away. Human interaction plays an important role in brain development and in attachment and bonding between parent and newborn (Figure 9-15).

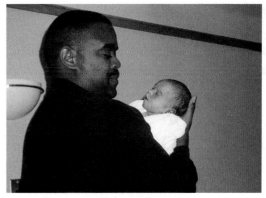

FIGURE 9-15 The newborn gazes intently at the father in the *en face position* (eye to eye), which promotes bonding.

NEUROLOGIC ASSESSMENT

The neurologic assessment is conducted to determine whether the newborn's nervous system is intact. It is important to obtain baseline information on general behaviors, including resting posture, cry, quality of muscle activity, and state of alertness.

Newborn tremors are common; however, they must be assessed to make sure that they are in the normal range and are not convulsions. Seizures may consist of excessive blinking, chewing, or swallowing movements. Whether the newborn's spontaneous movements are smooth or jerky and whether both sides move equally well are significant evaluations. Lack of good muscle tone may be caused by

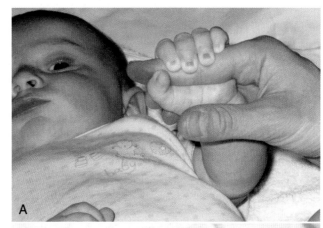

A

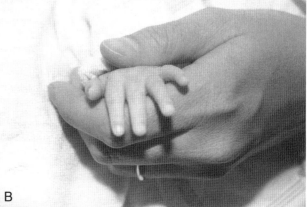

B

FIGURE 9-16 **Grasp reflex. A,** When the newborn's palm is touched, the hand closes into a tight fist in a term newborn. **B,** The preterm newborn does not respond with a firm grasp.

CNS immaturity, which is seen in preterm newborns (Figure 9-16). Some basic reflexes demonstrate neurologic function and an intact CNS (Table 9-6, Figure 9-17).

SCREENING

A **screening test** is used to detect the presence of an abnormal condition before symptoms appear. The purpose is not diagnostic because a positive screening

Table 9-5	Behavioral States of Newborns
STATE	**CHARACTERISTICS AND INTERVENTIONS**
Sleep State	
Quiet sleep	Difficult to awaken
Active sleep	Easily awakened; the best time to test hearing
Transitional State	
Drowsiness	Gentle rocking can prolong sleep Avoid abrupt movements Gentle whisper and touch can bring newborn to awake state
Awake State	
Quiet alert	Eyes are open and focused; minimal body activity Best time for parent-newborn interaction Best time to test responses and reflexes
Active alert	Precedes hunger cues Active body movements; increased heart rate; eyes are open but wander
Crying	Reaction to stimulus may be violent, indicating newborn needs a diaper change or may need to be fed or comforted; newborn should be picked up and consoled

Table **9-6**   Assessment of Reflexes and Senses of the Newborn

REFLEX OR SENSE	NORMAL FINDINGS	PRESENCE, DURATION, AND POTENTIAL PROBLEMS
Reflex		
Moro's (startle)	Elicited by sudden jarring, sudden movement, or a loud noise; newborn's response is extension and abduction of extremities, with a fanning of the fingers forming a C, followed by flexion of arms in an embracing motion.	Persistence of Moro's reflex past 6 months may indicate brain damage; strongest in first 2 months; asymmetric (unequal) Moro's reflex can be caused by an injury to the clavicle or brachial plexus.
Palmar grasp	Newborn will grasp any object that touches the palm and can hold on momentarily.	Fades at approximately 2 months; it is replaced by a voluntary movement by 8 months.
Plantar reflex	When the sole of the newborn's foot is stimulated, the toes curl downward.	Absence in term newborn indicates a spinal cord defect. Disappears after 1 year.
Babinski's reflex	Can be elicited by stroking one side of the sole from heel upward or across the ball of the foot; newborn's response is hyperextension and fanning of the toes.	Failure to respond properly may indicate CNS problem.
Tonic neck	Can be elicited when newborn is on back; when the newborn's head is turned quickly to one side, the extremities on that side extend and those on the opposite side flex; this is sometimes called the "fencing position."	Disappears by 4 months. Absence or asymmetry in term newborn indicates neurologic problem.
Stepping	When the newborn is held upright and one foot touches a flat surface, the newborn will step out with opposite foot.	Disappears after 4 weeks. Absence in term newborn may indicate neurologic problem.
Trunk incurvation	When the newborn is in a prone position, stroking the spine causes the trunk to turn to the stimulated side.	Absence may indicate CNS damage. Disappears at approximately 4 weeks.
Pupillary	Elicited by shining bright light into the eye; newborn response is constriction of the pupil.	Continues throughout life. Unequal constriction or fixed, dilated pupil is indicative of CNS damage and requires further assessment.
Blink	Stimulated by flashlight.	Absence indicates possible cataracts.
Sucking	Can be elicited by placing nipple or gloved finger in newborn's mouth.	Sucking is also stimulated by touching the lips. Continues through 6-8 months.
Rooting	Touching the cheeks or lips causes the newborn to turn the head toward the stimulus.	Lasts until 6 months.
Gag	On stimulation of the uvula, as during suctioning and sometimes during feeding; reverse peristalsis occurs.	Continues throughout life.
Sense		
Sight	At birth, the newborn can focus on an object 7-10 inches from the face and 4-6 inches above or to the side.	Newborns have preferences for human faces, moving objects, and bold, contrasting colors; newborn's visual alertness enhances eye-to-eye contact and maternal-newborn attachment; provides means for parent-newborn interaction.
Hearing	Responds to a variety of sounds, especially the range of the human voice; can locate the general direction of a sound.	The human voice provides a means to console the upset neonate (response demonstrates the value of this stimulus to the newborn).
Touch	Newborn response to touch used as a consoling means.	A newborn's lips are very sensitive to touch; a newborn can be soothed by touch, progressing from a crying to an active-alert or sleep state.
Smell	Newborns can smell sweet and sour odors.	A newborn can distinguish his or her mother's breast odor from other odors.

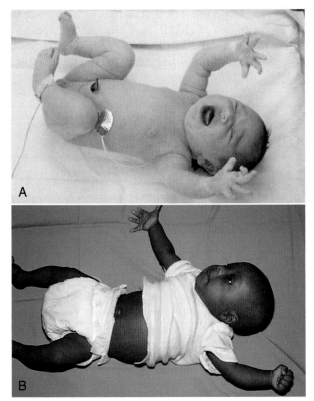

FIGURE 9-17 **Assessment of reflexes. A,** Moro's reflex. Sudden jarring of the bed causes extension and abduction (an embracing motion) of the arms and spreading of the fingers, with the index finger and the thumb forming a C shape. A unilateral (one-sided) response may indicate a fractured clavicle. Absence of the Moro's reflex may indicate a pathologic condition of the central nervous system. **B,** An abnormal Moro's reflex. Note the clenched fist of one hand that does not follow a symmetric embracing motion. This newborn requires a follow-up examination.

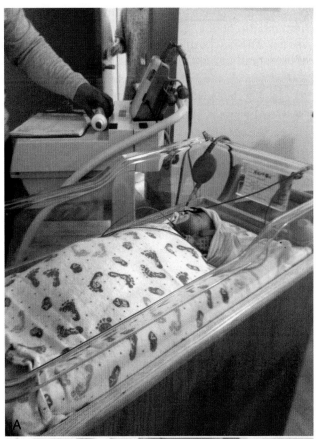

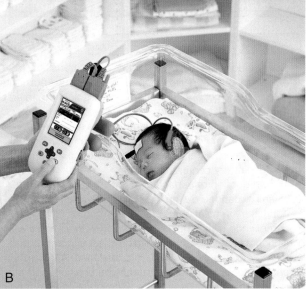

FIGURE 9-18 **A,** The nurse administers a hearing test in the newborn nursery. This test facilitates easy and accurate screening of all newborns for hearing impairment before hospital discharge. **B,** The ALGO hearing screener shows how the test is accomplished. 1. The screener sends a series of soft clicking sounds to the baby's ear. 2. The baby's brain responds with a specific brain wave pattern called the auditory brainstem response (ABR). 3. The screener automatically compares the baby's ABR to a stored template from infants with normal hearing. 4. The ALGO screener generates an immediate pass/refer result.

test indicates a need for further follow-up and specific diagnostic tests to confirm the diagnosis. The main purpose of screening tests is to enable early intervention if a possible health problem exists because waiting for signs and symptoms to occur increases risk for irreversible damage (Figure 9-18).

Newborn screening programs are state funded. Nurses need to be aware of laws and policies regarding newborn screening within their state, as well as the early symptoms of the diseases and treatment protocols so that they can educate parents. The optimum time for a screening test to be performed is before the fifth day of life in a healthy newborn. Standards for collecting, handling, and transporting screening specimens can be found online at www.marchofdimes.com/files/neonatal.pdf, or the nurse can contact the facility's clinical laboratory for this vital information.

Some states test for fewer than 10 conditions, whereas others test for more than 20 conditions. Screening for hypothyroidism and phenylketonuria is mandated in all states (Spahis & Bowers, 2006). **Phenylketonuria (PKU)** is a condition in which the newborn cannot metabolize phenylalanine (which is present in milk), and it accumulates in the blood,

→ Crying is good in the 1st 24hrs due to better oxygen perfusion & it releases fluid in the ears.

causing mental retardation. If treatment is begun in the first month of life, mental retardation can be prevented. The newborn, ideally, would receive feedings of breast milk or formula before the test is performed.

Treatment is discussed in Chapter 16. In May 2005, the U.S. Department of Health and Human Services suggested that all states screen for specific conditions (Table 9-7) and offered federal assistance as needed.

Table 9-7 Selected Newborn Screening Tests

AREAS AT RISK	NAME OF CONDITION SCREENED
Endocrine conditions	Congenital hypothyroidism Congenital adrenal hyperplasia
Other	Hearing impairment Cystic fibrosis Transferase-deficient galactosemia (classic)
Organic acid metabolism	Glutaric acidemia type 1 3-Hydroxy-3-methylglutaric aciduria Methylmalonic acidemia (vitamin B_{12} disorders)
Fatty acid metabolism	Trifunctional protein deficiency Carnitine uptake defect (carnitine transport defect)
Amino acid metabolism	Phenylketonuria, hyperphenylalaninemia Maple syrup urine disease Homocystinuria Tyrosinemia type 1
Hemoglobinopathies	Sickle cell anemia Thalassemia

Modified from Spahis, J., & Bowers, N. (2006). Navigating the maze of newborn screening. *MCN. The American Journal of Maternal Child Nursing, 31*(3), 190-196.

Get Ready for the NCLEX® Examination!

Key Points

- The newborn must make adaptations for transition to extrauterine life. To live independently, the newborn must establish pulmonary ventilation, which is accompanied by marked circulatory changes.
- After the umbilical cord is clamped, the newborn's respirations are initiated by a combination of chemical, sensory, thermal, and mechanical factors that stimulate the respiratory center in the brain.
- The production of surfactant is critical to keeping the alveoli expanded during expiration and to establish pulmonary ventilation. Surfactant promotes lung compliance, which helps the lungs fill with air more easily.
- During a vaginal birth, the fetus's chest is compressed, promoting drainage of fluid from the lungs. After birth, the chest returns (or recoils) to its natural position, and air replaces the fluid. Expansion of the lungs and clearing of fluid allow pulmonary circulation to take place.
- Extrauterine respiration, the increase in blood oxygen levels and increase in pulmonary blood flow, causes shifts in the pressures in the heart and results in closure of the ductus arteriosus, foramen ovale, and ductus venosus shortly after birth.
- At birth, the term newborn has weak cardiac and pyloric sphincters in the stomach and has bouts of reversed peristalsis. Thus, the neonate has a tendency for mild regurgitation or slight vomiting.

- During the first week of life, the liver is immature and may be slow to convert bilirubin from an indirect fat-soluble form to a water-soluble form that can be excreted in the urine and feces. The neonate's liver is also burdened with the destruction of red blood cells that are no longer needed, resulting in increased bilirubin levels in the blood. Therefore, visible jaundice is seen in many newborns on the third day of life.
- Newborns acquire passive immunity against bacterial and viral infections for which the mother has developed antibodies. This form of immunity lasts for approximately 3 to 5 months.
- Temperature regulation of the newborn is maintained by balancing the amount of heat produced with the amount of heat lost. It is easy for the newborn to lose heat through *evaporation, conduction, convection,* and *radiation.*
- Newborns are vulnerable to heat loss because they have thin skin, little subcutaneous fat, blood vessels close to the surface, and a large skin-surface area. Immediately after birth, newborns lose heat by evaporation because they are wet from amniotic fluid or from procedures such as bathing. In addition, heat loss can occur from radiation and convection because of the large body surface area compared with weight.
- The primary source of heat production when the newborn is chilled (cold stress) is the use of brown fat. If cold stress continues, acute problems such as hypoglycemia, acidosis, jaundice, and respiratory distress can develop.

- Acrocyanosis, the bluish discoloration of the hands and feet of the newborn is normal.
- Caput succedaneum is the general edema of the head, and cephalohematoma is subperiosteal hemorrhage; both can be caused by prolonged labor.
- Basic reflexes (sucking, rooting, grasp; Moro's; tonic neck) demonstrate an intact CNS.
- The Ballard scale is used to determine gestational age of the newborn.
- Newborn screening detects the presence of abnormal health conditions before signs and symptoms occur, enabling early intervention.

Additional Learning Resources

SG Go to your Study Guide on pages 489–490 for additional Review Questions for the NCLEX® Examination, Critical Thinking Clinical Situations, and other learning activities to help you master this chapter content.

 evolve Go to your Evolve website (http://evolve.elsevier.com/Leifer/maternity) for the following FREE learning resources:
- Animations
- Answer Guidelines for Critical Thinking Questions
- Answers and Rationales for Review Questions for the NCLEX® Examination
- Concept Map Creator
- Glossary with pronunciations in English and Spanish
- Patient Teaching Plans
- Skills Performance Checklists and more!

Online Resources
- www.advancesinneonatalcare.org
- www.neonatalnetwork.com
- www.parenting.com

Review Questions for the NCLEX® Examination

1. Many powerful stimuli send messages to the respiratory center of the neonates's brain. Clamping the umbilical cord is a powerful:
   1. Sensory stimulus
   2. Chemical stimulus
   3. Thermal stimulus
   4. Mechanical stimulus

2. Apnea in the newborn is defined as cessation of breathing for more than:
   1. 5 seconds
   2. 10 seconds
   3. 20 seconds
   4. 60 seconds

3. By thoroughly drying the newborn as quickly as possible after birth, the nurse prevents heat loss due to:
   1. Evaporation
   2. Conduction
   3. Convection
   4. Radiation

4. Which assessment in the newborn would require immediate attention in the first few hours after birth?
   1. A pause in breathing
   2. Nasal flaring
   3. Irregular respirations of 60 breaths/minute
   4. Sounds of moisture heard in the lungs

5. A nursing student is obtaining a newborn's temperature during phase 2 of assessment. The preferred route to obtain this reading is:
   1. Orally
   2. Rectally
   3. Tympanically
   4. Axillary

6. A collection of blood between the periosteum and a bone of the skull that it covers is called:
   1. Cephalhematoma
   2. Molding
   3. Caput succedaneum
   4. Craniosynostosis

7. Which newborn observation(s) would be considered normal? *(Select all that apply.)*
   1. The newborn grasps any object that touches the palm of the hand.
   2. Cyanosis appears in the hands and feet.
   3. Jaundice develops in the first 24 hours.
   4. Anterior fontanelle is flat and diamond shaped.
   5. White dots are present on the midline of the upper palate.

Critical Thinking Questions

1. A new father thinks the stockinette cap put on his baby's head at the time of birth is "ugly." How would you explain the reason for its placement? What else might you include in your explanation?

2. The newborn, 4 hours old, has his first stool. The infant's mother is concerned about the color of the stool and asks whether it is normal. How would you explain this type of stool to the mother?

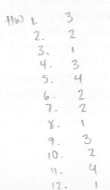

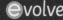
Objectives

1. Define key terms listed.
2. Discuss the nursing responsibilities concerning the care of the newborn infant.
3. Describe a neutral thermal environment.
4. Demonstrate three ways to hold a newborn.
5. Demonstrate the proper way to suction the newborn with a bulb syringe.
6. Describe newborn bathing and cord care to parents.
7. Interpret instructions for parents about newborn stools and voiding patterns.
8. Discuss care of the circumcised and uncircumcised penis.
9. Describe pain assessment and control in the newborn.
10. Explain the discharge care plan.
11. Discuss five aspects of newborn care that the mother should understand before discharge.

Key Terms

circumcision (sĭr-kŭm-SĬZH-ŭn, p. 197)
cord care (p. 186)
en face (p. 191)
kangaroo care (p. 188)

neutral thermal environment (p. 187)
ophthalmia neonatorum (p. 188)
retraction (rē-TRĂK-shŭn, p. 198)

THREE PHASES OF NEWBORN CARE

The nursing care of the newborn is directed toward promoting the physical well-being of the baby and supporting the family unit. The immediate care of the newborn takes place in the delivery room and is discussed in Chapter 7. Because numerous physiologic adaptations begin right after birth, immediate nursing care is very important. The first goal is to help the newborn make the transition to extrauterine life. The second goal is to assess and provide nursing care that supports the newborn's health status. The third goal is to teach the parents and family members how to care for and bond with the new baby.

Three phases of newborn care are discussed that span from the immediate neonatal period until the infant has stabilized in the transition to extrauterine life. The three phases of transition are:

Phase 1: Birth to 1 hour—first period of reactivity; takes place in delivery room (see Chapter 7)

Phase 2: One to 4 hours—may take place in the labor, delivery, recovery, and postpartum (LDRP) room, nursery, or parents' room; when the initial detailed health assessment is completed (see Chapter 9)

Phase 3: Four hours to discharge—second period of reactivity; takes place in mother's room and involves nursing interventions and family teaching

This chapter briefly reviews phases 1 and 2 and focuses on phase 3.

A clinical pathway indicates specific care given over a specified period that is related to a planned outcome. It includes nursing assessments, interventions, medical interventions, teaching, and discharge and follow-up care (Clinical Pathway 10-1).

PHASE 1 CARE: NURSING INTERVENTIONS

CLAMPING THE UMBILICAL CORD AND CORD CARE

The umbilical cord is initially white and gelatinous in appearance. It contains two umbilical arteries and one vein in the center of the umbilical cord. Deviations in the number of vessels in the cord could indicate a congenital anomaly and must be reported to the health care provider. The cord begins drying within 1 to 2 hours after birth. Bleeding from the cord or a foul odor should be reported immediately.

 Memory Jogger

Umbilical Vessels

An easy way to remember the number and types of umbilical vessels is to use the mnemonic *AVA*, which stands for *Artery, Vein, Artery.*

Clinical Pathway 10-1	Newborn		
ASSESSMENT	**BIRTH–1 HOUR (PHASE 1)**	**1-4 HOURS (PHASE 2)**	**4 HOURS–DISCHARGE (PHASE 3)**
Nursing assessment	Take vital signs with continuous electronic monitor. Determine Apgar score (see Table 7-7). Check weight. Assess reflexes. Take measurements. Assess activity. Calculate gestational age. Check for deviations or anomalies.	Take vital signs every 4 hours. Determine stabilization of temperature and circulation. Observe mucus production and need for suctioning. Check condition of umbilical cord. Check for deviations (detailed assessment). Assess tolerance of feeding. Assess voiding and stooling.	Check cord clamp and care. Assess vital signs. Monitor and record sleep-wake activity, feeding, intake, urinary and stool daily output.
Nursing interventions	Dry newborn. Weigh newborn. Apply identification (ID) bands and take footprints of newborn. Use radiant warmer and hat to prevent heat loss. Bulb suction as needed. Initiate breastfeeding. Assist with collection of blood specimens. Apply appropriate cord clamp. Enable bonding.	Wean from radiant warmer. Check oxygen saturation. Bathe, position newborn. Perform cord care per protocol. Keep diaper below cord area. Observe and support breastfeeding. Assess and promote bonding.	Obtain blood for screening tests. Swaddle newborn. Provide cord care per protocol. Discuss "back to sleep" positioning of newborn with parents. Complete birth certificate information.
Medical and other interventions	Administer prophylactic eye ointment or drops after baby makes eye contact with parents. Initiate breastfeeding. Wean from radiant warmer.	Administer hepatitis B immunization with parent consent. Administer vitamin K (phytonadione [AquaMEPHYTON]) intramuscularly.	Teach cord and circumcision care. Reinforce feeding technique. Ensure parents have proper car seat and instructions on its correct installation and use. Perform hearing screening test. Assist with circumcision if indicated and consented.
Teaching	Review ID bands and security procedures. Discuss parent bonding. Assist with breastfeeding. Review newborn appearance and reflexes.	Discuss feeding techniques. Review care of newborn and swaddling. Review behavior of newborn. Review handwashing and diaper handling. Support positive parenting behaviors. Review newborn's weight changes during first few weeks.	Review care of newborn. Include father and extended family in teaching plan. Discuss safety concerns and home environment. Identify community referral needs. Reinforce breastfeeding techniques. Provide written literature. Discuss use of breast pump.
Discharge and follow-up	Coordinate with social worker or case manager to determine family home needs and support system.	Discuss plans for immunization needs. Provide and discuss handout concerning newborn growth and development and follow-up care.	Provide Women, Infants, and Children (WIC) or clinic referral and lactation consultant. Document screening tests and immunizations given. Provide car seat information. Arrange return appointment for mother and newborn. Provide hotline referral number for questions.

*cord falls within 10 days
Umbilical cord care done
every time theres a diaper change

After the newborn is stabilized in phase 1 care, a disposable umbilical clamp is applied and the cord is cut to a shorter length. Before discharge, the parents are shown how to care for the umbilical cord stump at home. The cord clamp may be removed before discharge if the cord is dry and crisp, or it may be left on at discharge and discarded when the cord falls off, which usually occurs within 10 days. Parents are taught cord care, which may include dipping a cotton swab in isopropyl alcohol, triple dye, saline, or a solution prescribed by the health care provider and using it to clean around the base of the cord where it joins the skin. The cord stump is allowed to dry (Skill 10-1).

Studies have shown that newborns who have cord care involving the application of topical human breast milk, or dry care, take less time for cord separation and have fewer infection risks (Vural & Kisa, 2006).

Cleansing is done at every diaper change until the cord stump falls off. The nurse shows the parents how to fold the diaper below the level of the umbilicus so that it will not become wet with urine. A cord that is moist or red or has a discharge or a foul odor should be reported immediately to the health care provider.

IDENTIFICATION AND SECURITY

Matching identification (ID) bands are placed on the newborn's wrist and ankle and the mother's wrist in the delivery room. In some hospitals, the partner also receives a wrist band with matching numbers. For security reasons, many hospitals have either an umbilical clamp or ID wrist band with an electronic sensor attached that will sound an alarm if the newborn is taken out of the unit (Figure 10-1). The ID band is checked by the nurse and mother at any time the

---

Skill 10-1   Providing Umbilical Cord Care

PURPOSE

To assist the cord in drying and falling off.

Steps

1. Check umbilical clamp placement for tight closure. There should be no bleeding from the cord.
2. Keep cord dry and exposed to the air.
3. Assess the cord for presence of vessels.
4. Using an alcohol wipe, start from the base of the cord and gently wipe upward and outward.*
5. Lift the cord away from the infant's abdomen to facilitate cleansing of all areas.
6. Observe cord and abdominal area for redness, discharge, or foul odor.
7. Diaper infant, and be certain the upper end of diaper is folded down below the cord so it does not rub against the cord.
8. Document cord care and observations, solutions used to cleanse the area, condition of the cord, teaching of the parents, and their response.

※ Cord hasn't fallen off yet, one must do a sponge bath only!

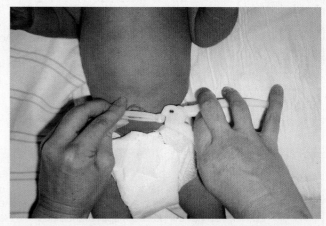

The nurse removes the umbilical cord clamp with a clamp remover before the newborn is discharged.

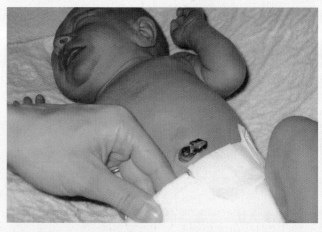

Note that the edge of the diaper is folded below the umbilical stump.

---

*Some hospitals use triple dye, alcohol, or other solutions per facility policy. Cord care is completed with every diaper change per facility protocol.

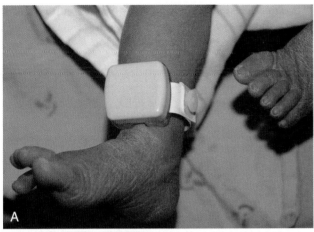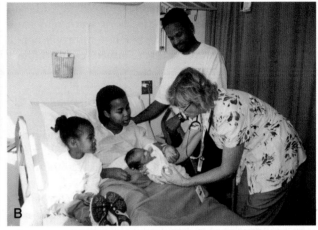

FIGURE 10-1 **A,** An identification (ID) band with an alarm sensor attached. Note the band on the right ankle has a sensor that will activate an alarm if the newborn is removed from the unit. **B,** The nurse compares the ID band of the newborn with the band on the mother's wrist as the father and sibling look on.

newborn is separated or returned to the mother and before discharge. The nurse and mother verify the ID bands together.

BIRTH CERTIFICATES

Birth certificates are completed before the infant is discharged or within 48 hours of birth. Birth certificates include vital data concerning the mother and infant that can be used for research and statistical purposes. Valid information can aid in improving public health strategies and formulating public health action plans. Ninety-nine percent of all births were registered on official birth certificates in 1998 (Northam & Knapp, 2006).

Birth certificate information is sent to the Bureau of Vital Statistics via computer. The data recorded on the birth certificate should be reviewed by the health care provider to increase the validity and reliability of information recorded. Birth certificates are required throughout the life of the child for admission to school, employment, travel, and so forth.

THERMOREGULATION

Maintenance of temperature—or thermoregulation—immediately after birth is discussed in Chapters 7 and 9. The technique of assessing temperature is reviewed in Chapter 9. Maintenance of a neutral thermal environment after birth aids the infant in achieving thermoregulation. A neutral thermal environment is maintenance of an environmental temperature at which oxygen consumption is minimal but adequate to maintain body temperature (Kenner & Lott, 2007). Strategies to conserve heat and to prevent cold stress in the newborn are important nursing responsibilities. Cold stress is discussed in Chapter 9.

The American Academy of Pediatrics (1997) defines normal rectal or axillary temperatures to be between 36.5° C and 37.5° C (97.7° F and 99.5° F). Hypothermia is classified as mild if the temperature is 36° C to 36.4° C (96.8° F to 97.5° F), moderate at 32.0° C to 35.9° C (89.6° F to 96.6° F), and severe if less than 32.6° C (90.7° F). Newborns are at greater risk for hypothermia than adults are because they have a higher body surface area to body mass ratio, higher metabolic rate with limited metabolic stores, and immature thermoregulation mechanism.

Although hypothermia can be a sign of a central nervous system (CNS) infection or metabolic anomaly, about 20% of all normal newborns are seen with hypothermia, and about 50% of newborns have one or more episodes of hypothermia in the first 72 hours of life (Li, Sun, & Neubauer, 2004). Hypothermia can cause increased cell metabolism, increased oxygen consumption, hypoglycemia, and other complications in the newborn and should be actively prevented. Strategies to conserve heat and to prevent cold stress are important nursing responsibilities.

In phase 1 care, the newborn is placed in a radiant warmer with a temperature probe on the abdomen until body temperature is stabilized. In phases 2 and 3 care, when the newborn is in the nursery or the mother's room, the baby's axillary temperature is recorded every 4 hours (see Skill 9-1). The newborn is wrapped warmly and placed in a bassinet. A hat is placed on the newborn's head to conserve heat because the head has a large surface area, and the newborn is dressed in a shirt and diaper only. When the newborn's temperature is stabilized, a bath may be given to remove excess blood and vernix. The bath does not need to remove all vernix because it provides some antimicrobial protection. Until the completion of the initial bath, the nurse should wear gloves and a cover gown when handling the newborn (see Appendices A and B). The room temperature should be maintained at 24° C to 25° C (75.2° F to 77° F). The newborn is weighed and measured on admission to the newborn nursery.

Skin-to-skin contact, with the newborn placed on the mother's naked chest, has been shown to be an effective temperature stabilizer (Galligan, 2006). The

*after skin to skin contact neonate can be weighed

infant is covered with a blanket and may wear a hat. Skin-to-skin (kangaroo care) is effective to warm a hypothermic infant when the mother's temperature is normal, her skin is dry, and she is relatively comfortable (Figure 10-2).

ADMINISTERING AN INTRAMUSCULAR INJECTION

The newborn should receive vitamin K (phytonadione [AquaMEPHYTON] 0.5 to 1 mg) (see Skill 7-8). It is given intramuscularly in the midanterior thigh (the vastus lateralis muscle) where the muscle development is adequate. Because newborns cannot synthesize vitamin K in the intestines without the presence of bacterial flora, they are deficient in clotting factors, and vitamin K must be administered as a prophylaxis to assist in clotting.

PROPHYLACTIC EYE CARE

The newborn can acquire an eye infection, such as gonorrhea or chlamydia, when passing through an infected birth canal. Prophylaxis against gonococcal ophthalmia neonatorum, an infection that can cause blindness, is required for all newborns. Erythromycin (Ilotycin) ophthalmic ointment is commonly used for prophylactic eye care because it produces less eye irritation than other eye medications and also destroys the *Chlamydia* organism. Ideally, a single-unit dose (new tube) of ointment is used. The ointment is placed so that it reaches all areas of the conjunctival sac (see Skill 7-9). It is recommended that eye prophylaxis be administered approximately 1 hour after birth to allow time for newborn-parent interaction without the newborn's vision being disturbed.

PHASE 2 CARE: ROUTINE NURSING INTERVENTIONS

WEIGHING AND MEASURING

Weight

The infant is weighed in the birthing room or when admitted to the nursery (Skill 10-2). Disposable paper is put on the scale, and the scale is balanced to zero according to its model. The unclothed infant is then placed on the scale. The nurse's hand should not touch the infant but should be kept just above him or her to prevent falls. The weight must be converted to grams for gestational age assessment. The normal term newborn weighs approximately 3402 g (7 lbs, 8 oz). The normal newborn may lose up to 10% of its birthweight in the first week (physiologic weight loss) and regains the birthweight by the tenth day. After the first week, the newborn typically gains 200 g (7 oz) per week (gestational age is discussed in Chapter 15).

Measurements

Three typical measurements are length, head circumference, and chest circumference. A disposable tape measure is used. The tape should not be pulled out from under the infant to avoid giving a paper cut. Measurements must also be noted in centimeters for gestational age assessment.

> **? Did You Know?**
>
> **Average Measurements of the Full-Term Infant**
>
> Weight: 3402 g (7 lbs, 8 oz)
> Length: 48-53 cm (19-21 inches)
> Head circumference: 33-35.5 cm (13-14 inches)
> Chest circumference: 33-35 cm (12-13 inches)

Length. There are several ways to measure length. Some facilities have a tape measure applied to the clear wall of a bassinet. The nurse places the infant's head at one end, extends the leg, and notes where the heel ends. Another method is to bring the infant to the bassinet or warmer with the scale paper. The paper is marked at the top of the head, the body and leg are extended, and the paper is marked where the foot is located. Length is measured between the marks. Still another method involves placing the zero end of the tape at the infant's head, extending the body and leg, and stretching the tape to the heel. The average length of the full-term newborn is 48 to 53 cm (19 to 21 inches).

Head Circumference. The fullest part of the infant's head is measured just above the eyebrows (see Skill 10-2). Molding of the head may affect the accuracy of the initial measurement. The average head

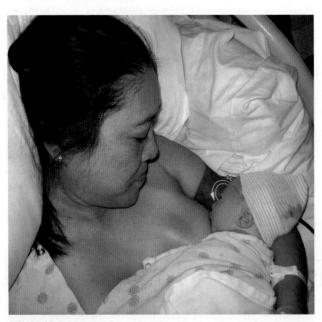

FIGURE 10-2 Skin-to-skin contact (kangaroo care), with the mother and infant's chest bare and with a blanket covering the mother and infant, is effective in warming a hypothermic infant and promotes bonding. It can be used any time after birth for term or preterm infants. Note the bloodstain on the hat of the newborn from the internal fetal monitor applied during labor.

PURPOSE

To obtain a baseline weight and measurement of the newborn infant.

Steps

Weight

1. Cover the scale with a barrier, such as a paper pad, to prevent conductive heat loss from a cool surface; this also helps prevent cross-contamination.
2. Balance scale to zero after a barrier is placed on the scale. If using a self-adjusting electronic scale, ensure the readout is at zero.
3. With the newborn in the supine position, place your hand above the newborn as a safety measure. (With active movements, the newborn could slide off the scale.)
4. Some electronic scales will read "stable" when an accurate weight is obtained. An electronic scale displays weight both in pounds and ounces and in grams.
5. Write the weight down immediately (such as on the paper covering scale). Document on the newborn's medical record after returning the newborn to the bassinet.
6. Compare the weight with previous weight and normal range of 3402 to 3997 g (7 lbs, 8 oz to 8 lbs, 13 oz).

Length

1. Place newborn in the supine position with the head at the upper edge of the ruler on the scale (can measure in the crib).
2. While holding the newborn so the head does not move, use your other hand to press the knee to extend the leg along the measuring device. Note the length at the bottom of the newborn's heel. Document in newborn's medical record.

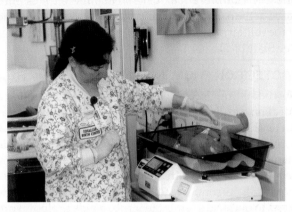

Weighing the newborn. Note the barrier placed under the newborn and the nurse's hand held above the newborn for safety. Gloves should be worn when handling the nude newborn.

Using Paper Tape Measure

1. Mark paper on which the newborn is lying at the top of the newborn's head and at the end of the extended leg. This method is useful when the newborn is extremely active.
2. Compare the length with normal range of 48 to 53 cm (19 to 21 inches) for a term newborn.
3. Remove the tape by rolling or lifting the newborn. Do not pull the tape from beneath the newborn because it could cut the newborn's skin.

Head and Chest Circumferences

1. Place tape under the head and over the prominent part of the occiput and above the ear and eyebrows. This allows measurement of the largest diameter of the head.
2. Move tape down to measure the chest at the level of the nipples. Measure on expiration.
3. Compare measurements with normal range for a term newborn: head, 33 to 35.5 cm (13 to 14 inches); chest, 30.5 to 33 cm (12 to 13 inches).

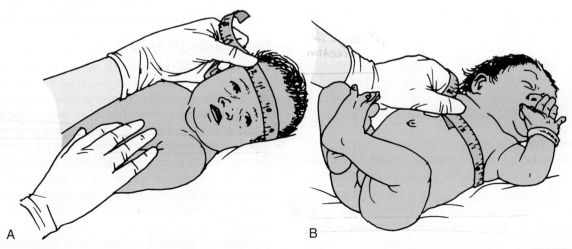

A, Measuring the head circumference. The tape is placed above the eyebrow and ear and around the occiput. B, Measuring the chest circumference. The tape is placed at the nipple line.

circumference of the full-term newborn is 33 to 35.5 cm (13 to 14 inches).

Chest Circumference. Chest circumference is measured at the nipple line. The average chest circumference of the full-term newborn is 30.5 to 33 cm (12 to 13 inches) (see Skill 10-2).

PROTECTION FROM INFECTION

Newborns are susceptible to infection, and prevention of infection constitutes a major part of nursing care and parent teaching. Cracks in the skin, particularly on the newborn's hands, feet, and umbilical cord, are especially vulnerable to infection. All newborns are also at risk for health–care-acquired infections. Many facilities require all personnel who have direct contact with newborns to perform a 3-minute scrub (hands to elbow) procedure at the beginning of each shift. The hands must always be cleaned, with either soap and water or an alcohol-based hand sanitizer, before and after contact with a newborn or any soiled surface. Alcohol-based hand sanitizers should be available for use by personnel, parents, and visitors. Avoiding cross-contamination is an important objective in newborn care.

Health Promotion

Measures to Protect the Newborn from Infection

- Persons who have direct contact with the newborn should be required to perform a 3-minute (up to the elbows) scrub at the beginning of each shift.
- All health care providers should wear clean attire before caring for the newborn.
- Caregivers should wash their hands again before touching the common nursery equipment or another newborn to avoid cross-contamination.
- Any person who has an infection should not be admitted to the maternal-newborn area.
- Every newborn should have his or her own individual bassinet and supplies.
- The umbilical cord area and any broken skin should be assessed daily for redness, warmth, or purulent discharge.
- If the mother has an infection, the nurse should consult with the health care provider to determine safety of mother-newborn contact.

Signs of newborn infection include poor feeding, lethargy, and periods of apnea. More obvious signs of infection are drainage, redness, and possible odor from the umbilical cord stump, eyes, or circumcision site.

Hepatitis B Vaccination

The American Academy of Pediatrics and the Centers for Disease Control and Prevention (AAP, 2009) recommend that all newborns receive their first vaccination against hepatitis B within 12 hours after birth regardless of the mother's hepatitis B surface antigen (HBsAg) status. It is important that newborns receive their second vaccination at approximately 1 month of age and their third one at 6 months of age.

ASSESSING AND MANAGING PAIN IN THE NEWBORN

The nurse is responsible for understanding physiologic and behavioral responses to pain in infants and for providing appropriate relief measures. Untreated pain in the preterm or term newborn or in early infancy can have long-term effects because pain pathways and structures required for long-term memory are well developed by 24 weeks' gestation.

Several pain assessment tools are available:

- **CRIES:** A 10-point scale used postoperatively in newborns at 32 or more weeks' gestation that assesses facial expression, cry, movement of arms and legs, consolability, and oxygen saturation (C = cry; R = requires oxygen; I = increased vital signs; E = expression on face; S = sleeplessness)
- **PIPP:** A preterm infant pain profile based on scales similar to the CRIES scale
- **NIPS:** A neonatal infant pain profile based on scales similar to the CRIES scale
- **N-PASS:** A neonatal pain, agitation, and sedation scale that considers the above criteria in addition to behavior and is a reliable and valid assessment tool, even for preterm infants on ventilators
- **FLACC:** The **F**ace expression, **L**eg movements, **A**rousal and activity, **C**ry high pitched, and **C**onsolability difficulty is rated on a 2-point scale that gives a score from 0-10 to rate newborn pain.

Unrelieved pain in the neonate can cause exhaustion and irritability and slow the healing process (Figure 10-3). Pharmacologic pain relief includes the use of morphine or fentanyl for severe pain or acetaminophen for mild pain. Nonpharmacologic pain relief includes touching, stroking, swaddling, and nonnutritive sucking (pacifiers). Administration of 25% oral dextrose during brief invasive procedures has been shown to be effective in relieving pain (Chermont, 2009). Reducing environmental stimuli and noise, nesting, hugging, gentle massage, warm blankets, and distraction can also be effective. Overstimulation should be avoided.

PROMOTION OF SAFETY

Parents should be taught ways to protect their newborn from injury. For example, never leave the newborn alone on the changing table or bed because the newborn can roll over and fall. Never prop a bottle because it increases the risk of aspiration, choking, dental caries, and otitis media. Always leave the side rails up on the crib when the parent is not at the bedside. Parents should be advised to obtain an infant car seat for vehicle transportation before discharge. Safety measures in the hospital include verification of mother and infant ID bands every time the mother and infant are separated or reunited, recognition of employees in the

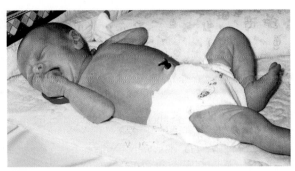

FIGURE 10-3 **Pain in the newborn.** Note the furrowed brow, clenched fist, irritability or cry, chin quiver, increased muscle tone and activity, tightly closed eyes, facial grimace, raised cheeks, deepened nasolabial fold, and open mouth. Diaphoresis; rapid, shallow respirations; and increased heart rate and blood pressure also can be observed in the neonate experiencing pain. Pain relief for the neonate during any medical procedure is important.

unit who wear photo ID badges, and placement of the infant bassinet near the mother's bed on rooming-in units.

⚠ Safety Alert

Precautions to Promote Newborn Safety

- Newborns should never be left unattended on a table or on a weighing scale.
- Newborns should be held for bottle feedings. Bottles should never be propped because of the potential for spitting up, aspirating, and choking. Propped bottles may also lead to otitis media (ear infection).
- Newborns should not be allowed to lose body heat.
- Newborns should be placed on their side after feeding to prevent aspiration.
- Newborns should be placed on their backs when put to sleep for the night.
- Extra linen or diapers should not be stored in the crib.

FACILITATION OF PARENT-NEWBORN ATTACHMENT AND NURSING INTERVENTIONS

Parent-newborn attachment is promoted by encouraging the family to be involved with the newborn, such as holding, feeding, and diapering. Nearly every contact the nurse has with the parents presents an opportunity for teaching that can promote their competence in newborn care.

The nurse needs to discuss newborn behaviors, identify newborn cues (see Chapter 9), and discuss with parents how to respond to them. Parents are more likely to respond to their newborn when they know the newborn's capabilities for interaction, such as hearing, touch, gaze, eye contact, and facial expressions. Parents need to know that most newborns respond positively to stroking, massaging, and cuddling. Mothers need to be encouraged to hold their newborn so that they can have eye-to-eye (**en face**) contact. Parents will want to know that talking or singing to the newborn will provide social stimulation, and siblings should be

given the opportunity to become acquainted with the newborn before discharge (Figure 10-4).

The brief hospital stay for many mothers requires the nurse to set priorities in newborn care. Teaching must begin as soon as the parents are ready to participate in the newborn's care. Rather than observing a bath demonstration, parents are encouraged to participate according to their ability as early as possible.

It is important for the nurse to continue to assess the newborn throughout the hospital stay. The newborn should be assessed and clinical findings recorded every 4 to 8 hours. Assessment includes vital signs, general appearance, skin integrity, color, fluid intake, voiding and stooling, activity (such as crying, irritability, or lethargy), and parent-newborn bonding.

The newborn is cleansed as needed and kept in dry clothes, and cord care is demonstrated. Cleaning the genitalia after each voiding and stool is important

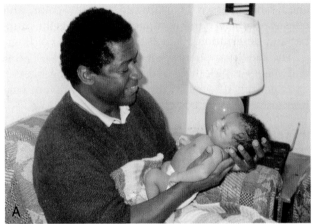

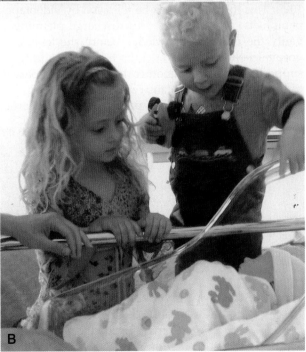

FIGURE 10-4 **A,** A father bonds with his newborn. **B,** Siblings need time to bond with the new family member.

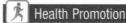

dehydration: ↑pulse, ↑temp, ~~sunken~~ fontanelles
sunken

because ammonia from the urine can rapidly irritate the newborn's skin. In the female newborn, it is important to clean from front to back or from the vagina toward the anus. See Skill 16-2 for instructions on obtaining a urine specimen when urinary tract problems are suspected.

During the first 24 hours of life, the newborn's skin color and sclera of the eyes are assessed for signs of jaundice. If the sclera appears more yellow (jaundiced) than at birth, a heel stick is likely to be performed to obtain the bilirubin level. If the bilirubin level rises above 10 to 12 mg/dL, the newborn may be given phototherapy (see Chapter 16).

The nurse should carefully monitor the newborn's amount and type of fluid intake. Breastfeeding is recorded according to how long and how vigorously the newborn sucks (see Chapter 11). Recording of intake includes the amount taken and tolerance for feedings (e.g., whether the newborn spits up formula and, if so, whether it was projectile or forceful). Stools should be assessed according to amount, color, and consistency. The nurse accurately documents the number and description of stools and number of voidings.

The newborn should not be overdressed. A shirt and diaper for clothing and a light receiving blanket usually are sufficient. A cap is useful to prevent heat loss from the large body surface area of the head.

PHASE 3 CARE

PARENT EDUCATION

Ideally, the nurse demonstrates holding, suctioning, bathing, and dressing of the newborn and then observes the mother or parents perform each procedure (Figure 10-5). This instruction may be followed by videotapes, pamphlets, group classes, and discharge planning to verify the mother's knowledge before she leaves the hospital. Follow-up calls after discharge lend additional support by providing another opportunity for parents to have their questions answered. Available help line numbers should be given to parents before discharge.

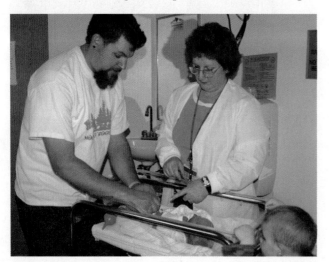

FIGURE 10-5 The nurse teaches a father the principles of cord care, diapering, and dressing his newborn.

Health Promotion

When to Call the Health Care Provider

Call the health care provider if any of the following signs is present:

- Axillary temperature greater than 38° C (100.4° F) or less than 36.1° C (97° F)
- Difficulty breathing or an absence of breathing for more than 20 seconds
- Changes in skin color: dusky appearance, blueness around mouth, or whites of eyes appearing yellow
- Discharge, bleeding, redness, or foul odor from cord
- Bleeding from circumcision site
- Redness, swelling, or discharge from eyes
- More than one episode of forceful or frequent vomiting
- Refusal to feed for two or more consecutive feedings
- Two or more green, watery stools or hard and infrequent stools
- No wet diapers in 18 hours or fewer than six voidings in a 24-hour period
- Inconsolable newborn: quieting techniques not effective or continuous high-pitched cry

Patient Teaching

Teaching Points: Parent Education Before Discharge

- Safe positioning of newborn to maintain an open airway and prevent sudden infant death syndrome (SIDS)
- Use of bulb syringe for suctioning to prevent aspiration
- Maintenance of temperature in clothing and bathing infant
- Cord care and prevention of infection
- The infant's capabilities to communicate needs
- The importance of face-to-face contact with the newborn
- Comforting techniques, including touch and swaddling
- Recognizing cue and needs of infant in providing consistent care
- Feeding (see Chapter 11)
- Importance of follow-up appointments for well-baby care
- Help line numbers available to parents to answer questions

The Interactive Bath

Initial skin care after the infant is stable involves washing the blood, amniotic fluid, and vernix from the skin. Until the infant's first bath and shampoo, the nurse wears gloves and a cover gown when handling the newborn.

Newborn care procedures, such as bathing, provide an excellent opportunity for assessment and teaching (Skill 10-3). The nurse can emphasize certain basic principles of care, including handwashing, cleansing the tub, organizing supplies, setting the water temperature, cleaning the creases in the infant's neck, and cleaning the eyes and ears. The use of cotton-tipped swabs should be avoided.

The baby bath is also a unique opportunity to assess parent-newborn interaction and to help the parent cope with the behavior cues and responses of the newborn to the warmth of the water, the touch of the washcloth, wrapping, drying, and dressing (Amy, 2001). The nurse can identify techniques of waking a sleepy newborn or calming an active newborn. Safety precautions can be emphasized, and the interactive nature of the bath can promote parent-newborn bonding.

An important consideration in skin cleansing is the preservation of the skin's pH. Alkaline soaps, oils, powder, and lotions are not advised because they alter the pH of the skin and provide a medium for bacterial growth. Therefore, plain water is best for the first 1 to 2 weeks of life. Patting the newborn dry rather than rubbing protects delicate skin.

Parents may be advised to give sponge baths until the cord stumps fall off and the umbilicus is well healed; then the newborn may have a tub bath.

Skill 10-3   Bathing the Newborn

PURPOSE

To cleanse the skin and interact with the newborn.

Steps

- Give sponge baths until the umbilical cord site and circumcision site are healed; tub baths can then begin.
- Give a bath between feedings at the most convenient time for the baby and family. A bath should not be given immediately after feeding.
- Complete baths are not necessary every day because specific areas are washed after diaper changes and spitting up milk.
- After the bath, the baby will likely want to sleep.

Sponge Bath

Note that the nurse wears gloves for the first bath of the newborn.

1. Just before the bath begins, test the bath water. It should feel warm to the inner wrist (approximately 36.7° C to 37.2° C [98° F to 99° F]).

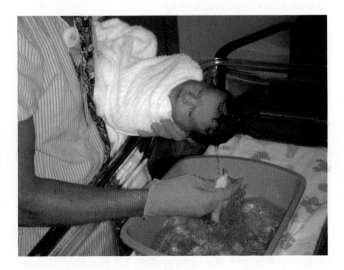

2. The bath will proceed from the cleanest to the most soiled area of the body: from eyes and face to the trunk and extremities and, finally, to the diaper area.
3. Carefully wash and dry each area to prevent heat loss.
4. Keep the baby warm by exposing only the area you are washing.
5. Wash the baby's face with clear water. Use a separate clean area of the washcloth (or use cotton ball) to wipe each eyelid. Use a clean area to wash the outer ear (do not put anything inside the ear or nose).
6. Wash behind the ears, where milk that is spit up may accumulate.
7. If necessary, clean the nose with a clean corner of the washcloth.
8. Put your hand under the baby's shoulders and lift slightly. This allows you to wash the creases of the neck.
9. Wash the vulva of a female newborn, wiping from front to back, to prevent contamination of the vagina or urethra by rectal content. In the male newborn, do not force back the foreskin of the uncircumcised penis. Clean the penis and scrotal area gently. It is important to clean under the scrotum and the folds of the scrotum.
10. The easiest way to wash the hair is to hold the baby in one arm using the football hold over the basin of water. Soap hair and rinse by pouring water from a container over the head. Then dry hair to prevent chilling.

Continued

Skill 10-3   Bathing the Newborn—cont'd

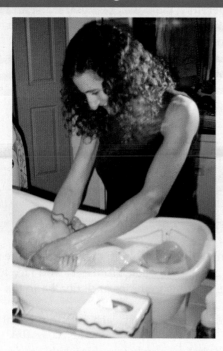

Tub Bath

1. Use a plastic tub or a clean sink for the bath.
2. Place a small blanket or pad at the bottom of the tub for comfort and to prevent slipping.
3. Place approximately 3 to 4 inches of warm water in the tub. The water temperature should be 36.7° C to 37.2° C (98° F to 99° F) and feel comfortably warm to the inner wrist.
4. Using a clean, dampened washcloth, wash the eyes and face with plain water.
5. The baby may seem frightened and cry when first put in the water. Holding the baby securely and talking with a soft voice will often help the baby adjust to the bath, which is a new experience.
6. Be certain all soap is rinsed off the baby before removing him or her from the tub.
7. Remove the newborn from the tub and immediately wrap in a dry towel.
8. With the baby in a football hold, gently shampoo the hair, rinse thoroughly with warm water, and dry with a clean towel.

Baths do not have to be given every day and can be given between meals at a time convenient for the family to get acquainted with the newborn. It is advisable to avoid baths just after feeding because excessive handling of the newborn could result in regurgitation.

Positioning and Holding the Newborn

Parents should be taught that the newborn has limited control of the head. Therefore, when positioned prone, the newborn may raise the head slightly and briefly only. Because of this, parents are taught that the newborn must be placed on a firm crib mattress and should not be placed in a prone position (lying on the stomach) when left alone. Most SIDS deaths occur while the newborn is in the prone position. The "back to sleep" motto reminds parents to place the newborn on its back when positioning for sleep.

Whenever the newborn is lifted up and held, the head must be supported because the head is larger than the rest of the body and the neck muscle strength is not well developed. There are four basic ways to hold the newborn (Figure 10-6). The cradle hold is commonly used during feeding. The newborn's head is cradled in the bend of the holder's elbow. This hold permits eye-to-eye contact, provides a sense of closeness and warmth, and frees one of the holder's hands to reach for objects needed, such as the formula bottle. The upright position is a way to hold the baby and feel

secure in supporting the head, upper back, and buttocks. It is an ideal position for burping the infant. In the football hold, approximately half of the newborn's body is supported by the holder's forearm, and the head and neck rest in the palm of the hand. This hold is ideal for shampooing and breastfeeding. A combination of basic infant holds is often used to provide warmth and closeness, allow eye-to-eye contact, and feed the infant. The colic hold is helpful in quieting a fussy newborn.

Nasal and Oral Suctioning

During the first few days of life, the newborn has increased amounts of mucus, and gentle suctioning with a bulb syringe may be indicated. The nurse demonstrates how to correctly use the bulb syringe in removing mucus from the mouth and nose (Skill 10-4). Parents should be asked to repeat the demonstration before discharge to confirm their understanding of the procedure. Parents are advised to wash the syringe thoroughly with soap and water after each use. A bulb syringe is often sent home with the parents.

Diapering and Diaper Rash

Newborns void and stool frequently, and diapers must be changed when wet or soiled. Clear water or premoistened wipes are appropriate for perianal cleansing. However, wipes that contain chemicals and

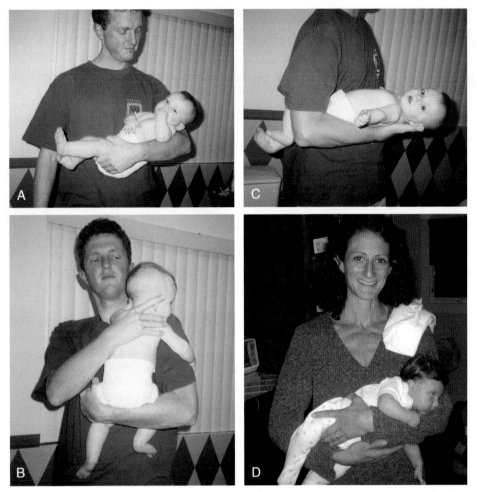

FIGURE 10-6 **Carrying an infant.** Cradle **(A)**, upright **(B)**, football **(C)**, and colic carry **(D)**.

fragrances can irritate the newborn's skin. Mild soap or mineral oil on a cotton pad may be helpful to remove some stool from the skin.

Diaper rash, or diaper dermatitis, is an acute inflammation of the skin as a reaction to contact with urine or feces or diaper friction, and develops rapidly if the area is not cleansed frequently. Whenever serious or prolonged diaper rash is noted, the presence of systemic symptoms such as fever or enlarged lymph glands should be documented and reported (Jackson, 2010). Topical barriers such as vitamins A and D (A&D) ointment or zinc oxide may be applied to the buttocks after washing and careful drying. An antifungal cream such as Nystatin may be recommended for dermatitis lasting more than 3 days and low potency glucocorticoids such as 1% hydrocortisone can be used beneath the topical barrier for 3-5 days if inflammation is noted. Bacitracin or Neomycin should be avoided because they are common allergens (Jackson, 2010). If disposable diapers are used, the newborn may develop a rash where the skin comes in contact with the plastic on the diaper. Because of

environmental concerns, some parents may prefer to use cloth diapers; therefore, nurses need to be able to discuss the advantages and disadvantages, as well as the care and disposal, of each.

Clothing

Parents are advised to dress the newborn for comfort and appropriately for the weather. In general, the newborn should wear a T-shirt, diaper, and a light-to-medium-weight stretch sleeper. Clothing should not be too warm or too snug in warm weather or too sparse in cold weather. Hats should be worn in cool weather or when in the sun; because of the newborn's delicate skin, care should be taken to protect the skin from sunburn.

The newborn's clothing should be washed with a mild soap. It is important to rinse the clothing thoroughly to remove all of the soap residue. The family should be advised to avoid detergents and laundry softeners because they can leave a residue that can irritate the newborn's skin.

During the first weeks, the newborn may prefer being swaddled (Skill 10-5). The newborn feels secure

- newborn rash acceptable usually goes away with one wk

Skill 10-4   Suctioning with a Bulb Syringe

   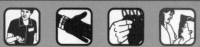

PURPOSE

To clear the airway of mucus.

Steps

1. Compress the ball of the bulb syringe.
2. Insert the narrow portion into the side of the mouth to avoid stimulating the gag reflex. Suction the mouth first to prevent inhalation and aspiration of mucus during a gasp reflex, which is stimulated by nasal suctioning.
3. Release the pressure on the ball of the bulb syringe and listen for the sound of mucus being suctioned.
4. Remove the bulb syringe and empty the contents into a receptacle.
5. Compress the bulb syringe and insert into one nostril, then release pressure on the bulb to suction out the mucus.
6. Remove the bulb syringe and empty it into a receptacle by compressing the bulb. Repeat for the other nostril.

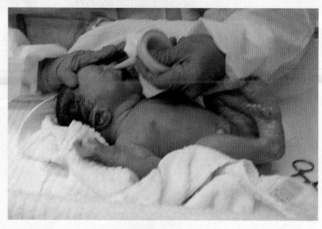

The bulb syringe should be readily available to suction mucus from the infant's mouth and nose. The bulb is compressed before insertion, then released to create sufficient suction to remove mucus. The syringe can be emptied into an emesis basin. The nurse should demonstrate the technique of suctioning with a bulb syringe and review cleaning and storage of the bulb syringe with the parents.

Skill 10-5   Swaddling the Newborn

PURPOSE

To provide warmth and a sense of security to the newborn.

Steps

1. Place a small blanket flat on the bed in the shape of a diamond, with the top corner folded down slightly.
2. Place the newborn with the shoulders at the upper edge of the blanket. The arm may be placed at the baby's side or positioned so the hand is near the mouth. Wrap the right corner of the blanket around the newborn and tuck it under the left side. Fold the left corner of the blanket over the newborn and tuck it under the right side of the infant.
3. Pull the bottom of the blanket up to the infant's chest and secure each corner around the newborn and under his or her back (snugly but not tightly).

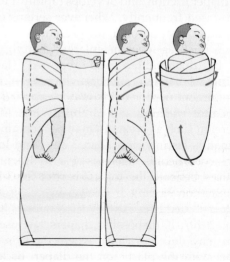

when wrapped snugly in a blanket, and the parents are able to cradle the newborn with confidence.

Circumcision

Circumcision is the surgical removal of the foreskin of the penis; parents decide whether to have their son circumcised. The decision is usually based on hygiene, religious beliefs, culture, or social norms. There is a general agreement that the newborn should be circumcised if the newborn has phimosis, a condition in which the foreskin is tight, obstructs the urinary stream, and cannot be retracted. The American Academy of Pediatrics does not recommend routine circumcisions but acknowledges that there are values and indications for this procedure. The infant should be physiologically stabilized before the circumcision is performed. Preterm infants are not candidates for elective circumcision at birth.

The circumcision of a Jewish newborn has importance as a religious custom. Among Orthodox Jews, it is performed by an ordained circumciser called a *mohel*. The ceremony, called the *bris*, is performed on the eighth day of life, often at home. The child is then officially named (Figure 10-7).

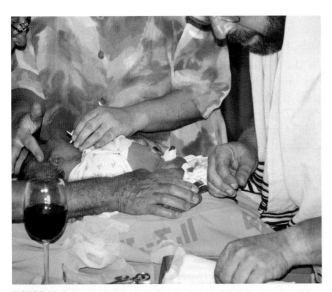

FIGURE 10-7 **A ritual circumcision.** In the Jewish faith, a circumcision is called a *bris milah* and is performed at home on the eighth day of life. It is performed by a specially trained individual called a *mohel* (seen in this picture wearing a tallit, or religious scarf). The person who restrains the newborn during the procedure is known as the *sandak* (pictured on the left); this honor is often bestowed on an elder in the family. A minimum of 10 adults must be present for the ceremony. The wine in the foreground is fed to the newborn by a nipple for pain relief during the procedure. The naming ceremony is often combined with the circumcision ceremony. Understanding and respecting the rituals and traditions of others is an integral part of cultural competence. Circumcisions performed in the hospital before discharge are usually performed by an obstetrician without the family present. Written instructions concerning the care of the circumcised penis should be given to the parents.

Different techniques are used for circumcision. Circumcision with the Yellen or Gomco clamp and the Plastibell are the most popular. Written consent from the mother is necessary before the procedure is performed in the hospital. The newborn is placed on a circumcision board. A dorsal penile nerve block or application of a topical analgesic is used for pain relief. The newborn may also be soothed with a glucose pacifier. Pain relief minimizes the changes in the normal newborn behavioral patterns, such as crying, irritability, and disturbed sleep. Nursing measures used are comfort techniques, such as stroking the newborn's head and talking to him or her (Box 10-1).

Immediately after the circumcision, a sterile gauze with petroleum jelly (Vaseline) or A&D ointment is applied to the penis. The nurse observes for bleeding every 15 minutes for the first hour and then every 30 minutes for the next 2 to 4 hours. If bleeding occurs, it should be reported immediately to the health care provider. Each time the diaper is changed, A&D ointment or petroleum jelly on sterile gauze should be applied to the penis to prevent the diaper from sticking to it. The circumcision wound usually heals in 3 to 5 days.

Two potential complications after a circumcision are infection and hemorrhage. The newborn should be closely monitored for pain, swelling, bleeding, and voiding. If slight bleeding occurs, the nurse applies gentle pressure to the site of bleeding with a folded sterile gauze pad or sprinkles on powdered Gelfoam (according to facility protocol).

If the Plastibell is used, no ointment is applied. Parents are informed that the Plastibell will fall off in approximately 4 to 8 days. If it remains longer, the physician should be notified. Occasionally, it may require manual removal by the clinician.

Box 10-1	Recommended Protocol for Pain Relief During Circumcision

PREOPERATIVE
- Oral acetaminophen 15 mg/kg
- Eutectic local anesthetic topical cream

DURING PROCEDURE
- Dorsal penile nerve block or lidocaine at midshaft of penis
- Use of sucrose pacifier
- Swaddling of upper body

POSTOPERATIVE
- Swaddling
- Assessment of pain using pain scale
- Oral acetaminophen 15 mg/kg every 6 hours as needed

Regarding Home Care of Circumcision

The nurse should provide the parents with written general instructions regarding the care of the circumcised penis:

- Keep area clean, and change the diaper often.
- Wash area with warm water. Do not use soap because it can be drying to the skin, or baby wipes because alcohol contained in the wipes can be irritating to the wound.
- Do not remove the yellow crust that forms on the wound.
- Apply the diaper loosely to prevent pressure on the circumcised area.
- Check that the newborn has at least six wet diapers per day.
- Report any redness, bleeding, or drainage to the health care provider.

Caring for the Uncircumcised Penis

The American Academy of Pediatrics issued a policy statement in 1999 stating that, although there are potential medical benefits of newborn male circumcision, the data are not sufficient to recommend routine neonatal circumcision. When a newborn is not circumcised, specific instructions concerning penile hygiene should be provided to the parents. These include:

- Avoid forceful retraction of the foreskin; tearing can cause adhesions and phimosis. (Retraction is the pulling back of the foreskin over the glans penis to expose the urinary meatus.)
- Wash the penis with only water during infancy; retraction of the foreskin is not necessary. Whitish lumps under the foreskin, known as smegma, are a normal shedding of skin cells.
- At toddler age, gentle retraction during bathing and drying can prevent accumulation of moisture under the foreskin. The foreskin should always be replaced to its normal position after retraction.
- The school-age child can be taught to retract the foreskin gently at least once a week during routine bathing.
- Full retraction of the foreskin may not be possible before puberty, and retraction must never be forced.

Cardiopulmonary Resuscitation

Families should be advised to learn basic cardiopulmonary resuscitation (CPR) and should be instructed to call 911 to summon emergency medical help if the newborn stops breathing. While on the telephone, they should simply report "My baby is not breathing" and then give pertinent information such as their name and address, especially if a cellular phone is used. Also, it is important not to hang up until instructed to do so by the dispatcher; if possible, continue rescue breathing while the dispatcher is speaking. CPR courses are taught by the American Heart Association and the American Red Cross.

CULTURAL BELIEFS AND PRACTICES IN NEWBORN CARE

Cultural beliefs and practices influence the type of care that parents give their newborns. People of Latin American or Filipino background may use a bellyband to protect the newborn against injury and sickness. They may also apply oils to the cord stump or tape a coin to the umbilicus to ward off evil spirits. People of Asian ancestry tend to pick up and carry the newborn as soon as he or she cries. Some Native American Indians still use cradleboards to carry their newborns. Breastfeeding is common in many cultures, and it is not unusual for women to continue to breastfeed until their children are 2 years of age. In many cultures, such as in Egypt, the newborn is swaddled. Cutting the newborn's nails is not done in some cultures; for example, some Vietnamese people believe that cutting the nails or hair will cause illness to the newborn. Some people of Latin American descent may avoid cutting the nails to avoid nearsightedness. In other cultures, breastfeeding is delayed because colostrum is considered bad.

Nurses must demonstrate a nonjudgmental attitude to families with cultural practices different from their own. If the practices are harmful to the newborn, the nurse should try to educate the families about the concerns related to the practice.

DISCHARGE AND FOLLOW-UP CARE

In the United States, laws require specific restraint systems to be used for infants and children in automobiles (Figure 10-8). The American Academy of Pediatrics (2004) recommends that all parents be advised concerning proper car seat use. The car seat in the vehicle should not move more than 1 inch in any direction, and the harness strap should be snug at the armpit level of the child. A rear-facing position in the back seat of the

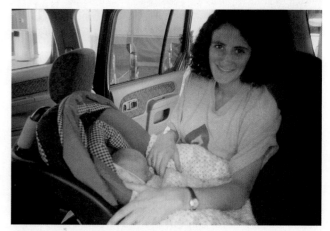

FIGURE 10-8 **A mother prepares to leave the birth facility.** The newborn is placed in a rear-facing car seat that is secured in the center of the back seat of the automobile. Car seats are specially designed for infants younger than 1 year or weighing less than 9 kg (20 lbs).

car is required for infants less than 9 kg (20 lbs) or younger than 1 year of age to prevent head injury from an accident that would cause sudden and forceful head flexion. A newborn should be placed in a newborn safety seat that reclines approximately 45 degrees to maintain an open airway. Car seats designed for children older than 1 year enable the child to sit more upright and should be placed in the middle of the rear seat. Special car seats are available for preterm newborns or children with special health needs. Special cushioned inserts are available to pad the area around the head and neck of the newborn, or a rolled towel can also offer head support.

Early discharge places the responsibility of health care for the newborn on the parents. Health care professionals must make every effort to provide instruction during their brief stay. Some institutions provide home care or head start programs for the care of the mother and newborn. Most pediatricians recommend that all newborns have a follow-up office visit within 7 days of discharge from the hospital. The parent should be instructed to return to the health care provider if the newborn develops fever, lethargy, irritability, poor feeding, signs of dehydration, or yellowing of the skin (jaundice).

The discharge nurse must make sure that the mother has at least a minimum "safety net" of the name and phone number of a clinic or private physician who will do follow-up visits with her and the baby. If she is breastfeeding, the mother should be given the name and phone number of a lactation consultant.

The American Academy of Pediatrics recommends that parents receive training to give them the ability and confidence to care for their newborn. Topics can include breastfeeding, bottle feeding, bowel and bladder patterns, cord care, skin care, signs of illness, car seat use, and follow-up care. Statistics have shown that effective parent counseling can change risk behaviors and prevent illness and injuries (Moyer, 2006).

Throughout the chapter, emphasis has been placed on continuous observation and assessment of the newborn and the planning of care that centers around the newborn's needs. In addition, parent education and discharge planning should be an integral part of the care plan. Developing a written care plan that incorporates nursing diagnoses and expected goals is helpful to assess the adequacy of the newborn's care and the family's ability to perform the care once the newborn has been discharged (Nursing Care Plan 10-1). The nurse should help the parents increase their awareness of community facilities available to them, including home care visits, when necessary.

Nursing Care Plan 10-1 Family Care Plan

Scenario
A woman has given birth to her second child. Her husband, older child, and mother are in the room. The grandmother tries to keep the sibling away from the newborn, and the woman states she was hoping to return to work and school but is not sure she should.

Selected Nursing Diagnosis
Risk for impaired parent/newborn/child attachment related to acceptance of newborn into family

Expected Outcomes	Nursing Interventions	Rationales
Healthy parent-newborn attachment will be evidenced by positive bonding behaviors between parent and newborn (talking to newborn, cuddling newborn, meeting newborn's needs, eye-to-eye contact, calling newborn by name, newborn looking into parents' faces or turning toward their voices).	Allow parents time to hold and interact with newborn as soon as possible after birth. Assess parents' and sibling's perceptions of newborn.	Immediate contact with the newborn is beneficial in initiating the bonding process. Provides baseline information that will assist in individualizing care plan. Parents and siblings who are excited about the newborn will attach easier to the newborn than those who have negative feelings toward the newborn.
	Assess for positive bonding behaviors between parents or sibling and newborn. Provide praise and reinforcement when they occur.	Positive reinforcement of a behavior increases the probability that the behavior will be repeated.
	Explain to parents that bonding may not occur instantaneously but grows over time.	Helps normalize feelings and relieves anxiety. When parents do not initially have overwhelming feelings of joy and acceptance of newborn or when sibling initially rejects newborn, parents often become anxious and need to know their feelings are not unusual.
	Describe behaviors that can be useful in enhancing the bonding process	Provides knowledge of activities that can be used to enhance bonding.

Continued

Nursing Care Plan 10-1   Family Care Plan—cont'd

Expected Outcomes	Nursing Interventions	Rationales
	(holding the newborn in the en face position, talking with the newborn, holding the newborn skin-to-skin, interacting during quiet alert stage).	
	Encourage extended family members to hold and interact with newborn, and provide reinforcement when positive bonding behaviors are observed.	Grandparents and other extended family members also need to be given the opportunity to bond with newborn.
Sibling will demonstrate acceptance of newborn (making positive statements about newborn, referring to self as big brother or sister, wanting to hold newborn or assisting with caring for newborn, talking to newborn).	Allow siblings to participate in care of newborn.	Provides feelings of enhanced self-esteem.
	Acknowledge sibling as big brother or sister.	Enhances self-esteem and helps sibling identify with new role.
	Instruct parents that behaviors of regression to earlier childhood stage are normal sibling responses to a new baby in the home.	Provides knowledge of normal coping behaviors that will decrease incidence of parents belittling or punishing sibling for reverting to earlier behaviors.
	Instruct parents to spend individualized time with older child and to encourage visitors to acknowledge and spend time interacting with sibling.	Decreases older child's feelings of being replaced or left out.
	Encourage parents to allow older sibling to attend and help open gifts at baby showers.	Provides older child with a sense of belonging and decreases feelings of jealousy about newborn getting presents.
	If sibling is early preschooler or younger, encourage parents to purchase a gift to give to the child from "baby" brother or sister.	Many young children will not understand that the baby cannot purchase gifts and thus will be thrilled that the baby cares enough about them to give a gift.
	Tell siblings what they are able to do that the baby cannot do because of his or her size and age.	Enhances self-esteem.
	If sibling is initially resentful of new baby, do not leave him or her alone in the same room.	Prevents injury from being inflicted on newborn by sibling.

Selected Nursing Diagnosis

Parental role conflict related to demands of fulfilling multiple roles (mother, wife, employee, and student)

Expected Outcomes	Nursing Interventions	Rationales
Patient will state she feels more comfortable about assuming parental role.	Encourage patient to verbalize concerns by using therapeutic communication techniques.	Having patient verbalize concerns provides baseline information for the development of a plan to address them. Therapeutic communication techniques such as broad opening statements encourage patients to share their thoughts, whereas techniques such as reflection and restating assist the patient in developing her own solutions for perceived problems.
Patient will describe a plan for incorporating the parental role into her life with the least amount of stress possible.	Reinforce parent skills necessary for caring for newborn.	Increased knowledge and improved ability to perform skills alleviate anxiety and enhance patient's confidence level in assuming parental role.
	Encourage the patient to evaluate current commitments and to determine whether any lifestyle changes can be made.	Often during times of stress, parents will exhibit less skill in problem solving and will exaggerate the problem, making it more than it really is. The nurse can assist in developing a

Nursing Care Plan 10-1	Family Care Plan—cont'd	
Expected Outcomes	**Nursing Interventions**	**Rationales**
		realistic perspective of the situation and goals to achieve desired outcome.
	Assist the patient in identifying nonessential activities or those she can delegate to others.	Reduces the current level of commitment and allows more time for interacting with the newborn.
	Assist patient in identifying support persons who are available.	Provides physical assistance and emotional support.
	Encourage patient and spouse to practice ongoing open communication to discuss changed role expectations and concerns.	Communication is an essential part of the marriage relationship and allows each partner to understand what the other is feeling and desiring.
	Encourage patient to allow for uninterrupted time with newborn each day.	Encourages bonding by allowing patient to focus all her attention on the newborn. Emphasizing this as a priority alleviates guilt of abandoning other tasks during this time.
	Encourage patient to plan at least two dates per month with spouse.	Spending uninterrupted time alone with spouse provides time to build the marriage relationship.
	Encourage patient to try to include something in her daily schedule that she enjoys.	Taking time to pamper self will help alleviate stress associated with increased responsibilities.
	Reassure patient that many women are able to successfully balance family duties and careers.	Provides hope and reassures patient that she is not alone in her situation.

Selected Nursing Diagnosis

Compromised family coping related to intergenerational and cultural conflicts regarding child rearing

Expected Outcomes	**Nursing Interventions**	**Rationales**
Family members will formulate a plan of mutually decided on boundaries for each of their roles as they relate to the newborn	Allow extended family members to visit frequently during hospitalization	Allows time for bonding with neonate and for the opportunity to assess family processes that may require intervention.
	Stress the significance of grandparents' and extended family members' involvement in the child's growth and development	In addition to providing love and support, they can pass on family traditions or cultural practices that can enrich the lives of family members.
	Discuss the importance of showing respect for one another and for not making critical remarks about another family member's behavior in front of the child.	As the child grows in understanding, he or she can experience confusion and emotional conflict when exposed to criticisms of loved ones.
Couple will verbalize that they feel comfortable expressing their desires to extended family members.	Encourage family members to discuss concerns and expectations regarding roles and child-rearing practices.	Establishing open communication provides a way of letting desires be known and allows for resolution of differences.
	Teach importance of communicating in a clear, concise manner.	Decreases misunderstandings.
	Reassure parents that they have the ultimate decision-making responsibilities regarding how to raise and care for newborn.	Helps alleviate guilt and provides parents with permission to act freely according to their desires when their desires differ from those of extended family members.
	Teach the importance of the couple maintaining a united front when communicating with extended family members.	Avoid assigning blame, which can damage relationships, and prevents others from having their way though manipulating the parents.
	Teach parents that there is often more than one way to accomplish something correctly, and unless an action is medically, emotionally, or	Allows for more flexibility in child rearing and for family members to interact in an individualized manner with the newborn. Increasing a

Continued

⭐ Nursing Care Plan 10-1	**Family Care Plan—cont'd**	
Expected Outcomes	**Nursing Interventions**	**Rationales**
	morally contraindicated, it is not harmful for children to be exposed to a variety of ideas and experiences.	child's exposure to new and different experiences can enhance learning.
	Assist family members in developing a mutually acceptable plan for their role in the newborn's life.	When conflicts occur, those emotionally involved often require the assistance of an outside party to view the situation in a realistic manner and to reach an agreeable resolution to the conflict.
	Refer to parenting and grandparenting classes.	Increases understanding of current trends in child-rearing practices and helps them learn important strategies that can enrich the life of the newborn.

Critical Thinking Questions

1. The oldest sibling of the newborn is crying and seeking attention. What suggestions would you give the mother to help the sibling bond with the newborn?
2. You have just completed a teaching session with the parents regarding how to care for their newborn. The parents state they do not think they can remember so much information. What can you do to help them feel better prepared for their newborn after discharge?

Get Ready for the NCLEX® Examination!

Key Points

- A clinical pathway is a tool used to indicate specific interdisciplinary care within a specified timeline that is related to a planned outcome. It includes activities such as nursing assessments, interventions, teaching, medical interventions, and discharge and follow-up care.
- Nursing care of the newborn is directed toward promoting physical well-being of the newborn and supporting the family unit.
- Nursing goals during phase 1, the immediate care of the newborn, include clearing the airway, clamping the cord, regulating body temperature, evaluating the cardiorespiratory function, Apgar scoring, identifying the newborn, recording information about the birth, and beginning the bonding process.
- Procedures carried out in phase 2 newborn care include the weight and measurement of the newborn, prophylactic eye care to protect the newborn from infection, intramuscular injection of vitamin K to prevent bleeding, cord care, and stabilization of the newborn's temperature.
- The first hepatitis B vaccination may be given within 12 hours after birth.
- Because of the mother's brief hospital stay, it is critical for nurses to use every opportunity to teach the mother and family how to care for the newborn, such as general hygiene, feeding, elimination, transporting, and when to call the health care provider.
- After the circumcision, the newborn is observed closely for signs of bleeding, inability to void, and infection.
- If the newborn is not circumcised, information concerning care of the uncircumcised penis should be given to the parents.
- Safety precautions must be emphasized to parents. The nurse should teach safety measures to avoid injury, such as never leaving the newborn alone on a table, proper positioning of the newborn, performing oral and nasal suctioning to clear the airway, preventing chilling or overheating of the newborn, and using an infant car seat when riding in a vehicle.
- The nurse should teach parents signs of illness in newborns, which include a temperature above 38° C (100.4° F), refusal of two or more consecutive feedings, lethargy, more than one episode of forceful vomiting, pallor, cyanosis, and absence of breathing for more than 20 seconds.
- Parent-newborn attachment is a process that needs encouragement for the development of newborn trust and bonding.
- At time of discharge, several areas of teaching should be assessed, preferably by an interactive review of the checklist that is given to the mother. The teaching provided should be documented.

Additional Learning Resources

SG Go to your Study Guide on pages 491–492 for additional Review Questions for the NCLEX® Examination, Critical Thinking Clinical Situations, and other learning activities to help you master this chapter content.

 evolve Go to your Evolve website (http://evolve.elsevier.com/Leifer/maternity) for the following FREE learning resources:
- Animations
- Answer Guidelines for Critical Thinking Questions
- Answers and Rationales for Review Questions for the NCLEX® Examination
- Concept Map Creator
- Glossary with pronunciations in English and Spanish
- Patient Teaching Plans
- Skills Performance Checklists and more!

Online Resources
- http://aappolicy.aappublications.org/cgi/content/full/pediatrics;105/2/454
- www.carseat.org
- www.natus.com
- www.ncast.org
- www.safekids.org
- www.vachss.com/guest_dispatches/neonatal_pain.html

Review Questions for the NCLEX® Examination

1. Phase 2 of newborn care typically lasts from:
   1. Birth to 1 hour
   2. 1 to 4 hours
   3. 4 hours to discharge
   4. After discharge

2. The nurse is preparing vitamin K (AquaMEPHYTON) for a newborn, which will be administered:
   1. Orally
   2. Rectally
   3. Subcutaneously
   4. Intramuscularly

3. The Centers for Disease Control and Prevention (CDC) and the American Academy of Pediatrics (2009) recommend that all newborns receive their first vaccination against hepatitis B:
   1. Within 12 hours after birth
   2. At approximately 1 month of age
   3. At 6 months of age
   4. No later than 12 months of age

4. Which statement made by the parents of a newborn would indicate the need for further teaching?
   1. "The newborn's clothing should be washed with mild soap."
   2. "I will place my newborn in the prone position for the best sleep."
   3. "My newborn should wear a hat in cool weather."
   4. "During the first weeks my newborn may prefer being swaddled."

5. Regarding caring for the newborn with an uncircumcised penis, parent education should include which instruction(s)? *(Select all that apply.)*
   1. Avoid forceful retraction.
   2. Wash with mild soap and water.
   3. Report appearance of whitish lumps under foreskin.
   4. By school age the child can be taught to retract the foreskin gently at least once a week during routine bathing.
   5. Full retraction of the foreskin may not be possible before puberty, and retraction must never be forced.

6. Individuals from which culture may avoid cutting the newborn's nails to prevent nearsightedness?
   1. Latin American
   2. Asian
   3. Filipino
   4. Native American

Critical Thinking Questions

1. Parents are receiving their discharge instructions for their first child. They asked for clarifications such as whether it is necessary to put the newborn in the car seat when it is "just a little way home" and when the umbilical cord will fall off. You know that these points have already been discussed. What factors could be involved with the lack of retention of your previous instructions?

2. Parents want to be prepared when they take their son home. They have observed the nurse suction the baby with a bulb syringe. They are visibly upset and ask you if something is wrong with their son. What should you tell them?

chapter 11

Newborn Feeding

http://evolve.elsevier.com/Leifer/maternity

Objectives

1. Define key terms listed.
2. Discuss the cultural influences related to the choice of breastfeeding or bottle feeding the newborn.
3. Explain the physiologic characteristics of lactation.
4. Discuss the dietary needs of the lactating mother.
5. Compare the nutrients of human milk with those of cow's milk.
6. Discuss breastfeeding in relation to advantages, care of the breasts, diet and fluids, newborn responses, and secretion of drugs in breast milk.
7. Compare various maternal and newborn positions used during breastfeeding.
8. Identify principles of breast pumping and milk storage.
9. Illustrate techniques of formula feeding.
10. Discuss the various types of formula and their preparation.
11. Explain nipple confusion.
12. Identify contraindications to breastfeeding.

Key Terms

colostrum (kă-LŎS-trŭm, p. 207)
engorgement (ĕn-GŎRJ-mĕnt, p. 206)
foremilk (p. 207)
galactogogues (găh-LĂK-tō-gŏgs, p. 204) *allows the "let-down reflex."*
hindmilk (HĪND-mĭlk, p. 207)
lactation (lăk-TĀ-shŭn, p. 206) *↑ production of milk*

latch-on technique (p. 211)
let-down reflex (p. 206)
milk-ejection reflex (p. 206)
oxytocin (ŏks-ē-TŌ-sĭn, p. 206)
prolactin (prō-LĂK-tĭn, p. 206)
satiety (să-TĪ-ĕ-tē, p. 208)

For many women, breastfeeding or bottle feeding the newborn is a satisfying but sometimes anxiety-provoking task. Besides providing essential nutrition, feeding is an important mechanism in the formation of the newborn's emotional development and the trusting relationship between the newborn and the mother or family. The decision whether to breastfeed or bottle (formula) feed is usually made during pregnancy.

Feeding the newborn should be an enjoyable and pleasurable task for both the newborn and the parent. It is a time when the parent and newborn can get to know each other. The nurse plays an important role in assisting the mother in either breastfeeding or bottle feeding her newborn. Education, including discussion of common concerns, will help the parents smoothly assume one of their important new tasks of parenting.

CULTURAL INFLUENCES

Cultural attitudes and beliefs vary about breastfeeding the newborn. Modesty and embarrassment may prevent the woman from breastfeeding in the hospital, and she may prefer to begin to breastfeed after she is home. This is often true of mothers from Asian and Muslim cultures. Mormon women believe that breastfeeding is an important part of motherhood. Mothers from some cultures believe that colostrum is unclean and therefore should not be given to newborns. Some recent or first-generation immigrants to the United States come from countries where breastfeeding is the norm and see formula as a symbol of a new way of life.

The hot-cold theory of health and illness is common to many cultures. Because the postpartum period is considered a "cold" condition, only approved "hot" foods are eaten after delivery. Chicken, honey, rice, and hot soup may be preferred, whereas salads and iced drinks will be refused even by a hungry mother. In some cultures, mothers use galactogogues (breast milk stimulators), and the nurse must be aware of such requests in the form of beer, brewer's yeast, or sesame tea.

Health care personnel who casually ask whether women are planning to breastfeed or bottle feed may imply that they are equal in value if the advantages and disadvantages are not carefully explained (Table 11-1). Americans value fast food and may not realize the ready convenience and low cost of breast milk compared with formula. When a mother plans to return to work after the birth of the baby, she may not know that her breast milk can be easily expressed,

[handwritten: & 24-72 hrs encourage breastfeeding]

Table 11-1   Advantages and Disadvantages of Breastfeeding and Bottle Feeding

ADVANTAGES	DISADVANTAGES
Breastfeeding: Mother	
Oxytocin release aids uterine involution.	Only mother can feed newborn unless milk is pumped
Strong mother-newborn bonding occurs with skin-to-skin contact.	and stored.
Nighttime feedings are less complicated.	Pumping breasts is time-consuming for working mothers.
Enforced rest periods occur.	Mother must be careful about taking medications.
It is convenient, always available, no preparation.	Some mothers are embarrassed by breast exposure.
It is cost-effective.	
It is emotionally satisfying.	
Progesterone-based contraception can be taken when	
breastfeeding less than every 2 hours.	
Breastfeeding: Newborn	
Immunologic properties help prevent infections.	HIV from infected mother may be transmitted to newborn
Breastfeeding meets nutritional needs.	via breast milk.
Presence of fatty acids and amino acids promotes neurologic	Drugs administered to the mother may pass through breast
development.	milk to the newborn and produce adverse effects.
Breast milk is easily digested.	
Breast milk contains less sodium and protein than cow's milk	
and puts less stress on newborn's kidneys.	
Calcium is better absorbed.	
It is the least allergenic food for newborn.	
Breastfeeding promotes development of facial muscles, jaw,	
and teeth.	
Infants are less likely to be overfed or obese.	
It produces less nitrogen waste, which provides less of a burden	
on kidneys.	
Breast milk has natural laxative effects.	
Others can participate in burping infant after feeding is complete.	
Bottle Feeding: Mother	
It allows more participation for family members.	It requires cleanliness in preparation.
It provides more freedom for mother.	It requires refrigeration and storage.
Feeding in public is less stressful.	It is more costly.
Mother does not have to worry about taking medications	
or modifying diet.	
Combined oral contraceptives can be resumed postpartum.	
Bottle Feeding: Newborn	
It allows easy monitoring of intake (know how much newborn	Formula may not provide natural fatty acids to promote
is taking).	neurologic development.
Formula takes longer to digest, so newborn eats less often.	Formula does not provide newborn with immune bodies
	to protect from infection as does human milk.
	Formula has more sodium to burden newborn's kidneys.
	Bottle feeding often does not provide skin-to-skin contact
	that nurtures bonding for both infant and mother.

[handwritten in left margin: HELPS prevent SIDS]

stored, and fed by bottle by the caregiver. Although one of the goals of *Healthy People 2010* was to have 75% of new mothers breastfeed, and the American Academy of Pediatrics (AAP, 2007) recommends breastfeeding as the optimum nutrition for newborns that should be continued through the first year and beyond, the final decision is with the parents. The nurse's role is to educate the parents concerning their choices, promote feelings of confidence and competence in feeding techniques, and accept the feeding choice of the parents. Nurses should be alert to mothers who need encouragement if they desire to breastfeed but who may not do so because of a lack of knowledge and support.

Success or failure that a mother achieves in breastfeeding may determine her feelings about being an adequate mother; therefore, the choice to breastfeed is an important one. The mother needs to be comfortable with what she is doing and enjoy the experience for breastfeeding to be successful.

Americans value breastfeeding as a natural right and have supported laws that allow breastfeeding in public. Knowledge of breastfeeding laws can create a more supportive breastfeeding environment. Nurses play an important role in supporting breastfeeding legislation and educating parents concerning their rights and resources. As of 2004, only two states, Oregon and Utah, had met the *Healthy People 2010* goals of having 75% of mothers' breastfeed (Centers for Disease Control and Prevention [CDC], 2005).

Laws that foster a supportive environment for breastfeeding may encourage mothers to breastfeed even when not at home. Breastfeeding-supportive laws include clarification that breastfeeding is not part of indecent exposure, lewd conduct, or sexual misconduct in public (National Conference of State Legislators, 2010). A federal bill, H.R. 2236, may have allowed breast pumps to be a deductible medical expense. The National Alliance for Breastfeeding Advocacy (NABA) collaborates with many organizations to promote a supportive social environment for breastfeeding. Currently, NABA is designing a universal logo that is posted at public sites, such as airports, to indicate protected breastfeeding sites, much like the universal logo for men's or women's restrooms.

MATERNAL NUTRITION DURING LACTATION

The mother must maintain her own nutritional stores while providing for the infant through breastfeeding. The mother needs 500 calories more than her nonpregnant diet each day, selected from the various major food groups. Protein intake should be 65 mg/day, and calcium intake should match pregnancy requirements. Vitamin supplements taken during pregnancy are often continued during lactation. It is recommended that 8 to 10 glasses of noncaffeinated liquids be consumed each day. Some foods eaten by the mother may change the taste of her breast milk or cause the infant to have gas. If a mother suspects a certain food she consumes is causing fussiness or gas in the infant, she can eliminate it from her diet for a few days to determine whether the infant has fewer problems.

Many drugs taken by the mother can be passed to the infant via breast milk and should be taken on the advice of a health care provider only. In some cases, timing the drug dose so that it passes its peak of activity before the infant is put to the breast can reduce the amount delivered to the infant. See Chapter 4 for drug-risk categories, Chapter 5 for specific nutritional needs for pregnant and lactating women, and Chapter 21 for common herbs used or contraindicated during lactation.

PHYSIOLOGY OF LACTATION

Lactation (the secretion of milk) is the end result of many interacting physiologic factors, including the development of breast tissue and duct system, primarily under the influence of hormones (estrogen,

progesterone, and human placental lactogen [hPL]). In addition, hPL stimulates the alveolar cells of the breast to begin lactogenesis (milk production), so that, by the later part of pregnancy, the breasts secrete colostrum, a thick, creamy fluid. After the birth of the newborn and the delivery of the placenta, the hormones estrogen, progesterone, and hPL decrease rapidly, causing a rapid increase of prolactin secretion. Prolactin, secreted from the anterior pituitary gland, stimulates milk production, which is then enhanced by newborn suckling. Suckling also causes the posterior pituitary to secrete oxytocin, producing the let-down reflex, or milk-ejection reflex, which causes the milk to be delivered from the alveoli (milk-producing sacs) through the duct system to the nipple (Figure 11-1). The mother usually feels a tingling in her breasts when this reflex occurs. The woman also often feels abdominal cramping because oxytocin stimulates the uterus to contract, which helps with postpartum uterine involution.

By the third or fourth postpartum day the prolactin effect on the breast tissue is evident, and the hormone is present in sufficient amounts to cause engorgement (congestion or distention) of the breasts. At this time,

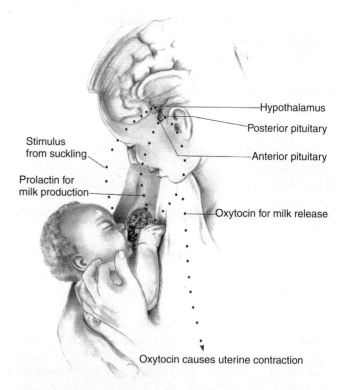

FIGURE 11-1 Effect of prolactin and oxytocin on milk production. The infant suckling on the breast stimulates nerve fibers in the areola of the nipple that travel to the hypothalamus. The hypothalamus stimulates the anterior pituitary to secrete prolactin; this stimulates milk production and stimulates the posterior pituitary to release oxytocin, which causes a let-down reflex, contracting the lobules in the breast and squeezing milk out into the nipple and to the infant. Oxytocin also helps contract the uterus.

milk begins to replace the colostrum. Once lactation has been established, suckling is the most important stimulus for the maintenance of milk production.

BREAST MILK   *Colostro*

Three types of milk are produced during the establishment of lactation: colostrum, transitional milk, and mature milk. Colostrum is produced for the first 3 or 4 postpartum days; it contains high levels of antibodies, protein, minerals, and fat-soluble vitamins. Although it is high in protein, it is fairly low in sugar and fat and is therefore easy to digest. It is rich in immunoglobulin (antibodies), which helps protect the newborn's gastrointestinal tract from infections. Therefore, colostrum helps establish the normal intestinal flora in the intestines, and its laxative effect speeds the passage of meconium.

Transitional milk comes in the period between colostrum and mature milk, which is about 5 days to 2 weeks. The composition of the milk changes, and lactose, fat, and calories increase. Mature milk, the final milk produced, looks similar to skim milk (somewhat bluish), which leads some mothers to question whether their milk is rich enough to give to their newborns. Nurses need to explain that mature milk contains approximately 22.5 kcal/oz and is just right to meet the newborn's needs (Table 11-2).

The percentage of calories derived from protein is lower in breast milk than in formulas, with a greater proportion of calories from carbohydrates in the form of lactose. The amount of fat in breast milk varies during the feeding; there is more fat present in the hindmilk, the milk produced at the end of the feeding, than at the beginning (foremilk).

Breast milk contains enzymes that aid digestion. **Lipase** in breast milk helps the newborn digest fat. **Fluoride** is present in breast milk if the mother drinks fluoridated water. However, a supplement of fluoride may be prescribed in the form of newborn vitamins with fluoride if the family uses bottled water or well water. Fluoride is needed for the development of healthy tooth enamel.

The immunologic benefits include protection against several bacterial and viral diseases, especially those of the respiratory and gastrointestinal tracts. **Lactoferrin,** which is secreted in human milk, is believed to play a part in controlling bacterial growth in the gastrointestinal tract. **Immunoglobulin A,** present in colostrum and breast milk, protects against the development of many allergies. Immunoglobulins to the poliomyelitis virus are also present in the breast milk of mothers who have a passive immunity to the virus (see Table 11-2). Breast milk also contains long-chain polyunsaturated fatty acids and amino acids that promote eye and neurologic development. The level of docosahexaenoic acid (DHA) (an omega-3 fatty acid) in breast milk is directly related to the amount of DHA ingested by the mother in her diet. Sources of omega-3 fatty acids include fish such as salmon, herring, mackerel, and lake trout and oils such as canola, hempseed, soy, walnut, and soybeans (see Chapter 5).

Table **11-2** Human Milk Versus Commercial Formula

NUTRIENT	HUMAN MILK	COW'S MILK-BASED FORMULA
Protein	Lower amount but sufficient; contains more lactalbumin (because easy digestible, provides ideal quantity)	Greater; contains more casein, which forms large curds that take longer to digest
Fat	Varies; lowest in morning and highest in afternoon; used rapidly because of enzyme lipase; easier to digest. Contains omega-3 fatty acids to promote neurologic development	Fat poorly absorbed (commercial formulas often add fat source such as corn oil)
Carbohydrate	Lactose higher (7%). Lactose improves absorption of calcium; also promotes growth of normal bacterial flora in intestines	Lactose less (4.8%). Some formulas add DHA and fatty acids
Iron	Small amount but better absorption than cow's milk. Lactoferrin in human milk enhances iron absorption	Small amount
Calcium, phosphorus, sodium, and potassium	Lower amount of these minerals; imposes a lower solute load on newborn's kidneys	Greater amount results in renal solute load
Immunoglobulins	IgA, IgG, IgM protect newborn from infections (diarrhea, respiratory infections, and gastroenteritis)	None
Antiallergic factors	Infants rarely allergic to human milk. May protect from development of allergies (less eczema in newborns)	Allergy to cow's milk possible

DHA, docosahexaenoic acid; *Ig,* immunoglobulin.

The World Health Organization (WHO) recommends adding DHA to formula feedings to benefit the central nervous system, cognitive, behavioral, and eye development of the newborn (Blanchard, 2006).

BREASTFEEDING

wash hands prior to breastfeeding to avoide infection to the breast and the infant!

PREPARING THE BREASTS

Flat or inverted nipples can be treated during pregnancy, but interventions can begin after birth. Flat nipples can be rolled between the mother's fingers just before feeding to help them become more erect so that the newborn can more easily grasp them. Hoffman's exercise can be started after the newborn is born. In Hoffman's exercise, the fingers are placed on the areola and gently pulled apart to stretch the tissue. This helps release adhesions that may cause the nipple to be inverted. The exercise is repeated with movement of the fingers around the areola. Babies can usually learn to breastfeed even if the nipple is not completely erect. Newer ultra thin nipple shields are artificial nipples, usually made of a soft, thin material and worn over the nipple of the mother's breast; they may be used in special cases such as nipple soreness or latch-on problems. However, prolonged use can result in decreased milk production because the maternal milk sinuses are not compressed adequately by the suckling newborn. Lengthy weaning of the infant to the natural breast nipple may also become a problem. The use of breast shields should be monitored by a lactation specialist.

Preparations for the mother include voiding, washing her hands, and assuming a comfortable position. The importance of the mother washing her hands before putting the newborn to the breast should be emphasized because the hands are the primary source for the spread of infection.

Many hospitals have a lactation specialist who is available to assist the woman in breastfeeding. On discharge, the mother should be given the telephone number of a referral group, such as the La Leche League, that will assist her with a telephone call if a problem arises. Lactation specialists also have private practices, making home visits for a consultation fee (Figure 11-2).

FREQUENCY AND LENGTH OF FEEDINGS

Because breast milk is digested more quickly than formula (usually within 2 hours), the newborn needs to be fed every 2 to 3 hours. Also, in the beginning, the newborn's stomach capacity is small. Newborns who are fed frequently during the daytime may, on average, have longer sleep periods during the night. Until meconium is passed, the newborn may consume 15 to 30 mL per feeding. By 1 week of age, the neonate will consume 60 to 90 mL during each feeding.

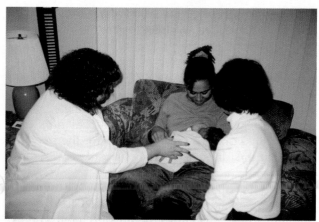

FIGURE 11-2 Lactation specialist visits the home to help the mother with breastfeeding technique.

mouth & tounge movements

Readiness for feeding can be determined by observing the newborn's behavior. Rooting, sucking, hand-to-mouth activity, crying, and alertness are clues that the newborn is hungry. *Crying is often a late sign of hunger.* Mothers often notice the sensation of the let-down reflex (tingling, fullness, stinging) or have milk leakage when they think of getting ready to nurse. This can also happen when they hear the newborn cry. The let-down reflex can be inhibited or stimulated by the mother's state of mind (embarrassment or anxiety about breastfeeding). Generally, the newborn is placed for approximately 15 minutes of suckling on the first breast, followed by the other breast until the infant is satisfied. The mother should allow the first breast to completely empty before placing the infant on the other breast. Parents should be informed that short pauses in suckling are normal during nursing.

The average time for breastfeeding is 15 to 20 minutes per breast. If the feedings are too short, the infant may get only the foremilk and will be hungry sooner if he or she does not get to the richer hindmilk. Engorgement can occur if milk is not removed from the breast, and milk production will decrease if suckling is not adequate to empty the breast. The infant should be burped after feeding. The next breastfeeding session should begin on the breast opposite the one started at the last session (alternate starting breasts). The mother should be taught to take her cues from the newborn to determine when the newborn is full, such as the slowing of the newborn's suckling pattern; the newborn falling asleep; and the mother's breasts feeling soft and empty, which indicates satiety (fullness to satisfaction).

The anxious mother may ask how she can tell whether the newborn is getting enough milk. The nurse can help the parent listen for sounds of swallowing as the newborn sucks and identify changes in behavior that indicate newborn satiety, such as falling asleep after breastfeeding. Having at least six wet diapers and several stools in a 24-hour period is also indicative of adequate intake. Palpating the breasts before and after breastfeeding will also reveal a change from firm, engorged breasts to soft, "empty" breasts after breastfeeding. These signs of successful breastfeeding will be reinforced by the weight gain the newborn shows after the first week and during the follow-up clinic visits.

TEACHING FEEDING TECHNIQUES

Positioning

Both the mother and the newborn must be comfortable during breastfeeding. Using different positions is important because this varies the pressure points on the nipple and areola, which helps prevent nipple soreness. The mother may prefer the **cradle hold, football hold,** or **side-lying position** (Figure 11-3).

Some mothers prefer to sit up in bed or in a chair and hold the infant in a cradle hold with the infant's head in the mother's antecubital area. To prevent fatigue, the infant's body can be supported by a pillow, and the mother's arm should be supported by pillows or the armrest of the chair. The newborn must be in a chest-to-chest position with the mother to avoid the need to turn the head to latch on to the nipple. Turning of the infant's head may interfere with swallowing and places pressure on the mother's nipple, which can result in discomfort.

With the football hold, the mother supports the newborn's head, with the body resting on pillows alongside her hip. This hold allows the mother to see the position of the newborn's mouth on the breast; this position is helpful for mothers with large breasts. This position also avoids pressure against an abdominal incision.

The side-lying position avoids pressure on the episiotomy or the abdominal incision from a cesarean birth. Pillows are placed behind the mother's back to increase her comfort. Folded blankets or pillows can be used to elevate the newborn to breast level so that there is no tension on the nipple. Pulling on the nipple can make it tender and sore. The newborn's head and body should directly face the breast (Figure 11-4).

Hand Position

Once the newborn is properly positioned, the mother should hold her hand in a C position, supporting the breast from below and placing her thumb above the nipple and her fingers below the areola. It is important for the newborn to get enough of the areola in his or her mouth; otherwise, suckling will be directly on the nipple. For the newborn to obtain milk from the breast, the jaws must compress the milk sinuses beneath the areola (Figure 11-5). The tongue should be visible between the lower gum and breast. The lips are widely flanged and sealed around the breast, with an absence of clicking sounds as the newborn sucks.

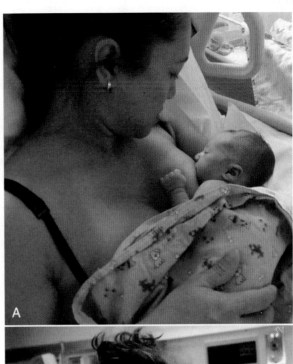
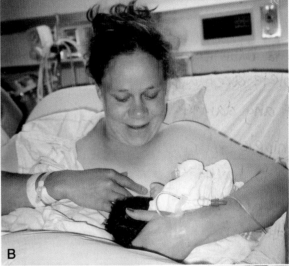
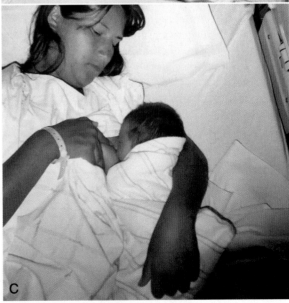

FIGURE 11-3 Positions commonly used in breastfeeding. A, Cradle hold. B, Football hold. C, Side-lying.

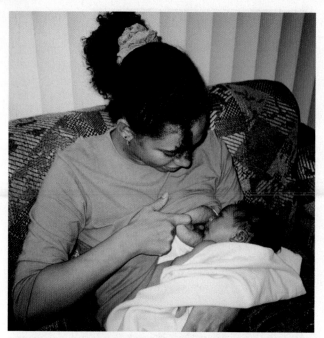

FIGURE 11-4 The mother indents breast tissue and draws the newborn close to latch on to the breast.

Because the newborn is a nose breather, make sure the newborn's nose is not blocked by breast tissue. For women with large breasts, the breast tissue can be indented by the finger away from the newborn's nose; however, care must be taken to avoid pulling the nipple out of the newborn's mouth. The mother can elevate the newborn's hips, which provides more breathing space.

Correct positioning before beginning to breastfeed is significant in getting a good start and preventing problems. Four separate elements that need consideration are (1) the alignment of both the mother's and newborn's bodies; (2) the position in which the mother holds the newborn; (3) the hand position for supporting the breasts; and (4) the newborn's mouth, lip, and tongue positions.

Sucking Patterns

Newborns have different sucking patterns when they breastfeed. Some newborns suck several times before swallowing, and others swallow with each suck. A soft sound indicates that the newborn is swallowing milk

⊛ have the baby cover the complete areola to prevent any damage to the nipple & for the baby to have a better chance to feed better.

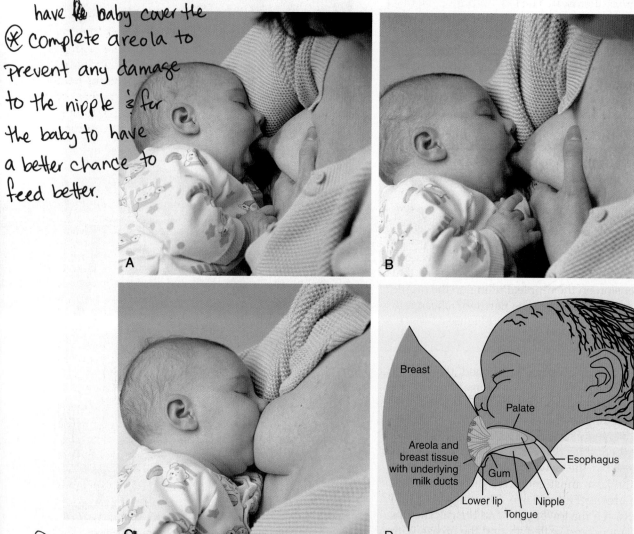

FIGURE 11-5 **Latching on. A,** The newborn responds to touch on the lips and opens the mouth wide. **B,** Once the baby's mouth is open, quickly pull newborn close to enable latch-on. **C,** The baby should have as much areola in his or her mouth as possible, not just the nipple. **D,** Correct attachment (latch-on) at breast.

(nutritive sucking). Noisy sucking, a clicking sound, or dimpling of the cheeks usually indicates improper mouth position and requires repositioning of the infant.

Initiating Breastfeeding

The ideal time to initiate breastfeeding is within 1 hour after birth, when the newborn is in the quiet-alert phase. After positioning the newborn to face the breast, the mother can slightly compress the breast and, with her thumb above and fingers below the areola, stroke or brush the nipple against the newborn's lower lip or stroke the mouth. This stimulates the rooting reflex, causing the newborn to turn toward the nipple. As the newborn's mouth opens wide, the mother quickly brings the newborn close to her so that the newborn can latch on to the areola (Skill 11-1). This is referred to as the latch-on technique. In other words, the mother guides the nipple into the newborn's mouth, pulling the baby close to her. As much of the areola as possible should be in the newborn's mouth to avoid sore nipples. Later, when her milk comes in, the mother can listen for the sound of swallowing (sometimes gulping) the milk (Clinical Pathway 11-1).

If the breasts are full, expressing some milk softens the breasts and makes it easier for the newborn to grasp the areola. Also, the breast can be softened by massage.

Removal from the Breast

The mother is taught to safely remove the newborn from the breast for burping, for switching to the other breast, and when the infant is finished being fed. To avoid trauma to the breast, the newborn should be removed properly. The mother should insert her finger into the corner of the newborn's mouth to break the suction, and then remove the breast quickly before the newborn begins to suck again. Downward pressure on the newborn's chin is another way to break the suction (Figure 11-6). The principles of teaching the mother how to breastfeed are listed in Table 11-3 and Nursing Care Plan 11-1 on p. 217.

Burping

Breastfed newborns, like formula-fed newborns, must be burped to remove swallowed air, which can make the newborn feel uncomfortable. The newborn should be burped to remove air in the middle and at the end of the feeding. The three ways commonly used to "bubble" the newborn are holding the newborn over the shoulder or face down on the lap, or sitting the newborn up while gently patting his or her back (Figure 11-7 on p. 214).

The Sleepy Infant

Some newborns are sleepy and need to be awakened for feedings until a routine of feeding on demand is established. To bring the infant to an alert state in preparation for feeding, the infant should be unwrapped, the diaper can be changed, the mother should hold the infant upright and talk softly to him or her, or she may provide a gentle massage of the back, palms, or soles of the feet. When the infant is awake, feeding will be more successful.

— Can remove or change diaper to stimulate the baby.

Skill 11-1   Breastfeeding Techniques

PURPOSE

To enable successful infant latch-on and sucking at breast.

Steps

1. Before putting the newborn to the breast, the mother should manually express a few drops of colostrum. This will make the nipple erect so the newborn can pull the nipple back into the mouth.
2. Body alignment is important. The body of the newborn should face the mother so that the head does not turn to latch on.
3. The mother should stroke the newborn's cheek or lower lip with the nipple. The newborn will turn toward the nipple and usually open the mouth. The mother can then bring the newborn closer to her body to aid in latching on.
4. Nursing begins with the opposite breast from the one started in the last nursing period. After the third day, it is important to have the newborn empty the first breast completely before changing to the other breast.
5. Before taking the newborn off of the breast, the mother should break the suction by putting a finger in the corner of the newborn's mouth or by pushing downward on the newborn's chin.
6. While the newborn is sucking, it is necessary to keep the breast away from the newborn's nose. Because newborns are nose breathers, they will let go of the nipple if they cannot breathe.
7. Document the ability of infant to latch on, the mother's focus and positioning of infant, and signs of satiety in the infant.

The Fussy Infant

Some infants awaken from sleep crying lustily, eliminating the opportunity to observe for early cues of hunger (Box 11-1 on p. 214). These infants must be calmed before successful feeding can be attempted. The infant is wrapped snugly (swaddled) and held close. The mother should talk calmly to the infant. When the infant calms, feeding can begin.

Stiffening and crying after feeding starts can indicate a sore mouth from thrush, gas, cramps, or some illness that requires a health care provider's intervention. Collaboration with a lactation consultant is advisable.

Evaluating Feeding Techniques

The nurse should observe the mother and infant during breastfeeding to evaluate her technique and offer individualized advice and teaching. Observations should include:

- *Infant position:* Is the infant's head in a neutral position and hands at midline? Is the infant's nose

Clinical Pathway 11-1	Breastfeeding		
ASSESSMENT	**1-8 HOURS**	**8-24 HOURS**	**24-48 HOURS**
Newborn	Newborn is sleepy. Newborn correctly latches onto breast. Note first void and meconium stool.	Newborn is more alert. Newborn has audible swallow.	Newborn is alert for all feedings. Newborn feeds every 2-3 hours during day and every 3-4 hours during night. Newborn has at least 6 wet diapers per day and 1-3 bowel movements (3 or more by day 7).
Mother	Mother rooms-in with newborn. Nipples are erect. Mother makes an informed choice between breastfeeding or bottle feeding for newborn.	Milk begins to come in. Mother is relaxed during feeding.	Mother recognizes hunger cues of newborn before cry. Breasts are soft after breastfeeding.
Medical and nursing interventions	Administer pain medication immediately after breastfeeding to minimize drug transfer by breast milk. Breastfeeding assessment and teaching should be documented on each shift to eliminate duplication or omission of essential details.	Avoid meperidine (Demerol) during breastfeeding. Codeine, fentanyl, methadone, and morphine are approved for use during lactation. Doxepin and benzodiazepines are contraindicated for breastfeeding mothers.	Consult social service or home care nurse as needed.
Teaching	Discuss breast and nipple care. Encourage skin-to-skin contact between mother and baby. Teach proper latch-on technique. Review frequency of feedings and length of time on each breast.	Notify lactation nurse to assist as needed. Check for nipple protrusion or tenderness. Discuss various breastfeeding positions. Review proper release of newborn's suction at breast by placing clean finger in corner of newborn's mouth. Discuss techniques that stimulate sucking, such as unwrapping newborn, stroking soles of feet.	Discuss resources for breast pump purchase or rental if needed. Discuss milk banking and technique of freezing and storing breast milk. Help mother identify audible swallow to determine nutritive sucking and milk intake. Discuss comforting techniques for fussy baby, such as swaddling or rocking. Discuss normal urine and stool output of neonate.
Discharge and follow-up	Discuss home needs and support system available to mother. Discuss ongoing care of nipples. Discourage use of ointments as indicated.	If discharged before 48 hours, offer follow-up at 7 days. Discuss plans for home care or return to work. Discuss minor problems of breastfeeding and remedies such as breast shields.	Before discharge give mother lactation consultant contact information and community resource list to take home. Give telephone number of advice nurse or clinic. Give return appointment to mother for her newborn. Ensure mother feels confident of feeding plan at time of discharge.

[Handwritten annotation next to "Mother" row: ⊛ need up to 500 calories more of intake]

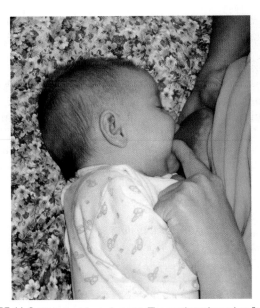

FIGURE 11-6 **Removal from breast**. The mother places her finger in the corner of the newborn's mouth to break the suction before removing the newborn from the breast.

unobstructed by the breast? Is the infant able to grasp the entire nipple to initiate breastfeeding?
- *Maternal focus:* Is the mother focused on the baby, undistracted by TV or conversation?
- *Technique:* Is the mother relaxed and unhurried? Does she take time to burp the infant or re-stimulate the infant when needed?
- *Satiety:* Is the infant relaxed or asleep after feeding? Are the mother's breasts soft after feeding? Does the mother position the infant in the bassinet after feeding?

SPECIAL BREASTFEEDING SITUATIONS

Multiple Births

Twins can be fed one at a time or simultaneously. The mother's body adjusts the milk supply to the greater demand. The mother may want to use the crisscross hold when nursing simultaneously. She will need help to position two infants at the breast in a cradle hold in each arm. She positions the first infant in a cradle hold, and then her helper positions the second infant at the

Table 11-3	Teaching the New Mother How to Breastfeed	
INSTRUCTION	**RATIONALE**
Wash hands before feeding; wash nipples with warm water, no soap.	Prevents infection of the newborn and breast; plain water prevents nipple cracking and irritation.
Position self (sitting or side-lying).	Alternating positions facilitates breast emptying and reduces nipple trauma.
Sit comfortably in chair or raised bed with back and arm support; hold newborn by cradle hold or football hold supported by pillows.	Pillow support of mother's back and arm and the newborn's body in any position reduces fatigue; newborn is more likely to remain in correct position for nursing.
Lie on side with pillow beneath head, arm above head; support newborn in side-lying position.	Side-lying position reduces fatigue and pressure on abdominal incision.
Turn body of newborn to face mother's breast.	Prevents pulling on nipple or poor position of mouth on nipple.
Stroke newborn's cheek with nipple.	Elicits rooting reflex to cause newborn to turn toward nipple and open mouth wide.
Newborn's mouth should cover entire areola.	Compresses ducts and lessens tension on nipples; suction is more even.
Avoid strict time limits for nursing; nurse at least 10 minutes before changing to other breast or longer if newborn is nursing vigorously.	Let-down reflex may take 5 minutes; a too-short feeding will give newborn foremilk only, not the hunger-satisfying hindmilk. Strict time limits do not prevent sore nipples.
Use safety pin on the bra strap as a reminder about which breast to start with at the next feeding.	Alternating which breast is used first increases milk production.
Lift newborn or breast slightly if breast tissue blocks nose.	Provides a small breathing space.
Break suction by placing finger in corner of newborn's mouth or indenting breast tissue.	Prevents nipple trauma.
Nurse newborn after birth and every 2-3 hours thereafter.	Early suckling stimulates oxytocin from mother's pituitary to contract her uterus and control bleeding. Breast milk is quickly digested. Early, regular, and frequent nursing reduces breast engorgement. Skin-to-skin contact promotes bonding.
Burp newborn halfway through and after feeding.	Rids stomach of air bubbles and reduces regurgitation.

From Leifer, G. (2010). *Introduction to maternity and pediatric nursing* (6th ed.). Philadelphia: Saunders.

other breast in the crook of her arm. Their bodies cross over each other. The infants and the mother's arms are supported with pillows.

Preterm Birth

Breastfeeding is especially good for a preterm infant because of the immunologic advantages. If the infant cannot nurse, the mother can pump her breasts and freeze the milk for gavage (tube) feedings. See Chapter 15 for further information on the preterm infant.

When nursing the preterm or small infant, the mother may prefer the cross cradle hold. She holds the infant's head with the hand opposite the breast that she will use to nurse. She uses the same arm to support the infant's body. The hand on the same side as the nursing breast is used to guide the breast toward the infant's mouth.

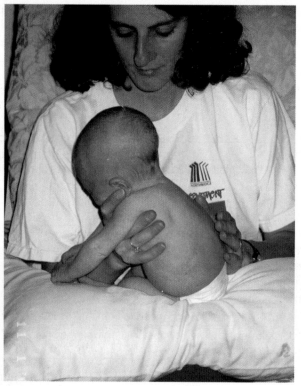

FIGURE 11-7 Burping the newborn. The mother can burp the newborn by holding the newborn in a sitting position on her lap, supporting the chin and chest, and gently patting the newborn's back. In this position, the mother can see the newborn's face in case of spit-up.

Box 11-1   Recognizing Hunger in Newborns
• Hand-to-mouth movements • Mouth and tongue movements • Sucking motions • Rooting movements • Clenched fists • Kicking of legs • Crying (a late sign of hunger; may result in shutdown and poor feeding if needs are not met)

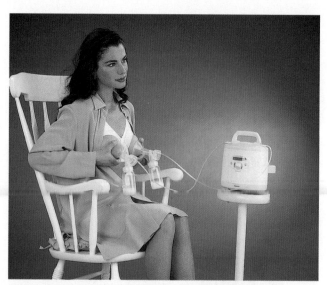

FIGURE 11-8 Breast pumping. The mother can pump both breasts at the same time or one at a time with an electric breast pump.

Delayed Feedings

When breastfeeding must be temporarily delayed, the mother should be taught how to pump her milk in order to resume full breastfeeding and avoid engorgement of the breasts (Figure 11-8).

Use of Breast Pump. Electric, battery operated and manual breast pumps are available for purchase or rental. Double breast pumps are also available to pump both breasts at the same time. If breastfeeding is delayed after delivery, pumping should start within 6 hours. Breast massage, application of heat, and moistening the breast before applying the suction before pumping can help start the process. The mother should pump her breasts as often as the infant would nurse, including some nighttime hours when the prolactin levels are high. Pumping sessions can last about 15 minutes. Excess pressure should be avoided, and the pump should be cleaned after each pumping session.

 Patient Teaching

Tips for Breast Pumping

- Find a quiet, private area with a comfortable chair.
- Wash hands and set up the pumping system.
- Spend a few minutes relaxing, looking at a picture of the newborn, or massaging breasts to nurture the let-down reflex.
- When finished pumping, store milk in a cooler or refrigerator and rinse the equipment well.
- Pumping can be repeated every 3 hours for a 15-minute session.

Supplemental Feedings and Nipple Confusion

Supplemental bottle feedings of formula or water should not be offered to the healthy newborn who is in the process of establishing breastfeeding success.

A form of "imprinting" may occur if a newborn is given a formula and finds it easy to obtain fluid from the nipple on the bottle with minimum effort. When the infant is then placed on the breast, more effort is needed to obtain the breast milk. As a result, the hungry infant may become irritable or fretful, which causes the mother to feel the baby is rejecting the breast in preference for the bottle. This is called *nipple confusion*. When lactation is firmly established after the neonatal period, the use of a pacifier to meet nonnutritional sucking needs will not cause nipple confusion (Jenik, Vain, Gorestein, & Jacobi, 2009). The neonate *should not* be given water between feedings. When the infant is fed breast milk from a bottle, a slow-flow nipple should be selected because a fast-flow nipple requires less effort by the newborn.

Storing and Freezing Breast Milk

Milk stored at room temperature over 4 hours has an increased potential for bacterial contamination. Various commercial containers are available for the storage of breast milk, each with advantages and disadvantages. The container should hold about as much milk as the infant will consume at one feeding and be tightly capped.

Milk may be safely stored in glass or hard plastic. Leukocytes may stick to the glass but are not destroyed. Several types of plastic bottles are available in stores. Clear, hard plastic bottles are made of polycarbonate; although little research is available, they are considered safe for storing and freezing milk. Dull or cloudy hard plastic bottles are polystyrene or milky white polypropylene. Polystyrene bottles are not designed for frozen milk storage. Polymers become unstable when heating after freezing. When used for freezing, polypropylene bottles alter the lysozyme, lactoferrin, and vitamin C content of breast milk. Polyethylene containers are usually clear plastic bags that may be at risk for puncture and invasion by microorganisms; some brands contain a special nylon between the polyethylene layers to reduce the puncture risk. The loss of lysozyme and fat is significant, and some valuable antibodies that adhere to polyethylene are lost to the infant. Plastic bottles or cups with the number 3, 6, or 7 embedded in the small triangle on the bottom of the bottle are not safe to reuse.

Milk can be thawed in the refrigerator for 5 days (best to preserve immunoglobulins) or by holding the container under running lukewarm water or placing it in a container of lukewarm water, rotating (not shaking) the bottle often. Microwaving is not advised because it destroys some immune factors and lysozyme contained in the milk, and the milk can develop hot spots because of uneven heating.

Milk can be stored in the refrigerator (4° C [39.2° F]) up to 5 days without significant changes occurring, in the refrigerator freezer for 2 weeks or in a deep freezer (−6.7° C [−20° F]) for up to 12 months. Freezing can destroy some antimicrobial factors in the breast milk.

For safe storage of breast milk in the hospital setting, breast milk may be stored in the hospital for feeding to infants in the NICU or hospitalized infants when the mother cannot room-in to breastfeed. It is very important to assure that pumped breast milk stored in hospital refrigerators is fed to the appropriate infants. To ensure breast milk safety, nursing responsibilities include:

- Maintain secure mother-infant identification per hospital policy.
- Hospital identification bands must be securely attached to mother and baby, be moisture proof, and contain the name and hospital ID number.
- The identification label on the bottle of stored breast milk must include date and time milk was expressed and thawed and mother/baby ID information.
- The ID bracelet of mother and baby must be verified with the identification label on the bottle of breast milk and documented on the chart.
- A separate refrigerator in the hospital unit should be dedicated to the exclusive use of breast milk storage.
- The temperature of the refrigerator should be checked each shift and be maintained at 35° F to 40° F (2° C to 4° C) (Huber, Blanco, & Davis, 2009).

Nipple Soreness

Nipple soreness is a common symptom in the early weeks of breastfeeding and may be a significant cause of abandoning breastfeeding in favor of bottled formula. Lanolin (Lansinoh) is an absorptive ointment that maintains internal moisture and is often used by mothers to prevent or treat nipple soreness. Breast milk has also been advocated as an "ointment" for sore nipples because it contains lysozymes that can prevent infection and aid in healing.

Newer thin-walled breast shields can facilitate breastfeeding until sore nipples heal. A lactation specialist is often available in most hospital settings for guidance in their use (Chertok, 2009). Cracked nipples that are infected with bacteria or yeast may require prescribed antibacterial ointments.

Nurses should discuss prevention and treatment of nipple soreness with all breastfeeding mothers. Proper positioning of the newborn at the breast and proper removal techniques are the best measures to prevent cracked nipples.

Breast Engorgement

Early, regular, and frequent nursing helps prevent engorgement. If engorgement does occur, and the breast and areola are tense and uncomfortable, the

Caused by the baby not sucking correctly or not positioned correctly.

mother can pump her breasts to get the milk flow started. Cold applications to the breast between feedings and heat just before feedings may help reduce discomfort. Manual massage of all segments of the breasts helps soften them and express milk downward toward the ducts. The mother cups her hand near the chest wall around the breast and firmly slides her fingers down toward the nipple, while rotating the hand and massaging the areas surrounding the breasts in order to make contact with all of the milk ducts. Massage stimulates the release of oxytocin that increases milk ejection. A supportive bra should be worn to increase comfort.

Complementary and Alternative Therapy During Breastfeeding

Some mothers use herbs such as alfalfa, dandelion, fennel, caraway, and anise to increase milk supply. Caraway tea is also popular for use in newborns with colic (Skidmore-Roth, 2009). Black walnut, parsley, and yarrow can decrease milk supply. Essential oils also play a role in breastfeeding. Oil of peppermint compresses, and cabbage leaves can relieve engorged breasts. See Chapter 21 for further information concerning complementary and alternative therapies.

Weaning

Mothers should be taught that gradual weaning is preferred to abrupt weaning. Abrupt weaning can cause engorgement, which increases the risk of mastitis. There is no ideal time to wean. The decision is based on cultural norms and practices; however, it is best to eliminate one feeding at a time. After a few days, a second feeding can be eliminated. It is advisable to eliminate the infant's favorite feeding last, which will likely be the bedtime or early morning feeding. The younger infant will likely need formula from a bottle, and the older infant may be weaned from the breast to a cup. Whole milk is not usually started before 1 year of age.

If the woman has to abruptly wean her baby, she should wear a firm supporting bra. Ice packs may provide comfort. She should avoid nipple stimulation.

CONTRAINDICATIONS FOR BREASTFEEDING

Maternal Illness

Some maternal illness may preclude breastfeeding a newborn. True galactosemia, untreated maternal active tuberculosis, active herpes lesions on the breast, maternal drug abuse, maternal chemotherapy, and active HIV infection are contraindications to breastfeeding (Weil, 2010). Because many drugs pass through breast milk, any medications the mother is taking must be evaluated concerning its effect on the newborn. Certain drugs, such as levodopa, barbiturates,

antihistamines, pyridoxine, estrogens, androgens, and bromocriptine, decrease the breast milk volume.

Infectious Diseases and Breastfeeding

The only absolute contraindication to breastfeeding is infection with human immunodeficiency virus (HIV) and human T-lymphotrophic virus (HTLV 1 and 2). HIV infection is a contraindication to breastfeeding because it can be transmitted to the infant via breast milk. The HTLV 1 and 2 viruses are retroviruses that can also be passed to the newborn via breast milk, and breastfeeding is also contraindicated. Maternal hepatitis A infection is *not* a contraindication to breastfeeding. The infant can receive immunoglobulin and hepatitis A vaccine therapy. Infants of hepatitis B virus (HBV)–positive mothers should receive HBV vaccine therapy before discharge and can breastfeed the baby. In mothers who are infected with the hepatitis C virus, breastfeeding is contraindicated in the presence of liver failure. In mothers infected with the herpes simplex virus or the varicella zoster virus, breastfeeding is contraindicated when lesions are present on the breast.

Mothers who have active tuberculosis (TB) must be isolated from their newborn infants, but infants can be fed breast milk that is pumped because the breast milk does not contain the tubercle bacilli.

Immunizations and Breastfeeding

Breastfeeding is not a contraindication for the administration of any vaccine, except for the smallpox vaccination. Most live virus vaccines have not shown evidence of being excreted in breast milk (CDC, 2006). A woman who does not breastfeed should wear a supportive bra; breast binders are not advised. Tenderness and leakage usually disappear in 7 to 14 days (Nursing Care Plan 11-1).

FORMULA FEEDING

Parents need to be assured that commercially prepared formula provides adequate nutrition for the newborn. Parents should be advised that the physician or nurse-midwife can select a formula appropriate for the newborn. Closeness and warmth that occur during breastfeeding should also be a part of bottle feeding (Figure 11-9). Under no circumstances should a bottle be propped for infant feeding because this practice does not support parent-infant bonding and carries a high risk for aspiration. An advantage of bottle feeding is that both parents can share in this caring experience with their newborn. Mothers who choose to bottle feed should not be made to feel guilty by health care providers. Breast milk or formula is the only nourishment needed for the first 6 months of life. The newborn is not capable of digesting solid food in the first few months of life.

Scenario

A mother is breastfeeding her day-old newborn for the first time. She appears anxious and says she is not sure she is doing it right.

Selected Nursing Diagnosis

Ineffective breastfeeding related to maternal anxiety and sleepy newborn

Expected Outcomes	Nursing Interventions	Rationales
Patient will express confidence in ability to breastfeed.	Initiate breastfeeding as soon as possible after delivery.	Promotes bonding and initiates sucking while newborn is in the quiet-alert stage, which often occurs in the first hour after delivery.
	Assess and record effectiveness of each breastfeeding session.	Identifies problem areas that require intervention.
	Encourage patient to relax during feedings. Inform her that breastfeeding is something that is a learned behavior for both mother and baby.	When the patient is tense, the newborn senses her anxiety and often becomes fussy. Letting the patient know breastfeeding does not always happen instantaneously helps reduce anxiety.
	Teach mother techniques for breastfeeding and positioning.	Knowledge increases confidence and decreases anxieties.
Newborn will latch on and effectively suck (evidenced by audible swallows) for 10-15 minutes on each breast.	Teach mother normal newborn behaviors during breastfeeding (e.g., intermittent sucking).	Anticipatory guidance helps mother realize behaviors are normal.
	Encourage mother to ask questions and to verbalize concerns.	Allows the nurse to provide needed information and to clear up any misconceptions or misunderstandings.
	Provide positive reinforcement for correct breastfeeding practices.	Enhances self-esteem and builds confidence.
Newborn will appear satisfied for 2-3 hours after each feeding.	Teach ways to stimulate newborn and increase alertness (unwrap or undress newborn, provide skin-to-skin contact, massage newborn, change diaper, hold in upright position, talk to newborn, burp frequently).	When first establishing breastfeeding, the newborn needs to be awakened every 2-3 hours to feed. It is important to stimulate babies so they are awake and alert enough to breastfeed effectively.
	Initiate a lactation consultant referral.	Reinforces prior teaching and provides additional information that may help establish effective breastfeeding. Often hearing information from an "expert" will decrease anxiety.

Selected Nursing Diagnosis

Imbalanced nutrition: less than body requirements related to knowledge deficit of mother regarding maternal nutritional needs

Expected Outcomes	Nursing Interventions	Rationales
Newborn will not lose more than 10% of birth weight in the first week and will then show steady weight gain consistent with normal newborn growth curve.	Assess patient's current knowledge level of dietary needs while breastfeeding and how to determine whether newborn is getting enough nutrients.	Provides baseline information for the development of an individualized teaching plan.
	Teach patient the importance of not dieting while breastfeeding and that breastfeeding women usually return to prepregnancy weight sooner than those who bottle feed.	After delivery, women are often anxious to return to prepregnancy weight but need to be reminded that if they reduce food intake, they are reducing the nutrients available to their baby.
Patient will be able to correctly describe maternal dietary requirements while breastfeeding.	Teach patient that 500 additional calories are needed per day to produce adequate milk for the newborn.	Increased knowledge increases compliance with dietary requirements.
	Teach patient the importance of using a food guide pyramid when preparing foods.	A food guide provides a quick resource to ensure adequate intake of nutritional foods and allows individuals to accommodate cultural dietary preferences.
	Teach patient to increase fluid intake to approximately 2 quarts (64 oz) per day.	Provides sufficient fluid for milk production and maternal needs.
	Instruct patient to continue taking prenatal vitamins.	Ensures adequate vitamin intake to meet needs of both mother and newborn.
Newborn will appear satisfied after feeding for 2-3 hours and have at least six wet diapers per day.	Teach patient ways to know newborn is getting enough milk (appears satisfied after feedings, at least six wet diapers per day, adequate weight gain, etc.).	Allows prompt intervention if breastfeeding is not meeting newborn's nutritional needs.
	Teach importance of taking newborn to all well-baby appointments.	Assesses normal growth patterns and nutritional status.

Continued

Expected Outcomes	Nursing Interventions	Rationales
	Refer to Women, Infants, and Children (WIC) program if woman qualifies.	WIC is a federally subsidized food program that offers nutritional classes for breastfeeding mothers and provides food vouchers enabling them to obtain nutritional food items.
	Refer to dietitian as needed.	Patients who are on medically indicated diets may need specialized instruction on specific modifications needed while breastfeeding.

Selected Nursing Diagnosis

Acute pain related to improper latch-on, cracked nipples, breast engorgement, or mastitis

Expected Outcomes	Nursing Interventions	Rationales
Patient will state that she is not experiencing nipple or breast pain.	Determine presence of nipple and breast discomfort, engorgement, and impaired nipple integrity at every feeding.	Determines whether intervention is required.
	Assist with correct positioning (football hold, cradle hold, or side-lying) with newborn's body and face turned toward the breast and with mouth surrounding nipple and areola. Support with pillows as needed.	Incorrect positioning can cause nipples to crack and blister. When the areola is not in the newborn's mouth, milk ducts are not being adequately compressed. Pillows help decrease maternal fatigue and aid in maintaining correct newborn positioning.
	Teach patient to alternate newborn's position with each feeding.	Avoids constant pressure in the same area of breast tissue.
	Teach mother to stroke newborn's cheek with nipple.	Initiates rooting reflex in which newborn turns toward the nipple and opens mouth widely so entire nipple and areola can be inserted.
	Instruct patient to break suction by inserting finger into newborn's mouth before pulling newborn away from the breast.	Decreases risk of injury to nipples.
	Instruct patient to feed newborn every 2-3 hours for a minimum of 10-15 minutes each breast.	Frequent feedings help prevent engorgement.
	Teach patient to begin new feeding with the breast that was last used at prior feeding (a safety pin on the bra strap can be a helpful reminder).	Ensures each breast is emptied completely a minimum of every other feeding. When the newborn initially starts to feed, sucking is more aggressive because of hunger; it may not be as strong while on the second breast.
	Instruct parent to avoid bottle feeding commercial formula and feeding water or juice between, or as an alternate to, breastfeeding.	When the breast is not emptied at regular intervals, engorgement can occur.
Patient will have no cracking, blistering, or bleeding on nipples.	Instruct patient to cleanse nipples with water only.	Soap can dry out nipples, making them more prone to cracking.
	Instruct patient to apply a small amount of breast milk to nipples after each feeding and to allow nipples to air dry.	Breast milk is beneficial in protecting and restoring the skin integrity of the breast.
	Instruct patient to use breast pads in bra.	Absorbs moisture from leaking breasts. Nipples that are exposed to moisture for prolonged periods are more prone to cracking.
Breasts will be soft, nontender, and without redness or excessive warmth.	Instruct patient to report fever, localized breast redness and tenderness, headache, or nausea and vomiting with generalized aching to health care provider.	These are signs and symptoms of mastitis, which will require antibiotic therapy.
	Instruct patient to use cool compresses between feedings and warm compresses immediately before feedings.	Alleviates discomfort of engorgement. Cool compresses are soothing, and warm compresses stimulate the let-down reflex.
	Administer analgesics as ordered and needed (specify medication, dosage, route, and frequency to individualize for your patient).	Reduces pain sensations. To ensure maximum benefit, medications should be administered before feeding or feeding should start after peak of action of medication.

Critical Thinking Questions

1. You are caring for a non–English-speaking woman who needs information concerning breast care. The father of the baby, who is bilingual, is at the bedside. Is it appropriate to ask him to interpret the instructions?
2. A first-time mother wants to breastfeed but states she is instead thinking about bottle feeding her infant because she is worried she may not have enough milk to meet the needs of the infant. What can you tell her to increase her confidence in breastfeeding her infant?

! Safety Alert

Tips for Safe Bottle Feeding

- Always check the expiration date on the formula container; do not buy formula that has expired.
- Wash hands thoroughly before preparing formula.
- Wash top of can with detergent and hot water before opening it.
- Use a clean can opener to open can and wash between uses. Check the can opener for food or rust spots before using it again.
- Have a clean container (dishpan) reserved for washing all things used for feeding newborn. Squeeze soapy water through nipple holes, then rinse several times.
- Follow the product directions precisely when mixing formula.
- Heat bottle of formula, if necessary, by running warm water over it. (Most newborns are just as content with their formula unheated. Be consistent in your choice.)
- Test temperature by shaking a few drops on your inner wrist, not just feeling the bottle.
- Do not heat bottle in a microwave oven; the liquid often warms unevenly unless stirred. The container may remain cool even though the formula is hot enough to burn the newborn.
- Opened containers of liquid formula should be tightly covered and stored in the refrigerator for no longer than is designated on the label.
- Once a formula can is opened or formula is mixed, use it right away or refrigerate because bacteria multiply rapidly at warm temperatures.
- Carry filled bottles away from home in an insulated bag or cooler with ice packs inside.
- Milk should not be saved for the next feeding if the newborn does not empty the bottle. Organisms will grow, and the newborn can develop diarrhea (infection).
- Newborn infants should not be given bottles of water because hyponatremia may result.
- Honey should not be given to infants younger than 12 months of age because it increases the risk of infant botulism. Sorbitol-containing prune, pear, or apple juice may be given for mild constipation (Langan, 2006).

TYPES OF FORMULAS

Commercial formulas are available in different forms: **powder,** which is combined with water; **concentrated liquid,** which is diluted with an equal amount of water; and **ready-to-feed formula,** which requires no dilution. The powder is less expensive and easy to prepare. The ready-to-feed type is the most expensive but has the advantage of not needing refrigeration or preparation (other than removing the bottle cap) (Table 11-4).

Commercially Prepared Formulas

Milk-based formulas are used for the average newborn. Soy-based formulas are used for newborns with lactose intolerance or galactosemia. Newborns with protein allergies and fat malabsorption are given protein

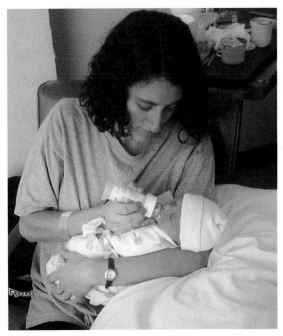

FIGURE 11-9 **Bottle feeding the newborn**. The mother holds the newborn in a semi-upright position in a cradle hold. The nipple should be kept full of formula to reduce the amount of air the newborn swallows. A pillow supports the mother's elbow. Holding the newborn close promotes bonding just as breastfeeding does.

hydrolysate-based formulas. Both milk- and soy-based formulas are designed to be similar to breast milk in terms of protein, carbohydrate, fat, and mineral content. Formulas given to term newborns are designed to contain 20 kcal/oz when prepared according to directions. Vitamin and mineral supplements are usually added to commercially prepared formulas (Table 11-5).

FORMULA PREPARATION

It is important to teach parents that formulas must be prepared according to directions. When too little water is added, the formula may be too concentrated and cause diarrhea, electrolyte imbalance, or both. If the formula is prepared with more water than suggested, the formula may be too weak and the newborn will receive insufficient calories and nutrients, which can result in growth retardation.

Bottles and nipples should be washed in warm, soapy water with a nipple and bottlebrush and rinsed well. Boiling the bottles, nipples, or water used for preparation may not be necessary unless the safety of the water supply is in doubt. Boiling the water used to prepare formulas for the newborn for 2 minutes is recommended (WHO, 2007). A 24-hour supply of formula can be prepared according to directions and refrigerated for use. Single-feeding powder packets are available when the family is traveling and does not have refrigeration facilities, or a ready-to-feed formula may be used.

Prepared formula should remain at room temperature for no longer than 2 hours before use because

Table 11-4 Common Milk Preparations for the First Year

MILK PREPARATION	ADVANTAGES	DISADVANTAGES
Human breast milk	No preparation needed; nonallergenic; provides antibodies	Lifestyle or illness of mother may influence availability
Prepared, ready-to-feed formula	No preparation needed; no refrigeration needed before opening bottle	Expensive
Formula concentrate	Easy to prepare; can prepare one bottle at a time or a maximum of one day's feeding at a time	Must be refrigerated after preparation Must use accurate proportions; safe water supply necessary to dilute concentrate (water from a natural well may have a high mineral concentration)
Formula powder	Least expensive formula; lasts up to 1 month once opened	Necessitates accurate measurement; necessitates safe water supply and must be shaken thoroughly to dissolve powder

Table 11-5 Commercially Prepared Formulas

INFANT FORMULAS	BRAND NAME	WHEY/CASEIN RATIO
Standard formula	Enfamil Lipil	60:40
Iron fortified cow's milk–based formula with DHA and ARA	Good Start Supreme Similac Advance	100:0 48:52
Modified cow's milk-based protein (partially hydrolyzed)	Enfamil Gentlease-Lipil Good Start Supreme Gentle Infant Formula Similac Sensitive (kosher)	60:40 100:0 60:40 48:52
Organic cow's milk-based	Similac organic, Bright Beginnings organic	48:52

SPECIALTY FORMULAS	BRAND NAME	PROTEIN/NUTRIENT CONTENT
Cow's milk-based with rice starch added	Enfamil AR Lipil Similac Sensitive RS	Contains rice starch without adding calories
Lactose free	Similac Sensitive Enfamil Gentlease	May contain palm olein to enhance calcium absorption
With prebiotics or probiotics	Similac EarlyShield Bright Beginnings Nestle Good Start Natural Cultures (100% whey protein)	Contains prebiotics (oligosaccharides) Contains *Bifidobacterium* (*Bifidobacterium animalis* subsp lactis) cultures; probiotics
Iron-fortified soy-based	Bright Beginnings Soy Enfamil Prosobee Lipil Isomil Advance	Soy protein isolate Soy protein and methionine Soy protein isolate
Extensively hydrolyzed milk protein formulas	Similac Alimentum Nutramigen Pregestimil	Casein hydrolysate Lactose and sucrose free Casein hydrolysate and free amino acids
Amino acid–based Elemental formula	Elecare Neocate	Free l-amino acids
Electrolyte solution	Pedialyte Lytren Enfalyte	Electrolytes and rice syrup as carbohydrate source 115 mg sodium, 98 mg potassium

Data from Abbot Laboratories http://abbotnutrition.com/products; Bright Beginnings www.brightbeginnings.com/professionals; Mead Johnson www.meadjohnson.com; Nestle www.nestle-infantnutrition.com; Ouwehand, A. (2007). Antibacterial effects of probiotics. *Journal of Nutrition, 137*(1), 7945-7975; Gottesman, M. (2008). Choosing the right infant formula. *Advance for Nurse Practitioners, 16*(5), 47-51; and Kleinman, R. (Ed.). (2004). *Pediatric nutrition handbook* (5th ed.). Elk Grove Village, IL: American Academy of Pediatrics; and Leifer, G. (2010). *Introduction to maternity and pediatric nursing* (6th ed.). Philadelphia: Saunders.
NOTE: Other formulas are available for specific conditions such as maple syrup urine disease, homocystinuria, phenylketonuria (PKU), etc.
ARA, arachidonic acid; *DHA*, docosahexaenoic acid.

of bacterial growth. Whether to warm or not warm the formula is up to the parents. Parents should be advised not to warm the formula in a microwave oven. Rather, the bottle should be placed in a container of warm water. The temperature of the formula should be tested on the inside of the parent's wrist. The rate of nipple flow should be in drops when the bottle is inverted. Newborns who tire easily do better with a soft, pliable nipple, whereas a vigorously sucking newborn should be

Box 11-2   Guidelines for Safe Formula Preparation

- Wash hands before preparation.
- Clean or sterilize feeding equipment with soap and water.
- Boil water for 2 minutes before reconstituting powdered formula.
- Bottled water is not considered sterile unless labeled.
- Never use vitamin or electrolyte enhanced water to prepare powdered formula.
- Cool formula and refrigerate promptly.
- Use prepared formula within 24 hours.
- For outdoor trips, use formula placed in cooler within 2 hours.

Data from WHO. (2007). *Safe preparation, storage, and handling of powdered infant formula: guidelines.* Geneva, Switzerland: Author; and Eby, A. (2009). Metabolic alkalosis after using enhanced water to dilute formulas. *MCN. The American Journal of Maternal Child Nursing, 34*(5), 290-295.

given a slow-flow nipple. Formula that remains in the bottle after feeding should be discarded because it has mixed with saliva, which can be a medium for bacterial growth (Box 11-2).

TEACHING BOTTLE-FEEDING TECHNIQUES

Positioning

Placing the newborn in a semi-upright cradle position allows the mother to hold the newborn close in a face-to-face position (Skill 11-2). The bottle should be held in a manner to keep the nipple full of formula at all times to reduce the amount of air swallowed. Bottles made with an angled neck are available to help keep the nipple filled with fluid.

Burping

The newborn should be burped, or bubbled, frequently (see Figure 11-7). After feeding, the newborn should be placed on the side and propped with a rolled blanket. This position lessens the chance of aspiration if more bubbles of air come up with the spitting up of formula.

Frequency

The newborn should not be kept on a rigid schedule; rather, the mother should take cues from the newborn that he or she is hungry. Most newborns are formula

---

Skill 11-2   Bottle Feeding the Infant

PURPOSE

To enable safe ingestion of nutrients necessary for growth and development.

Steps

1. Verify formula prescribed and expiration date on the bottle.
2. When preparing formula for use, be sure to carefully follow the directions for dilution. Do not add water to ready-feed formulas.
3. Change diaper and provide cord care. Wash and sanitize hands.
4. Select an appropriate nipple: cross-cut nipples offer rapid feedings, single-hole nipples offer regular milk flow, and preemie nipples are softer and require less sucking effort.
5. The nipple hole should be just large enough so that milk flows in drops when the bottle is inverted.
6. When the nipple hole is too large, the infant can eat too fast and regurgitate or overeat.
7. If formula runs out of the side of the mouth during infant feeding, the nipple holes may be too large. The nipple should be discarded and replaced with a different one.
8. When opening a ready-to-feed bottle (you should hear a "pop" to indicate bottle was unopened), place the selected nipple on the bottle and tighten securely. Use room temperature formula.
9. Hold infant in cradle position with infant's head slightly elevated above the body (see Figure 11-3).
10. Touch infant's lips with nipple and gently insert nipple along infant's tongue. Hold bottle so nipple is *always* full of formula.
11. Feed infant slowly. Stop to "burp or bubble" infant after 1 to 1½ ounces (30 to 45 mL) and at end of feeding.
12. The newborn should be held close and cuddled to facilitate bonding. Stroking and talking during feeding promotes pleasure and relaxation for the newborn and the parent. The infant should *never* be prop fed or fed while lying flat in bed because aspiration of formula can occur.
13. To burp the infant, sit the infant on your lap with his or her body leaning slightly forward. Support the head and gently pat the middle or upper back (see Figure 11-7).
14. Place the infant in the crib in Fowler's position after feeding.
15. Leftover formula should be discarded because microorganisms from the infant's mouth grow rapidly in warm formulas.
16. Document the amount taken, type of formula, any regurgitation, sucking strength, and parent teaching that was provided.

fed every 3 to 4 hours. In a few weeks, the newborn may skip a feeding, which may occur during the night.

The mother should be cautioned not to prop the bottle and leave the baby alone. Newborns are more likely to regurgitate, aspirate, and choke when the bottle is propped. In addition, propping the bottle increases the danger of ear infections and does not promote bonding.

Although the mother's intentions may be good, she should not coax the newborn to finish the milk in the bottle at each feeding. This can result in overfeeding the newborn, which can result in regurgitation. Overfeeding can cause excessive weight gain.

Avoiding Nursing Caries

Teach parents not to give newborns or infants a bottle of milk or juice as a pacifier to suck on at will. The liquid can pool in the mouth for a long time, promote the growth of bacteria, and lead to dental cavities (nursing caries).

DISCHARGE PLANNING

Discharge planning begins on admission or even earlier, when parents attend childbirth classes. Because mothers and infants are discharged quickly after birth, self-care and infant care teaching often must begin before the mother is psychologically ready to learn. Some birth facilities use *clinical pathways* (also called care maps, care paths, or multidisciplinary action plans [MAPs]) to ensure that important care and teaching are not overlooked (see Chapter 1). These plans guide the nurse in identifying areas of special need that require referral, as well as a means to keep up with the many facets of routine care needed after birth. The nurse must take every opportunity to teach during the short birth facility stay. Ample written materials for both new mother and infant care should be provided to refresh the memory of parents who may be tired and uncomfortable when teaching occurs.

Nurses should recommend the best websites that contain accurate and complete information. Websites recommended for patients should be presented at the appropriate reading level. Many women turn to the Internet for information and support about breastfeeding and other health issues; therefore, nurses should evaluate websites before recommending them for patient use. Evaluation of websites should include credibility, updated and unbiased information, related link sites, interactivity, and evidence-based information (Weber, Derrico, Yoon, & Sherwill-Navarro, 2010).

Get Ready for the NCLEX® Examination!

Key Points

- The newborn should be breastfed as soon as possible after birth and 8 to 12 times a day in the first months of life.
- Parents are provided with information about breastfeeding and formula feeding so that they can make a choice based on facts.
- Mothers are advised that a positive attitude toward breastfeeding is important in achieving success. In addition, mothers are advised that the size of the breasts is not related to breast milk production.
- Advantages of breastfeeding include that it is easier to digest; provides immune factors; and results in fewer allergies, respiratory tract infections, and gastrointestinal problems. Also, breastfed newborns are less likely to be obese.
- Frequent stimulation and emptying of the breasts are the best way to maintain or increase breast milk production.
- Adequacy of breast milk intake is determined by an audible swallow, sleep after feeding, at least six wet diapers per day, and a steady weight gain after the first week of life.
- Frequent and regular breastfeeding can prevent breast engorgement.
- If breastfeeding is delayed, breast pumping can maintain the milk supply and avoid engorgement.
- The composition of commercial formulas is based on the composition of human milk.
- The diet of a lactating mother requires an additional 500 calories per day over the nonpregnant diet, an increased fluid intake, and calcium-rich foods.
- Three basic types of commercial formulas are powder, which is combined with water; concentrated liquid, which is diluted with an equal amount of water; and formula that is ready to feed.
- Bottle-feeding techniques include keeping the nipple full of formula at all times to reduce swallowing air; burping the newborn regularly; feeding the newborn when hungry rather than on a rigid schedule; and not forcing the newborn to empty the bottle if not hungry, which will encourage obesity.
- Nursing caries can be prevented by teaching the parent not to put the infant to bed with a bottle of milk or juice or offering a bottle of milk or juice to suck on at will.

Additional Learning Resources

SG   Go to your Study Guide on pages 493–494 for additional Review Questions for the NCLEX® Examination, Critical Thinking Clinical Situations, and other learning activities to help you master this chapter content.

evolve Go to your Evolve website (http://evolve.elsevier.com/Leifer/
maternity) for the following FREE learning resources:

- Animations
- Answer Guidelines for Critical Thinking Questions
- Answers and Rationales for Review Questions for the NCLEX®
  Examination
- Concept Map Creator
- Glossary with pronunciations in English and Spanish
- Patient Teaching Plans
- Skills Performance Checklists and more!

Online Resources

- www.aap.org/healthtopics/breastfeeding.cfm
- www.breastfeedingbasics.com
- www.cdc.gov/breastfeeding
- www.educationupdate.com/archives/2005/June/html/Med-Omega.html
- www.lalecheleague.org
- www.nlm.nih.gov/medlineplus/breastfeeding.html

Review Questions for the NCLEX® Examination

1. A new mother asks the nurse how many more calories she
   requires each day than in her pre-pregnant diet while
   breastfeeding her newborn. The nurse correctly responds:
   1. 300 calories each day
   2. 500 calories each day
   3. 1000 calories each day
   4. 1500 calories each day

2. The component in breast milk that helps the newborn
   digest fat is:
   1. Lipase
   2. Fluoride
   3. Lactoferrin
   4. Immunoglobulin A

3. The average time for breastfeeding is:
   1. 5 to 10 minutes per breast
   2. 10 to 15 minutes per breast
   3. 15 to 20 minutes per breast
   4. 20 to 30 minutes per breast

4. Which position for breastfeeding a newborn in the
   immediate postpartum period would be the most
   comfortable for both a patient with an episiotomy and
   a patient with an abdominal incision?
   1. Cradle hold
   2. Football hold
   3. Side-lying hold
   4. Cross-cradle hold

5. Principles of storing and freezing breast milk include:
   (Select all that apply.)
   1. Breast milk can be safely stored in glass.
   2. Breast milk can be stored in the refrigerator up to 48
      hours.
   3. Freezing breast milk can destroy some antimicrobial
      factors.
   4. Microwaving breast milk is not advised.

6. Which immunization is contraindicated for the
   breastfeeding mother?
   1. Rubella vaccine
   2. Hepatitis B vaccine
   3. Influenza vaccine
   4. Smallpox vaccine

7. If a postpartum mother informs the nurse that she has
   decided to formula-feed her newborn, which type of
   formula is the least expensive as well as easy to
   prepare?
   1. Ready-to-feed formula
   2. Concentrated liquid formula
   3. Powder formula
   4. Formulas are priced equally

8. The nurse is caring for a postpartum woman that
   follows the hot-cold theory of health and illness. Which
   food(s) would likely be included in this patient's dietary
   intake during the postpartum period? *(Select all that
   apply.)*
   1. Iced tea
   2. Chicken
   3. Honey
   4. Salad
   5. Soup

Critical Thinking Questions

1. A discharged mother, 2 days postpartum, calls the
   postpartum unit with questions about breastfeeding her
   newborn daughter. She is concerned that her baby is not
   getting enough milk because her daughter "cries a lot and
   seems hungry." The mother sounds anxious and upset.
   What would you tell her?

2. A mother is formula feeding her newborn for the first
   time and asks for a nurse to help her. Her baby has just
   spit up some formula, and she wonders what she is doing
   wrong. What questions would help you assess the
   situation?

chapter

12

Postpartum Assessment and Nursing Care

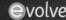volve

http://evolve.elsevier.com/Leifer/maternity

Objectives

1. Define key terms listed.
2. Describe the postpartum period.
3. Explain the involution of the uterus, and describe changes in the fundal position.
4. Explain the cause of afterpains.
5. Distinguish between the characteristics of lochia rubra, lochia serosa, and lochia alba.
6. Explain how to assess the postpartum woman's perineum.
7. Describe two ways in which the fluid accumulated during pregnancy is eliminated during the postpartum period.
8. Explain the importance of monitoring the vital signs during the first 24 hours postpartum.
9. List three factors that influence urinary retention after delivery.
10. Discuss three factors that contribute to postpartum constipation.
11. List two significant events that occur as a result of changes in the endocrine system.
12. Explain the factors involved in the woman's weight loss after birth.
13. Interpret Rubin's taking-in and taking-hold phases.
14. Explain the psychological alteration called *postpartum blues*.
15. Demonstrate three ways to prepare the sibling for the new family member.
16. Present two ways to encourage parent-newborn attachment.
17. Explain why early ambulation is encouraged.
18. Review the importance of Kegel (perineal tightening) exercises.
19. Describe five danger signs that the woman should report after discharge from the hospital.

Key Terms

afterpains (p. 228)
diaphoresis (dĭ-ă-fŏ-RĒ-sĭs, p. 231)
diastasis recti (dĭ-ĂS-tā-sĭs RĔK-tĭ, p. 230)
diuresis (dĭ-ŭr-Ē-sĭs, p. 231)
episiotomy (ĕ-pēz-ē-ŎT-ō-mē, p. 229)
exfoliation (ĕks-fō-lē-Ā-shŭn, p. 226)
Homans' sign (p. 230)
involution (ĭn-vō-LOO-shŭn, p. 226)
letting-go phase (p. 234)
lochia alba (LŌ-kē-ă ĂL-bă, p. 228)

(R) test!

lochia rubra (ROO-bră, p. 228)
lochia serosa (sĕr-Ō-să, p. 228)
postpartum blues (p. 234)
postpartum fatigue (p. 245)
puerperium (pū-ĕr-PĒ-rē-ŭm, p. 224)
REEDA scale (p. 229)
sitz bath (p. 241)
subinvolution (sŭb-ĭn-vō-LOO-shŭn, p. 227)
taking-hold phase (p. 234)
taking-in phase (p. 234)

The postpartum period, or puerperium, is the 6-week interval from childbirth to the return of the uterus and other organs to a prepregnant state. An arbitrary time frame divides the period into the immediate postpartum (first 24 hours), early postpartum (first week), and late postpartum (second to sixth weeks). Care during this time presents a challenge to nurses. With the short hospital stay, the time must be well planned to assist in maternal recovery, newborn care, family preparation, and intensive patient teaching. Many hospitals offer extended postpartum care by home visits, hospital outpatient clinic visits, and telephone communication to assist the woman and family during the postpartum recovery period (Clinical Pathway 12-1).

GOALS OF POSTPARTUM CARE

The main goals in postpartum care are to assist and support the woman's recovery to the prepregnant state and identify deviations from the norm; educate the mother about her own self-care, newborn feeding, and newborn care; and promote bonding between the newborn and family. During the first 1 to 2 postpartum hours (i.e., the fourth stage of

Clinical Pathway 12-1   Postpartum Care

ASSESSMENT	1–8 HOURS	8–24 HOURS	24–48 HOURS
Assessment	Assess q15 minute 1st hour; q30 minute 2nd hour then q4h: Fundus for firmness, level Lochia for color, amount, clots Bladder for voiding Perineum for sutures, bruising, hemorrhoids Breasts for softness, colostrum Vital signs (compare to baseline) Pain	Assess q4h: Fundus Breasts, nipples Newborn latch-on Colostrum Feeding technique for breast or bottle Vital signs (compare to baseline) Pain Homans' sign Bonding Perineal healing Lochia	Assess: Breasts for softness, nipples, latch-on of newborn Feeding techniques and positioning Newborn care Hand hygiene Fundus q8h Perineal state Lochia Vital signs Family interaction
Teaching	Teach fundal massage, application of perineal pads, breastfeeding techniques. Discuss afterpains and pain management. Request assistance for first ambulation. Discuss orthostatic hypotension.	Explain cord care, bulb suctioning, circumcision care, newborn feeding techniques. Advise on maternal diet. Stress need for periods of rest.	Discuss: Maternal role Perineal care Newborn feeding Maternal diet Home setting and problems Support systems Plans to resume outside work Newborn care options Family planning Return of normal bowel function and the influence of medication on constipation
Medical and nursing interventions	Administer: Straight catheterization if unable to void Medications as ordered Stool softener if ordered Hep-Lock IV when taking oral fluids	Provide as needed: RhoGAM Hematocrit test Stool softener if no bowel movement Topical analgesics for sutures Medicine for pain Lactation nurse assistance	Provide shower and assistance with ambulation. Explain information and screening tests. Give return clinic appointments for mother and newborn. Assess bowel movements and diet. Provide discharge medication for pain, stool softener, lanolin for nipples. Provide community referral to WIC program if qualified.
Discharge and follow-up plan	Discuss understanding of postpartum care and newborn care. Identify support person and culturally specific needs.	Check that birth certificate is completed. Provide referral for birth records. Discuss home care. Discuss need for follow-up care for mother and newborn. Assess bonding. Discuss role of siblings and husband or partner. Administer immunizations if needed (e.g., Rubella).	Review discharge instructions for breast care, perineal care, family planning, newborn feeding, resumption of sexual activity, postpartum exercises, diet. Provide telephone resources. Review family and support system. Provide prescriptions as needed. Give appropriate gift pack and picture of newborn, as available.

IV, intravenous; *RhoGAM,* Rh₀(D) immune globulin; *WIC,* Women, Infants, and Children.

labor), the woman is closely observed and assessed because it is a critical time to prevent the dangers of hemorrhage and hypovolemic shock. When her condition is stabilized, the woman may be moved to a postpartum unit.

To provide high-quality care, the nurse must be knowledgeable about the physical and emotional physiology of postpartum adaptation. After the initial dangers of **hemorrhage** and **shock** have passed, the primary postpartum danger is **infection.** The uterine cavity is easily accessible to microorganisms from the exterior. Also, the site where the placenta was attached is an open wound and can be easily infected.

The clinical pathway includes nursing assessments, teaching, medical and nursing interventions, discharge, and follow-up care for the postpartum woman. By indicating specific care and progress of the woman and newborn within a specified timeline that is related to a planned outcome, the nurse can clearly identify deviations from normal so they can be treated. The nurse documents the care and reports variation in progress during the postpartum period.

💬 Communication

Confirm That the Patient Understands

To verify that the woman (or family) understands what the nurse has told her, have the woman repeat the teaching in her own words. A nod may indicate courtesy, not understanding, when the primary language and culture of the nurse and family are different.

PHYSIOLOGIC CHANGES AND NURSING INTERVENTIONS

CHANGES IN THE REPRODUCTIVE SYSTEM

Involution of the Uterus

 Involution refers to the changes that the reproductive organs (particularly the uterus) undergo after birth of the newborn to return to the pre-pregnant size and condition. The process begins after the expulsion of the placenta with uterine muscle contractions. Immediately after birth, the placental site contracts to a size less than half its original diameter. During contractions, the uterine muscles act like living ligatures and compress the blood vessels, which control and reduce the amount of blood loss (Figure 12-1). A unique healing process, called *exfoliation*, enables the placental site to heal without scarring. In exfoliation, necrotic tissue is sloughed off of the superficial tissues, leaving a smooth surface of endometrial tissue. This unique reparative process ensures that future fertilized ova will implant in an unscarred uterus. Endometrial regeneration is completed within 16 days (Oats & Abraham, 2010), except for the placental site, where regeneration is not complete until 6 weeks postpartum.

The uterus undergoes a rapid reduction in size and weight. The uterus weighs approximately 1000 g (2.2 lb) immediately after birth. It decreases to 500 g (1.1 lb) during the first week and 340 g (12 oz) by 2 weeks postpartum. The rate of decrease varies with the size of the newborn and the number of previous pregnancies. The primary cause of involution is the sudden withdrawal of estrogen and progesterone, which triggers the release of proteolytic enzymes into the endometrium. This release

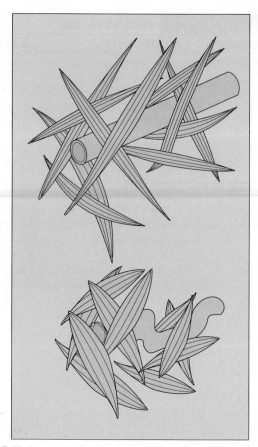

FIGURE 12-1 The uterine muscles form a "living ligature" to occlude blood vessels.

causes the protein material within the endometrial cells to be broken down into substances that can be excreted in the urine. The number of muscle cells does not change during involution, but the size of each cell is markedly reduced.

Factors that can slow uterine involution include (1) prolonged labor, (2) incomplete expulsion of placenta and membranes, (3) anesthesia, (4) previous labors, and (5) a distended (full) bladder. Factors that can enhance involution include (1) uncomplicated labor and birth, (2) breastfeeding, and (3) early, frequent ambulation.

The cervix after birth is soft. By 18 hours, it has regained its form. The cervical os (dilated to 10 cm during labor) gradually closes within 2 weeks. The external os never regains its original appearance; after childbirth, it appears as a slit instead of a circle.

Descent of the Uterine Fundus

Fundal height is measured in centimeters (or fingerbreadths) in relation to the umbilicus (Skill 12-1). It is used to assess the rate of uterine involution. The usual progression of uterine descent into the pelvis is 1 cm (about one fingerbreadth) a day. After delivery (especially when an oxytocin drug is

Skill 12-1   Assessing and Massaging the Uterine Fundus

PURPOSE
To prevent excessive postpartum bleeding.

Steps

1. Ask the woman to empty her bladder if she has not voided recently. (A full bladder contributes to uterine relaxation and subinvolution.)
2. Have the woman assume supine position with knees slightly flexed (relaxes abdominal muscles).
3. Apply a lower perineal pad, and observe lochia as fundus is palpated.
4. Determine uterine firmness. Cup one hand above the symphysis pubis to support the lower uterine segment; with the other hand, palpate abdomen until top of fundus is located. Determine whether firm (if not, massage lightly until firm).
5. Determine height of fundus. Measure height of top of fundus in fingerbreadths above, below, or at umbilicus.

6. Determine whether fundus is in midline (deviation typically indicates full bladder). Observe for firmness of fundus.
7. If the fundus is not firm, massage the fundus in a circular motion with the flat surface of the fingers of the dominant hand.
8. Document the consistency and location of fundus. Consistency is recorded as "fundus firm with massage" or "fundus boggy." Record fundal height (e.g., U2 or U2 fingerbreadths below or above umbilicus).

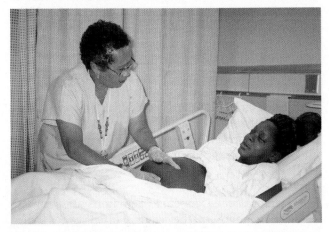

The nurse measures the fundus of the postpartum patient.

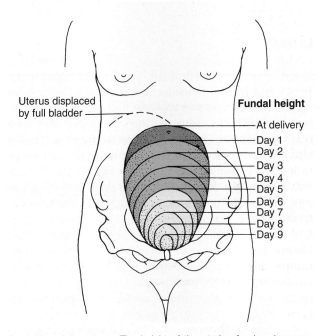

Involution of the uterus. The height of the uterine fundus decreases approximately 1 cm per day until it is no longer palpable at 10 days' postpartum.

administered after the expulsion of the placenta), the fundus of the uterus is firm and may be approximately at the level of the umbilicus or just below. Breastfeeding enhances involution because sucking stimulates the release of oxytocin from the posterior pituitary gland. The uterus is contracted to the size of a large grapefruit. By 10 days' postpartum, it should not be abdominally palpable. A full (distended) bladder can push the uterus up and cause it to deviate to one side (usually the right side) and interfere with involution. If blood clots collect within the uterus, contractions stop, and the fundus of the uterus may rise and feel soft or boggy. This atony results in increased bleeding. Massage may be needed. A uterus deviating from the midline usually requires emptying of the bladder in order for involution to continue.

At 6 weeks after delivery, the uterus is approximately pre-pregnant size. Subinvolution is the failure of the uterus to return to the pre-pregnant state and is most commonly caused by retained placental fragments.

Afterpains

Intermittent uterine contractions, which represent relaxation and contraction of the muscle fibers, cause uterine cramping and are called *afterpains*. Afterpains occur for the first 2 or 3 days' postpartum. The hormone oxytocin, released by the posterior pituitary gland, strengthens uterine contractions, compressing blood vessels and preventing excessive blood loss. If the mother breastfeeds, infant suckling stimulates oxytocin release. Therefore, the mother often notices the afterpains when she breastfeeds her newborn. Women who have had previous pregnancies often have stronger afterpains because the contraction of the uterine muscles is not sustained because of decreased muscle tone. Nonsteroidal antiinflammatory medications such as ibuprofen are more effective than acetaminophen or propoxyphene in relieving afterpains for most women (Gabbe, Niebyl, & Simpson, 2007). Ibuprofen is safe for nursing mothers (Gabbe, Niebyl, & Simpson, 2007).

Lochia

Lochia is postpartum vaginal discharge. It contains blood from the placental site, particles of necrotic decidua, and mucus. Lochia normally has a fleshy odor similar to that of menstrual flow. The quantity of lochia rapidly diminishes and becomes moderate and then scant. Lochia is the heaviest during the first 1 or 2 hours after birth. Initial lochia is bright red and commonly called lochia rubra (lasts 1 to 3 days); it may contain small clots. The vaginal flow then pales and becomes pink to brown after approximately 3 days; this is called lochia serosa. Lochia serosa should not contain clots and can last up to 27 days in some women (Gabbe, Niebyl, & Simpson, 2007). Typically, by 10 days' postpartum, the vaginal discharge often becomes yellow to white and is called lochia alba. Lochia alba may continue, on average, to the sixth week postpartum (Table 12-1).

Estimating the amount of lochial flow by observation is difficult. Many facilities use perineal pads that have cold or warm packs in them. These pads absorb less lochia, which must be considered when estimating the amount of blood loss. If a mother has excessive lochia, a clean pad should be applied and checked within 15 minutes. The number of perineal pads applied during a given period should be counted or the pads weighed to help determine the amount of vaginal discharge. One gram of weight equals 1 mL of blood. In addition, the woman's fundus should be checked for firmness. Nurses often estimate the amount of lochia in terms of the approximate size of the area soiled in 1 hour (Skill 12-2).

The amount of lochia is less after a cesarean birth. Breastfeeding or the use of oral contraceptives does not affect lochial flow. Lochia is briefly heavier when the mother ambulates because blood that has pooled in her vagina is discharged when she assumes an upright position. The gush of blood can be anxiety provoking to the woman and should not be confused with a postpartum hemorrhage. Excessive lochia rubra early in the postpartum period may suggest bleeding as a result of retained fragments of the placenta or membranes. Recurrence of bleeding in 7 to 10 days after birth suggests bleeding from the placenta site but may be the result of normal sloughing (Gabbe, Niebyl, & Simpson, 2007). After 3 to 4 weeks, late bleeding may also be caused by infection or subinvolution. Continued lochia serosa or alba suggests infection (endometritis) and is often accompanied by fever, pain, or abdominal tenderness and an offensive, foul odor to the lochia. Any abnormal lochia pattern should be documented and reported. Ultrasound is one of the diagnostic methods that can be used to confirm the cause of postpartum bleeding.

Assessment of uterine firmness, location, and position in relation to the midline (see Skill 12-1) is performed at routine intervals. A poorly contracted (soft, boggy) uterus should be massaged until firm to prevent hemorrhage. It is essential not to push down on an uncontracted uterus to avoid inverting it.

Vagina

The vagina usually appears edematous and bruised, and the opening in the vagina often gapes when intraabdominal pressure is increased, such as by

Table 12-1	Normal and Abnormal Characteristics of Lochia			
LOCHIA TYPE	**TIME**	**NORMAL LOCHIA**		**ABNORMAL LOCHIA**
Lochia rubra	Days 1-3	Bright red, bloody consistency; fleshy odor; temporary increase during breastfeeding and on rising		Numerous large clots; foul smell; saturation of perineal pad in 1 hour or less
Lochia serosa	Usually days 4-9 (can last to 27 days)	Pinkish brown; serosanguineous consistency		Foul smell; saturation of perineal pad in 1 hour or less
Lochia alba	Day 10 to approximately sixth week	Creamy white; fleshy odor		Foul smell; persistent lochial discharge over 3 weeks; return to pink or red discharge

Skill 12-2   Assessing Lochia

PURPOSE

To determine normal progress of the postpartum period.

Steps

1. Assess lochia for quantity. A guideline to estimate and document the amount of flow on the menstrual pad in 1 hour is as follows (see illustration):
   a. **Scant:** less than a 2-inch (5-cm) stain
   b. **Light:** less than a 4-inch (10-cm) stain
   c. **Moderate**: less than a 6-inch (15-cm) stain
   d. **Large** or heavy: larger than a 6-inch stain or one pad saturated within 2 hours
   e. **Excessive**: saturation of a perineal pad within 15 minutes
2. Assess lochia for type and characteristics. In first 3 days, normal lochia has fleshy odor with small clots with red or reddish brown color. Abnormal lochia has foul odor, large clots, and saturated pad with bright red color.

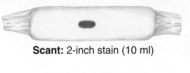
Scant: 2-inch stain (10 ml)

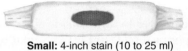
Small: 4-inch stain (10 to 25 ml)

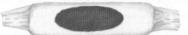
Moderate: 6-inch stain (25 to 50 ml)

Large: >6-inch stain (50 to 80 ml)

Estimating the volume of lochia on the perineal pad. Different brands of peripads absorb in different patterns. The nurse should be familiar with the pattern of the peripad used at the facility to standardize documentation.

coughing. By the third postpartum week, the vagina resumes the appearance of the pre-pregnant state, with some relaxation of tissue. The rugae, or vaginal folds, disappear during pregnancy, and the walls of the vagina become smooth. The rugae reappear within 3 weeks postpartum. Within 6 weeks, the vagina has almost regained its pre-pregnancy form. Breastfeeding mothers, in particular, may have vaginal dryness and discomfort during sexual intercourse. A water-soluble vaginal lubricant such as K-Y Jelly makes intercourse more comfortable. Dryness usually disappears when ovulation and menstruation return.

Perineum

The perineum has been stretched and thinned to accommodate the size of the newborn. The pelvic floor muscles are overstretched and weak. The appearance of the perineum varies greatly, depending on the type and extent of the laceration(s) or episiotomy (cut in the perineum). The soft tissues of the perineum are often edematous and bruised.

The nurse puts on clean gloves before assessing the perineum to prevent contact with vaginal blood flow. The perineum is assessed for the type and amount of vaginal discharge, unusual swelling, discoloration, healing of the tissues, and discomfort (Skill 12-3). If an episiotomy was performed, the state of healing is

assessed by the REEDA scale, a mnemonic for *Redness*, *Edema*, *Ecchymosis* (bruising), *Discharge*, and *Approximation* of the wound. Foul odor accompanied by drainage indicates infection; further examination of the incision and area of warmth and tenderness should be performed. Hemorrhoids, if present, are assessed for size, number, and discomfort. During the assessment, the nurse asks the woman about relief obtained from comfort measures (sitz bath, warm or cold applications, and medications). The nurse should record his or her findings.

Studies have shown a positive response to cold sitz baths (Gabbe, Niebyl, & Simpson, 2007). Occasionally, the cause of perineal pain is prolapsed hemorrhoids. Witch-hazel pads, astringent pads, suppositories, or local anesthetic sprays are helpful. Healing usually takes place within 6 weeks. Daily perineal care is described in Skill 12-4.

CHANGES IN THE MUSCULOSKELETAL SYSTEM

Muscles and Joints

During the first few days, levels of the hormone **relaxin** decrease and ligaments and cartilage of the pelvis begin to return to the pre-pregnancy state. With the delivery of the placenta, the effect of **progesterone** on muscle tone is removed. Therefore, muscle tone begins to be restored throughout the body. In particular, the

discoloration = blueish & numbness = inform physician.

Skill 12-3   Assessing the Perineum

PURPOSE

To observe perineal trauma, hemorrhoids, and status of healing.

Steps

1. Ask the mother to turn on side and flex upper leg, lower perineal pad, and lift up upper buttock; if necessary, use flashlight to inspect perineum.
2. Observe for edema, bruising, and hematoma.
3. Examine episiotomy or laceration for REEDA (*R*edness, *E*dema, *E*cchymosis, *D*ischarge, and *A*pproximation).
4. Observe hemorrhoids for extent of edema (can interfere with bowel elimination).
5. Apply clean peripad.
6. Dispose of soiled contents in appropriate waste container and wash hands.
7. Document findings. Report abnormal findings.

Skill 12-4   How to Perform Perineal Care

PURPOSE

To promote healing and prevent infection.

Steps

1. Gather supplies needed, such as bottle with warm water, peripad, and prescribed ointments.
2. Help the woman to bathroom.
3. Instruct the woman to wash her hands before and after perineal care.
4. Remove soiled pad from front to back; discard in waste container.
5. Squeeze peri bottle or pour warm water or cleansing solution over perineum without opening labia.
6. Pat dry with tissue. Use each tissue one time; pat from front to back, then discard tissue.
7. Apply medicated spray, ointment, or pad, as directed. Do not apply perineal pad for 1 to 2 minutes (otherwise, medication will be absorbed in pad).
8. Apply clean perineal pad from front to back, touching only sides and outside of pad to lessen risk of infection.
9. Do not flush toilet until the woman is standing upright; otherwise, the flushing water can spray on perineum.
10. Always perform perineal care after each voiding or stool, or at least every 4 hours during puerperium.
11. Report clots, increase in lochia flow, or excessive abdominal cramping.
12. Document care, findings, and teaching.

tone in the **rectus abdominis muscles** and the pubococcygeal muscle is restored. The abdominal muscles, including the rectus abdominis muscles, may be separated, and **diastasis recti** can occur (Figure 12-2). Special exercises can strengthen the abdominal wall. Women need to be advised that with proper diet, exercise, and rest, the abdominal muscle tone is usually regained more rapidly. Good body mechanics and correct posture are important to help relieve low back pain. Kegel exercises help the pubococcygeal muscle (muscle that aids bowel and bladder control) to regain normal function (see Chapter 5).

A generalized decrease in bone mineralization occurs after birth. This bone loss is not affected by calcium intake or exercise but returns to normal within 18 months (Gabbe, Niebyl, & Simpson, 2007).

Lower Extremities

Venous stasis, particularly during the later part of pregnancy, contributes to the risk of blood clots (thrombosis) forming in the lower extremities. By passively dorsiflexing the woman's feet, the nurse determines whether there is pain in the calf (a positive **Homans' sign**) (Figure 12-3). This may be an early sign of venous thrombosis and should be reported. In addition, the nurse inspects the legs for redness, swelling, and warmth.

CHANGES IN THE CARDIOVASCULAR SYSTEM

Dramatic changes to the maternal cardiovascular system occur in the postpartum period. During pregnancy, an approximately 50% increase in circulating blood volume occurs (hypervolemia), which allows the woman to tolerate considerable blood loss at birth

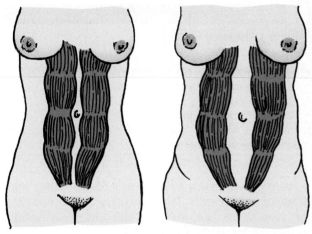

FIGURE 12-2 Diastasis recti occurs when the longitudinal muscles of the abdomen separate during pregnancy.

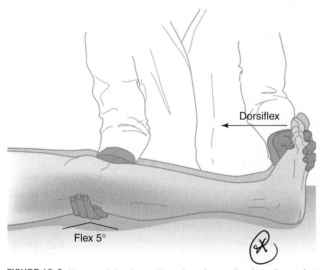

Dorsiflex

Flex 5°

FIGURE 12-3 Homans' sign is positive when the mother has discomfort on sharp dorsiflexion of the foot. A positive Homans' sign should be promptly reported.

without adverse effects. Many women lose at least 200 to 500 mL of blood during vaginal births and approximately twice as much during cesarean births. Readjustments in the maternal vasculature after childbirth are rapid. During postpartum adaptation, dramatic and immediate changes take place in the circulating blood volume that prevent hypovolemia from normal blood loss during delivery. These changes include (1) elimination of the placenta, which diverts 500 to 750 mL of blood flow into the maternal systemic circulation; (2) rapid reduction of the size of the uterus, which puts more blood in the systemic circulation; (3) increase of blood flow to the vena cava from elimination of compression by the gravid uterus; and (4) mobilization of body fluids accumulated during pregnancy. Cardiac output may remain increased for 1 year or more (Gabbe, Niebyl, & Simpson, 2007). A healthy woman's body can make these changes, but a woman with a heart disorder can encounter problems.

Excess blood volume, which is necessary during pregnancy, is removed to help the woman's body return to the pre-pregnant state. This excess is disposed of in two ways: (1) diuresis (increased excretion of urine), in which a daily urinary output can be as much as 3000 mL; and (2) diaphoresis (profuse perspiration).

Blood Values

During the first 72 hours after childbirth, the loss in plasma volume is greater than that in the number of red blood cells (RBCs). This results in a temporary rise in the hematocrit and hemoglobin levels. Any excess will gradually disappear in accordance with the RBC life span. The normal levels are achieved within 2 to 4 weeks' postpartum. The excess body fluids are excreted by the kidneys, which cause a marked increase in daily urinary output. **Leukocytosis,** an increase in the white blood cell count to 15,000/mm^3 or more, occurs immediately after birth in women without infection; the levels return to normal within 10 days.

WBC will be elevated up to ten days post. partum

Blood Coagulation

Blood clotting factors that increased during pregnancy tend to remain elevated during the initial postpartum period. Fibrinogen levels may return to normal within 2 weeks of delivery. This fact, along with trauma, immobility, and infection, predisposes the woman to the development of a **thromboembolism** (one of the leading causes of maternal death is an embolus or thrombus). To decrease this risk, early and frequent ambulation is essential. Dyspnea (difficulty breathing) and tachypnea (rapid breathing) are hallmark signs of pulmonary embolus and require immediate medical intervention.

Varicose veins that have developed during pregnancy usually diminish during the puerperium because the venous stasis that was caused by the gravid uterine compression (pressure of the uterus on pelvic blood vessels) decreases. In addition, progesterone level is decreased, which during pregnancy is largely responsible for a decrease in smooth muscle tone.

Orthostatic Hypotension

Resistance to the blood flow in the vessels of the pelvis decreases after birth. As a result, the woman's blood pressure falls when she sits upright or stands, and she may complain of feeling dizzy, lightheaded, or faint. Guidance and assistance are needed during early ambulation to prevent injury.

Postpartum Diaphoresis

Diaphoresis (perspiration) is the elimination of excess fluid through the skin. It is the body's way of getting rid of excess fluid accumulated during pregnancy. Profuse diaphoresis (excessive sweating) often occurs at night. This adjustment has implications for nursing care. Showers, frequent changes of clothing, and adequate fluid intake are important for the woman's comfort.

VITAL SIGNS

Temperature

The woman's temperature during the first 24 hours after delivery may rise to 38° C (100.4° F) as a result of the dehydration and exertion of labor. After the first 24 hours, the woman should be **afebrile,** and any temperature greater than 38° C suggests infection. An elevated temperature that persists longer than 24 hours or that exceeds 38° C should be reported to the physician or nurse-midwife. A short-term elevation on the second or third postpartum day can occur as a result of breast engorgement.

Pulse

The heart rate often decreases to a rate of 50 to 60 beats/min (**bradycardia,** or slow pulse) for the first 6 to 8 days' postpartum. An elevated heart rate may indicate undue blood loss, infection, pain, anxiety, or cardiac disease.

Blood Pressure

Blood pressure readings should remain stable after birth. A decrease in blood pressure may be related to excessive blood loss. Blood pressure elevation—especially when accompanied by a headache—suggests gestational hypertension and indicates the need for further evaluation (see Chapter 13).

CHANGES IN THE URINARY SYSTEM

The **bladder** of the postpartum woman has increased in capacity and has lost some of its muscle tone. In addition, during the birth, the urethra, bladder, and tissue around the urinary meatus may become edematous and traumatized. Urination is also impeded by anesthetic drugs. The diminished awareness of the need to urinate may result in decreased sensitivity to fluid pressure, and the woman may not feel an urge to void. This is important to remember because the bladder fills rapidly as a result of intravenous fluids administered during labor and after birth. With bladder distention, the uterus is displaced (often over to one side, usually the right) and has a reduced ability to contract. When the uterus fails to contract, blood vessels are free to bleed. Therefore, it is important that the nurse monitor the woman for voiding. The urinary output in the early postpartum period can be great (diuresis). Tenderness over the costovertebral angle, fever, urinary retention, and dysuria with urinary frequency signify potential urinary infection, and further evaluation is necessary. Glomerular filtration may remain elevated for up to 8 weeks postpartum.

Safety Alert

Signs of a Distended Bladder

- Fundus above umbilicus or above baseline level
- Fundus over to side, displaced from midline
- Bulge of bladder above symphysis pubis
- Excessive lochia
- Tenderness over bladder area
- Frequent voidings of less than 150 mL of urine, indicating urinary retention with overflow

Mild proteinuria may occur as a result of the breakdown of uterine cells. The urine may also test positive for acetone or ketones from dehydration during a prolonged labor. Lactosuria may occur in breastfeeding women as a result of the lactation process. Normal status returns by 4 weeks' postpartum. The following measures may help a woman urinate:

- Provide privacy (but monitor woman for safety).
- Run water in the sink.
- Have woman use peri bottle to squirt warm water over the perineal area to aid in relaxing the sphincter (be sure to measure the water used so that urinary output can be accurately documented).

CHANGES IN THE GASTROINTESTINAL SYSTEM

The woman is frequently hungry and thirsty after the birth of her newborn because of energy expended and the long period of fluid or food restriction during labor. The woman is typically offered solid food after she has shown she can tolerate liquids. Constipation may occur during the postpartum period for the following reasons: (1) decreased peristalsis caused by the lingering relaxing effects of progesterone; (2) stretched abdominal muscles, making it more difficult to bear down to expel the stool; (3) limited food and fluid intake; (4) soreness and swelling of the perineum and hemorrhoids; and (5) fear of pain. If an episiotomy were performed, a stool softener such as Docusate sodium or a gentle laxative such as MiraLAX would be prescribed to avoid the discomfort of straining. A bowel movement is expected within 3 days after delivery.

Nutrition is important for the woman's gastrointestinal tract to function properly. The woman should be encouraged to eat three well-balanced meals and maintain adequate calcium and phosphorus intake if she is breastfeeding. A high-fluid and high-fiber intake is recommended to reduce constipation. While breastfeeding, she is advised to increase her caloric intake by 500 calories per day above the pre-pregnancy requirements. In addition, she is encouraged to increase her daily fluid intake to increase her milk supply.

The hospital's dietitian is consulted to manage cultural aspects of postpartum nutrition. Laboratory values are often determined at the 2- or 6-week postpartum examination to detect whether anemia has persisted or developed.

CHANGES IN THE NERVOUS SYSTEM

Neurologic changes during the postpartum period result from a reversal of maternal adaptations to pregnancy and trauma from the birth process.

Elimination of physiologic edema through diuresis that follows childbirth relieves carpal tunnel syndrome by easing the compression on the median nerves in the wrists. Headaches require careful assessment because gestational hypertension can continue to cause headaches in the postpartum period.

CHANGES IN THE INTEGUMENTARY SYSTEM

During pregnancy, many skin changes occur as a result of an increase in hormones. After childbirth, the skin gradually reverts to the pre-pregnancy state. The melanocyte-stimulating hormone (MSH) levels, which cause hyperpigmentation during pregnancy, decrease rapidly after childbirth. This is particularly noticeable when the mask of pregnancy (chloasma) and linea nigra disappear. Also, spider nevi and palmar erythema that develop as the result of increased estrogen levels gradually disappear. **Striae gravidarum** (stretch marks), which develop on the abdomen, thighs, and breasts, gradually fade to become less noticeable silvery lines but do not disappear completely. Hair growth slows, and some hair loss may be experienced in the first months after delivery, but it typically returns to normal without intervention.

CHANGES IN THE ENDOCRINE SYSTEM

After the expulsion of the placenta, estrogen and progesterone levels decrease. If the mother is bottle feeding, estrogen levels begin to rise to follicular levels approximately 3 weeks after delivery, which allow the return of menses. Often the first menses is anovulatory. Return to pre-pregnancy levels of estrogen and progesterone is slower in breastfeeding women. Lactation is initiated as levels of prolactin increase, and, with increased breastfeeding, the prolactin level rises further. In nonlactating women, the prolactin level declines and reaches the pre-pregnancy level by 14 days' postpartum. The dramatic change (drastic drop in hormones) in the endocrine system allows two significant events to occur: lactation (milk secretion) begins with the newborn suckling, and the menstrual cycle function returns.

Lactation (the secretion of milk) is the end result of many interacting factors (see Chapter 11). After delivery, estrogen, progesterone, and human placental lactogen (hPL) (all prolactin-inhibiting agents) decrease rapidly, causing a brisk increase in prolactin secretion. Once lactation has been established, suckling is the most important stimulus for the maintenance of milk production and ejection. **Prolactin,** secreted by the anterior pituitary gland, promotes milk production by stimulating the alveolar cells of the breast, and **oxytocin,** secreted by the posterior pituitary, triggers the ejection of milk as the newborn sucks. Oxytocin also stimulates uterine contractions (afterpains) felt by the mother.

By the third day after delivery, the prolactin effect on the breast tissue is evident, and the hormone is present in sufficient quantity to cause breast engorgement. The breasts become distended, firm, tender, and warm. At this time, milk, which is thin and bluish, begins to replace the colostrum (premilk).

If the woman does not wish to breastfeed her newborn, she should avoid any breast stimulation, including newborn suckling, pumping the breasts, or allowing warm water to flow on the breasts during showers. Prolactin levels drop rapidly. Palpation of the breast on the second or third day will likely reveal **engorgement.** The breasts become distended (swollen), firm, tender, and warm to touch (due to vasocongestion). Breast engorgement is primarily caused by the temporary congestion of veins and lymphatics rather than by an accumulation of milk. Engorgement spontaneously resolves, and discomfort usually decreases within 24 to 36 hours. A snug, supportive bra worn for 72 hours, ice packs, and mild analgesics may be used to relieve breast discomfort. If suckling has never begun and nipple stimulation is avoided, lactation ceases within a few days to a week. Breastfeeding is discussed in detail in Chapter 11.

Resumption of Ovulation and Menstruation

Most nonlactating mothers resume menstruation within 3 months after childbirth. Breastfeeding delays the return of ovulation and menstruation. Ovulation may return within 1 month in nonlactating women and up to 6 months in lactating women. Many lactating women resume menstruation within 6 months, although some do not menstruate as long as they nurse their newborns at least 10 to 12 times in a 24-hour period. The first menstrual flow is often greater than normal for both nursing and non-nursing mothers. The woman should be advised that it is possible to ovulate and become pregnant before her menstrual periods are established. In other words, breastfeeding is not an effective contraception method. The woman should be encouraged to discuss family planning with her health care provider.

WEIGHT LOSS

Immediately after delivery, the woman's weight decreases by approximately 4.5 to 5.8 kg (10 to 13 lbs). This weight loss is accounted for by the removal of the fetus, placenta, and amniotic fluid. An additional 2.3 to 3.6 kg (5 to 8 lbs) are lost during the early postpartum period as a result of diuresis and diaphoresis. An additional 0.9 to 1.4 kg (2 to 3 lbs) is lost via lochia and involution in the first week postpartum (Blackburn, 2007).

During pregnancy, the woman's body stores 2.3 to 3.2 kg (5 to 7 lbs) of fat for lactation needs. The breastfeeding mother gradually uses this fat store over the first 6 months, and she often returns to her approximate pre-pregnancy weight. Some women tend to retain some of the excess weight gained during pregnancy. Therefore, women are encouraged to perform postpartum exercises to lose the excess weight gained during pregnancy and to increase the strength and tone of various muscles in their bodies. Aerobic exercise has no adverse effects on breastfeeding (Gabbe, Niebyl, & Simpson, 2007).

PSYCHOLOGICAL CHANGES AND NURSING INTERVENTIONS

Mood swings are common during the postpartum period. The rapid decline of hormones such as progesterone and estrogen is believed to contribute to the emotional upset. Other factors related to emotional reactions are conflict about the maternal role and personal insecurity. Women who have economic or family problems usually demonstrate more stress in response to motherhood. In addition, past fetal losses or pregnancy failures contribute to postpartum emotional problems. Physical discomforts such as a painful perineum, afterpains, breast engorgement, and fatigue all contribute to negative postpartum reactions and should be promptly managed to promote comfort in the postpartum phase.

PHASES OF MATERNAL ADAPTATION

Maternal adaptation has been described by Rubin (1984) as a series of three phases (Box 12-1). The taking-in phase begins immediately after birth and lasts for a few hours to approximately 2 days' postpartum. This phase is characterized by passive, dependent behavior. The woman focuses on her own needs and is concerned about the overall health of her newborn. The mother often repeatedly reviews her labor and birth experience.

The taking-hold phase is the second maternal phase, when the woman is ready to assert her independence. She becomes the initiator and is ready to participate independently in newborn care. She often becomes exhausted in her new role and verbalizes anxiety about it.

The third stage is the letting-go phase. In this stage, the woman assumes her position in the home and her new maternal role. Sometimes, demands placed on her may lead to feelings of mild depression.

ATTAINMENT OF THE MATERNAL ROLE

Maternal role attainment is the process by which the woman learns mothering behaviors and becomes comfortable with her identity as a mother. As the bond between the newborn and mother forms, the mother and newborn grow to know each other.

Box 12-1   Phases of Postpartum Adaptation

Phase 1: Taking in. Mother is passive and willing to let others do for her. Conversation centers on her birth experience. Mother has great interest in her infant but is willing to let others handle the care and has little interest in learning. Primary focus is on recovery from birth and her need for food, fluids, and deep restorative sleep.

Phase 2: Taking hold. Mother begins to initiate action and becomes interested in caring for the infant. She becomes critical of her "performance." She has increased concern about her body's functions and assumes responsibility for self-care needs. This phase is ideal for teaching.

Phase 3: Letting go. Mothers, and often fathers or partners, work through giving up their previous lifestyle and family arrangements to incorporate the new infant. Many mothers must give up their ideal of their birth experience and reconcile it with what really occurred. They give up the fantasy child so they can accept the real child.

Adapted from Rubin, R. (1984). *Maternal identity and the maternal experience.* New York: Springer.

Maternal role attainment occurs in four stages. These four stages correspond to those identified by Rubin (1984). In the **anticipatory stage,** which occurs during pregnancy, the woman looks to role models of how to be a mother. In the **formal stage,** which begins when the newborn is born, the mother is still influenced by the guidance of others. The **informal stage** begins when the mother starts to make her own choices about mothering, and she begins to find her own style. In the **personal stage,** the mother does what she is comfortable with in the role of mother. This stage occurs from 3 to 10 months after delivery. Social support, the mother's age, her personality traits, and her socioeconomic status all influence her success in assuming the mothering role.

The transition to motherhood is a complex behavioral process. Today's new mothers tend to be less dependent and are better able to assume the self-care responsibilities because of factors such as the reduced amount of medications received during labor, early ambulation, rooming-in, and increased support from the father, significant other, or family.

Parents who are ill-prepared for the changes in relationships, lifestyle, and roles associated with the integration of the newborn in the family have more difficulty making the necessary transition. The woman's immaturity, minimum exposure of the mother to the baby in the days after birth, lack of a support system, or ill health also can interfere with maternal role attainment.

POSTPARTUM BLUES

Postpartum blues occur in approximately 70% of women during the first few days after birth and generally last up to 10 days. This state is characterized by tearfulness, insomnia, lack of appetite, and a feeling of being disappointed. Psychological adjustments and hormonal factors are thought to contribute, and discomfort, anxiety, anger, and fatigue seem to play a part. There is no obstetric, social, personality, or economic factor that predisposes a woman to developing postpartum blues. It is possible that altered function of central neurotransmitters and hypothalamic-pituitary-thyroid interaction may be involved. However, rapid role changes and new responsibilities play a major role (Gabbe, Niebyl, & Simpson, 2007). Rest, empathy, and supportive care are the primary management strategies (Table 12-2). Teaching relaxation techniques,

Table 12-2	How to Develop an Individualized Postpartum Blues and Depression Care Map

Step 1: List all findings in data collection concerning patient assessment.
Step 2: From the patient data collection, choose an appropriate NANDA-I diagnosis.
Step 3: Code each of the assessment findings: *A* = requires ongoing assessment;
                T = requires teaching;
                I = requires intervention.
Step 4: Develop appropriate actions.

FINDINGS	INTERVENTIONS
Physiologic Factors	
Hormonal changes *(T)*	Teach that hormonal changes can result in negative feelings.
Fatigue from long labor and newborn feeding schedule *(I)*	Provide rest periods; use nursery at night and as needed.
Alteration in comfort *(I)*	Provide comfort measures: analgesics, positioning, ice packs, etc.
Vital signs within normal limits *(A)* Moderate lochia rubra with firm fundus at umbilicus at midline *(A)* Voiding without difficulty *(A)*	
Breastfeeding ineffective because of poor latch-on *(I, T)*	Teach proper breastfeeding techniques, assist with breastfeeding as needed, and refer to lactation consultant.
Individual Sociocultural Factors	
No extended family close by *(I)* Decreased social support because of recent relocation *(I)* Supportive husband or partner Economically stable	Encourage frequent contact with family by phone and e-mail. Provide information on community programs, parenting classes, and support groups.
Individual Spiritual Factors	
States, "If I had faith in God, I wouldn't feel this way" *(I)*	Make a referral to have hospital chaplain visit.
States she believes in God but feels disconnected from fellow believers because of not deciding on a church to join since move *(I)*	Provide a list of local places of worship.
Nursing diagnosis: *Ineffective individual coping* related to effects of postpartum blues or depression	
Developmental Factors	
Assuming new role of mother *(I)*	Encourage positive bonding behaviors through teaching and positive reinforcement
Identifying newborn as separate being *(I)*	Demonstrate normal newborn care. Encourage patient to verbalize feelings and concerns regarding new role. Encourage patient to ask questions. Let patient know that bonding occurs over time and may not be immediate. Encourage active participation in caring for newborn and provide positive reinforcement
Individual Psychological Factors	
Expressing feelings of being "down" *(A)* Frequent crying *(A)*	At each contact, determine and document mood (facial expressions, actions, verbal statements).
Verbalizes guilt about not being "happy" *(A)*	Encourage patient to share feelings regarding parenting role and newborn by using active listening techniques.

Continued

Table 12-2	How to Develop an Individualized Postpartum Blues and Depression Care Map—cont'd	
FINDINGS	**INTERVENTIONS**
Individual Psychological Factors—cont'd	
Flat affect (A)	Encourage patient to describe how she is feeling and how long she has had these feelings to rule out long-term depression that may need more immediate and more intense interventions.* If symptoms of depression are present, report to charge nurse or physician.
Withdrawn (A, T, I)	Encourage patient to share concerns, correct any misconceptions, and provide interventions needed to alleviate said concerns.
Expresses feelings of inadequacy (A, I)	Teach patient that new mothers often have feelings of inadequacy when adapting to new role.
Methodically cares for newborn without signs of positive bonding behaviors (A, I)	At each contact, assess and document bonding behaviors.
Anxiety from ineffective breastfeeding and feelings of not being able to care for newborn (A, T, I)	Teach patient that postpartum blues affects up to 80% of new mothers. Teach patient that postpartum blues is a self-limiting condition and should resolve within 2 weeks. Teach patient that if postpartum blues lasts longer than 2 weeks or if she has feelings of wanting to harm herself or others, she should contact her physician immediately.* Explore coping mechanisms that have been helpful to the patient in the past, and encourage her to use these. Explain what postpartum blues is to husband or partner and ways to be supportive during this time. Teach signs and symptoms of depression. Refer to support group or obtain social service consult.

*Long-term depression and postpartum depression may require psychotherapy, antidepressants, or inpatient psychological treatment.

increasing confidence in self-care and newborn care, and promoting communication between the woman and her partner are essential nursing responsibilities. Postpartum support groups may be available in the community. Postpartum depression is discussed in Chapter 17.

Providing support, anticipatory guidance, and reassurance that her feelings are experienced by many mothers is helpful. If the woman continues to feel depressed or has intense mood swings, further evaluation by the health care provider is necessary.

CARE MANAGEMENT AFTER DELIVERY

Nursing assessment during the first 1- to 2-hour recovery period requires close monitoring every 15 minutes for vital signs (blood pressure, pulse, and respirations), fundal location and consistency, and amount of bleeding. If the woman's status is stable, these assessments are made less frequently, usually every 30 minutes for 1 hour and then hourly for at least 2 hours. The infant may be put to the breast, and the initial parent-infant bonding process begins. After the initial 1- to 2-hour assessments, the woman who is going to the traditional postpartum unit is transferred by wheelchair or gurney to her room. In hospitals that have a labor,

delivery, recovery, and postpartum (LDRP) unit, the woman remains in the same room for the entire experience. With dyad or couplet care (the nurse cares for mother and newborn), the report is given to that nurse. In the traditional setting, an applicable report is given to a nursery nurse and a postpartum nurse. A physical assessment, including the measurement of vital signs, is performed on admission to the postpartum unit. Also at this time, the woman's knowledge level about self-care and newborn care is determined.

The care plan incorporates nursing strategies to assist the mother and family in learning about self-care and care of the newborn. The family and siblings can visit the mother and newborn while in the facility. The basics of postpartum care (e.g., perineal care) are explained. The mother is encouraged to ask questions about her and the baby's care. Nursing efforts during postpartum are directed toward the parents' knowledge, expectations, anticipatory guidance, and teaching. Discharge planning is begun by using every contact with the mother to fulfill the teaching and learning goals.

The routine physical assessment focuses on the woman's general appearance, breasts, reproductive tract, bladder and bowel elimination, and any specific physical or psychological problems.

CULTURAL CONSIDERATIONS

The nurse needs to explore cultural differences and practices concerning postpartum recovery. Cultural rituals, taboos, and traditions need to be respected. It is not uncommon for the woman to receive special foods and herbs that are believed to promote recovery. For some women, the time after childbirth (postpartum period) is a special time when others attend to their needs. For example, some groups of women from China and Southeast Asia view the first month after birth as a period for relative confinement and rest. Female family members perform the household duties and participate in the newborn's care. Rooming-in after birth may not be compatible with some cultural beliefs. In contrast, in the American culture, women often perform light tasks soon after their discharge from the hospital.

One of the most common non-Western beliefs is the humoral theory of maintaining a balance between hot and cold. Because blood is considered "hot," loss of blood during labor and delivery leaves the woman in a "cold" state, thus requiring "warm" items to restore balance, such as hot baths and warm water. In even the hottest weather, drinking ice water and staying in an air-conditioned room are rejected after birth by some cultures. In other cultures, such as Mexican American, bathing and hair washing are contraindicated for 40 days after delivery. Therefore, the new mother may refuse to shower the day after giving birth. This 40-day period corresponds somewhat to the modified activity recommended in traditional Western medicine. Non-Western health care practices may also have rituals related to the disposal of the umbilical cord and placenta.

Birth control practices vary among cultures and must be considered when discussing family planning. The nurse must be sensitive to the various practices and recognize that some women may feel distressed when they are told to ambulate early and participate in newborn and self-care activities. The nurse should incorporate cultural practices of the patient in the care plan (Nursing Care Plan 12-1).

 Nursing Care Plan 12-1 | **Cultural Considerations for Postpartum Care**

Scenario

A mother is 1 day postpartum. She does not speak English well and appears anxious. When encouraged by the nurse to ambulate and shower, the woman cries.

Selected Nursing Diagnosis

Decisional conflict related to desire to please health care workers and desire to engage in cultural rituals and practice

Expected Outcomes	Nursing Interventions	Rationales
Patient will participate with nurse in developing a culturally congruent individualized plan for obstetric care.	Assess cultural rituals and practices that are important to the patient by interview, with an interpreter if necessary or with a birth plan questionnaire.	Information obtained aids in the development of a culturally congruent individualized care plan.
	Provide a warm, friendly environment.	Relieves anxiety and conveys a message of acceptance.
Patient will freely verbalize her desires when asked to participate in culturally incongruent practices.	Explain to patient that she has the right to verbalize any disagreement with the way care is being delivered and to request that the care include culturally specific rituals and practices.	Patient and support persons are more likely to disagree and make requests when they are informed it is acceptable to do so.
	Allow patient to engage in cultural rituals or practices whenever it is medically safe to do so.	Allowing patient to engage in activities can be comforting and can enhance coping abilities.
Patient will express satisfaction with the care received during her hospitalization.	Whenever possible, provide choices to patient (e.g., "Would you like to take a shower now or would you prefer to wait?").	Allows patient to choose culturally acceptable ways of doing things without feeling like she is being disrespectful to health care providers.

Selected Nursing Diagnosis

Impaired verbal communication related to effects of language barrier

Expected Outcomes	Nursing Interventions	Rationales
Patient and support persons will have all essential information communicated to them in a manner they can understand.	Whenever possible, assign a nurse who speaks the same language as the patient.	Allows direct communication between nurse and patient.
	Obtain an interpreter or use a support person. If patient feels uncomfortable answering questions when using an interpreter who knows her, provide a hospital interpreter and inform the patient that all information will be kept confidential.	Ensures that correct information is obtained and conveyed.

Continued

Expected Outcomes	Nursing Interventions	Rationales
	Ask permission to use the support person or family member to interpret. Inform patient that she has the right to refuse to answer any question when she does not want the interpreter to know the answer.	Patients have a right to privacy regarding health care matters, so they need to give permission for information to be shared with someone they know. Persons in some cultures believe they must answer all questions to maintain respect, so they need to be told it is acceptable to keep information confidential.
	Ask permission before using children to interpret and use only if another interpreter is not available.	In some cultures, it is not acceptable for children to know more than their parents.
	Obtain hospital interpreters as needed (preferably a woman); inform patient that all information will remain confidential.	When patients feel uncomfortable discussing health care information with support persons, or when support persons do not speak the dominant language, a hospital interpreter is needed to translate information. Most women prefer to discuss intimate matters with other women.
	In the absence of an interpreter, provide a questionnaire in the patient's native language to be given on admission that includes essential assessment information that can be answered with numbers, yes/no answers, or multiple choice answers.	This can be compared with an identical questionnaire that is written in English and the dominant language of the patient to provide important assessment data that can be charted in English on the medical record.
Patient and support person will have all of their questions answered.	Assess for patient's and support person's nonverbal signs of needs or concerns.	Facial expressions or tone of voice used as the patient and support person interact can be clues that they have questions or concerns.
	Write down or memorize short yes/no questions and simple commands you can use to communicate with the patient and support person.	Allows for quick assessments to be made in the absence of an interpreter. It is important to remember that some patients may respond "yes" even when they do not understand the question; therefore, it is important to look for congruence between the verbal response and nonverbal responses or behaviors.
Health care providers will become aware of all needs of patient and support person as they arise.	Assess ability to read and provide literature to patient in her native language if appropriate.	If patient can read written information, it can be an effective way of communicating when verbal communication is impaired.
	Use pictures, diagrams, or body signals to communicate.	Can be an effective way to convey information or directions in the absence of an interpreter.

Selected Nursing Diagnosis

Fear related to unfamiliarity of the dominant culture's environment and childbirth practices

Expected Outcomes	Nursing Interventions	Rationales
Patient will freely express her feelings and concerns.	Orient patient to the environment, equipment, procedures, routines, and anticipatory guidance of what she can expect. Use interpreter as needed.	Knowledge reduces fears and can clear up misconceptions that may be contributing to fear.
Patient will verbalize and use coping strategies to alleviate fears.	Use events to identify or estimate when things will occur (e.g., before sunset, after lunch).	Many cultures rely on events rather than a clock to determine time. When patients can anticipate approximate time frames, fear and anxiety can be reduced.
	Encourage family members to visit and stay with patient.	Provides support to the patient.
Patient will state she is less afraid.	Encourage patient to express fears and concerns.	Provides the opportunity to correct misconceptions or misunderstandings.

★ Nursing Care Plan 12-1	Cultural Considerations for Postpartum Care—cont'd	
Expected Outcomes	**Nursing Interventions**	**Rationales**
	Assess childbirth and newborn cultural practices and rituals that are important to patient. Unless these practices are contraindicated or unsafe, allow patient to participate in those that are important to her.	Provides insight into cultural belief system, which can be used to individualize a care plan. Participating in cultural practices can provide feelings of security, which help alleviate fear.
	Maintain a nonjudgmental attitude toward cultural practices that are safe to implement.	Conveys feelings of acceptance and decreases patient's fears of not acting in expected manner.
	Provide scientific rationale for practices that are contraindicated or unsafe.	Knowledge allows patients to make informed decisions about adopting safer practices.
	Develop mutually acceptable compromises when cultural practices are contraindicated or unsafe.	Can increase compliance with adopting safer practices.
Patient will have relaxed facial expressions.	Provide patient and support person with frequent encouragement.	Increases patient's feelings of well-being and self-worth.

Critical Thinking Questions

1. A mother tells you that she refused to give her newborn to the technician, who wanted to bring the infant to the nursery for routine screening tests, because the technician was not wearing a name badge. How should you respond?
2. You are assigned to care for a woman who gave birth yesterday. She refuses to get out of bed or take a shower. How should you respond?

POSTPARTUM CHECK

The postpartum check, which can be remembered by the mnemonic *BUBBLE-HE,* includes assessment of the *B*reasts, *U*terus, *B*ladder, *B*owel, *L*ochia, *E*pisiotomy (perineum), *H*omans' sign, and *E*motions (psyche) (Table 12-3). The Homans' sign checks for the development of blood clots in the lower extremities. The emotional status includes bonding between parents and infant.

In addition to these specific assessments, observation and recording of vital signs, pain, hydration status, the woman's ability to ambulate, and the ability to care for her newborn should also be included. When performing the postpartum check, the nurse explains that the reason for the assessment is to rule out any deviation from normal. In addition, the nurse teaches the woman how to assess the height and firmness of the uterus (Table 12-4). Because of early discharge,

Table 12-3   Postpartum Assessment

ASSESSMENT	RECORDING
Breasts and nipples	Signs of engorgement, tenderness, lactation
Uterus	Fundal height, location, and consistency
Bladder	Output amount, frequency, and discomfort
Bowel	If or when patient had bowel movement
Lochia	Amount, color, presence of clots, and odor
Episiotomy	Edema, hematoma, signs of episiotomy or laceration healing, or signs of inflammation (REEDA scale)
Homans' sign	Edema, redness, tenderness, warmth of legs, and Homans' sign (positive or negative)
Emotional status	General attitude, sense of satisfaction, level of fatigue
Hydration	Amount of fluid intake, tissue turgor
Ambulation	If patient was dizzy or faint when up and about; frequency of ambulation
Vital signs	Temperature, pulse rate, respirations, and blood pressure
General condition	Color of skin and mucous membranes, coping ability
Pain or discomfort	Location and degree of discomfort, pain management strategies
Parenting	Mother's reaction to newborn

Table 12-4	Assessment of the Uterine Fundus	
FINDING	**CHARACTERISTIC**	**NURSING INTERVENTION**
Fundus is firmly contracted and at level of umbilicus.	Fundus feels like a hard grapefruit.	Instruct woman how to massage fundus.
Fundus is soft and boggy.	Fundus is difficult to locate and soft.	Support lower uterine. Segment and massage fundus until firm. Apply slight pressure to expel clots. Notify health care provider if fundus remains soft or if a trickle of bright red blood continues after fundus is firm.
Fundus is displaced from midline or above level of umbilicus.	Fundus may be firm but above level of umbilicus and not in midline.	Assess bladder for distention. Assist mother to void or catheterize and recheck fundus. Document findings.

the woman is encouraged to continue this assessment when at home. If the uterus appears relaxed or boggy during the assessment, the uterus should be massaged until it is firm and remains firm. When the uterus is massaged, it is important not to be too vigorous because this may cause overstimulation, which can result in uterine atony (loss of muscular tone of the uterus) and hemorrhage.

On completion of the postpartum check, the nurse documents the findings and promptly reports any abnormal findings. In addition to the usual postpartum assessments, the post-cesarean mother must also be assessed as a postoperative patient. Care of the woman after a cesarean birth is discussed in Chapter 14. Breast care and breastfeeding are discussed in Chapter 11.

AMBULATION

Early and frequent ambulation is essential to reduce the risk of infection or thrombosis (clot formation). Early ambulation also reduces the chance that respiratory, circulatory, gastrointestinal, or urinary problems will develop and promotes the rapid return of strength. The woman is advised to ask the nurse to be with her when she gets out of bed for the first time. Women who have lost a large amount of blood are more apt to feel faint because of the decrease in blood volume.

POSTPARTUM CHILL

Women often experience a shaking, uncontrollable chill immediately after birth. The exact cause is unknown, but it may be related to a nervous response or to vasomotor changes rather than the coldness of the delivery or recovery room. If the chill is not followed by an elevated temperature, it is of no clinical significance. The woman should be covered with a warm blanket or have a hot drink and be reassured that the chill is a common experience after birth. After the first 24 hours, chill and fever may indicate infection, and the woman should have further evaluation.

PROMOTING COMFORT

Most women have some degree of discomfort during the first few postpartum days. Common causes of discomfort include episiotomy, hemorrhoids, afterpains, and breast engorgement. Nursing interventions are intended to reduce the discomfort and allow the woman to take care of herself and her baby. Nonpharmacologic measures are used, either alone or in combination with pharmacologic interventions.

Nursing Interventions

Simple interventions that can decrease the discomfort associated with perineal trauma and hemorrhoids include encouraging the woman to lie on her side whenever possible and to use a pillow when sitting. Other interventions include applying an ice pack, moist or dry heat, or topical applications (if ordered); cleansing the perineum with a squeeze bottle (see Skill 12-4); and taking a warm shower or a sitz bath (Skill 12-5).

Application of Cold to the Perineum. An ice pack is often intermittently applied to the episiotomy in the first few hours after birth to reduce edema and numb the tissues, which can promote comfort. Commercial chemical ice packs are commonly used. Inexpensive ice bags can be made by filling a disposable glove with ice and then taping or securing the glove at the wrist opening to prevent water leakage as the ice melts. An ice pack is most effective during the first 24 hours after delivery.

The nurse should teach the woman about the purpose of the ice pack and its preparation at home if swelling is present. The woman is advised to cover the ice pack with a towel to prevent damage to skin integrity.

Application of Heat to the Perineum. Heat can also be used to decrease the woman's discomfort. Heat increases circulation to the perineal area and relaxes the tissues. Either moist or dry heat can be applied after the first 24 hours.

Skill 12-5   Assisting with a Sitz Bath

PURPOSE

To aid healing of perineum through application of moist heat or cold.*

Steps

1. Provide privacy.
2. Assess the woman's condition and analyze appropriateness of procedure.
3. Assemble equipment: sitz bath, clean towel, and clean perineal pad.
4. Place sitz bath on toilet seat; turn on flow of water.
5. Help the woman remove pad and sit in flow of water for 20 minutes.
6. When completed, help woman pat perineum dry; apply clean perineal pad (front to back).
7. Assist woman in returning to the room (then to the chair or bed).

8. Document that sitz bath was taken, condition of woman, and condition of perineum.

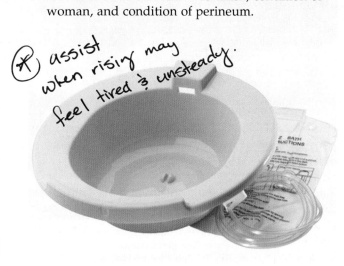

(handwritten note) ⓧ assist when rising may feel tired & unsteady.

*Cool water may reduce pain caused by edema on first day postpartum. Warm water may increase circulation and promote healing after the first day.

Sitz Bath. A sitz bath is an effective method of applying moist heat or cold to the perineum. It provides comfort, promotes healing, and reduces the incidence of infection. It is supplied as a plastic, disposable basin that fits inside the toilet. The sitz bath should not last longer than 20 minutes. Because of the soothing effect of the warm water and the sitting position, the woman may feel extremely tired and unsteady on her feet afterward and may need help getting into bed.

The nurse encourages the woman to clean a portable sitz bath basin or the tub before using it when she is home and to have the temperature of the water at approximately 38° C to 40.5° C (100° F to 105° F) when warm water is used. Cold moisture numbs nerve endings and causes vasoconstriction, which can reduce edema and hematoma. The use of a sitz bath is described in Skill 12-5.

Topical Anesthetic Application. Topical anesthetics (e.g., benzocaine [Americaine] or benzocaine and menthol [Dermoplast]) are given to relieve perineal discomfort. Sprays, dibucaine ointment, or witch hazel pads are commonly used to relieve hemorrhoidal discomfort. The woman is advised to apply the topical medication after a sitz bath or after using a heat lamp and to wait 1 to 2 minutes before applying the perineal pad, or much of the medication will be absorbed into the pad rather than stay on the perineal tissues.

FAMILY ADJUSTMENT AND DEVELOPMENT OF ATTACHMENT

PARTNER BONDING

The advancement from a generally farming society to a high-technology industrial economy has changed family and social interactions. Extended families often live far apart. Two-career families result in both partners working and both contributing to the nurturing of the family. The nurse should be sensitive to the roles of each parent, which may be nontraditional.

Responsibilities are often negotiated. The partner should be included in all teaching sessions involving newborn care and feeding. Partners often attend prenatal classes with the mother, are present at delivery as a primary coach, and must be included in follow-up care. Adaptation of the partner parallels that of the mother. Bonding actually begins prenatally when the father or partner feels the fetus move or hears the heartbeat.

Engrossment is the keen awareness and interest in the newborn, characterized by holding the newborn *en face*; studying and touching features; accepting and expressing unique resemblances of the newborn to family or themselves; and feeling pride, elation, and increased self-esteem (Figure 12-4). The reality is established when the partner participates in newborn care. A stage of conflict may follow when the partner may resent the time the mother spends focused on

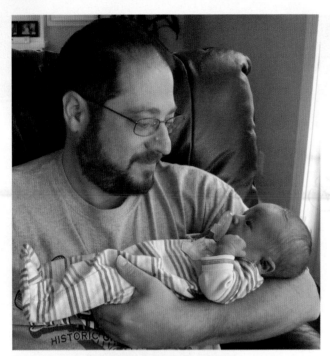

FIGURE 12-4 **Engrossment.** Intense interest in this newborn is shown as the baby is placed in the en face position (eye-to-eye contact) and unique features are studied. This helps the bonding process.

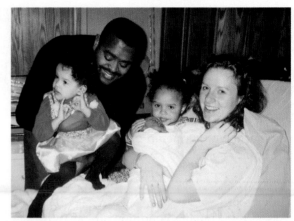

FIGURE 12-5 Siblings benefit from visiting the mother and newborn in the hospital setting. Early involvement helps in the adjustment process.

Box 12-2	Sibling Preparation for the New Family Member

- Encourage the child to feel the fetus move.
- Give simple, concise explanations about the expected baby.
- Take the child along on a prenatal visit to the clinic or physician.
- Make changes in sleeping arrangements before the birth of the baby.
- Get a special new bed for the sibling.
- Increase the father's involvement with the child (seems to be directly related to better adjustment to separation from mother and baby).
- Give a gift to the child at the time of the baby's homecoming.
- Involve the child in the baby's care whenever possible.
- Praise the child for independent activities, such as getting dressed.

the newborn; the partner may seek recognition or feel excluded. Adjustment and transition occur when the partner is able to increase interaction with the newborn and understand that there will be time set aside for partner interaction as well. Family crises can be prevented by helping the parents incorporate the newborn into their modified lifestyle and helping them communicate personal and family issues and needs. The role of siblings and grandparents may need to be reestablished. The availability of social support and community resources should be explored and telephone numbers for support and advice given to parents.

SIBLING ADJUSTMENT

Sibling response to the birth of a new sister or brother depends on their age and development. Younger siblings may consider the newborn to be competition and may fear that they will be replaced in the parents' affections. Experts believe that children benefit from seeing the mother and newborn in the hospital setting (Figure 12-5). Early involvement can help reduce the older child's anxiety, jealousy, and rivalry toward the newborn (Box 12-2). Behaviors that may surface include regression to more infantile behaviors such as thumb sucking. Some may show jealousy and frustration when they see the mother holding or feeding the newborn and miss how it feels to be the baby. Special time must be taken by both parents and grandparents to give attention to older siblings.

GRANDPARENT INVOLVEMENT

The involvement of grandparents with grandchildren depends on many factors. One of the most significant factors is proximity. Grandparents who live nearby often develop a strong attachment that involves sharing love, which adds security for the grandchildren (Figure 12-6). However, parenting practices change from one generation to the next, and this may bring conflict in child rearing. Attending classes, especially for grandparents, should be encouraged. In some cultures, the grandparents are expected to be with the new mother for the first 1 to 3 months to both help with the household duties and care for the new baby.

PROMOTING PARENT-NEWBORN BONDING

Bonding and attachment are processes that produce an affectionate and emotional commitment between two individuals. This process is intense during the early post-birth period. The newborn, when alert, is able to elicit a strong positive response from the mother

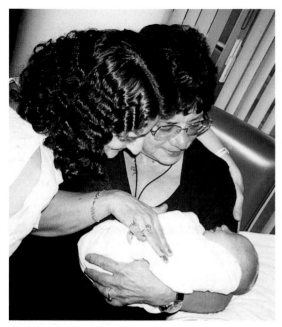

FIGURE 12-6 The daughter's arm around her mother shows how proud she is to introduce her newborn to Grandma. Grandmothers can reinforce cultural customs, help with infant care, and assist with household tasks.

by making eye contact with her. Touch is important and elicits a positive response from the mother and stimulates the newborn. Mothers are observed using a high-pitched voice as they comfort the newborn, which causes newborns to become more alert and turn toward the mother. The attachment process is usually progressive over time. It is made easier with positive newborn behaviors, such as sucking, smiling, clinging by the grasp reflex, and eye-to-eye contact. During the postpartum stay, the nurse is responsible for monitoring that attachment is developing between family members and the newborn. Promoting and facilitating parental attachment are important. The nurse must recognize that the attachment process is strengthened through the use of sensual responses between the parents and newborn. Every positive interaction between parent and newborn intensifies the attachment (Box 12-3).

Evidence-Based Practice

Signs of Positive Parent-Newborn Attachment

- Holds newborn close while feeding
- Makes eye contact with newborn
- Speaks and sings to newborn
- Identifies physical characteristics to admire about newborn
- Assigns meaning to newborn's actions such as grasp reflex ("The baby is holding my finger.")
- Identifies newborn by name
- Not upset with newborn stooling
- Strokes and massages newborn as newborn becomes quiet and relaxed

Box 12-3   Strategies for Promoting Parent-Newborn Attachment

- Encourage eye-to-eye contact. Advise parent to position newborn so they can look at each other. Optimum gazing distance for newborn is 7 to 10 inches.
- Encourage touch; parent's touch usually progresses from fingertip exploration to open palm caress; the mother may then enfold the baby in her arms; this is followed by stroking newborn, picking up newborn, and holding newborn close; the newborn will become quiet and relaxed; touch facilitates attachment.
- Encourage mother to inspect her newborn. Inspection fosters identification and allows mother to replace a fantasized newborn with a real newborn.
- Advise mother to talk about her newborn; verbalization about the newborn allows the parent to identify with the newborn ("Look, the baby has my ears.").
- Encourage cuddling the newborn; holding the newborn close and feeling the warmth initiates a positive experience for the mother; it is self-quieting and consoling to the newborn.
- Encourage care-taking activities; the mother's participation in newborn care often increases her competence and satisfaction ("I bathed our baby today.").

EARLY DISCHARGE PLANNING AND HEALTH PROMOTION

Discharge planning is especially important with the current length of hospital stay. The woman's greatest need is education to prepare her to care for herself and her newborn (Table 12-5). The woman must know how to prevent introducing infection to the still-unhealed uterus and episiotomy before discharge. She must be made aware of the danger signs and, if they occur, know to call the physician, nurse-midwife, or clinic.

Patient Teaching

Postpartum Danger Signs

After discharge, the woman should contact her physician or nurse-midwife if any of the following develops:
- Sudden persistent or spiking fever
- Change in vaginal discharge: increased amount, change to earlier color (bright red bleeding), offensive odor
- Pain or tenderness in abdomen or pelvic area
- Localized pain, redness, swelling, or warm area in calf
- Localized area of pain, redness, or swelling in breast
- Frequency, urgency, or burning on urination
- Continued postpartum depression
- Persistent perineal pain

Nursing efforts are directed toward assessing the couple's knowledge and expectations. The nurse should provide the parents with the opportunity to engage in newborn care while in the hospital to build confidence, allay fears, and ask questions. Referral

Table **12-5** **Postpartum Discharge Instructions**

KNOWLEDGE AND SKILLS	INSTRUCTIONS
Rest, sleep	Plan at least 1 rest period daily; rest when the newborn is sleeping; if you have other small children at home, explore possibility of having family member, neighbor, or community agency relieve you. Try to get a good night's sleep.
Hygiene	You can take sitz baths and showers; remember to continue to cleanse your perineum from front to back; if you had episiotomy, all stitches will be absorbed. Do not use douches until you return for your postpartum checkup.
Return to work	Avoid household tasks that require heavy lifting for at least 3 weeks after birth. You are encouraged not to return to an outside job for at least 3 weeks (6 weeks is better), not only for your health, but also to enjoy and bond with the baby.
Exercise and daily activities	Limit the number of stairs you climb to 1 flight a day for first week; if you can, have the baby downstairs with you during the day (avoid going up and down stairs to check on baby); in the second week, expand your activity.
Sexual intercourse	Sexual intercourse is safe as soon as your vaginal discharge has turned white and your episiotomy (if any) has healed (about 3 weeks after giving birth). Use a lubricant (contraceptive foam or gel) to aid your comfort because your hormonal balance has not completely returned.
Contraception	You can start using contraception when you begin having sexual intercourse; oral contraceptives are begun about 2-3 weeks after delivery; breastfeeding is not an effective birth control method. Be sure to use protection because you can become pregnant even before you have your first period.
Follow-up	Return to your physician or nurse-midwife 2-6 weeks after birth; notify your physician or nurse-midwife if your temperature is 38° C (100.4° F) or if you notice an increase in vaginal discharge greater than 1 pad per hour, if lochia becomes bright red, or if it ceases and returns. It is very important that you attend your follow-up examination as scheduled; this visit will make sure that you are recovering normally and that you do not have problems; plan to return for the postpartum checkup in 6 weeks.
Newborn care	Know how to: • Take the baby's temperature • Give the baby a bath • Feed and burp the baby • Care for the baby's umbilical cord • Care for the baby's circumcision (if applicable) • Recognize baby's normal sleeping and crying patterns Plan to take the baby for the 6-week checkup. Have a list of instructions of when to take your baby to the physician. Review newborn immunization plan. Have a car seat (rental or own) for your baby to ride in a car.

for postpartum home visits or hotline resources may be indicated. Parents need to discuss relationships, their return to work schedules, and their roles in transition to parenthood. The nurse should guide the parents in understanding newborn behavior and growth and development patterns. Before actual discharge, the nurse spends time with the woman or couple to teach them and determine whether they have any last-minute questions (see Nursing Care Plan 12-1). This may be done by the primary nurse, case manager, or, in some facilities, a perinatal educator. The use of a clinical path for timelines and a maternal-newborn teaching checklist can serve as a documentation tool and ensures that all mothers are provided similar key information. The

nurse often reviews the pamphlet or hospital-prepared discharge literature that explains what women are encouraged to do and not do for the stated period. The woman is informed whether videos on newborn bathing, cord and circumcision care, breast or formula feeding, and cardiopulmonary resuscitation (CPR) are available on loan or for purchase in the hospital gift shop. She also receives information about local agencies or support groups that can help them in parenting. When possible, literature should be provided in the patient's language of preference.

The woman should have a scheduled appointment for her 2- or 6-week postpartum examination and her newborn's first well-baby examination. Follow-up telephone calls and home visits allow for clarification and an opportunity to answer any questions. Many postpartum hospital units provide the woman with the telephone number, and she is encouraged to call if she has any questions, no matter how simple. The woman should be alerted to danger signs to report.

RESUMPTION OF NORMAL ACTIVITIES

Women often ask what they may or may not do once they are home. They are advised to increase their activities gradually and avoid fatigue. They are instructed to avoid heavy lifting and excessive stair climbing for the 6-week recovery period. Most women resume practically all activities by 4 to 5 weeks' postpartum. Current maternity leave provisions may enable the mother to delay returning to work outside of the home until after the 6-week postpartum period. When the woman can assume the duties of her previous position will vary, depending on the type of work and the normalcy of the postpartum recovery. Cultural factors also influence when normal activities are resumed.

RESUMPTION OF SEXUAL INTERCOURSE

Sexual intercourse can safely be resumed when lochia has ceased, the episiotomy incision has healed, and the woman feels ready. The time varies from 2 to 6 weeks' postpartum. If the woman had an extensive episiotomy or a laceration, she may want to wait for the perineum to heal. The first postpartum intercourse may be somewhat uncomfortable. This is partly attributable to dryness and diminished vaginal lubrication. Women are advised to use a water-soluble vaginal lubricant. Patience and gentleness by the partner are important factors for the woman and should be discussed with both before discharge. A position that puts less strain on the woman's perineum is helpful (woman on top or woman on her side). Couples may be frustrated if there is decreased libido because of hormonal changes that may persist for a few months. Breastfeeding mothers should be forewarned that during orgasm, milk may spurt from the nipples because of the release of oxytocin. Nursing the newborn before lovemaking may reduce the chance of milk release. Other factors that may inhibit satisfactory sexual experience include the baby's crying and sleep deprivation.

POSTPARTUM FATIGUE

Postpartum assessment should include evaluation for fatigue. In today's modern lifestyle, the woman often works throughout her pregnancy, rooms in with the newborn, and returns home in 48 hours or less to take on full household responsibilities. There may be little opportunity to rest and adapt to the postpartum phase. Postpartum fatigue is defined as an overwhelming, sustained sense of exhaustion and decreased capacity for physical and mental work. Most women start to experience fatigue during pregnancy, and it sometimes persists for more than a year after delivery. After delivery, most people inquire and comment about the baby; in the United States, few inquire about the mother's fatigue. The stresses of labor and hormonal changes, wound healing, and establishment of breastfeeding contribute to the development of fatigue in the early postpartum days. Continuing sleep difficulties, child care responsibilities, and lack of assistance contribute to longer term fatigue that can interfere with the return to full pre-pregnancy functioning. Nursing intervention is challenged by the short hospital stay of postpartum women.

Some anticipatory counseling concerning preventive techniques should be given to all new mothers before discharge. Plans to minimize fatigue could include using the side-lying position for breastfeeding, avoiding telephone interruptions with use of an answering machine, and using Internet resources for stress management techniques. Assessment for fatigue should continue during all postpartum mother and baby clinic visits.

FAMILY PLANNING

Although the decision is the couple's, they are encouraged to discuss the use of various contraceptives during their hospital stay. The nurse can provide information about options for family planning (see Chapter 19) before the woman's discharge from the hospital. The nurse should stress that ovulation often resumes before the first menses, and pregnancy can occur. Mothers who breastfeed exclusively may ovulate and menstruate later than women who breastfeed less frequently, but contraception should resume by 6 months' postpartum. Oral contraceptives can be started 3 weeks after delivery in nonlactating women and as soon as lactation is well established in breastfeeding women. Progestin-only contraceptives have been used for contraception after birth and have shown to enhance the quality and duration of lactation. However, progestin-only contraceptives may be contraindicated in Hispanic women who have gestational diabetes because of the risk of developing type 2 diabetes (Gabbe, Niebyl, & Simpson, 2007).

POSTPARTUM EXERCISES

Persistent maternal musculoskeletal and cardiovascular changes can present potential problems for the woman who exercises. The hormonal effects on connective tissue are not reversed until approximately 6 weeks' postpartum. Until that time, the risk of injury is still present. For the woman with an uneventful birth, deep breathing, abdominal exercise for diastasis recti muscles, Kegel exercises, and pelvic tilts can be started on the first or second postpartum day.

Walking is an ideal exercise. The woman's return to more vigorous fitness activities should be monitored according to individual responses and past fitness activities. Many hospitals and other facilities sponsor exercise classes for the postpartum woman.

Kegel Exercises

Kegel (perineal tightening) exercises are advised for the prenatal and the postpartum period. These exercises are encouraged to strengthen and tone the muscles of the pelvic floor. It is commonly believed that these exercises decrease stress incontinence, speed recovery, and increase sexual response. After a vaginal delivery, these muscles are often weaker than before birth, but tone can be regained with Kegel exercises. In performing these exercises, the woman contracts the pelvic floor muscles. The woman pulls up her entire pelvic floor, as if trying to suck up water with her vagina. She then bears down, as if trying to push the imaginary water out. In doing this, she is also using abdominal muscles. The woman should feel a tightening of the muscles around the anal sphincter, vagina, and urethra. This is done to promote healing of perineal tissues, increase the strength of the muscles, and increase urinary control. The woman is advised that doing perineal tightening exercises is beneficial throughout her life.

Pelvic Tilt

The pelvic tilt is helpful for good postural alignment and relief of strain on the lower back. It can be done in a sitting or standing position. With her arms stretched out, the woman tightens her abdominal and buttock muscles, arches her back, and then flattens her back against the wall (if standing) or chair (if sitting). This exercise strengthens back muscles and lessens back discomfort (see Chapter 5). This exercise is helpful beyond the postpartum period.

SPECIAL IMMUNIZATIONS

Most immunizations are not contraindicated during the postpartum phase, even if the mother is breastfeeding (Centers for Disease Control and Prevention, 2008).

Rubella Vaccine

Women who have a rubella titer of less than 1:10 are given the rubella vaccine during the postpartum period to protect their next fetus from fetal malformations. The nurse must make certain that these women understand the purpose of the rubella vaccine and that they must not get pregnant for the next 3 months.

Rh$_o$(D) Immune Globulin

Women who are Rh negative and meet specific criteria (see Chapter 13) should receive Rh$_o$(D) immune globulin (RhoGAM) within 72 hours' postpartum. RhoGAM prevents the development of antibodies that would destroy fetal RBCs in subsequent pregnancies. In 2004, Rhophylac was approved by the FDA and is used in many hospitals to replace RhoGAM. It is derived from human plasma and never contained thimerosal (mercury). Rhophylac can be given IM or IV but cannot be given at the same time as other vaccines.

Get Ready for the NCLEX® Examination!

Key Points

- The postpartum period (puerperium) is the 6-week period after childbirth. During the early postpartum period, dramatic physiologic changes are made that result in the return of the body systems to the pre-pregnant state.
- Partners should be included in teaching newborn care and feeding.
- After childbirth, the woman is at great risk for hemorrhage; therefore, the woman is monitored very closely during the first few hours. These assessments are critical; however, the overall observations and interventions are focused on wellness.
- Uterine involution is the process by which the uterus returns to its pre-pregnant state.
- Postpartum assessment (postpartum checks) is made frequently to determine the woman's response to recovery. The checks include the assessment of the level and firmness of the uterine fundus; the amount, color, and odor of the lochia; condition of the perineum, episiotomy, and hemorrhoids; hydration; adequate bladder emptying; and psychological responses.
- Lochia is the name given to vaginal flow after childbirth. The flow is lochia rubra (red) for the first 1 to 3 days, lochia serosa (pink to brown) during days 4 to 9, and lochia alba (yellow to white) until approximately 6 weeks' postpartum.
- A hypercoagulable state exists during the puerperium, increasing the risk of venous thromboembolism.
- Postpartum blues is a common occurrence during the first 10 days after delivery. Nurses can offer supportive care and management strategies.
- Various comfort measures are used to alleviate pain from tissue trauma that occurs during birth, episiotomy, afterpains, and breast tenderness. Nursing interventions include ice packs and administration of analgesics as necessary.

- Ways to prevent infection during the postpartum period include adequate perineal care: cleansing the perineum after each voiding and defecation and always wiping from front to back (urinary meatus toward anus).
- Counseling and guidance that help new mothers and their families make adjustments to the newborn, deal with sibling responses, and react positively with grandparents are important nursing interventions.
- Self-care teaching is an integral part of postpartum nursing. With the brief hospital stay, follow-up by telephone and home visits are a welcome trend. All women are advised to return for their 2- or 6-week visit to be sure their recovery is uneventful.
- Discharge planning includes the assessment of the woman's knowledge of self-care and newborn care. In addition, she is taught to report excessive vaginal bleeding, lochia with a foul odor, or increase in discharge; pain in the calf of the leg, which may be accompanied by redness, swelling, or warmth; pain, redness, or warmth of breasts in breastfeeding mothers; fever; pain, burning, or difficulty in urination; and abdominal or pelvic tenderness. Resumption of sexual intercourse and family planning are discussed with the couple.
- Anticipatory counseling to minimize postpartum fatigue should be offered to all new mothers.
- Information concerning support groups and telephone lines for questions or concerns should be given before discharge.

Additional Learning Resources

SG Go to your Study Guide on pages 495–496 for additional Review Questions for the NCLEX® Examination, Critical Thinking Clinical Situations, and other learning activities to help you master this chapter content.

 Go to your Evolve website (http://evolve.elsevier.com/Leifer/maternity) for the following FREE learning resources:
- Animations
- Answer Guidelines for Critical Thinking Questions
- Answers and Rationales for Review Questions for the NCLEX® Examination
- Concept Map Creator
- Glossary with pronunciations in English and Spanish
- Patient Teaching Plans
- Skills Performance Checklists and more!

Online Resources
- www.askhrsa.gov
- www.CDC.gov
- www.chss.iup.edu/postpartum
- www.cnn.com/HEALTH/library/PR/00142.html
- www.estronaut.com/a/post_partum_fatigue.htm
- www.medbroadcast.com/conditions
- www.postpartum.net

Review Questions for the NCLEX® Examination

1. The correct order for the phases of lochia during the postpartum period is:
   1. Lochia rubra, lochia alba, lochia serosa
   2. Lochia serosa, lochia rubra, lochia alba
   3. Lochia rubra, lochia serosa, lochia alba
   4. Lochia alba, lochia rubra, lochia serosa

2. Which changes are expected to occur during the initial postpartum period? *(Select all that apply.)*
   1. Rise in the hematocrit
   2. Decrease in daily urinary output
   3. Increase in white blood cell count to 15,000/mm^3
   4. Increased fibrinogen levels

3. The nurse is caring for a postpartum patient 24 hours following delivery. Which assessment made by the nurse requires immediate attention?
   1. Heart rate of 50 beats/minute
   2. Profuse diaphoresis
   3. Sluggish bowel sounds
   4. Decrease in blood pressure to 80/56

4. According to Rubin (1984), the taking hold phase is the second maternal phase and is characterized by:
   1. The woman's readiness to assert independence
   2. Passive, dependent behavior
   3. The woman focusing on her own needs
   4. The woman's concern about the overall health of the newborn

5. When assessing the amount of lochia present on the perineal pad of a postpartum woman, after it has been applied for 1 hour, the nurse notes a 5-inch stain. Documentation should indicate quantity as a:
   1. Scant amount
   2. Light amount
   3. Moderate amount
   4. Large amount

6. Postpartum blues occur in approximately 70% of women during the first few days after birth and generally lasts up to 10 days. This state is characterized by which trait(s)? *(Select all that apply.)*
   1. Tearfulness
   2. Suicidal thoughts
   3. Lack of appetite
   4. Insomnia
   5. Hallucinations

7. Put the stages of maternal role attainment in the correct order from first to last.
   1. Personal stage
   2. Anticipatory stage
   3. Formal stage
   4. Informal stage

Critical Thinking Questions

Mrs. E is a 30-year-old Para 6 Gravida 4 who delivered a full-term baby boy weighing 8 pounds. She had a NSVD with no episiotomy or tears. She is now 8 hours' postpartum and is very dependent, asking the nurse to change the baby's diaper and talking on her cell phone, telling her friends her birth story. Her temperature is 99.4° F, pulse is 70, respirations 20, and her blood pressure is 126/80. She is voiding well, her breasts are slightly engorged, and she has lochia rubra. The infant has been alert, active, and has breastfed well. She asks the nurse whether she can wait until her menstruation returns before starting contraception.

1. Assess her vital signs.

2. Where would you expect to find the fundus now?

3. Is Mrs. E in the taking-in, taking-hold, or letting-go phase postpartum? Why do you think that?

4. What are the teaching priorities for today? Before discharge?

5. How can you facilitate attachment to the newborn?

6. What advice will you give her concerning when her menstruation will return and when she can start contraception?

chapter

13

Health Problems Complicating Pregnancy

Evolve

Objectives

1. Define key terms listed.
2. Discuss three causes of spontaneous abortion.
3. Describe ectopic pregnancy.
4. Describe placenta previa, and state the characteristic symptom.
5. Explain five nursing measures for the care of a woman who is hemorrhaging.
6. Compare two types of abruptio placentae.
7. Review the cause of coagulation defects in pregnancy.
8. List five causes of high-risk pregnancies and three leading causes of maternal death.
9. Recognize four factors that increase the risk for gestational hypertension.
10. Discuss three signs that a pregnant hypertensive woman should report immediately to her physician.
11. Identify the antihypertensive drug most commonly given to women with gestational hypertension and its antidote.
12. Compare the effects of the physiologic changes in pregnancy related to thromboembolic disease.
13. Discuss heart disease in pregnancy.
14. Explain hyperemesis gravidarum.
15. Explain three ways diabetes mellitus affects pregnancy.
16. Review four aspects of self-care for the diabetic woman.
17. Describe rubella and its consequences in pregnancy.
18. Identify the changes that occur in pregnancy that predispose the woman to urinary tract infections.
19. Discuss the cause and prevention of toxoplasmosis.
20. Describe three self-care measures for a pregnant woman with a urinary tract infection.
21. Describe how the use of nicotine, alcohol, and recreational drugs can affect the fetus.
22. Discuss the effects of substance abuse on women's health.
23. Relate the impact of pregnancy on the woman's response to bioterrorist agent exposure and treatment protocols.
24. Recognize the effects of drugs used to treat bioterrorist infections on the developing fetus.
25. Identify signs of fetal demise.
26. Recognize stages of grieving and nursing interventions that can assist parents in dealing with fetal loss.

Key Terms

abortion (ă-BŎR-shŭn, p. 250)
abruptio placentae (ă b-RŬP-shē-ō plă -SĔN-tē, p. 256)
cervical cerclage (sĕr-KLĂZH, p. 252)
disseminated intravascular coagulation (DIC) (dĭ-SĔM-ĭ-NĀT-ĕd ĭn-tră -VĂS-cū-lă r kō-ă g-ū-LĀ-shŭn, p. 257)
eclampsia (ĕ-KLĂMP-sē-ă, p. 259)
ectopic pregnancy (ĕk-TŎ P-ĭk, p. 253)
gestational diabetes mellitus (GDM) (jĕs-TĀ-shŭn-ă l dī-ă -BĒ-tēz MĔL-ĭ-tŭs, p. 271)
gestational hypertension (GH) (p. 259)
gestational trophoblastic disease (trŏf-ō-BLĂS-tĭk, p. 254)
HELLP syndrome (p. 259)

hydatidiform mole (hī-dă -TĬD-ĭ-fŏrm mōl, p. 254)
hyperemesis gravidarum (hī-pĕr-ĕm-Ē-sĭs gră v-ĭ-DĂR-ŭm, p. 268)
incompetent cervix (ĭn-KŎ M-pĕ-tĕnt SĔR-vĭks, p. 252)
isoimmunization (p. 258)
macrosomia (mă k-rō-SŌ-mē-ă, p. 269)
placenta previa (plă -SĔN-tă PRĒ-vē-ă, p. 254)
preeclampsia (prē-ĕ-KLĂMP-sē-ă, p. 259)
pregestational diabetic (prē-jĕs-TĀ-shŭn-ă l dī-ă -BĔT-ĭk, p. 269)
RhoGAM (p. 258)
TORCH infections (p. 272)

Health problems during pregnancy can significantly affect pregnancy outcome. Some of these conditions develop as a result of the pregnancy state, whereas others are health problems that were present before pregnancy. This chapter discusses a wide variety of disorders, all of which have at least one thing in common: their occurrence during pregnancy puts the woman and her fetus at risk. For women whose pregnancies are at risk, focused prenatal care provides necessary health teaching for the promotion of health and prevention of illness. Prompt identification, assessment, and management of the problems are essential to the successful outcome of the pregnancy and the well-being of the newborn. The leading disorders of pregnancy that result in maternal death are hypertension, embolism, hemorrhage, and infection.

EFFECTS OF A HIGH-RISK PREGNANCY ON THE FAMILY

Normal pregnancy can be a crisis because it is a time of significant change and growth. The woman with a complicated pregnancy has stressors beyond those of the normal pregnancy. Her family is also affected by the pregnancy and impending birth. Many new noninvasive technologies are on the horizon to detect problem pregnancies and enable early diagnosis and treatment, which may help prevent perinatal loss. The woman should be instructed to return to the health care provider if she notices any of the danger signs listed in Box 13-1.

DISRUPTION OF USUAL ROLES

The woman who has a difficult pregnancy often must remain on bed rest at home or in the hospital, sometimes for several weeks. Others must assume her usual roles in the family, in addition to fulfilling their own obligations. Finding caregivers for young children in the family may be difficult if extended family lives far away. Placing the children in day care may not be an option if financial problems exist. Nurses can help families adjust to these disruptions by identifying sources of support to help maintain reasonably normal household functions.

FINANCIAL DIFFICULTIES

Many women work outside of the home, and their salary may stop if they cannot work for an extended period. At the same time, their medical costs are rising. Social service referrals may help the family cope with their expenses.

DELAYED ATTACHMENT TO THE INFANT

Pregnancy normally involves gradual acceptance of and emotional attachment to the fetus, especially after the woman feels fetal movement. Fathers feel a similar attachment, although at a slower pace. The woman who has a high-risk pregnancy often halts planning

---

Box **13-1**   **Danger Signs in Pregnancy**

- Sudden gush of fluid from vagina
- Vaginal bleeding
- Abdominal pain
- Persistent vomiting
- Epigastric pain
- Edema of face and hands
- Severe, persistent headache
- Blurred vision or dizziness
- Chills with fever over 38° C (100.4° F)
- Painful urination or reduced urinary output

---

for the child and may withdraw emotionally to protect herself from pain and loss if the outcome is poor.

BLEEDING DISORDERS

Bleeding during pregnancy is abnormal, and its cause should be investigated. Maternal blood loss decreases oxygen-carrying capacity, which predisposes the woman and fetus to risks. Approximately 15% of the maternal cardiac output (1 L/min) flows through the placental bed at term; unchecked bleeding can therefore be fatal.

Bleeding occurs in about 25% of first-trimester pregnancies, and the woman is at increased risk of preterm labor or abruption (Lykke, Dideriksen, Lidegaard, & Langhoff-Roos, 2010). Nosebleeds during pregnancy can be a predictor of postpartum hemorrhage and should be reported (Dugan-Kim, Connell, Sitka, Wong, & Gossett, 2009). Early in pregnancy, the most common causes of bleeding are spontaneous abortion, cervical polyps, uterine fibroids, ectopic pregnancy, and hydatidiform mole. Frequent causes of bleeding late in pregnancy include placenta previa and abruptio placentae. Disseminated intravascular coagulation (DIC) can occur as the result of a coagulation defect. Postpartum hemorrhage is discussed in Chapter 17.

BLEEDING IN EARLY PREGNANCY
ABORTION

Abortion is the intentional or unintentional ending of a pregnancy before 20 weeks' gestation, the point of viability. *Miscarriage* is a lay term applied to a spontaneous abortion. Abortion can be induced as a result of artificial or mechanical means for therapeutic or elective reasons.

Classification and Management of Abortions

Spontaneous abortions typically occur because of some maternal illness or genetic defect that has occurred in the fetus. Approximately 15% of all pregnancies terminate in spontaneous abortions. The majority of these abortions occur before the twelfth week of gestation. Specific causes may include:

- Genetic defects
- Defective ovum or sperm
- Defective implantation
- Uterine fibroids (benign uterine tumors; see Chapter 20)
- Maternal factors, including chronic conditions, acute infections, nutritional deficiencies, abnormalities of maternal reproductive organs, and endocrine deficiencies

Blood group dyscrasias (ABO and Rh) can also cause an abortion. Psychological and physical trauma has also been implicated as a cause. The use of an abdominal seat belt without a shoulder restraint in an automobile can cause placental separation and

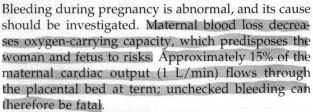

Handwritten margin note (left side, vertical): Rh (+) trait is more dominant than the negative

abortion because of the flexion of the body and displacement of the uterus in a car accident. Proper restraint of the upper and lower body in a moving automobile is very important (see Figure 5-9).

An induced abortion may be performed for the selective termination of a multifetal pregnancy. Often artificial reproductive technology (ART) or "fertility pills" result in multifetal pregnancies that, without intervention, can end in premature delivery and neonatal damage or loss.

Counseling the woman and family after an abortion is very important. Once the woman has had a spontaneous abortion, she often asks, "What are my chances of carrying another baby to term?" For the woman and her family, regardless of whether the pregnancy was planned, the loss is often accompanied by a certain degree of guilt. Many women go through the same grieving process as that caused by other types of personal loss. In some women, the grief response may be intensified if the abortion follows infertility treatments.

When symptoms of abortion such as bleeding and cramping occur, ultrasound scanning may be used to detect the presence of a gestational sac and assess if there is a developing embryo or live fetus. The woman is usually asked to abstain from sexual intercourse and placed on bed rest. If the abortion (loss of the products of conception) appears to be imminent, the woman is hospitalized. Intravenous therapy is started to replace the fluid loss. Blood transfusions usually are not necessary, but surgical intervention such as dilation and evacuation (D&E), formerly called dilation and curettage (D&C), may be necessary to remove the remainder of the products of conception to stop the bleeding. If the pregnancy is beyond 12 weeks' gestation, an induction of labor may be done to expel a dead fetus.

After an abortion, the Rh-negative woman should receive $Rh_o(D)$ immune globulin (RhoGAM) to protect her from isoimmunization. If the abortion is not after 12 weeks' gestation, MICRhoGAM is used.

Abortions are clinically classified according to the symptoms and whether the products of conception are partially or completely retained or expelled (Figure 13-1, Table 13-1).

Nursing Interventions

"Spotting" is common during pregnancy, especially after intercourse or exercise, because the highly vascular cervix is easily traumatized. However, occasional spotting does not necessarily indicate a pathologic problem. When a woman is admitted to the hospital for bleeding during pregnancy, nursing responsibilities include:

- Monitoring vital signs
- Observing for signs of shock, pallor, cold clammy skin, restlessness, and perspiration
- Weighing perineal pads to accurately determine the amount of bleeding

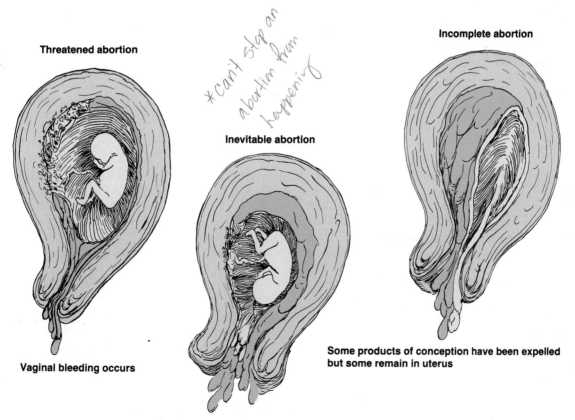

Threatened abortion

Vaginal bleeding occurs

*Can't stop an abortion from happening

Inevitable abortion

Membranes rupture and cervix dilates

Incomplete abortion

Some products of conception have been expelled but some remain in uterus

FIGURE 13-1 Three types of spontaneous abortion.

- Preparing for intravenous therapy
- Assessing fetal heart rate
- Having oxygen equipment available
- Obtaining a history and laboratory reports
- Providing emotional support to the woman and family

INCOMPETENT CERVIX

A woman is said to have an incompetent cervix when the cervix dilates without perceivable contractions, resulting in the products of conception being expelled early in pregnancy. In other words, the internal os of the cervix dilates because it is incapable of supporting the increasing weight and pressure of the growing fetus. For a fetus to be carried to term, the woman's cervix may need to be reinforced surgically with a heavy ligature placed submucosally around the cervix. This technique is called the **Shirodkar procedure.** If a heavy silk purse-string suture is used, the technique is called a **McDonald's procedure.** These procedures are known as cervical cerclage. When the pregnancy reaches term or labor begins, the suture is cut and labor

[handwritten margin notes: "Pt will stay on bed rest until delivery day"]

[handwritten left margin note: "→ More than 1 pad changed in 1 hr is not normal."]

| Table 13-1 | Comparison of Types and Management of Spontaneous Abortion (Miscarriage)* |

TYPE	CRAMPS	BLEEDING	TISSUE PASSED	CERVICAL OPENING	UTERINE SIZE	NURSING MANAGEMENT
Threatened	Slight (with or without cramps)	Slight to moderate (bleeding ceases)	None	Closed	Commensurate with date	Bed rest, sedation,† avoidance of coitus, ultrasound; observe amount of bleeding (save pads); woman to gradually increase activity; perform pregnancy tests; give Rh₀(D) immune globulin (RhoGAM) within 72 hours if indicated
Inevitable	Moderate	Moderate to severe	None	Open, with membranes or tissues bulging	Commensurate with date	Bed rest, sedation; transfusion may be indicated; observe amount of bleeding, color (save pads); give RhoGAM if indicated
Incomplete	Severe	Severe and continuous	Placental or fetal tissue	Open, with tissue in cervical canal or passage of tissue	Smaller than date	Bed rest, sedation; observe to determine how much tissue is passed; save all available tissue; carefully record vital signs; dilation and evacuation (D&E) as necessary; give RhoGAM if indicated
Complete	None	Minimal	Complete placenta and fetus	Closed, with no tissue in cervical canal	Smaller than date	Observe to determine if all tissue is passed (save pads); give RhoGAM if indicated
Missed	None; no life felt	Brownish discharge	None; prolonged retention of tissue	Closed	Smaller than expected	No specific treatment available; oxytocin may be used to induce labor and delivery; check for coagulation defect (DIC)
Recurrent (habitual)						Comprehensive and conservative care essential in early months; cerclage surgery performed if necessary for incompetent cervix

DIC, disseminated intravascular coagulation.

*Psychologically, many patients experience a grief period and have fears of inability and inadequacy as a woman. They express anxiety over the next pregnancy or ability to conceive again.

†Drugs are kept to a minimum to safeguard the fetus.

is allowed to progress or a cesarean birth is accomplished. If the woman has a history of repeated late abortion in the second trimester, the cervix is dilated 3 to 4 cm, and the membranes are intact, she may be a candidate for a cerclage to help the pregnancy reach term. When cerclage is in place, the mother must be taught the importance of notifying the health care provider at the first sign of labor, such as ruptured membranes or labor pains, to avoid complications such as a ruptured uterus.

ECTOPIC PREGNANCY

Ectopic pregnancy refers to an abnormal implantation of the fertilized ovum outside of the uterine cavity (Figure 13-2). Implantation occurs most commonly in some portion of the fallopian tube. Other sites, although rare, include the ovary, the abdominal cavity, and the cervix. Because the fallopian tube is not anatomically suited for implantation, the trophoblast cells erode the blood vessels and weaken the tissue, resulting in tube rupture. The tubal rupture can cause a fatal hemorrhage. Predisposing conditions include any factor that affects tubal patency, ciliary action, and contractility. Two prominent causes are partial tubal occlusion from pelvic inflammatory disease (PID) and the use of a contraceptive intrauterine device (IUD). The incidence of ectopic pregnancy is increasing but mortality is decreasing due to better diagnostic methods and technology. The nurse must be alert to symptoms of hemorrhage and shock and be prepared to act quickly to minimize blood loss and hasten maternal stabilization.

Assessment and Management

A combined use of transvaginal ultrasound examination and assessment of the hormonal levels of progesterone and beta-human chorionic gonadotropin (β-hCG) is used in the early detection of an ectopic pregnancy. The vaginal probe ultrasound will show an empty uterus and may show the site of an ectopic pregnancy. Characteristically, the woman misses one or two menstrual periods and then may have stabbing pain in either lower abdominal quadrant. These signs may or may not be followed by dark red or brown vaginal spotting. Shoulder pain caused by blood irritating the diaphragm or phrenic nerve is a common symptom. The signs of shock that develop are out of proportion to the clinical blood loss because most of the blood lost is hidden within the abdominal cavity. This is one obstetric complication in which rapid surgical treatment can save the woman's life.

Management of tubal pregnancy depends on whether the tube is intact or ruptured. If the tube is intact and hCG levels are declining, it indicates spontaneous regression of the tubal pregnancy. Methotrexate, a chemotherapeutic agent that interferes with cell reproduction, may be used to inhibit cell division in the developing embryo. The primary reason for medical management is preserving the fallopian tube to increase the chance of a future pregnancy. A woman who is receiving methotrexate therapy must avoid alcohol consumption and vitamins containing folic acid to prevent a toxic response to the drug. Photosensitivity is common with methotrexate therapy, so the woman should be counseled to protect herself from sun exposure.

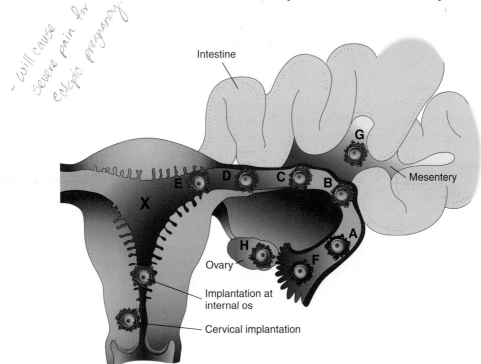

FIGURE 13-2 **Various implantation sites in ectopic pregnancy.** *A through F are tubal pregnancies that are most common. G is an abdominal pregnancy. H is the ovary where ovulation occurs. X indicates the wall of the uterus where normal implantation should occur.*

Surgical management of an unruptured tubal pregnancy may involve a linear salpingostomy, which is done to salvage the tube. A laparoscopic salpingectomy (removal of the tube) is performed when the tube is ruptured to control bleeding and prevent hypovolemic shock. Future pregnancy can occur with one tube remaining. Replacement of fluid loss and maintenance of electrolytes are essential aspects of treatment. Psychological support to help the woman and family deal with emotions and to answer questions about future pregnancies should be part of the nursing care plan.

GESTATIONAL TROPHOBLASTIC DISEASE

Gestational trophoblastic disease includes hydatidiform mole, invasive mole, and choriocarcinoma. Hydatidiform mole (molar pregnancy) is a condition in which the trophoblastic tissue proliferates and the chorionic villi of the placenta become swollen and fluid filled, taking on the appearance of grapelike clusters (Figure 13-3). Molar pregnancies are classified into two types: complete and partial. Chromosome banding and enzyme analysis have demonstrated that, in the complete mole, all genetic material is paternally derived. The mechanism of the loss of the genetic material from the ovum is unknown. No inner cell mass develops embryonically, and there is no fetal vascularization, which explains the avascular villi (vesicles). With partial mole, genetic material is maintained but the fetus is abnormal and usually aborts. The mole is distinguished from an abortion in that the mole shows trophoblastic proliferation. Some moles may develop into choriocarcinoma.

The cause is unknown, but the incidence increases with maternal age and parity. In the United States, this condition is fairly rare, occurring in approximately 1 in every 1000 pregnancies.

Assessment and Management
Early pregnancy appears normal. Then as gestation progresses, the uterus begins to grow rapidly because of the rapid proliferation of the trophoblastic cells.

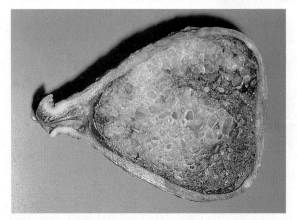

FIGURE 13-3 **Gestational trophoblastic disease.** Note the grapelike masses within the uterus containing a hydatidiform mole.

However, in 20% of the moles the uterus is found to be smaller than expected. Vaginal bleeding occurs in 84% of cases, which often is brownish (like prune juice), as well as excessive vomiting (hyperemesis gravidarum), most likely because the serum hCG levels are higher than in normal pregnancy. Symptoms of gestational hypertension (GH) occur before 24 weeks, which strongly suggests a molar pregnancy. Serial β-hCG levels and ultrasound are the primary diagnostic tools and can reveal the characteristic pattern of vesicles by the twelfth week of gestation (Goldstein, Baron, & Berkowitz, 2010).

Treatment begins with the evacuation of the mole by suction aspiration. Follow-up care is extremely critical for these women because of the great risk of choriocarcinoma (cancerous growth). Continued assessment includes hCG levels and ultrasound scans of the abdomen. Continued rising hCG levels are abnormal. If malignant cells are found, chemotherapy for choriocarcinoma may be started. If therapy is ineffective, metastasis is often rapid. Administration of RhoGAM to women who are Rh negative is necessary to prevent isoimmunization (see p. 258).

The woman is monitored for a year; if the hCG serum titers are within normal limits, the woman may be assured that she is healthy. The woman often takes oral contraceptives to prevent another pregnancy and to allow the hCG levels to return to normal. If the woman becomes pregnant immediately, it would make it impossible to monitor the decline in hCG, which is the significant part of follow-up care. Psychological support should be provided in relation to the pregnancy loss, and another pregnancy should be delayed for at least 1 year. Subsequent pregnancies should be normal because there is a low risk of recurrence.

BLEEDING IN LATE PREGNANCY
Vaginal bleeding, if slight, may be caused by the increased vascularization of the cervix, cervical polyps, or cervicitis. However, the major causes of bleeding in the second and third trimesters are placenta previa, abruptio placentae, and DIC.

PLACENTA PREVIA
Placenta previa occurs when the placenta abnormally implants near or over the cervical os instead of in the fundus of the uterus. The degree to which the internal cervical os is covered by the placenta determines how the placenta previa is classified (Figure 13-4). Two main dangers are hemorrhage for the mother and premature delivery or fetal demise.

Placenta previa occurs in approximately 1 in 200 live births (Gabbe, Niebyl, & Simpson, 2007). Defective vascularity of the decidua or previous infection in the upper uterine segment increases the risk of placenta previa. Uterine scarring from previous cesarean births, previous placenta previa, endometritis,

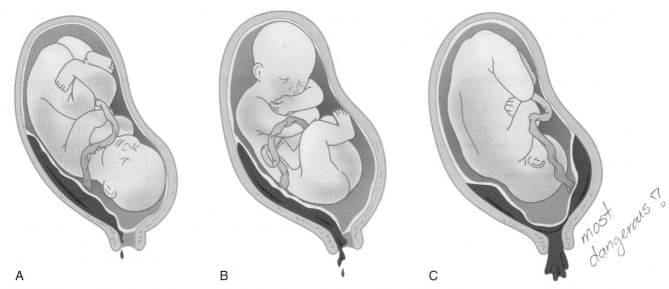

most dangerous?

FIGURE 13-4 **Three classifications of placenta previa. A,** Low; placenta barely extends to cervical os. **B,** Partial; placenta partially covers cervical os. **C,** Complete; placenta completely covers cervical os.

multifetal gestation, or multiple births increase the risk. Because the lower uterine segment is not as well vascularized as the upper segment, the placenta must cover a larger area for adequate function.

Assessment and Management

Placenta previa can be diagnosed before bleeding occurs in the third trimester because of the current routine practice of performing second-trimester ultrasound for detection of fetal anomalies. Women shown to be at risk for placenta previa at this time can have a repeat ultrasound performed at 28 and 35 weeks' gestation. Placenta previa should be suspected with the onset of painless bleeding occurring after 24 weeks' gestation. Painless bleeding results from the separation of the placenta from the uterus (that part of the placenta that is near, or covering, the internal cervical os). It most often occurs in the third trimester as the cervix begins to open in preparation for childbirth. Bleeding may be intermittent or in gushes. The bleeding can be extensive and can prove to be fatal. An abnormal fetal presentation may coexist in 15% to 20% of cases; therefore, a breech or transverse presentation should suggest the possibility of placenta previa.

The woman diagnosed with placenta previa must be closely monitored for the amount and character of blood loss. Vital signs, fetal heart rate, and activity are documented. Diagnosis is confirmed by ultrasound. Digital examinations (vaginal examinations) are strictly prohibited when a pregnant woman is bleeding because severe hemorrhage may result from the examination. A "double setup" vaginal examination may be performed by taking the woman to the operating room prepared for an immediate cesarean birth. However, this is required less often because of accurate ultrasound techniques available.

Management depends on the classification of previa and gestational age of the fetus. If the gestational age is less than 36 weeks and bleeding is slight, the woman is hospitalized for observation, placed on bed rest, and closely monitored. Blood count, type, and cross-match for blood and Rh factor are performed. Magnesium sulfate or other tocolytic drugs may be administered to prolong pregnancy if bleeding is not active (a tocolytic drug is a drug that stops labor contractions). The woman is told to notify the nurse immediately if she feels fluid escaping from the vagina. Vital signs are taken frequently, and external fetal monitoring is performed. Intravenous fluids may be given. Once the bleeding has subsided, the woman may be managed at home provided the following criteria are met:

- Woman understands her condition and that she must remain on bed rest and avoid coitus.
- Woman has around-the-clock transportation and communication available.
- Woman is compliant with oral tocolytic therapy.
- Woman has a hematocrit level above 30% to have some reserve in case of significant bleeding.
- Woman is able to be followed closely (e.g., ultrasound, nonstress test, and biophysical profiles).

If bleeding is heavy, an immediate cesarean birth is performed. The woman and family are kept informed during the monitoring or preparation for surgery.

Potential Complications

The main complications are hemorrhage for the woman and prematurity hypoxia or death for the fetus. Immediate postpartum hemorrhage often accompanies this condition because the surface area of attachment is greater than usual and the site of placental implantation in the lower uterine segment does not contract well after the placenta is expelled.

Hemorrhage can cause hypovolemic shock and death. Postpartum infection may also occur because of the closeness of the placental site to the cervix and vagina. Therefore, the woman is closely monitored postnatally for bleeding and infection.

(handwritten margin note: can lead to hypovolemic shock)

☼ ABRUPTIO PLACENTAE

Abruptio placentae is the premature separation of the placenta. Separation can be partial or total detachment of a normally implanted placenta and occurs after the twentieth week of pregnancy, usually during the third trimester (Table 13-2). The bleeding is accompanied by pain.

Risk factors for abruptio placentae include maternal hypertension, prior abruption, high parity, blunt abdominal trauma, multifetal gestation, social drug use that causes vasoconstriction (particularly cocaine), cigarette smoking, hydramnios, and infection of the chorion. Researchers have suggested that placental abruption can result from degenerative changes in the small arteries that supply the intervillous space, resulting in thrombosis, decidual degeneration (causing a retroplacental hematoma), and separation of the placenta. Some placental separations are mild and produce few symptoms. In other instances, the bleeding is severe, and both fetal and maternal compromise may occur. The degree of compromise depends on the extent of the separation and the amount of blood loss.

Abruptio placentae are subdivided into the following two types (Figure 13-5):

1. **Marginal or partial separation of the placenta:** This type usually has external drainage of blood through the cervix.
2. **Complete separation of the placenta:** This type allows blood to be trapped behind the placenta, and bleeding may or may not be evident. However, the woman will be in severe pain and the uterus will feel rigid and tender.

(handwritten margin note: fetal death due to)

Complications

If the blood gets into the muscles of the uterus, it may be difficult for the uterus to contract after the delivery of the newborn and placenta. Also, trapping of the blood may release thromboplastin into the maternal circulation. Thromboplastin release can result in DIC, which can be life threatening to the woman.

(handwritten note: loook for excessive bleeding)

Assessment and Management

Classic symptoms of abruptio placentae are dark red vaginal bleeding, uterine rigidity, severe abdominal pain, maternal hypovolemia, and signs of fetal distress. Management includes assessment for excessive bleeding; continuous fetal monitoring; a coagulation profile; and laboratory workup, including blood type and cross-match. Blood for transfusion is made available. The woman is prepared for a cesarean birth or an immediate vaginal delivery (whichever is quicker) if the

(handwritten left margin vertical note: d- celling fetus = give O2 for min. HR below 100beats/min not working = stat. C-section)

Table 13-2   Differentiation Between Placenta Previa and Abruptio Placentae*

SIGNS	PLACENTA PREVIA	ABRUPTIO PLACENTAE
Placenta location	Lower third of uterus; detected by transvaginal ultrasound	Normal
Onset	Frequently "quiet" for first episode of bleeding	"Stormy" in moderate to severe abruptions
Placenta	Palpable	Nonpalpable
Pain	None; painless bleeding (most significant sign)	May be cramplike to severe
Abdomen and uterus	Soft, not tender; may be contracting normally	May be tender to rigid
Bleeding	External, bright red bleeding; shock with excessive bleeding	External and/or internal, either bright or dark blood; may be signs of shock that are out of proportion to bleeding
Abdomen and uterus	Soft, not tender, may be contracting normally	May be tender to rigid
Bleeding	External, bright red bleeding; shock with excessive bleeding	External and/or internal, either bright or dark blood; woman may have signs of shock that are out of proportion to bleeding
Blood pressure	Usually normal; with excessive bleeding, hypovolemic shock can occur	History of hypertension and toxemia; postabruption hypovolemic shock can occur
Fetal death	Depends on fetal maturity and amount of blood loss	Fetal distress or fetal death may occur
Coagulation defect	Not usually a problem	Coagulation defect (DIC) with moderate to severe abruption can be a complication

DIC, disseminated intravascular coagulation.
*Some placental separations are mild and produce few or no symptoms; these separations are detected when the placenta is inspected after delivery.

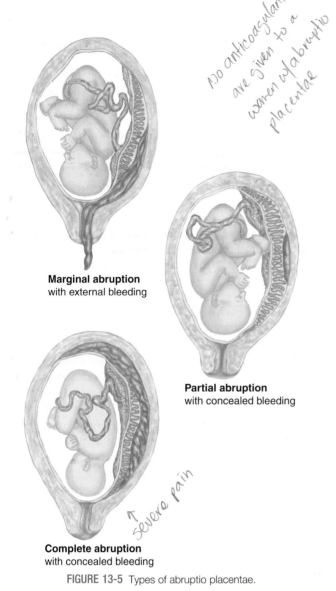

Marginal abruption
with external bleeding

Partial abruption
with concealed bleeding

Complete abruption
with concealed bleeding

(handwritten annotations: "No anticoagulants are given to a women w/abruptio placentae" and "↑ severe pain")

FIGURE 13-5 Types of abruptio placentae.

hemorrhage is severe or if fetal distress is evident. In Rh-negative women who have either placenta previa or abruptio placentae, the administration of RhoGAM is indicated (Box 13-2). Continuous monitoring for DIC is part of the care plan. A hysterectomy may be required in some cases. Surgery is contraindicated when uncontrollable bleeding and abnormal coagulation are present.

DISSEMINATED INTRAVASCULAR COAGULATION

Disseminated intravascular coagulation (DIC) is a condition in which a coagulation defect prevents blood from clotting. This results from overstimulation of the normal coagulation process. Massive, rapid fibrin formation results. This condition causes the widespread appearance of small thrombi in the small blood vessels. Factors that prevent coagulation and factors that stimulate coagulation are activated at the same time. DIC is a life-threatening condition that occurs with some complications of pregnancy such as abruptio placenta,

fetal death, amniotic fluid embolism, HELLP syndrome, and sepsis.

Assessment and Management

Because of the amount of intravascular clotting, the blood platelets and clotting factors are depleted. The process of clot lysis can have an anticoagulant effect. The following clinical problems may occur:
- Tendency toward generalized bleeding (because the clotting factors are depleted)
- Ischemia of the vital organs (caused by thrombi obstruction in the blood vessels)
- Severe anemia (resulting from excessive bleeding)

DIC does not occur as the primary disorder but rather occurs secondary to another complication. It should be suspected in women with abruptio placentae, GH, retained dead fetus, hydatidiform mole, hemorrhagic shock, and septic abortion. In addition, infection can activate the coagulation pathway. This disorder can often be resolved by correcting the underlying cause, which may require terminating the pregnancy to stop the production of thromboplastin; administering blood replacement products to maintain circulatory volume; and providing intensive supportive care, including monitoring vital signs, monitoring intake and output, and administering oxygen. The platelet count and fibrinogen level are monitored closely. Replacing depleted clotting factors, including platelets, fibrinogen, and coagulation factors, by frozen plasma or cryoprecipitate may be required. Heparin is contraindicated in DIC because it will increase bleeding.

The nurse can help in the early diagnosis of DIC by being alert to signs of bleeding and vascular occlusion.

Box 13-2	Care of the Pregnant Woman with Excessive Bleeding

- Estimate and document blood loss.
- Monitor vital signs frequently.
- Monitor intake and output.
- Assess presence and character of:
  - Pain
  - Uterine tenderness
  - Abdominal and uterine rigidity
- Have woman's blood typed and cross-matched.
- Monitor and maintain intravenous infusion.
- Observe for signs of shock.
- Prepare woman for surgery if indicated.
- If bleeding is in the third trimester of pregnancy:
  - Monitor fetal heart tones.
  - Monitor labor contractions.
  - Assess whether woman's vaginal examination should be omitted.
- Administer oxygen by mask.
- Monitor coagulation profile test studies.
- Prepare for newborn resuscitation.

Bleeding from the gums or injection sites, epistaxis, and petechiae on the skin are signs that DIC may be developing. Providing emotional support for the woman and her family is an important part of nursing care.

BLOOD INCOMPATIBILITY (ISOIMMUNIZATION)

The placenta, an organ that develops during pregnancy, allows maternal and fetal blood to exchange oxygen and waste products without actually mixing together. However, small leaks may occur and allow fetal blood to enter the mother's circulation during pregnancy. Fetal blood can also enter the mother's blood circulation when the placenta detaches at birth.

If fetal and maternal blood types are compatible, no problem occurs. However, if the fetal and maternal blood types differ, the mother's body produces antibodies to destroy foreign fetal red blood cells (RBCs). Rh or ABO **incompatibility** can occur. The phenomenon in which the Rh-negative mother develops antibodies against the Rh-positive fetus is called isoimmunization.

Rh Incompatibility

Individuals may or may not have the Rh blood factor on their erythrocytes. If they have the factor, they are Rh positive; if not, they are Rh negative. An Rh-positive person can receive Rh-negative blood if all other factors are compatible because, in Rh-negative blood, the Rh factor is absent. However, if the woman is Rh negative and the fetus is Rh positive, Rh incompatibility exists. The Rh-positive blood type is a dominant trait. This means that if the father of a fetus is Rh positive and the mother is Rh negative, there is a good chance that the newborn will be Rh positive. If fetal Rh-positive blood leaks into the mother's circulation, her body may respond by making antibodies to destroy the Rh-positive erythrocytes, and the antibodies will be returned to fetal circulation and destroy fetal RBCs. The first Rh-positive newborn is rarely affected seriously. However, each time the woman is exposed to Rh-positive blood, such as during childbirth,

amniocentesis, or abortion, her body will produce more antibodies. In future pregnancies, these antibodies in the maternal circulation will cross the placenta and cause hemolysis of the Rh-positive blood cells of the fetus. This is called *erythroblastosis fetalis* (Figure 13-6) (see Chapter 16).

The formation of anti-Rh antibodies can be prevented by giving Rh₀(D) immune globulin (RhoGAM) to the Rh-negative woman at 28 weeks' gestation and within 72 hours after birth of an Rh-positive newborn. RhoGAM can be given to the Rh-negative woman as late as 14 to 28 days' postpartum if not administered earlier, but to be effective it must be given before immune antibodies are developed (Gabbe, Niebyl, & Simpson, 2007). If the woman becomes sensitized (or develops antibodies) to destroy Rh-positive blood cells, the fetus can become anemic, develop heart failure, and die in utero. Several tests can be performed to determine whether too many fetal erythrocytes are being destroyed and to assess the status of the fetus. The tests include the Coombs' test, which determines whether the woman is sensitized and has antibody formation.

At the first prenatal visit, the Rh-negative blood type of a pregnant woman is identified, and antibody titers are monitored throughout pregnancy. Amniocentesis can determine whether fetal hemolysis is present. Intrauterine blood transfusions can be performed to prevent fetal death and prolong the pregnancy until the fetus is more mature. A Doppler ultrasound focused on the middle cerebral artery of the fetus may predict fetal anemia as well as or better than an amniocentesis (Oepkes, Seaward, & Vandenbussche, 2006) (see Chapter 5).

ABO Incompatibility

ABO incompatibility can occur if the woman has group O blood and the fetus has group A, group B, or group AB blood. Anti-A and anti-B antibodies are usually already present in the woman's body. However, fewer of these antibodies cross the placenta than those associated with Rh problems, so treatment

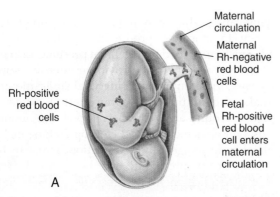

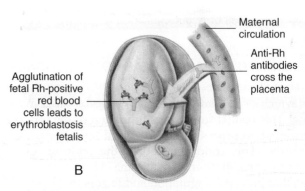

FIGURE 13-6 **Erythroblastosis fetalis. A,** A few fetal Rh-positive red blood cells enter the circulation of the Rh-negative mother at birth, causing the mother to produce antibodies against Rh-positive blood cells. **B,** The Rh-positive antibodies from the maternal circulation then cross the placenta, enter the fetal circulation, and destroy the fetal Rh-positive blood cells.

during pregnancy is not required. However, unlike the Rh problem, the newborn is often affected during the first pregnancy. The newborn may develop jaundice within the first 24 hours. Phototherapy is usually sufficient to reduce the bilirubin level in ABO incompatibility (see Chapter 16).

CARDIOVASCULAR DISORDERS *@ work load ↑ during preg.*

GESTATIONAL HYPERTENSION

Hypertensive disease in pregnancy complicates 12% to 20% of pregnancies (American College of Obstetricians and Gynecologists [ACOG], 2001). It is directly responsible for a significant number of maternal deaths. Maternal hypertension also is a significant cause of perinatal death. With preexisting hypertension during pregnancy, treatment is aimed at controlling hypertension; in gestational hypertension (GH), the disease process is closely monitored to prevent complications to the mother and fetus.

Classification and Risk Factors

In GH (formerly known as pregnancy-induced hypertension [PIH]), clinical subsets of the disease are recognized and traditionally have been given distinct labels related to the end-organ effects. Traditional labels include preeclampsia, when renal involvement leads to proteinuria; eclampsia, when central nervous system involvement leads to seizures and chronic hypertension with superimposed eclampsia (Table 13-3); and the HELLP syndrome, when the disease is dominated by hematologic and hepatic clinical manifestations. The ACOG has suggested that such terminology not be used to define separate disease entities but rather manifestations of the same disorder (Perry, & Hockenberry, 2009).

Pathophysiology of Preeclampsia

The pathology of GH is thought to start with placental implantation, although major signs may not be evident until 20 weeks' gestation. There is gradual loss of resistance to angiotensin II (the resistance normally exists during pregnancy and is the reason that normal pregnancies do not cause an increase in blood pressure). The loss of resistance to angiotensin II results in changes in the ratio of the prostaglandins prostacyclin and thromboxane. Prostacyclin is a vasodilator, and thromboxane is a vasoconstrictor with platelet aggregating effects. When resistance to angiotensin II is decreased, thromboxane becomes dominant and the resulting vasospasms are the cause of the pathologic condition and symptoms seen in GH. Because the prostaglandin hormones are produced by the placenta, the condition reverses when the placenta is removed (or the pregnancy is terminated).

Vasospasm is a well-established component of preeclampsia and is likely a major cause of most of the serious end-organ effects or alterations in function. Vasospasm in the arterioles (blood vessels) leads to an increase in blood pressure and, ultimately, a decrease in blood flow to the uterus and placenta. Renal vascular changes result in the lowering of the renal blood flow, lowering of the renal glomerular filtration rate, and, ultimately, proteinuria and oliguria. Sodium is retained, resulting in edema. Edema causes a decrease in intravascular volume that results in thicker blood and a rise in hematocrit levels. Central nervous system changes may include cell damage related to vasospasms and cerebral edema, resulting in headaches and visual disturbances. Hepatic alterations include enlargement of the liver and tension on the liver capsule. These alterations cause epigastric pain, which often precedes seizures.

Severe preeclampsia or eclampsia has been associated with serious complications, such as cerebrovascular accidents (stroke), acute renal failure, abruptio placentae, DIC, and fetal and maternal death. The HELLP syndrome is found in approximately 10% of severe preeclamptic conditions. In women who exhibit the HELLP syndrome, the onset of seizures may be abrupt.

Table 13-3	Types of Hypertension in Pregnancy	
TYPE	**DESCRIPTION**	
Gestational hypertension (GH)	Previously known as pregnancy-induced hypertension; blood pressure exceeding 140/90 mm Hg starts after the twentieth week of pregnancy and does not include proteinuria; blood pressure usually returns to normal by 6 weeks' postpartum	
Preeclampsia	GH with proteinuria present	
Eclampsia	Preeclampsia with related seizures	
Chronic hypertension	High blood pressure that occurs before pregnancy or before the twentieth week of pregnancy; hypertension usually lasts more than 42 days' postpartum	
Preeclampsia with superimposed chronic hypertension	Chronic hypertension that has new occurrence of proteinuria or occurrence of thrombocytopenia and increased liver enzymes	

Modified from American College of Obstetricians and Gynecologists. (2002). ACOG practice bulletin. Diagnosis and management of pre-eclampsia and eclampsia. *Obstetrics and Gynecology*, 99(1), 159-167; and National Institutes of Health. (2001). *National blood pressure workshop on blood pressure education*. Bethesda, MD: Author.

> ### Memory Jogger
>
> #### HELLP Syndrome
>
> HELLP syndrome is a variant of chronic hypertension with superimposed eclampsia. Hematologic abnormalities exist with severe gestational hypertension. HELLP is a mnemonic that stands for: ↙ ↓ of RBC
>
> **H:** Hemolysis, resulting in anemia and jaundice
>
> **EL:** Elevated liver enzymes, resulting in elevated alanine aminotransferase (ALT; or aspartate transaminase [AST]), epigastric pain, and nausea and vomiting
>
> **LP:** Low platelets, resulting in thrombocytopenia, abnormal bleeding and clotting time, bleeding gums, petechiae, and possibly DIC

A generalized vasospasm results in poor tissue perfusion, decreased vascular resistance with subsequent blood pressure elevation, and increased endothelial cell permeability. This allows excessive intravascular protein and fluid loss. Vascular endothelial cell injury can trigger coagulation pathways as well, resulting in abnormalities in bleeding and clotting.

An immunologic response may also trigger preeclampsia. The cause may be the presence of a foreign body in the form of a placenta or a fetus, which may explain why first-time pregnancies, pregnancy with a different partner (new genetic material), or multifetal pregnancies are at greatest risk for preeclampsia.

As preeclampsia progresses, the uteroplacental perfusion is further reduced and fetal blood flow is decreased, with constriction of the umbilical vessels. With uteroplacental changes, the risk for **abruptio placentae** is increased.

Effects on the Fetus

The decrease in placental function resulting from maternal vascular spasm in preeclampsia is associated with poor fetal outcome. Fetal complications include intrauterine growth restriction (IUGR) and fetal distress caused by hypoxia. Preterm birth may result

because the definitive treatment in worsening preeclampsia is termination of the pregnancy.

In HELLP syndrome, hemolysis may be caused by fragmentation of blood cells as they pass through damaged blood vessels. Elevated liver enzymes occur when fibrin deposits obstruct blood flow to the liver. Liver distention causes epigastric pain. When platelets collect at the site of vascular damage, thrombocytopenia develops. Transfusion may be indicated if the platelet count is below $20,000/mm^3$. Other presenting symptoms include nausea, vomiting, and malaise. Later symptoms are hematuria, jaundice, and generalized abdominal pain. HELLP syndrome can complicate pregnancy and the postpartum recovery period. Remember that a woman's condition can change quickly from mild to severe GH (Table 13-4). Table 13-5 presents nursing interventions and criteria used to determine the severity of GH.

Assessment and Management

Women who have GH develop before 34 weeks' gestation are screened for the presence of antiphospholipid antibodies. If antibodies are present, there is an increased risk of recurrent severe GH in subsequent pregnancies. For the woman with mild GH, conservative outpatient management is appropriate. Close monitoring of blood pressure and proteinuria and an evaluation of renal and hepatic function and platelet count are critical. Antepartum assessment of fetal well-being and serial ultrasound are also important in the management of GH. The woman at home must have telephone contact and readily available transportation to the hospital. The woman can be taught self-care management and how to count fetal kicks.

If the woman has only mild blood pressure elevations, minimal proteinuria, and no evidence of either end-organ damage or fetal compromise, delivery may be delayed until a favorable ripened cervix is present before labor is induced. Pregnancy in women with GH should not go beyond 40 weeks' gestation because of the risk of placental insufficiency.

Table **13-4** Criteria for Severe Preeclampsia	
SIGNS	**OBSERVATIONS**
Epigastric pain	Nausea, pain
Blood pressure elevation	Systolic of 160 mm Hg or diastolic of 110 mm Hg on two occasions, 6 hours apart
Proteinuria	$\geq$5 g in 24 hours, or 3 to 4+ on dipstick
Oliguria	<400 mL of urine in 24 hours
Cerebral or visual disturbances	Headache, scotomata or blurred vision, altered level of consciousness
Impaired liver function	Altered liver function tests, upper right quadrant or epigastric pain, increased risk for coagulation defects and hypoglycemia
Thrombocytopenia	Platelet count of $150,000/mm^3$; may drop to $100,000/mm^3$
Pulmonary signs	Pulmonary edema, cyanosis
Development of HELLP syndrome	Hemolysis, elevated liver enzymes, and low platelets

[handwritten margin note: - usually means that have GH will have preterm babies. due]

Table **13-5**	Nursing Care Related to Mild to Moderate Gestational Hypertension
NURSING INTERVENTIONS	**RATIONALES**
Restrict activity with frequent rest periods.	Rest promotes increased diuresis and decreases blood pressure and edema; strict bed rest is not recommended.
Weigh at the same time each day, preferably in early morning with empty bladder.	Weight change indicates increase or decrease in fluid retention (is not diagnostic of gestational hypertension [GH]).
Take blood pressure every 4 hours.	Blood pressure increase is indicative of greater severity of disease.
Assess fetal heart rate (FHR) frequently or monitor FHR continuously with electronic fetal monitor.	Assesses fetal well-being or fetal compromise.
Check urine for protein every 4 hours.	Assesses for preeclampsia.
Assess 24-hours fluid intake and hourly urinary output.	Assesses adequate kidney function.
Test for deep tendon reflexes (DTRs) for hyperreactivity.	Assesses muscle and nerve irritability.
Inquire about presence of headache, visual disturbance, and epigastric pain.	Checks for signs that are indicative of increasing disease severity.
Assess for signs of labor such as frequency and strength of contractions.	Medication prescribed for GH may slow or stop labor.
Assess anxieties and concerns.	Anxiety can increase blood pressure.
Attempt to reduce sensory stimulation.	Reduces neuromuscular irritability.
Check protein dietary intake.	Protein provides appropriate nutrients.
Assess need for sedation.	Sedation provides rest and reduces blood pressure.
Assess fetal kick count daily.	Determines status of fetus.
Check for completeness of emergency tray or equipment in woman's room and for drugs.	Have all necessary equipment readily available for emergency.

Termination of the pregnancy is considered in women who have severe GH at 32 to 34 weeks' gestation. The woman should maintain adequate diet and fluid intakes. Strict bed rest is no longer advocated, but restriction of activity is recommended.

Clinical manifestations of GH such as maternal oliguria, renal failure, and HELLP syndrome are reasons for an expedient delivery. When the woman is hospitalized for delivery, parenteral magnesium sulfate is usually given to prevent seizures. A continuous infusion is administered by a controlled infusion device. Intramuscular magnesium sulfate is not used because absorption cannot be controlled as readily as with intravenous administration, and tissue necrosis can occur. Magnesium sulfate therapy does not usually cause fetal heart rate problems but can cause respiratory depression after birth, so the nursery nurse should be notified that magnesium sulfate was given to the mother. Infusion of magnesium sulfate should be discontinued if the woman has loss of deep tendon reflexes (DTRs), respiratory rate less than 12 breaths/minute, and a decrease in urinary output to less than 30 mL/hour. When magnesium sulfate overdose (toxicity) occurs, calcium gluconate (10 mL of a 10% solution) is given intravenously over a 2-minute period to reverse the overdose. Respiratory ventilation support may be needed. Magnesium sulfate is an effective anticonvulsant; however, it does relax uterine muscles and stops labor.

When hypertensive therapy is indicated, intravenous hydralazine or labetalol is most often used (ACOG, 2001). Care must be taken to avoid reducing blood pressure to levels that will cause a decrease in maternal-placental perfusion. Angiotensin-converting enzyme (ACE) inhibitors should be avoided. Blood pressure and vital signs should be closely monitored.

Vaginal birth is preferred over cesarean birth, even for a woman with severe GH, although the decision to deliver by cesarean birth rather than a long induction may be best for some women.

Prenatal Nursing Assessment and Management

A major goal of prenatal care is early detection of GH before the condition progresses in severity. Recording the woman's weight, taking her blood pressure, and performing urinalysis are of the utmost importance during each prenatal visit. Blood pressure is affected by maternal position and measurement techniques; therefore, consistency is important. Blood pressure should ideally be taken after a period of rest, and the woman should be placed in a semi-Fowler's position with the arm at heart level. If the blood pressure is elevated, the woman should be allowed to relax; the measurement is then repeated (Skill 13-1). DTRs are evaluated, assessing the biceps, patellar reflexes, and ankle clonus. The nurse should report any abnormal findings. Proteinuria is determined by urine dipstick testing with a clean-catch midstream specimen. If the

-body feels flushed

Skill 13-1   Blood Pressure Measurement During Pregnancy

PURPOSE
To obtain an accurate blood pressure reading.

Steps

1. The woman should be seated with the arm resting at heart level.
2. Measure the blood pressure in the same arm at each assessment.
3. Use the appropriate size of blood pressure cuff (covering 75% to 80% of arm).
4. Wrap the blood pressure cuff snugly around the arm.
5. Inflation and deflation should be smooth and slow.
6. Record first appearance of sound.
7. Use the Korotkoff phase V (disappearance of sound) as the diastolic reading.*
8. Take two readings a few hours apart when blood pressure measurements are abnormal or borderline.

*American College of Obstetricians and Gynecologists. (2002). ACOG practice bulletin. Diagnosis and management of pre-eclampsia and eclampsia. *Obstetrics and Gynecology, 99*(1), 159-167.

protein is greater than 1+ on two or more occasions, further evaluation should be performed. The nurse asks the woman questions about significant subjective signs, such as frontal headache or epigastric pain. Edema is no longer considered a reliable diagnostic criterion for GH because it appears in many normal pregnancies (Gabbe, Niebyl, & Simpson, 2007). The nurse should promptly report any change observed in the woman's condition.

Because the woman may feel well, she may not understand the need for the close monitoring necessary in GH. Some women with GH (or preeclampsia) are comparatively symptom free and may have little or no noticeable discomforts. Remember, a mild form of GH may rapidly progress to a severe form, including seizures. Once severity of GH worsens, hospitalization is required and appropriate nursing management must be carried out.

Education for Self-Care
Although hypertension in pregnancy is often defined as a blood pressure of 140/90 mm Hg or greater in a previously normotensive woman, knowing the baseline blood pressure is essential. A systolic increase of 30 mm Hg and diastolic increase of 15 mm Hg above her baseline place the woman in a high-risk category. Therefore, if blood pressure was 90/60 mm Hg before pregnancy, a reading of 120/80 mm Hg indicates a risk for this patient. The same blood pressure elevation in a woman with chronic hypertension places the woman at risk for preeclampsia. The management of GH depends on the severity of the symptoms, the aggressiveness of the physician, and the understanding and compliance of the patient. Careful teaching, guidance, and compliance are critical to the woman, the developing fetus, and her family. In a woman who practices complementary or

alternative medical (CAM) therapies, the use of calcium is thought to decrease the severity of GH (Villar, Merialdi, Gulmezoglu, et al., 2003), and vitamins C and E and fish oils are often used to counter the antioxidative stress of preeclampsia.

Home Management
In early GH, if the woman is well informed and conscientious in carrying out the medical and nursing instructions (e.g., reports headaches, visual disturbances, or epigastric pain), management may be provided on an outpatient basis. Care is directed toward reducing hypertension and restoring normal kidney function. Requirements to remain at home include available telephone communication, transportation available at all times, and commitment to frequent clinic visits. Home visits by a perinatal nurse may take the place of the woman coming to some of the prenatal clinic visits.

Patient Teaching

Home Care of Mild Gestational Hypertension

- Restricted activity
- Rest on left side
- Daily blood pressure in same arm and position
- Daily weight
- Daily urine dipstick test for protein
- Fetal kicks and uterine activity monitored
- Diet with increased protein

Sufficient rest while in a left lateral position is important because it decreases pressure on the vena cava and increases both the renal and placental blood flow, which, in turn, decreases edema and blood pressure. A well-balanced diet is advised, with sufficient protein to replace protein lost in urine. Sodium should not be restricted; however, excessive intake of foods with high amounts of sodium, such as pickles, olives, and tortilla chips, should be avoided.

Attention is given to the woman's emotional and physical support while at home. Restricted activity may be difficult for a mother if she has small children. The fact that the woman usually feels well makes education especially important to ensure she takes precautions that will help avoid hospitalization. The woman and family must be taught to take a blood pressure reading each day; to perform a urine dipstick test for protein; and to record the results, including fetal and uterine activity and daily weight. The nurse can help the woman mobilize her support systems and use available community resources.

Hospitalization and Management of Preeclampsia and Eclampsia

Hospitalization for the woman with GH may be vital to control symptoms and stabilize the disease. If GH is worsening, the woman is placed in a quiet room and positioned on her left side to maintain optimum placental blood flow and to keep her as quiet and unstimulated as possible. This plan reduces the neuromuscular irritability and the potential for seizures. Rest is a key component of her care; for some women, the presence of a supportive person is helpful. Efforts should be made to reduce her anxiety because anxiety can further increase her blood pressure. Blood pressure is taken frequently. Urine is evaluated every 4 hours for protein and specific gravity, and accurate intake and output are recorded. Placement of a Foley catheter helps reduce the degree of renal compromise. DTRs are evaluated by eliciting the patellar reflex (response is graded from 0, no response observed, to +4, a brisk response). Clonus (a rapid alternating of involuntary contraction and relaxation of a muscle) is observed. A 5 + response is extreme neuromuscular irritation indicating a risk for an impending seizure. The nurse also assesses subjective symptoms by asking the woman if she has epigastric pain (upper abdomen), nausea or vomiting, blurred or abnormal vision, and headache. These symptoms are signs of worsening GH and possible impending seizure. Medications may be indicated to prevent seizures.

Nursing interventions include applying padding and raising side rails to protect the patient from injury or falling out of bed in case seizures occur. Nursing assessments must be continuous. In addition to MgSO₄, other types of medications used in the treatment of GH include sedatives, antihypertensives, and anticonvulsants (Nursing Care Plan 13-1).

The fetal status is determined by appropriate tests for fetal well-being. Uteroplacental perfusion is decreased with GH; therefore, the fetus can be in jeopardy.

Monitoring Magnesium Levels

When magnesium sulfate is used to treat preeclampsia, the woman must be monitored for signs of increased magnesium levels, which includes diminished reflexes, decreased respiratory rate, drooling, and difficulty swallowing.

Emergency Care

Emergency equipment and drugs should be kept at the patient's bedside. These include an oral airway, bag-valve-mask resuscitator (Ambu-Bag), oxygen, and suction equipment; ophthalmoscope; and medications such as MgSO₄, calcium gluconate, and cardiac stimulants. Oxygen saturation may be measured by pulse oximetry, and electrocardiographic (ECG) monitoring may be performed. Invasive hemodynamic monitoring with a flow-directed (Swan-Ganz) arterial catheter may be indicated and the woman transferred to an intensive care unit.

Fortunately, convulsions occur in only 5% of GH patients. However, every nurse should know that a rise in blood pressure level, epigastric pain, severe headache, apprehension, twitching, and hyperirritability of the muscles often precede a seizure. During a seizure, the nurse should protect the woman from injury without using force. If possible, the woman's head may be turned to the side to prevent aspiration of mucus and vomitus. Labor may progress rapidly at this time, and newborns have been born suddenly during a seizure episode. After the seizure, an airway may be inserted and oxygen administered. The nurse notifies the physician, records the description of the seizure and its after effects, takes vital signs, and evaluates the fetus. Providing information and support to the family is important.

When the seizures are controlled, labor may be induced or a cesarean birth performed if the woman does not go into labor spontaneously. Nursing care at this time includes continuous monitoring of the woman and fetus. All stimuli, such as noise and bright lights, should be reduced to lessen electrical charges to neurons. It is important to remember that the woman can have seizures up to 48 hours after delivery, and, therefore, careful postpartum assessment is essential.

CHRONIC HYPERTENSIVE DISEASE

Chronic hypertension is defined as blood pressure of 140/90 mm Hg or higher before pregnancy or before 20 weeks' gestation. The goal of care is to prevent the development of preeclampsia and ensure normal fetal growth and development. Antihypertensive medication is rarely prescribed for blood pressures below 160/100 mm Hg. Nursing responsibilities include educating the woman about self-care, including diet, exercise, and required record keeping.

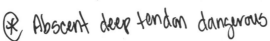

Scenario

A woman is admitted with signs of mild gestational hypertension (GH), and plans are made for discharge to the home with careful follow-up monitoring. The woman asks what she can do to avoid further complications and problems.

Selected Nursing Diagnosis

Deficient knowledge related to home care of mild GH

Expected Outcomes	Nursing Interventions	Rationales
Patient will restate correct home care measures related to GH.	Ask patient what she knows about hypertension during pregnancy; include family members if present.	Allows the nurse to build on woman's existing knowledge, reinforcing it and correcting any misunderstandings of the woman or family.
Patient will keep prescribed prenatal appointments.	Teach the woman the importance of keeping prenatal appointments, which will be more frequent because she has mild GH.	GH can quickly become more severe between prenatal care visits. If the woman understands why she should keep appointments, she is more likely to do so.
	Reinforce to the woman the prescribed measures to care for herself at home:	If woman understands these measures to limit the severity of GH, she may be more motivated to maintain them.
	Remain on bed rest, spending most of the time on her side (may walk to the bathroom and eat meals at table in most cases).	Bed rest reduces the flow of blood to the skeletal muscles, thus making more available to placenta; this enhances fetal oxygenation.
	Eat a well-balanced, high-protein diet; limit high-sodium foods such as potato chips, salted nuts, pickles, and many snack foods; include high-fiber foods and at least eight glasses of noncaffeinated drinks each day; consider food preferences and economic restraints when helping the woman choose appropriate foods.	Women with GH lose protein in their urine, which must be replaced to maintain nutrition and fluid balance; severe sodium restriction may increase severity of GH, but a high sodium intake may worsen hypertension and decrease the woman's blood volume; fiber and fluids help reduce constipation, which is more likely when activity is restricted.
	Discuss quiet activities the woman enjoys that can be done while she is on bed rest.	Bed rest can lead to boredom, and the woman may not maintain the prescribed activity if she is unaware of which activities she can do.
	Teach the woman to report signs that indicate worsening GH promptly: headache; visual disturbances (blurring, flashes of light, "spots" before the eyes); gastrointestinal symptoms (nausea, pain); worsening edema, especially of the face and fingers; noticeable drop in urinary output.	GH can worsen despite careful home management and patient compliance; if the woman has these symptoms, she needs to be evaluated and possibly hospitalized to prevent progression to eclampsia.

Selected Nursing Diagnosis

Ineffective therapeutic regimen management related to GH

Expected Outcomes	Nursing Interventions	Rationales
Blood pressure will remain within normal limits.	Monitor and record baseline vital signs.	Compare baseline data to changes that may indicate fetus is in jeopardy.
Fetal heart rate will remain in a reassuring pattern.	Monitor changes in fetal heart rate (FHR).	FHR reflects fetal status.
Patient will not have peripheral facial and abdominal edema.	Monitor urine protein (proteinuria).	Urine protein of 3 or more may be a sign of impending eclampsia.
Weight gain will be within normal limits.	Monitor weight gain and fluid intake and output and edema above the waist.	Weight gain exceeding 0.5 kg (1 lbs) per week is indicative of GH. Urinary output of less than 30 mL/hour may indicate renal shutdown. Edema may indicate increasing complications.
Seizures will not occur.	With severe preeclampsia, keep the room quiet with minimum stimulation in environment.	Environmental stimulants can precipitate seizure.

Critical Thinking Questions

1. A woman in the prenatal clinic states that high blood pressure runs in her family, and she has been taking medication for a slightly elevated blood pressure for many years. She states she has had most success with the medication she is currently taking (atenolol) and would like to continue this regimen during her pregnancy. What is your best response?
2. What factors need to be considered and included when developing a teaching plan for a woman with GH?

Chronic Hypertension with Superimposed Preeclampsia

Some women with chronic hypertension develop preeclampsia, and careful management is essential because they may rapidly progress to eclampsia.

Postpartum Management

For the first 48 hours' postpartum, careful monitoring is critical. After 48 hours, the maternal assessments are decreased to every 4 to 8 hours if the mother is stable. The Foley catheter is removed, and the woman is encouraged to ambulate and give independent care to her newborn. Return of blood pressure to baseline levels usually occurs within 2 weeks. For women with chronic hypertension, lifestyle changes to improve long-term health should be discussed. Because $MgSO_4$ relaxes the smooth muscle of the uterus, uterine tone must be monitored and the fundus massaged to prevent postpartum bleeding. In breastfeeding mothers who require antihypertensive therapy, methyldopa is the preferred medication.

THROMBOEMBOLIC DISEASE

Physiologic changes in pregnancy significantly increase the risk of superficial thrombophlebitis, deep vein thrombosis (DVT), and pulmonary embolism. This is dramatically evidenced by the fact that pulmonary embolism is one of the leading causes of maternal death (ACOG, 2001). It is essential that health care providers identify high-risk women and use methods to treat the condition in an effective and expedient manner. A thrombus is the collection of platelets and fibrin on the wall of a blood vessel that impedes blood flow through the vessel. A thrombus can enlarge as more platelets and fibrin are added, can detach and flow through the circulation, and can land in the lung. This is called an **embolus.** A thrombus on the wall of a vessel that causes inflammation is called **thrombophlebitis.**

Risk Factors

Venous stasis is a well-recognized component of pregnancy. Venous distensibility, increased blood volume, vena cava compression by the gravid uterus, lower extremity edema, and worsening of varicose veins are all evidence of venous stasis as pregnancy advances. Normal changes in the coagulability and fibrinolysis activity during pregnancy place all patients at risk. Vessel wall injury can occur from cesarean birth and postpartum infections such as endometritis. Women who used oral contraceptives before becoming pregnant and those who have jobs in which they sit for long periods are at risk. Other women at risk are those older than 30 years and those who are obese. Early ambulation is the primary prevention for this condition.

Assessment and Management

A number of conditions during pregnancy mimic thrombosis. Symptoms of superficial thrombosis and DVT vary, but the woman generally complains of sudden pain with swelling in the extremity. There may be warmth and redness at the site. Pain in the calf of the leg when the foot is passively dorsiflexed is a positive **Homans' sign.**

One of the most commonly used diagnostic methods is Doppler scanning of the deep veins. Magnetic resonance imaging (MRI) is also used with accuracy to identify thrombi in symptomatic patients. The symptoms associated with pulmonary embolism are dyspnea, chest pain, hemoptysis, and tachycardia.

Superficial thrombosis is treated with moist heat and elevation of the extremity. Early ambulation is encouraged. Elastic support stockings are worn when the woman walks. Early ambulation, range-of-motion exercises, and avoidance of placing pressure behind the knees are ways of preventing thrombus formation. Alternative methods of venous thrombosis prophylaxis include mechanical methods, such as compression stockings. Heparin is usually given but must be carefully monitored because of the increased risk of hemorrhage after birth. Women should be advised to avoid sitting with their legs crossed at the knee and should elevate their legs frequently when sitting. If their work requires standing for long periods, they should wear elastic support hose that cover the entire leg.

Treatment of DVT in postpartum women is intravenous heparin followed by warfarin sodium (Coumadin). Warfarin is contraindicated during pregnancy. Women receiving heparin should be carefully monitored for evidence of hematuria and easy bruising. Periodic laboratory checks of prothrombin time are necessary. Warfarin does not pass into breast milk and can be taken by breastfeeding mothers.

HEART DISEASE

Pregnancy results in increased cardiac output, heart rate, blood volume, and stroke volume. These changes can tax the cardiac functioning of a woman with heart disease. The nurse must have a sound understanding of the normal cardiovascular adaptations during pregnancy because the additional burden on an already compromised heart can result in maternal heart failure and place the newborn at risk for hypoxia, IUGR, and prematurity. The overall incidence of heart disease in pregnancy is 1%.

Effects of Pregnancy on Heart Disease

The hemodynamic changes that occur during pregnancy have a profound effect on the woman with heart disease. Each of these changes increases the work of the heart, and their combined effect may exceed the functional capacity of a damaged heart. Drugs used for some cardiac conditions, such as warfarin, propranolol, and some diuretics, may be contraindicated in pregnancy.

At some periods during pregnancy, the danger to the woman with a cardiac condition is especially great. The woman must be closely monitored during the early prenatal period when circulatory adaptation occurs. Febrile illness should be reported and promptly treated. Special risks are present during labor and delivery. During labor, every uterine contraction shifts 300 to 500 mL of blood from the uterus and placenta into the maternal bloodstream, increasing cardiac output by 15% to 20%, possibly overloading the heart, which may trigger congestive heart failure. During the second stage of labor, maternal pushing taxes the heart. Immediately after birth of the newborn and placental expulsion, the obstructive effect of the pregnant uterus on the vena cava disappears, and there is a sudden shift of blood (up to 1000 mL) from the lower extremities and from the placenta into the systemic circulation. This large and abrupt increase in blood volume may be more than the woman with cardiac disease can manage. During the postpartum period, approximately 4 to 5 days after birth, decreased peripheral resistance and pulmonary embolism are two major problems that can occur in the woman with a heart problem.

Assessment and Management

Many of the symptoms of cardiac illness such as shortness of breath with activity, weight gain, edema, and cardiac murmurs can be symptoms normally found in adaptation to pregnancy. However, a careful history of the woman with heart disease may reveal the symptoms are out of proportion to the stage of pregnancy. Diagnosis is usually established by transthoracic echocardiography. A chest X-ray examination or standard ECG will not provide specific information needed to treat the pregnant woman.

Most cardiac problems can be managed during pregnancy. However, some preexisting heart conditions may be a contraindication for a planned pregnancy because of the associated high mortality rate. These conditions include pulmonary hypertension, aortic coarctation, a history of myocardial infarction, and uncorrected tetralogy of Fallot. (The student should consult a medical text for a more complete discussion of these cardiac conditions.) Women with known cardiac conditions should be carefully counseled concerning the risks involved in pregnancy, labor, and delivery. A multidisciplinary approach to care includes the obstetrician, cardiologist, perinatologist, anesthesiologist, dietitian, and labor and delivery nurse.

Modifications of antepartum care are based on minimizing stress to the heart. The nurse should help the woman identify her normal activities and advise her

to notify her health care provider if she becomes unable to perform them, which may indicate cardiac decompensation. Because cardiac challenges occur slowly during pregnancy, symptoms of decompensation may also gradually appear. The woman with a cardiac problem is scheduled to be seen more often than one with a normal pregnancy, and fetal assessment tests may be indicated. A nursing responsibility includes being alert to symptoms of cardiac decompensation and educating the mother concerning her care plan. Rest periods, adequate sleep, and activity restrictions are essential. Referral to support groups may aid in coping with psychological stress.

The nurse should review the pharmacologic information concerning any medications administered to the pregnant patient. Dietary restrictions are based on individual patient need. If sodium restriction is needed, it should not be less than 2.5 g/day, and potassium levels must be monitored to prevent hypokalemia if diuretics are part of prescribed therapy. The woman with a cardiac history who is receiving anticoagulant therapy may need to restrict foods high in vitamin K, such as raw, dark green, leafy vegetables. A registered dietitian should be consulted when caring for a pregnant woman with cardiac problems to help design a culturally and medically appropriate dietary plan. The modified approach to management of labor and delivery for a pregnant woman with a cardiac problem is listed in Box 13-3. Student nurses and licensed nurses are usually certified in cardiopulmonary resuscitation (CPR) but should be aware of modifications required for the pregnant patient (Skill 13-2).

ANEMIA

Because of the increased blood volume during pregnancy, hemoglobin and hematocrit levels will fall below normal; they return to normal levels approximately 6 weeks' postpartum. Anemia is a reduced ability of the blood to carry oxygen to the cells.

Box 13-3	**Intrapartum Care Plan for a Woman with Cardiac Disease**

- Understand impact of cardiac problem on stresses of labor and delivery.
- Avoid prolonged labor.
- Induce if cervix is ripe only.
- Maintain stable vital signs.
- Avoid pain and pain responses by epidural analgesia with narcotic medication.
- Prophylactic antibiotics are prescribed when risk for endocarditis is present.
- Avoid maternal pushing; use forceps or vacuum extraction.
- Use intravenous fluid replacement as needed.

[handwritten margin note: Report SOB, dyspnea, fatigue, edema]

Skill 13-2 Modification of Standard Cardiopulmonary Resuscitation (CPR) For Pregnant Women

PURPOSE
To provide CPR without injury to mother or fetus.

Steps
1. Displace uterus laterally by placing a wedge or rolled blanket under one hip (to prevent supine hypotensive syndrome).*
2. If defibrillation is used, place the paddles one rib interspace higher than usual (because of the normal heart displacement by the enlarged term uterus).
3. Give chest compressions at a point slightly higher on the sternum (because the term uterus displaces the diaphragm to a higher position).
4. Do not use abdominal thrusts.
5. Determine resting uterine tone after CPR of a pregnant woman.
6. Perform hemodynamic monitoring after CPR.
7. Maintain continuous electronic fetal monitoring (EFM).

*American Heart Association. (2005). 2005 Guidelines for cardiopulmonary resuscitation and emergency cardiovascular care. *Circulation, 112*(24 Suppl), IV-19–IV-24; and Emad, A., & Gardner, M. (2007). Cardiopulmonary resuscitation in pregnancy. *Obstetrics & Gynecology Clinics of North America 34*(3), 585-597.

In pregnancy, anemia is defined by hemoglobin levels less than 10 g/dL and hematocrit levels below 30%. Women with anemia tire easily, are susceptible to infection, and are at an increased risk for pregnancy complications such as preterm delivery. Four types of anemia are significant during pregnancy: two nutritional anemias (iron deficiency anemia and folic acid deficiency anemia) and two anemias resulting from genetic disorders (sickle cell disease and thalassemia).

Iron Deficiency Anemia
With the expansion of plasma volume and use of iron by the fetus to build hemoglobin, it becomes difficult for women to replace the iron losses by nutrition alone. Frequent use of antacids decreases dietary iron absorption and predisposes the woman to the development of anemia. A serum iron concentration of less than 60 mg/dL with less than 16% transferrin saturation is laboratory confirmation of iron deficiency anemia (Oats & Abraham, 2010). Dietary sources of iron include meat, fish, chicken, and green leafy vegetables. Iron supplements—60 mg/day of elemental iron or 300 mg/day of ferrous sulfate—are commonly used to meet the needs of pregnancy and maintain iron stores. Vitamin C and zinc are often given to enhance the absorption of iron. It is necessary to advise the woman about the gastrointestinal effects of iron, including nausea and vomiting; epigastric discomfort; abdominal cramping; black, tarry stools; and constipation. In cultures where carbohydrates are the mainstay of the diet, iron supplementation may be required because cereals contain phylates, which prevent iron absorption (Oats & Abraham, 2010).

Folic Acid Deficiency Anemia
The need for folic acid increases considerably during pregnancy. Folic acid deficiency anemia may result from inadequate intake, poor absorption, or drug interactions. Poor cooking habits (e.g., cooking with large amounts of water) can also destroy the folic acid content of foods and can lead to folic acid deficiency. Folic acid deficiency is seen in women with vitamin B12 deficiency. Women who are strict vegetarians should be evaluated for this type of anemia.

Folic acid deficiency is associated with neural tube defects. Three common neural tube defects are anencephaly, spina bifida, and encephalocele. Recommendations from the U.S. Public Health Services are that all women of childbearing age take 0.4 mg of folic acid daily. Foods high in folic acid include dark green leafy vegetables, citrus fruits, beans, yeast, and fortified breakfast cereals.

Sickle Cell Anemia

Sickle cell anemia is an inherited disorder caused by the presence of abnormal hemoglobin in the blood. This abnormal hemoglobin causes the sickling of red blood cells (abnormal sickle shape). Approximately 1 in 11 African Americans in North America has the sickle cell trait; however, less than 1% have sickle cell anemia. Prenatally, women with sickle cell anemia are taught to prevent hypoxia, dehydration, infection, and fatigue to avoid developing a sickle cell crisis. In a sickle cell crisis, cells clump together and result in a blockage of vessels and infarcts in organs. If blockage to the placental circulation occurs, fetal compromise and even fetal death can ensue.

This disorder increases the risk for spontaneous abortion, IUGR, and stillbirth.

To safeguard against complications such as a sickle cell crisis in individuals with sickle cell disease, the following measures should be considered during labor: (1) oxygen supplementation to the mother, (2) administration of intravenous fluids, (3) adequate fetal monitoring, (4) maternal hemoglobin monitoring, and (5) administration of prophylactic antibiotics if operative delivery is necessary or if urinary tract infection is present (Oats & Abraham, 2010). Iron supplementation is rarely necessary, but folate supplements are advised during pregnancy. The goal of care is to prevent sickle cell crisis.

Thalassemia

Thalassemia is a genetic defect that causes abnormal hemoglobin, resulting in hemolysis and anemia. Iron supplementation may cause an iron overload in a woman with the disorder. Some infections can reduce erythrocyte production and accelerate destruction and should be treated promptly.

GASTROINTESTINAL DISORDER

HYPEREMESIS GRAVIDARUM

Mild nausea with or without vomiting occurs during normal pregnancy and usually disappears by the twelfth week, when the body adapts to the pregnant state. When vomiting persists, however, causing serious dehydration, starvation, and excessive weight loss before the twentieth week of pregnancy, the condition is called hyperemesis gravidarum (excessive vomiting of pregnancy). No single cause has been identified; however, endocrine imbalance and the slow motility of the gastrointestinal system during pregnancy are possible contributing factors. The highest incidence of hyperemesis gravidarum occurs with the first pregnancy, multifetal pregnancy, and hydatidiform mole and in women with a history of psychiatric disorders. Conditions such as pancreatitis, hepatitis, and thyroid disease should be ruled out. The fetus is at risk for IUGR if this condition persists.

Assessment and Management

Excessive vomiting, when it occurs over a prolonged period, may cause the woman to be dehydrated and results in electrolyte imbalances. Severe potassium loss may alter cardiac function, and fetal loss may be a risk. The woman may need to be hospitalized, and an intravenous infusion is started and continued until vomiting ceases. In some cases, intravenous therapy can be managed as home care. Correcting fluid and electrolyte imbalances is important in the treatment. All oral intake of food and fluids is stopped until the woman can retain fluid in small amounts. Vitamin and mineral supplements or steroids may be prescribed, and total

parenteral nutrition (TPN) is considered. A record of oral intake and urinary and stool output is maintained. Weight loss and ketonuria suggest that the woman's fat stores are being used to nourish the fetus and to meet the woman's energy needs. Low-fat frequent feedings, positioning, and other techniques to reduce nausea are used. Drugs such as pyridoxine, meclizine, diphenhydramine, and metoclopramide are often prescribed with good results (Tan, Khine, Vallikkannu, & Omar, 2010). PPIs such as Omeprazole have been found to be safe to administer in early pregnancy (Pasternak & Hviid, 2010). The pregnancy safety classification of drugs should be reviewed before administration. The home health nurse and dietitian are important members of the health care team. Good oral hygiene and weight monitoring are essential nursing interventions.

The nurse who is caring for a woman with hyperemesis gravidarum should demonstrate patience and understanding. The nursing assessment includes listening to the woman's conversation for clues to what triggers her nausea or vomiting. Usually after 48 hours of hospitalization, the woman's condition will improve and small amounts of food may be tolerated. The woman should return frequently to the clinic for assessments. CAM therapies such as wrist acupressure bands, herbal tea, ginger root, and vitamin B$_6$ are popular treatments (see Chapter 21).

ENDOCRINE DISORDERS

DIABETES MELLITUS

Diabetes mellitus is an endocrine disorder of carbohydrate metabolism. It is characterized by hyperglycemia (elevated blood sugar) resulting from the inadequate production or ineffective use of insulin. When insulin is insufficient or ineffective, glucose accumulates in the bloodstream and hyperglycemia results. Hyperglycemia causes an increase of intracellular fluid in the vascular system, resulting in an expanded blood volume. This causes the kidneys to excrete large amounts of urine (polyuria) in an attempt to regulate excess blood volume and to excrete the unusable glucose (glycosuria). Then the body tries to compensate for its inability to convert carbohydrate (glucose) into energy by burning protein (muscle) and fats, the end products of which are ketones and fatty acids. When ketones and fatty acids are in excess quantity, **ketoacidosis** is produced. Because of the breakdown of muscle and fat tissue, weight loss occurs. This causes the body to be in a state of starvation and compels the person to eat excessively; thus, **polyphagia** occurs. As this continues, vascular changes occur, affecting the heart, eyes, and kidneys. Any problem in carbohydrate metabolism before pregnancy is increased during pregnancy. If a woman has the potential for developing diabetes mellitus, pregnancy may trigger gestational diabetes mellitus (GDM) (London, Ladewig, Ball, & Bindler, 2006).

[handwritten note top left: - eating fruits for breakfast is bad because it stays in body as sugar. if their is a big gap between meals.]

[handwritten note top right: 125 bld sugar after eating / 90 bld sugar when waking up]

Classification

Pregestational diabetes mellitus is the label given to type 1 or type 2 diabetes that existed before pregnancy. GDM refers to glucose intolerance first recognized during pregnancy; it usually resolves after birth, although the woman is at risk of developing diabetes later in life. Box 13-4 classifies diabetes mellitus based on the cause. A classification of diabetes mellitus in relation to the extent of the disease—White's classification of diabetes in pregnancy—lists the duration of the illness and the extent of existing organ damage (London, Ladewig, Ball, & Bindler, 2006).

Effect of Pregnancy on Diabetes

Pregnancy has been called a *diabetogenic* state in which the need for glucose is increased, creating a resistance to insulin. It is important to remember that maternal insulin does not cross the placenta. Therefore, by the tenth week of gestation, the fetus is obligated to secrete his or her own insulin to use glucose obtained from the mother.

During the first trimester of pregnancy, maternal glucose levels decrease as a result of increased fetal demands of rapid cell division. In addition, during the first trimester, the woman experiences nausea and vomiting and decreased food intake, further decreasing her glucose levels. During the second and third trimesters, rising levels of hormones (e.g., estrogen, progesterone, human placental lactogen, cortisol, and insulinase) increase insulin resistance through their actions as insulin antagonists. These effects are more pronounced during the second and third trimesters because the concentration of the hormones is greater. Insulin resistance allows more maternal glucose to be available to the fetus. Periods of hyperglycemia may occur for which the diabetic mother will need an increased insulin supply. Hyperglycemia in the fetus results in rapid fetal growth (macrosomia). Control of maternal glucose levels is vital to a good pregnancy outcome.

[handwritten note left margin: can't produce insulin]

[handwritten note right margin: usually overweight / have hormone imbalances]

Box 13-4 Types of Diabetes Mellitus

Type 1 diabetes: Usually caused by pathologic condition of the pancreas, resulting in an insulin deficiency.
Type 2 diabetes: Usually caused by insulin resistance. This type of diabetes has a strong genetic predisposition.
Pregestational diabetes: Type 1 or 2 diabetes that exists before pregnancy occurs.
Gestational diabetes mellitus (GDM): Glucose intolerance with onset during pregnancy. In true GDM, glucose usually returns to normal by 6 weeks after pregnancy.

Modified from American College of Obstetricians and Gynecologists. (2003). Report of the expert committee on the diagnosis and classification of diabetes mellitus. *Diabetes Care, 26*(Suppl 1), S5-S20; and American Diabetes Association. (2007). Position statement: Standards of medical care in diabetes. *Diabetes Care, 30*(Suppl1), S4-S41.

During labor, with the increased energy needs, the diabetic woman may require more insulin. An abrupt decrease in insulin requirement occurs after birth, resulting from a decrease in levels of the insulin antagonist hormones formerly produced by the placenta. Maternal tissues quickly regain their nonpregnancy sensitivity to insulin. For the nonlactating woman, pre-pregnancy insulin-carbohydrate balance returns in approximately 7 to 10 days. Lactation uses maternal glucose; therefore, the breastfeeding mother's insulin requirements remain lower.

PREGESTATIONAL DIABETES MELLITUS

When the known diabetic becomes pregnant, she is referred to as a pregestational diabetic. Pregestational diabetics may have either type 1 (insulin-dependent) or type 2 (non-insulin-dependent) diabetes. The diabetogenic state of pregnancy imposed on the compromised metabolic system has significant implications. Pregnancy will affect glycemic control. In addition, pregnancy may accelerate the progress of vascular complications. Oral hypoglycemics cannot be taken during pregnancy because of their potential adverse effect on the developing fetus. *[handwritten asterisk symbol in margin]*

During the first trimester, with the fetus using glucose, the mother's blood glucose levels are usually reduced, and she may need less insulin. Insulin dosage for the well-controlled diabetic may need to be adjusted to avoid hypoglycemia (low blood glucose). Insulin resistance continues to rise until the last few weeks of pregnancy. Blood pressure and blood glucose levels must be maintained within normal ranges to prevent complications to the mother and newborn.

Risks and Complications

Maternal hyperglycemia in the first trimester of pregnancy can cause fetal anomalies. In the second and third trimesters, glucose, but not insulin, crosses the placental barrier. The fetus responds to the excess glucose by secreting additional insulin. Macrosomia and impaired fetal lung functions can occur. At birth, the infant is at risk because the high insulin production remains when the maternal glucose transfer ends, and hypoglycemia can result in the newborn.

The pregnant diabetic woman is at risk for several complications. The severity of the risk is related to the woman's glycemic control before and during the pregnancy. Maternal and fetal complications that commonly occur with the diabetic pregnancy are listed in Box 13-5. New techniques for monitoring glucose levels, delivering insulin, and monitoring the fetus can reduce perinatal mortality.

Preconceptional Counseling

A woman with pregestational diabetes mellitus should be counseled before a planned pregnancy regarding need for glycemic control, high-risk management of

[handwritten note bottom: ✗ snack and eat every 2-3hr to prevent bolus of sugar.]

Box 13-5	Maternal Diabetes Mellitus: Risks to Mother and Fetus

- Spontaneous abortion increases with diabetes mellitus; the risk is related to poor glycemic control.
- Infections may increase in pregnant diabetic women (urinary tract and vaginal infections increase because of glucose in the urine); any alteration in carbohydrate metabolism alters the body's resistance to infection.
- Hydramnios may increase, possibly because of increased fetal urination resulting from fetal hyperglycemia, causing overdistention of the uterus, premature rupture of membranes, preterm labor, and hemorrhage.
- Gestational hypertension increases, with the highest incidence in women with preexisting vascular changes caused by diabetes.
- Ketoacidosis occurs most often in the second and third trimesters, when the diabetogenic effect of pregnancy is the greatest as insulin resistance increases; it is commonly a result of untreated hyperglycemia, inappropriate dosage, or maternal infections. Ketoacidosis occurring during pregnancy can lead to fetal complications, even fetal death.
- Hypoglycemia increases even with strict glycemic control; hypoglycemia can be caused by overdose of insulin, skipped or late meals, or increased exercise. During the first trimester, severe hypoglycemia can cause congenital fetal defects. Hypoglycemia in the newborn can occur 2 to 4 hours after birth and requires immediate intervention.
- Hyperglycemia can cause excessive fetal growth (macrosomia) (see Chapter 15).
- Respiratory distress syndrome can occur in the newborn because high levels of insulin interfere with surfactant production in the lungs.
- Polycythemia in the newborn can occur because a maternal high glycosylated hemoglobin level occurs in poorly controlled diabetes mellitus; glycosylated hemoglobin does not release oxygen easily, and the resulting fetal hypoxia causes the fetus to develop polycythemia (too many red blood cells in the blood).

status and support system are assessed along with her knowledge of diabetes to determine her teaching needs. A thorough physical examination is performed to assess the woman's health status. A baseline ECG is performed to check her cardiovascular status. In addition to routine prenatal care, the diabetic woman needs special assessments and management at home and in the hospital.

 Patient Teaching

Self-Care for the Woman with Diabetes Mellitus

Symptoms of hypoglycemia and ketoacidosis: The pregnant diabetic woman must be able to recognize symptoms that indicate a change in glucose levels. She should be advised to check her capillary blood glucose level to see whether it is above or below normal. In addition, she should always carry a snack as a fast source of glucose. She should be advised to drink milk when possible to avoid a rebound of hyperglycemia.

Travel: If insulin is required, the woman should keep it refrigerated as needed while she is traveling. She should wear a bracelet that identifies her as being diabetic.

Cesarean birth: The woman should be advised of an increased possibility of a cesarean birth.

Hospitalization: The woman should be advised that she may be hospitalized two or three times during her pregnancy if evaluation of glucose levels or adjustment of her insulin levels is necessary.

Fetal monitoring: The woman should be advised that fetal status will be periodically assessed during pregnancy.

Smoking: The woman who smokes should be advised about the harmful effects of smoking on both the maternal vascular system and the development of the fetus.

Strict adherence to diet: The woman should understand that during pregnancy, for the well-being of the fetus, she must adhere to her diet.

Careful monitoring of glucose levels at home: The woman should be advised that reliability in her daily record of glucose levels is important in her care.

Exercise: Exercise should be carefully monitored.

the pregnancy, and postpartum follow-up care. The partner should be included in counseling to discuss careful family planning, the financial costs of frequent maternal-fetal monitoring, and need for compliance. Often the woman may be a well-controlled diabetic before pregnancy who finds that the physiology of pregnancy places special demands on her body; some medications used for glucose control cannot be used during pregnancy, and, therefore, modifications of care and close monitoring become necessary.

Assessment and Management

In large measure, the effective management of a diabetic pregnancy depends on the woman's adherence to the devised care plan (monitoring diet, exercise, and insulin administration). The woman's emotional

Diet. The recommended diet is based on blood glucose levels and individualized to meet cultural and lifestyle needs as well as fetal and metabolic requirements. The average diet may be 30 to 35 kcal/kg of body weight in the first trimester and 35 kcal/kg in the second and third trimesters, with carefully planned snacks. A large bedtime snack is recommended to prevent nighttime hypoglycemia. Forty percent to 50% of calories should be complex, high-fiber carbohydrates; 20% comes from protein, and 30% to 40% from fats (ACOG, 2005). The woman is taught signs of hypoglycemia and hyperglycemia and home care of such events. The woman is encouraged to eliminate empty calories in the form of sweets from her diet. Vitamins and folic acid supplementation in the form of prenatal vitamins are recommended, as with all pregnancies. A dietitian or nutritionist is an important part of the health care team and can help the woman develop appropriate individualized diet plans.

Nutrition Considerations

Simple Carbohydrates for Self-Treatment of Hypoglycemia (<60 mg/dL Blood Glucose)

- 4 oz unsweetened fruit juice
- 4 oz regular soda
- 5 Lifesaver candies
- 2-3 glucose tablets

Blood glucose should be reassessed to determine response.

Modified from American Diabetes Association. (2000). *Medical management of pregnancy complicated by diabetes* (3rd ed.). Alexandria, VA: Author.

Exercise. Individually prescribed exercise according to the pre-pregnant lifestyle is recommended. Proper exercise enables muscle activity to help normalize glucose levels.

Caused by hormones produced by placenta

GESTATIONAL DIABETES MELLITUS

Gestational diabetes mellitus (GDM) is diabetes mellitus defined as carbohydrate intolerance of variable severity, with the first recognition during the pregnancy. Pregnancy uncovers the diabetic tendencies of asymptomatic women by the insulin resistance that occurs during gestation. Women with GDM may have only an impaired tolerance to glucose, and others may have a mild form of the disorder. Some women with GDM exhibit the classic signs of diabetes, including excessive thirst, hunger, urination, and weakness. The routine urinalysis showing glucose (glycosuria) during a prenatal visit is usually the first indication of diabetes. Diagnosis of GDM is important, however, because even mild diabetes causes increased risks for the newborn. Because gestational diabetes develops after the first trimester, the risk of congenital malformation and spontaneous abortion is less than with pregestational diabetes.

Diet often controls gestational diabetes; however, 10% to 15% of women with GDM will require insulin to maintain glycemic control. In gestational diabetes, the problem is evidenced after 20 weeks' gestation, and, therefore, fetal malformation will not occur if oral hypoglycemics are used and the woman is closely monitored (Major, 2010). The symptoms of diabetes may disappear a few weeks after the birth of the newborn. However, as many as 35% to 50% of women with gestational diabetes will show further deterioration of carbohydrate metabolism in the next 15 years of life. Because of this, the woman and her family should be well educated in the recognition of signs and symptoms of diabetes and dietary management for hypoglycemia.

Screening During Pregnancy

The ACOG recommends that all pregnant women be screened for gestational diabetes. A glucose challenge test (a screening test) commonly given for gestational diabetes is the 50-g, 1-hour diabetes challenge test. It is not necessary to follow any special diet before the test. If the plasma glucose 1 hour after ingesting 50 g glucose is greater than 140 mg/dL, a follow-up oral glucose tolerance test is performed for more accurate evaluation. The usual time to screen is between 24 and 28 weeks' gestation. Because the renal threshold is lower during pregnancy, glucose may spill into the urine. Therefore, glycosuria is not considered diagnostic for diabetes but does indicate the need for further evaluation. Care of the newborn of a diabetic mother is discussed in Chapter 16.

Glucose Monitoring

The goal of glucose monitoring is to maintain a level between 80 and 120 mg/dL, the latter being a postprandial (after meals) level. The evaluation of glycemic control is based on a glycosylated hemoglobin (**HbA1c**) level. This measurement is based on the fact that glucose attaches to hemoglobin A (HbA); measuring the amount of glucose-attached HbA determines the glycemic control for the preceding 2 to 3 months. An HbA_{1c} level obtained at the first prenatal visit provides an estimated risk for diabetic-related problems in the first trimester. A measurement of under 7% is acceptable, but levels of 7.2% to 9.1% is associated with a 14% increased risk of fetal malformation (Major, 2010). Monthly levels are assessed throughout pregnancy. Monitoring daily blood glucose levels at home can be accomplished with a glucose monitor. Some models can be downloaded to a personal computer and communicated to the clinic nurse. Blood glucose should be measured before meals and 2 hours after meals until stable; a regular regimen should then be instituted.

Elective induction of labor may be planned between 38 and 40 weeks' gestation in a well-controlled diabetic woman. Close glucose monitoring during labor and postpartum is essential. Cesarean birth is common because of cephalopelvic disproportion caused by fetal **macrosomia** (increased fetal size). The postpartum patient taking oral hypoglycemics can safely breastfeed because exposure through breast milk is limited (Major, 2010).

Fetal Surveillance

Prenatal fetal assessment is essential during pregnancy and labor. Some tests that may be performed during the last trimester include a biophysical profile, serum alpha-fetoprotein (AFP), amniocentesis, a nonstress test, and kick counts to assess fetal activity. See Chapter 5 for fetal assessment tests.

Emotional Support and Communication

Empowering the woman to make as many decisions as possible concerning home care, diet selection, and exercise regimen will promote compliance and prevent her from feeling her pregnancy is an illness and a negative experience. Involving the multidisciplinary health care team in meeting the needs of the woman and including the family in the teaching program are essential for a positive outcome.

INFECTIONS

Maternal infections known as the TORCH infections are those infectious diseases identified as teratogenic, which cause harm to the embryo and developing fetus. They are *T*oxoplasmosis, *R*ubella, *C*ytomegalovirus (CMV), and *H*erpesvirus type 2. Some identify the "*O*" as *other infections*. Although the acronym *TORCH* is useful to identify congenital risks, it does not include all of the major infections that pose risks to the mother and newborn (Table 13-6). The mnemonic *Storch*[6] has been recommended as a modification of the TORCH mnemonic. *Storch* is a German term for stork, which is associated with pregnancy, and the H[6] takes the place of the "O" for other diseases. *Storch*[6] specifically adds syphilis, herpes, human immunodeficiency virus (HIV), human papillomavirus, human parvovirus, and hepatitis C. Selected sexually transmitted infections and other infections are discussed in Chapter 20.

URINARY TRACT INFECTIONS

Urinary tract infections (UTIs) affect 5% to 20% of pregnant women. During pregnancy, anatomic changes in the urinary tract predispose women to infections. The growing uterus compresses both ureters, which decrease the flow to the bladder, thereby causing urinary stasis. The incidence of glycosuria (glucose in the urine) is increased, which favors bacterial growth and development of UTIs. Progesterone relaxes the bladder muscle, causing delayed emptying and urinary stasis. The organism most commonly found in UTIs during pregnancy is *Escherichia coli* because the urinary meatus is near the rectum in women.

Three clinical types of UTI during pregnancy are asymptomatic infection, bladder infection (cystitis), and kidney infection (pyelonephritis). Some asymptomatic women with a UTI may develop pyelonephritis. A laboratory examination of the urine may show bacteriuria, pyuria, and hematuria. The symptoms and signs of UTI vary with the site and degree of infection. The significant symptoms are dysuria, increased frequency of urination, urgency, and

---

Box 13-6   Patient Education Concerning Urinary Tract Infections

- Explain the method of obtaining a clean-catch, midstream-voided urine specimen.
- Instruct the woman to cleanse her perineal area from front to back to avoid vaginal contamination with *Escherichia coli.*
- Explain to the woman the predisposing causes of urinary tract infection (UTI) during pregnancy and how to recognize symptoms.
- Encourage an increase in fluid intake to decrease risk of infection.
- Suggest the following: (1) a source of vitamin C daily to promote healing; (2) a glass of cranberry juice at bedtime to acidify urine; and (3) avoidance of coffee, tea, alcohol, and spices, which are potential bladder irritants.
- Counsel the woman to empty her bladder frequently and never ignore her urge to void.
- If drugs are ordered, explain the importance of maintaining medication schedules to keep blood levels stable.
- Instruct the woman to keep all appointments with the clinic or physician.

---

hematuria. Backache, elevated temperature, and tenderness over the kidney area occur with pyelonephritis. Septic shock and death, though rare, can occur with severe kidney infections. Teaching the importance of adequate hydration, perineal hygiene, prompt voiding, and signs of UTI is essential to the care plan (Box 13-6).

Bacteriuria

All pregnant women should have a urine culture no later than 35 to 37 weeks' gestation for group B beta-hemolytic streptococci (GBS). A positive GBS culture from a clean-catch midstream urine specimen requires prompt treatment with oral antibiotics to prevent UTI and decrease the risk for neonatal infection.

— if not treated baby will become septic

Assessment and Management

The woman should be asked at each prenatal visit whether she has any signs or symptoms of UTI. If symptoms are present, a clean-catch urine specimen for microanalysis, culture, and sensitivity tests should be ordered. The nurse instructs the woman on how to obtain the clean-catch specimen by first cleaning and drying the perineal area. Then the woman should hold her labia apart and collect the specimen midstream without touching the skin. The specimen is analyzed for bacteria count, after which a diagnosis is made. If diagnosis is positive, antibiotics are started; after the course is completed, a urine culture may be repeated to verify response to treatment. Women with positive GBS cultures are given antibiotics during the labor and delivery process.

Table 13-6   Infections Known to Be Harmful to the Fetus

ORGANISM AND INFECTION	MATERNAL EFFECTS	FETAL OR NEWBORN EFFECTS
Rubella	Rubella antibody titer <1:10 indicates susceptibility to rubella. Teratogenic virus is contracted through nasopharyngeal secretions; highly contagious; virus is present in the blood. Vaccine is contraindicated during pregnancy.	Cardiac anomalies; deafness, microcephaly, cataracts; heart disorder; IUGR; psychomotor retardation if mother has rubella in first 4 weeks of pregnancy.
Toxoplasmosis (protozoa *Toxoplasma gondii*)	Most women are asymptomatic. Acquired by eating raw meat or contact with cat feces; pregnant women should avoid cat litter boxes and garden soil, cook meat thoroughly, wash fruits and vegetables, and wash hands thoroughly. Detected by enzyme-linked immunosorbent assay (ELISA) antibody testing.	Central nervous system and ocular damage; severity varies with gestation; growth retardation. Sulfadiazine, pyrimethamine, and leukovorin may be used to treat the infected newborn.
Herpes simplex virus (HSV)	Primary maternal infection is transmitted by intimate mucocutaneous contact; highly contagious. It is associated with increased spontaneous abortion and preterm labor. Antiviral therapy may be indicated. Women with a prior history of herpes should deliver vaginally only if no genital lesions are present at the time of labor. Once delivered, mother and newborn can be together as long as direct contact with lesions is avoided. Mother may breastfeed if no lesions are present on breast.	50% of newborns born vaginally to mothers with primary infection will have HSV infection; mortality rate is 50%-60%; causes central nervous system and eye problems, jaundice, and respiratory distress.
Cytomegalovirus (CMV) (member of the herpes group)	Transmission of virus may be sexual or by body fluids. Transmission of CMV to fetus can occur at time of vaginal delivery. Diagnosis by isolation of virus from endocervical secretions, ELISA, complement fixation tests.	Preterm birth, IUGR, mental retardation, deafness, or blindness; no effective treatment available.
Group B beta-hemolytic streptococcus (GBS)	Organism is found in woman's rectum, vagina, cervix, throat, and saliva. Woman is usually asymptomatic, but newborn is infected through contact with vaginal secretions at birth. Linked to preterm labor and infection. Women are screened during pregnancy to see if they are GBS carriers; positive vaginal cultures at 35-37 weeks' gestation are treated with penicillin during labor. Positive GBS urinalysis is treated prenatally. If membranes have been ruptured for more than 18 hours, also treated prophylactically with penicillin.	GBS can be fatal for newborn; newborn can have early-onset GBS (within 12 hours after birth) or late-onset GBS infection after 7 days of age. Neurologic impairment may occur; pneumonia, sepsis, respiratory distress, apnea, meningitis.
Syphilis (spirochete *Treponema pallidum*)	Diagnosed by the Venereal Disease Research Laboratory (VDRL) test or Rapid Plasma Reagin (RPR) test. Can be passed through placenta to fetus. Untreated cases can cause abortion, stillbirth; penicillin is treatment of choice.	Congenital syphilis can cause multiple neonatal and development problems.

IUGR, intrauterine growth restriction.

 Medication Safety Alert

Some Antibiotics Are Contraindicated in Pregnancy

Penicillin and erythromycin are considered safe during pregnancy, but sulfonamides and nitrofurantoin are not (Crider, Cleves, Reefhuis, Berry, Hobbs, & Hu, 2009).

BACTERIAL VAGINOSIS

Hormonal changes, pregnancy, and antibiotic therapy are usually the cause of bacterial vaginosis (BV). BV is associated with preterm pregnancy, premature rupture of the membranes, and postpartum infections. Symptoms include a thin grey vaginal discharge with a foul fishy odor. Oral metronidazole or clindamycin is the drug of choice to treat BV.

SUBSTANCE ABUSE

The use of illegal drugs, tobacco, and alcohol during pregnancy can seriously affect fetal development and pregnancy outcome. The newborn is at greatest risk during the first trimester; however, these substances can be damaging to the fetus throughout the pregnancy (Table 13-7). Substances taken intravenously or intranasally are most likely to cross the placental barrier, and a lifestyle that includes substance abuse by the mother is often associated with poor nutrition and poor prenatal care, which also affect pregnancy outcome. Nurses must be alert to history or physical signs of substance abuse to ensure a positive pregnancy outcome.

ACCIDENTS DURING PREGNANCY

Motor vehicle accidents are the most common cause of trauma during pregnancy. Blunt trauma to the abdomen can cause abruptio placentae and fetal death.

Falls sometimes occur in late pregnancy when balance is altered and the abdomen protrudes. In minor injuries, the fetus is protected by the bony pelvis; muscle layers of the abdomen and uterus; and the amniotic fluid, which distributes the force of the blow equally in all directions. Serious blunt trauma or penetrating wounds can cause shock, preterm labor, or spontaneous abortion. Prevention of injury can be accomplished by patient education concerning fall prevention, posture, shoes, and the proper wearing of seatbelts when riding in a car (see Chapter 10). In case of severe injury, the ABCs (airway, breathing, circulation) of general life support of the mother are a priority. The pregnant woman should be positioned on the left side to prevent vena caval hypotension syndrome. Oxygen is administered, and the fetal heart rate is monitored. If the uterus is damaged, it may be repaired or a cesarean birth may be indicated. Monitoring for at least 24 hours is indicated when major trauma occurs. Normal changes associated with pregnancy will alter assessments of the woman (Criddle, 2009) (Box 13-7).

Table 13-7   Substance Abuse

SUBSTANCE	MATERNAL EFFECTS	FETAL OR NEWBORN EFFECTS
Tobacco (including passive smoking)	Nicotine crosses placenta and is a vasoconstrictor, causing fetal hypoxia; carbon monoxide effect inactivates hemoglobin, resulting in increased hypoxia of fetus.	IUGR, preterm birth, fetal malformation, neurologic defects
Alcohol (central nervous system [CNS] depressant)	There is no established safe level of alcohol intake during pregnancy. Mother should refrain from regular or heavy alcohol intake; alcohol crosses placental barrier and retards cell organization and growth. Increases risk for spontaneous abortion, abruptio placentae.	Growth retardation, CNS impairment, facial anomalies, mental deficiencies, irritability
Cocaine (crack) (powerful stimulant)	Crosses placenta; causes euphoria (sense of well-being). Generalized hypertension, tachycardia, vasoconstriction, resulting in abruptio placentae and abortion; preterm birth causes anoxia and hyperglycemia; lifestyle of the user places pregnancy at risk.	Causes preterm delivery, tachycardia, fetal hyperactivity, IUGR, poor feeding reflexes, irritability, and difficulty consoling. Crosses into breast milk and will affect the suckling newborn
Heroin (opiate drug related to morphine)	Drug is taken parenterally; therefore woman is likely to be exposed to HIV and other blood-borne infections. Increases risks for premature rupture of membranes, abruptio placentae, malnutrition, anemia, abortion; withdrawal causes fetal hypoxia.	Hyperactivity, high-pitched cry, continuous need for sucking, tremulousness, seizures, disrupted sleep-wake cycles, lack of response to cuddling
Amphetamines ("speed," "crystal," "meth")	Malnutrition causes withdrawal symptoms, anxiety, paranoia.	Risk for anomalies, cardiac problems; can be born with withdrawal symptoms
Sedatives, tranquilizers	Cause CNS depression.	Seizures, delayed lung maturity
Marijuana ("grass," "pot")	Often used with other drugs associated with decreased appetite and poor nutrition.	Possible prematurity, IUGR, sensitivity to light

HIV, human immunodeficiency virus; *IUGR,* intrauterine growth restriction.

BIOTERRORISM EXPOSURE AND PREGNANCY

Pregnancy may alter the metabolism and elimination of drugs. Pregnancy must be evaluated in relation to the gestational age of the fetus. The effects of emerging bioterrorist infections during pregnancy may be different than in the nonpregnant woman. Pregnancy increases the susceptibility to infectious disease, and the death risk is also increased. Delayed gastric emptying and decreased gastrointestinal motility that normally occur during pregnancy influence absorption of oral medication. A decrease in gastric acid secretion during pregnancy may also affect absorption of oral medications. The increased cardiac output that normally occurs during pregnancy may increase absorption of intramuscular medications, whereas decreased blood flow in lower extremities during the third trimester can decrease absorption in these areas. Fat-soluble drugs may distribute faster in the pregnant woman, but concentration of proteins available for binding may result in higher than normal free, unbound drug in the circulating blood. The liver is responsible for most drug metabolism, and enzyme activity is decreased in pregnancy. These factors

indicate that the safe dose of medications given to a nonpregnant woman may not be safe for a woman who is pregnant.

The pregnant woman's immune response is thought to be similar to that of the nonpregnant woman. In bioterrorism emergencies, protecting the life of the mother is the priority. When a life-threatening risk is associated with a bioterrorism agent, a vaccine may be advised regardless of the pregnancy status (Cono, Cragon, Jamieson, & Rasmussen, 2006). The risk of a specific vaccine must be weighed against the risk for the illness and death from the infectious exposure. Close fetal monitoring is required until the woman has recovered from the exposure.

The changes in the immune system of the pregnant woman that occur in order to enable her body to tolerate the "foreign substance" of the fetus make her more susceptible to some infectious diseases and to respond with a more severe type of illness than the nonpregnant woman. All drug books contain information concerning standardized classification of drug safety during pregnancy, ranging from A (no demonstrated fetal risk) to D (evidence of fetal risk, but benefit may outweigh the risk) and X (use in pregnant women is contraindicated). The U.S. Food and Drug Administration classification for bioterrorism medical countermeasures is listed in Table 13-8.

LOSS OF EXPECTED BIRTH EXPERIENCE

Couples rarely anticipate problems when they begin a pregnancy. Most have specific expectations about how their pregnancy, particularly the birth, will proceed. A high-risk pregnancy may result in the loss of their expected experience. If the loss is during early pregnancy, they may be unable to attend childbirth

Box 13-7	The Influence of Pregnancy on Trauma Response and Assessment

- Displacement of the bladder, spleen, and bowel by the enlarged uterus causes them to be at increased risk for rupture.
- In the third trimester, stretching of the peritoneum makes signs of peritoneal irritation (rebound tenderness) difficult to elicit.
- Abdominal palpation is difficult due to enlarged uterus.
- Normal $PaCO_2$ is normally lower during pregnancy and cannot be used as a sensitive indicator of respiratory distress.
- Displacement of diaphragm and reduced lung residual capacity normal in pregnancy increases risk for hypoxia.
- Peripheral vasodilation is normal in pregnancy and may mask early external signs of shock.
- Glomerular filtration rate of kidney is normally increased during pregnancy, making urine output not a reliable indicator of impending shock.
- Esophageal sphincter relaxes, and gastric emptying is normally delayed during pregnancy, increasing risk for aspiration.
- Increased blood volume normal during pregnancy may cause swelling of the nose, pharynx, and trachea, resulting in difficult intubation, epistaxis, and shortness of breath.
- Blood clotting factors are normally increased during pregnancy, resulting in increased risk for thrombophlebitis.
- Injury to the uterus that has an increased blood flow can cause significant blood loss.
- Trauma can cause complications of pregnancy such as abruptio placenta or ruptured uterus.

Table 13-8	Food and Drug Administration Classification for Bioterrorism Countermeasures in Pregnancy	

MEDICATION	CATEGORY	BIOTERRORISM AGENT USE
Amoxicillin	B	Anthrax
Botulism antitoxin	C	Botulism
Cidofovir	C	Vaccinia and monkeypox
Ciprofloxacin	C	Anthrax, plague, and tularemia
Penicillin	B	Anthrax
Vaccinia immune globulin	C	Vaccinia

Data from Cono, J., Cragon, J., Jamieson, D., & Rasmussen, S. (2006). Prophylaxis and treatment of pregnant women for emerging infections and bioterrorism emergencies. *Emerging Infectious Diseases, 12*(11), 1631-1636.

preparation classes or to have a vaginal birth. Perinatal loss shatters the hopes of human life and severs a unique attachment between mother and fetus. Parents exhibit mourning behaviors associated with the various stages of the grieving process. As they work with the parents, health care providers must address aspects of the grieving process.

PREGNANCY LOSS: GRIEF AND BEREAVEMENT

The incidence of perinatal loss after 20 weeks' gestation in the United States is 6.8 per 1000 total births, with 50% occurring before 28 weeks' gestation (CDC, 2009). The cause can be physiologic; maladaptation, such as eclampsia or placenta previa; birth defects; or exposure to teratogens during pregnancy. Contributing to these figures is perinatal loss due to procedures such as assisted reproductive technology, amniocentesis, infections, and paternal exposure to teratogenic pesticides.

The release of thromboplastin from the dead fetus triggers the maternal clotting mechanisms. Maternal fibrinogen levels fall, and the risk of developing DIC increases. An abdominal X-ray film will reveal the Spalding's sign (overriding of fetal cranial bones), and fetal heart tones are absent. Induction of labor is typically started. Fetal and placental studies may be done after delivery to determine the cause of the fetal loss and to provide information and parent counseling.

Because of the dependency of the growing fetus and the newborn on the parents, a unique attachment is created. The parents begin to focus their hopes and dreams on the fetus and, at birth, the newborn. When the fetus or newborn dies, the hopes and dreams are shattered. The terms *grief* and *mourning* are often used interchangeably. The types of perinatal loss include abortion (miscarriage), fetal and neonatal death, sudden infant death syndrome (SIDS), and fetal anomalies.

Acceptance of the loss is difficult for many people. Parents may feel devastated and feel an intense emotional trauma. The behaviors that a couple exhibit while mourning may be associated with the various stages of grieving. Often the first stage is **denial.** Many are in shock and denial, and their behavior is characterized by numbness and impaired decision-making ability, rather than intense feelings about their loss. The second stage is **anger.** Parents begin to look for answers and often talk about the events that led up to and occurred during the time of death. They may project their anger on significant others or on health care providers and may have feelings of guilt. Behavior is characterized as intermittent crying, loss of appetite, and insomnia. **Bargaining,** the third stage, depends on the couple's preparation for the death of the fetus. They may express their feelings by statements such as, "I wish I could change what I did, and maybe it would not have happened." Behavior may be characterized by disorganization or wishing things were different. The fourth stage is **depression.** With the loss of a fetus, it may appear in 24 to 48 hours. Parents may feel fatigued, withdraw from their relatives and friends, and feel powerless. Behavior is characterized by verbalization of sad memories. By talking through their feelings, they begin to face the reality of the loss and begin to integrate it into their lives. In the fifth stage, **acceptance,** parents may begin to accept the reality of the loss and begin to participate in daily routine activities. Parents need to be asked whether they want health care providers to call clergy to assist them through the pain of the loss. Referral to community support groups may be helpful (Nursing Care Plan 13-2).

Some facilities have a checklist to make sure health care providers address important aspects of grieving as they work with the parents. The checklist might include:

- Allow the woman and her partner to remain together as much as they wish. Provide a private room if possible.
- Allow the couple to show their emotions freely and accept their crying and depression.
- Develop a plan to allow the same nurse to care for the woman to increase support for her and her family.
- Let the woman decide whether she wants sedation.
- Let the woman decide whether she prefers to be in another unit. If in the same unit, assign her a room away from the new mothers with babies.
- Offer a memento, such as a card with footprints, crib card, identification band, or possibly a lock of hair (Figure 13-7).
- Give the couple an opportunity to see and hold the stillborn if they choose. Prepare the couple for the appearance of the baby. Be truthful in your descriptions, such as "The baby is blue."

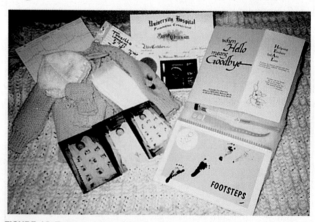

FIGURE 13-7 This "memory kit" includes a picture of the newborn, clothing, death certificate, footprints, identification band, fetal monitor printout, and ultrasound picture.

- Support the parents' choice. Some parents will want to dress the baby.
- Provide the couple with educational material.
- Provide information about community support groups, including their telephone numbers.

- Refer parents to a religious support group or, if they attend a particular church, ask whether they would like someone in that church to be contacted.
- Discuss further care of the baby, including their religious or cultural rituals.

⭐ Nursing Care Plan 13-2   The Family Experiencing Early Pregnancy Loss

Scenario

A woman is admitted at 18 weeks' gestation and within a few hours delivers a fetus that does not survive. The woman asks what she has done wrong to cause this loss.

Selected Nursing Diagnosis

Grieving related to loss of anticipated infant

Expected Outcomes	Nursing Interventions	Rationales
Patient and family will express grief to significant others.	Promote expression of grief by providing privacy, eliminating time restrictions, allowing support persons of choice to visit, and recognizing individualized grief expressions and cultural norms.	Grief is an individual process and people react to it in different ways; these measures encourage woman and family to express grief and begin resolving it.
Patient and family will complete each stage of the grieving process within individual time frames.	Use the four stages of grief and related behaviors as a basis for nursing interventions: *Stage 1:* shock and disbelief at loss; characterized by numbness, apathy, impaired decision making *Stage 2:* seeking answers for why loss happened; characterized by crying, tears, guilt, loss of appetite, insomnia, blame placing *Stage 3:* disorganization; characterized by feelings of purposelessness and malaise; gradual resumption of normal activities *Stage 4:* reorganization; characterized by sad memories, but daily functioning returns	Knowledge of normal stages of grieving helps the nurse identify whether it is progressing normally or whether any family member has dysfunctional grieving. Stages help the nurse better interpret patient's behavior; for example, blame placing is a normal part of grieving and is not necessarily directed at the nurse or caregivers; allows the nurse to reassure the patient that feelings are normal without diminishing the intensity of their feelings.
	Use open communication techniques such as: Quiet presence Expression of sympathy ("I'm sorry this happened.") Open-ended statements ("This must be really sad for you.") Reflection of patient's expressed feelings ("You feel guilty because you didn't stay in bed constantly?")	Presence, empathy, and open communication encourage the family to express feelings about the loss, which is the first step in resolving them. Refer as needed to community agency or multidisciplinary health care team.
	Reinforce explanations given by the health care provider or others (e.g., what the problem was, why it occurred); use simple language.	Grieving people often do not hear or understand explanations the first time they are given because their concentration is impaired.

Critical Thinking Questions

1. What steps should you, as a nurse, take to assist the woman in dealing with the loss of pregnancy?
2. How should you formulate questions to foster communication with the patient?

Get Ready for the NCLEX® Examination!

Key Points

- The causes of bleeding in early pregnancy include abortion, ectopic pregnancy, and hydatidiform mole. Later in pregnancy, two major causes of bleeding are placenta previa and abruptio placentae.
- Ectopic pregnancy, an abnormal implantation of the fertilized ovum outside of the uterine cavity, can be fatal to the woman without prompt management. Implantation usually occurs in the fallopian tube, and tubal rupture and hemorrhage can occur. With a transvaginal ultrasound probe, detection of ectopic pregnancy can be made earlier and with accuracy, thereby preventing a fatal hemorrhage.
- Two main dangers of placenta previa are hemorrhage for the mother and prematurity for the fetus.
- Placenta previa should be suspected in the last half of pregnancy when there is painless bleeding, which may be intermittent or in gushes. Manual vaginal examination is contraindicated in bleeding of late pregnancy.
- Abruptio placentae is premature separation of the normal placenta and can be partial or total. Classic symptoms of the disorder are dark red vaginal bleeding, uterine rigidity, severe abdominal pain, and fetal distress. If the blood is trapped behind the placenta (concealed bleeding), it can make it difficult for the uterus to contract. Also, trapping the blood may release thromboplastin into the maternal bloodstream and initiate DIC.
- Rh incompatibility is an antigen-antibody sensitization. Rh-negative women can be exposed to fetal Rh-positive red blood cells in many ways (e.g., through amniocentesis, abortion, and as the placenta separates after birth). To protect against maternal formation of antibodies against Rh-positive fetal blood, RhoGAM is given.
- GH is a multisystem disease. The major target organs are the cardiovascular system, kidneys, and the uteroplacental bed.
- The two cardinal signs of GH are hypertension and proteinuria. The definitive treatment for GH, if the disease is worsening, is termination of the pregnancy (delivery of the fetus).
- During hospitalization, MgSO₄ is given to prevent seizures in GH. The antidote, calcium gluconate, should be readily available at the woman's bedside.
- Methyldopa is the drug of choice to treat GH. ACE inhibitors should be avoided.
- The HELLP syndrome is manifested by Hemolysis, Elevated Liver enzymes (transaminase), and Low Platelet count (thrombocytopenia). It is a variant of severe GH.
- Thromboembolic disease places pregnancy at risk and can endanger the woman's life. Physiologic changes that occur during pregnancy increase the risks, including venous distensibility, vena cava compression, and venous stasis of the lower extremities. With slowing of blood flow, blood stasis occurs, and a clot may form and attach itself to a blood vessel; if the embolus breaks off and travels to the lungs, it can be life threatening unless treated promptly.
- The hemodynamic changes that occur during pregnancy can have a profound effect on the woman with heart disease. These changes (e.g., increased cardiac output) may exceed the limited functional capacity of a damaged heart. Management includes additional rest, activity restriction, infection control, and diet modification.
- MgSO₄ is the drug of choice to treat eclamptic convulsions.
- Iron deficiency anemia is a common disorder of pregnancy. With the expansion of plasma volume and use of iron by the fetus, it is difficult for many women to replace iron by diet alone; therefore, ferrous sulfate is often given as a dietary supplement during pregnancy. Vitamin C and zinc should be taken to enhance the absorption of iron.
- Folic acid deficiency anemia may result from inadequate folic acid intake. Folic acid deficiency increases the risk of neural tube defects; therefore, 0.4 mg of folic acid daily should be taken by all women of childbearing age.
- Hyperemesis gravidarum occurs when excessive vomiting persists and causes serious dehydration, starvation, and electrolyte imbalance. Liquids and solid food are withheld until tolerated, and intravenous infusions are administered.
- A woman who is previously known to have diabetes is classified as having pregestational diabetes. When onset occurs or is first diagnosed during pregnancy, the woman is classified as having GDM.
- Complications that commonly occur in the woman with pregestational diabetes include spontaneous abortion, infections, GH, macrosomia, hypoglycemia, and ketoacidosis. Glycemic control is critical to the well-being of the newborn.
- GDM becomes apparent due to the metabolic demands of pregnancy.
- Insulin is used in treating diabetes in pregnancy when diet alone does not provide glucose control. Oral hypoglycemics are not used during the first trimester because they cross the placental barrier and can cause fetal anomalies.
- Maternal infections, known as the *TORCH infections*, are those infections that can be harmful (teratogenic) to the embryo and fetus. These include toxoplasmosis, rubella, cytomegalovirus, and herpesvirus.

Additional Learning Resources

SG Go to your Study Guide on pages 497–498 for additional Review Questions for the NCLEX® Examination, Critical Thinking Clinical Situations, and other learning activities to help you master this chapter content.

*e*volve Go to your Evolve website (http://evolve.elsevier.com/Leifer/maternity) for the following FREE learning resources:
- Animations
- Answer Guidelines for Critical Thinking Questions
- Answers and Rationales for Review Questions for the NCLEX® Examination
- Concept Map Creator
- Glossary with pronunciations in English and Spanish
- Patient Teaching Plans
- Skills Performance Checklists and more!

Online Resources

- www.acog.org
- www.cdc.gov/groupBstrep
- www.phf.org

Review Questions for the NCLEX® Examination

1. Education for a woman following diagnosis of gestational trophoblastic disease would include: *(Select all that apply.)*
   1. The hCG titers will be monitored for a year.
   2. Pregnancy can be attempted as soon as hCG levels begin to decrease.
   3. Subsequent pregnancies should be normal because there is a low risk of recurrence.
   4. Treatment begins with the evacuation of the mole by suction aspiration.

2. A condition resulting from overstimulation of the normal coagulation process in which a coagulation defect prevents blood from clotting is:
   1. Abruptio placentae
   2. Thrombocytopenia
   3. Eclampsia
   4. Disseminated intravascular coagulation (DIC)

3. A pregnant woman in the thirtieth week of gestation is diagnosed with gestational hypertension (GH). Which statement made by the woman indicates a need for further education regarding management of GH?
   1. "I should maintain an adequate diet and fluid intake."
   2. "I will remain on strict bed rest for the remainder of my pregnancy."
   3. "I must have a mode of transportation available at all times."
   4. "I should not restrict sodium."

4. A pregnant woman with a cardiac history is receiving anticoagulant therapy and has been instructed to restrict foods high in vitamin K. Which food should the nurse instruct the woman to restrict?
   1. Spinach
   2. Cheese
   3. Chicken
   4. Bananas

5. The highest incidence of hyperemesis gravidarum occurs with:
   1. Adolescent pregnancies
   2. First pregnancies
   3. Advanced maternal age
   4. Gestational diabetes

6. The goal of glucose monitoring in a woman with gestational diabetes is to maintain a level between:
   1. 60 and 80 mg/dL
   2. 80 and 120 mg/dL
   3. 100 and 130 mg/dL
   4. 120 and 140 mg/dL

7. A pregnant woman is diagnosed with bacterial vaginosis (BV). The drug of choice to treat BV is:
   1. Clindamycin
   2. Amoxicillin
   3. Topical hydrocortisone
   4. Tetracycline

8. Management of placenta previa depends on which characteristic(s)? *(Select all that apply.)*
   1. Maternal age
   2. Classification of previa
   3. Fetal heart rate
   4. Gestational age of the fetus
   5. Maternal vital signs

Critical Thinking Questions

1. A woman has been diagnosed with mild GH. Her blood pressure is 140 mm Hg systolic and 90 mm Hg diastolic, urine showed 1 + protein, and ankle edema is present. What type of home conditions must she have to stay home and not be hospitalized?

2. A woman is 8 weeks pregnant and has started to have vaginal bleeding. She has not had abdominal cramps and has not passed tissue. She asks you if she has lost her baby. What do you know about her clinical situation, including her symptoms, that will guide your answer?

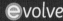
Objectives

1. Define key terms listed.
2. Discuss four factors associated with preterm labor.
3. Describe two major nursing assessments of a woman in preterm labor.
4. Explain why tocolytic agents are used in preterm labor.
5. Interpret the term *premature rupture of membranes*.
6. Identify two complications of premature rupture of membranes.
7. Differentiate between hypotonic and hypertonic uterine dysfunction.
8. Name and describe the three different types of breech presentation.
9. List two potential complications of a breech birth.
10. Explain the term *cephalopelvic disproportion* (CPD), and discuss the nursing management of CPD.
11. Define and identify three common methods used to induce labor.
12. Explain why an episiotomy is performed, and name two basic types of episiotomies.
13. Describe three types of lacerations that can occur during the birth process.
14. List two indications for using forceps to deliver the fetus.
15. Describe vacuum extraction.
16. Define precipitate labor, and describe two nursing actions that should be taken to safeguard the baby.
17. Review the most common cause of rupture of the uterus during labor.
18. Describe umbilical cord prolapse, and state two associated potential complications.
19. List three potential complications of multifetal pregnancy.
20. Discuss five indications for a cesarean birth.
21. Describe the preoperative and postoperative care of a woman who is undergoing a cesarean birth.
22. Discuss the rationale for vaginal birth after a prior cesarean birth.

Key Terms

amnioinfusion (ăm-nē-ō-ĭn-FŪ-zhăn, p. 294)
amniotomy (ăm-nē-ŎT-ŏ-mē, p. 290)
augmentation of labor (ăwg-mĕn-TĀ-shŭn, p. 289)
Bishop score (p. 290)
caput chignon (kap′ət′shĕn′yän, p. 293)
cephalopelvic disproportion (CPD) (sĕf-ă-lō-PĔL-vĭc dĭs-prō-PŌR-shŭn, p. 286)
cesarean birth (sĕ-ZĀR-ē-ăn, p. 295)
chorioamnionitis (kō-rē-ō-ăm-nē-ō-NĪ-tĭs, p. 284)
dysfunctional labor (p. 285)
dystocia (dĭs-TŌ-sē-ă, p. 284)
episiotomy (ĕ-pēz-ē-ŎT-ō-mē, p. 291)
external version (p. 287)
fern test (p. 284)
forceps (p. 292)
hydramnios (hī-DRĂM-nē-ŏs, p. 293)

hypertonic uterine dysfunction (hī-pĕr-TŎN-ĭk Ū-tĕr-ĭn, p. 285)
hypotonic uterine dysfunction (hī-pō-TŎN-ĭk, p. 285)
induction of labor (p. 289)
multifetal pregnancy (mŭl-tē-FĒ-tăl, p. 294)
Nitrazine paper test (NĪ-tră-zēn, p. 284)
oligohydramnios (p. 294)
oxytocin (ŏks-ē-TŌ-sĭn, p. 290)
precipitate labor (prē-SĬP-ĭ-tāt, p. 293)
preterm labor (p. 280)
prolapsed umbilical cord (PRŌ-lăpst ŭm-BĬL-ĭ-kăl, p. 294)
prostaglandin (PGE₂) gel (p. 290)
tocolytic agents (tō-kō-LĬT-ĭk, p. 283)
trial of labor after cesarean (TOLAC) (p. 300)
uterine rupture (p. 293)
vaginal birth after cesarean (VBAC) (p. 300)

Labor and birth usually progress with few problems. However, when complications occur during labor, they can have devastating effects on the maternal-fetal outcome. Health care providers must quickly and accurately identify the nature of the problems and intervene to reduce or limit detrimental effects on the mother and newborn. This chapter discusses high-risk intrapartum care. Nursing care is incorporated throughout the chapter.

PRETERM LABOR

Preterm labor is defined as the onset of labor between 20 and 37 weeks' gestation. It occurs in approximately 12% of pregnancies and accounts for most perinatal deaths not resulting from congenital anomalies. Preterm labor and premature rupture of membranes are the two most common factors that lead to preterm birth. Preterm birth has great significance for society because of the high rate of perinatal deaths and the excessive financial cost of caring for the preterm newborns. One of the *Healthy People 2020* (U.S. Department of Health and Human Services, 2010) goals is for 90% of all pregnant women to have prenatal care starting in the first trimester and to reduce preterm labor and delivery. Early prenatal care makes it possible for the woman to reduce or eliminate some risk factors that contribute to preterm labor.

> **! Safety Alert**
>
> **Risk Factors for Preterm Labor**
>
> - History of preterm delivery
> - Multifetal pregnancy
> - Bacterial vaginosis
> - Short cervix
> - Fetal abnormality
> - Hydramnios
> - Substance abuse →cocaine & meth mostly.
> - Trauma or surgery during pregnancy
> - Periodontal dental disease → (absess on teeth possibly)
> - Fibronectin in vaginal secretions between 22 and 37 weeks' gestation
> - Alkaline phosphatase level greater than 90th percentile
> - Alpha-fetoprotein level greater than 90th percentile
> - Increased estriol level in urine after 32 weeks' gestation

The criteria for diagnosing preterm labor include:
- Gestation between 20 and 37 weeks is considered preterm
- Late preterm is between 34 and 36 completed weeks of gestation
- Documented uterine contractions every 5 to 10 minutes lasting for at least 30 seconds and persisting for more than 1 hour
- Cervical dilation more than 2.5 cm and 75% effaced

ASSOCIATED FACTORS

The exact cause of preterm labor is unclear; however, several risk factors are known. Because epidemiologic data have shown some risk factors to be avoidable, there are some promising avenues for both prevention and treatment. Increased risk factors include poor prenatal care; infections, including periodontal (dental) infections; nutritional status; and sociodemographics (socioeconomic status, race, and lifestyle). Preterm labor, followed by preterm birth, has been associated with maternal anemia; urinary tract infection; cigarette smoking; and use of alcohol, cocaine, and other substances, all of which are potentially avoidable risk factors. In addition, alterations in maternal vaginal flora by pathogenic organisms (e.g., *Chlamydia* or *Trichomonas* organisms, bacterial vaginosis) are associated with preterm labor. The risk of spontaneous preterm birth increases as the length of the cervix decreases. The length of the cervix can be measured by transvaginal ultrasound.

SIGNS AND SYMPTOMS

Clinical manifestations of preterm labor are more subtle than for term labor. Health care providers and pregnant women need to know the warning signs of preterm labor. The health care provider should be notified of the following signs or symptoms:
- Uterine cramping (menstrual-like cramps)
- Abdominal cramping (with or without nausea, vomiting, or diarrhea)
- Any vaginal bleeding
- Change in vaginal discharge
- Vaginal or pelvic pressure
- Low back pain
- Thigh pain (intermittent or persistent)

ASSESSMENT AND MANAGEMENT

Early prenatal care and education about prevention and the warning signs of preterm labor are extremely important to prevent preterm birth. The nurse should review the signs and symptoms that place a woman at risk for preterm labor and emphasize the importance of reporting the signs for prompt care in order to delay the newborn's birth until the fetal lungs are mature enough for extrauterine life. Open communication between the woman, nurse, and other health team members is essential for collaborative care and successful prevention of preterm births. Once the woman has been identified as at high risk for preterm labor, the use of various strategies and more intense surveillance allows earlier identification and intervention for preterm labor.

When amniotic membrane integrity is lost, a protein in the amniotic fluid, called **fibronectin,** will be found in vaginal secretions. A vaginal swab for fetal fibronectin can help the physician decide which women should be treated most aggressively to stop preterm labor (Gabbe, Niebyl, & Simpson, 2007).

Infection is associated with preterm births. Identification and eradication of offending microorganisms that cause inflammation in the lower reproductive tract lessen the inflammatory response and provide a healthier cervix, thereby decreasing the incidence of preterm labor. Antibiotics may be prescribed prophylactically for women at risk for preterm labor, with premature rupture of the membranes, or with group B streptococcal cervical cultures.

The physician may order uterine activity monitoring at home for women at risk for preterm labor. The monitor assesses contractions only; it does not assess fetal heart rate. In the delivery unit, the pediatrician should be present to assist in assessment and resuscitation of the preterm newborn, and equipment and a working incubator for transportation to the neonatal intensive care unit (NICU) should also be available.

Stopping Preterm Labor

Once the woman is admitted to the hospital and the diagnosis of preterm labor is made, management focuses on stopping the uterine activity (contractions) before the cervix dilates beyond 3 cm, or "the point of no return." The initial measures to stop preterm labor include identifying and treating any infection, restricting activity, ensuring hydration, and using tocolytic drugs (Table 14-1). The woman is placed on modified bed rest with bathroom privileges and is encouraged to maintain a lateral position. Assessment of uterine activity by palpation provides valuable information. The nurse communicates with the woman to help reduce her anxiety and concerns about fetal well-being and birth. Anxiety produces high levels of circulating catecholamines, which may induce further uterine activity. Explaining the planned care and procedures can reduce the patient's fear of the unknown. Some drugs used as tocolytics may have an effect on carbohydrate metabolism and are used with caution in the diabetic patient.

Tocolytics should not be used in women who are hemorrhaging because vasodilation may increase bleeding. If signs of fetal distress are noted, tocolytics may not be used if adequate survival therapy is available in the NICU. Tocolytics are usually not effective in a cervical dilation of 5 cm or more.

Table 14-1 Drugs Used to Stop Preterm Labor (Tocolytics)

TOCOLYTIC DRUG	ADVERSE EFFECTS	COMMENTS
Ritodrine (Yutopar) (β-adrenergic agonist)	Cardiovascular: maternal and fetal tachycardia Pulmonary: shortness of breath, chest pain, pulmonary edema, tachypnea Gastrointestinal: nausea, vomiting, diarrhea, ileus Central nervous system: tremors, jitteriness, restlessness, apprehension Metabolic alterations: hyperglycemia, hypokalemia, hypocalcemia	Approved by FDA but not in popular use. Side effects are dose related and more prominent during increases in the infusion rate than during maintenance therapy. ECG clearance suggested; hypertension and uncontrolled diabetes mellitus are contraindications.
Magnesium sulfate	Depression of deep tendon reflexes, respiratory depression, cardiac arrest (usually at serum magnesium levels >12 mg/dL) Less serious side effects: lethargy, weakness, visual blurring, headache, sensation of heat, nausea, vomiting, constipation, oliguria Fetal-neonatal effects: reduced heart rate variability, hypotonia	Adverse effects are dose related, occurring at higher serum levels. FHR and maternal vital signs must be monitored during labor and postpartum.
Indomethacin (prostaglandin synthesis inhibitor)	Epigastric pain, gastrointestinal bleeding; increased risk for bleeding; dizziness. Fetal effects: may have constriction of ductus arteriosus and decreased urinary output; decreased urinary output is associated with oligohydramnios, which may result in cord compression Respiratory distress syndrome	Not used after 32 weeks' gestation or for more than 48-72 hours. Observe for maternal bleeding and adverse FHR patterns.
Nifedipine (Procardia) (calcium channel blocker)	Maternal flushing, transient tachycardia, hypotension; use with magnesium sulfate can cause serious hypotension and low calcium levels	Monitor for hypotension and increased serum glucose levels in those with diabetes.
Terbutaline (Brethine) (β-adrenergic agonist)	Tachycardia; monitor vital signs Shortness of breath; may cause hyperglycemia	Approved for investigational use and is widely used. Must not be used longer than 48 to 72 hours (FDA 2011)
Corticosteroids	Increased blood sugar	Given to accelerate production of surfactant, increase fetal lung maturity, and prevent neonatal intracranial hemorrhage
Betamethasone, dexamethasone	Monitor mother and newborn closely: mother for pulmonary edema and hyperglycemia, and newborn for heart rate changes	Given to mother 24-48 hours before birth of preterm newborn (<34 weeks of gestation) because it can hasten lung maturity

Data from Clayton, B.D., Stock, Y.N., & Cooper, S.E. (2010). *Basic pharmacology for nurses* (15th ed.). St. Louis: Mosby; Creasy, R., Resnik, R., Iams, J., Lockwood, C., & Moore, T. (2008). *Creasy & Resnik's maternal-fetal medicine* (6th ed.). Philadelphia: Saunders; London, M., Ladewig, P., Ball, J., & Bindler, R. (2006). *Maternal & child nursing* (2nd ed.). Upper Saddle River, NJ: Prentice Hall; American Congress of Obstetricians and Gynecologists. (2003). Management of preterm labor. *International Journal of Gynecology & Obstetrics, 101*, 1039–1047.
ECG, electrocardiogram.

The woman should be asked to report any vaginal discharge (color, consistency, and odor). Baseline maternal vital signs are important and may provide clues of infection. Tachycardia and elevation of temperature can be early signs of amniotic fluid infection.

Fetal surveillance includes external fetal monitoring; fetal tachycardia of more than 160 beats/minute may indicate infection or distress. Fetal movement and biophysical profile assessment with the nonstress test (NST) provide information about fetal well-being. Special fetal assessment tests can be performed, such as measuring lecithin/sphingomyelin (L/S) ratio to determine fetal lung maturity.

Resting in the lateral position increases blood flow to the uterus and may decrease uterine activity. Strict bed rest may have some adverse side effects, which include muscle atrophy, bone loss, changes in cardiac output, decreased gastric motility, and gastric reflux. In addition, bed rest may result in depression and anxiety in the woman.

Hydration is encouraged, and intravenous fluids are often administered to increase vascular volume and prevent dehydration. The pituitary gland responds to dehydration by secreting antidiuretic hormone and oxytocin. Therefore, preventing dehydration will prevent oxytocin from being released. A baseline admission complete blood count is useful for determining whether there has been a decrease in the hemoglobin and hematocrit levels.

Use of tocolytic agents is an additional measure undertaken to stop uterine activity. The goal of tocolytic therapy is to delay delivery until steroids can hasten lung maturity of the fetus. Several drugs can be used, but none is without side effects. The nurse must know the adverse effects of the drug given and monitor the woman for their possible appearance. β-Adrenergic-agonist drugs such as terbutaline (Brethine) are often used as tocolytics. Terbutaline should not be used for longer than 48-72 hours and should not be used for home or maintenance therapy to prevent preterm labor. Terbutaline therapy may result in adverse effects to both the mother and fetus (FDA, 2011). Propranolol should be available to reverse adverse effects. Magnesium sulfate is also an effective tocolytic, and calcium gluconate 10% should be available to aid in reversing any toxic effects. Nursing responsibilities with this drug include hourly monitoring of maternal vital signs and oxygen saturation. Indocin (indomethacin) is a prostaglandin synthesis inhibitor that can be used as a tocolytic drug. Indocin can prolong maternal bleeding time, and the woman should be observed for unusual bruising. Fetal monitoring is essential when Indocin is used because it may have adverse effects on the fetus if used for more than 48 hours. Calcium antagonists, such as nifedipine (Procardia), reduce smooth muscle contractions of the uterus, and the woman must be monitored for hypotension (Iams, Romero, & Creasy, 2009).

Chapter 13 discusses the nurse's role regarding assessment for magnesium sulfate toxicity. Intervention for magnesium sulfate administration is the same as when given to prevent seizures in gestational hypertension.

Promotion of Fetal Lung Maturity
Promotion of fetal lung maturity is a goal in management because respiratory distress syndrome (RDS) is a common problem in preterm newborns. Respiratory distress can be reduced if steroids, such as betamethasone or dexamethasone, are given to the mother at least 24 to 48 hours before the birth of a newborn who is less than 34 weeks' gestation. After birth, preterm newborns are commonly treated prophylactically with surfactant therapy to reduce the risk of RDS.

NURSING CARE RELATED TO PHARMACOLOGIC THERAPY
All tocolytic therapies have maternal risks; therefore, continuous assessment for effects of the drugs is indicated during administration. Intravenous tocolytics are given according to the institution's protocol. Accurate intake and output, bilateral breath sounds, changes in vital signs, and mental status are closely monitored to identify early signs of fluid overload and pulmonary edema. If the woman is receiving β-adrenergic-agonist drugs such as Terbutaline, a heart rate of 120 beats/minute or greater, or a decrease in blood pressure to less than 90/40 mm Hg, should be immediately reported to the health care provider. These findings may indicate profound hemodynamic changes, including decreased ventricular filling time, decreased cardiac output, and myocardial infarction may occur if the drug is not discontinued. A pulse oximeter and arterial blood gas results may be used to determine maternal oxygenation and acid-base balance. The woman may be placed in the Fowler's position and given oxygen as needed. Tocolytic therapy is discontinued if the woman has chest pain or shortness of breath. When corticosteroids are given, the nurse must observe for fluid retention and pulmonary edema. Indomethacin can constrict the ductus arteriosus in the fetus and reduces amniotic fluid by reducing fetal kidney function. Careful fetal monitoring is essential. Side effects of magnesium sulfate include a feeling of warmth, headache, nausea, and lethargy. Nifedipine and magnesium sulfate cannot be used together because low maternal calcium levels may occur. Progesterone therapy is under study for use as a tocolytic (ACOG, 2003).

HOME CARE MANAGEMENT
If the woman meets appropriate criteria, the primary health care provider may consider home care (see Chapter 18). There is evidence that using the home uterine activity monitor (HUAM) is effective in

└ Procardia - to stop contractions, but edu. on ↑ risk of hypotension

[margin handwritten note: water broke too soon!]

decreasing preterm births in a select group of women. Detecting contractions or contraction frequency before cervical changes occur makes HUAM worthwhile.

PREMATURE RUPTURE OF MEMBRANES

Spontaneous rupture of the amniotic sac more than 1 hour before onset of true labor is referred to as premature rupture of membranes (PROMs). Rupture of the membranes before 37 weeks' gestation is known as preterm premature rupture of the membranes (PPROMs). The exact cause is unknown, but there are several risk factors.

Infection for both the mother and the fetus is the major risk; when membranes are ruptured, microorganisms from the vagina can ascend into the amniotic sac. Compression of the umbilical cord can occur as a result of the loss of amniotic fluid. Prolapse of the cord can also occur, which results in fetal distress. Because amniotic fluid is slightly alkaline, confirmation that the vaginal fluid is amniotic fluid can be obtained by a Nitrazine paper test, which it will turn blue-green on contact with amniotic fluid (Skill 14-1). Examination of the fluid under a microscope (fern test) will also show a ferning pattern as the fluid dries.

MANAGEMENT

Treatment depends on the duration of gestation and whether evidence of infection or fetal or maternal compromise is present. For many women near term, PROM signifies the imminent onset of true labor. If pregnancy is at or near term and the cervix is soft and with some dilation and effacement, then augmentation of labor may be started a few hours after rupture. If the woman is not at term, the risk of infection or preterm birth is weighed against the risks of an induction by oxytocin or a cesarean birth (Nursing Care Plan 14-1 on p. 300).

Infection of the amniotic sac, called chorioamnionitis, may be caused by prematurely ruptured membranes because the barrier to the uterine cavity is broken.

The risk of infection increases if the membranes have been ruptured for more than 18 hours.

Management will likely consist of bed rest with bathroom privileges and observation for infection, NST, and daily assessment for fetal compromise. Antibiotics are given to reduce infection and steroids to hasten fetal lung development (Table 14-2).

The woman may remain in the hospital until birth; however, if there is no sign of infection or fetal compromise, she may return home and self-monitor. Preparation for nursing management includes:

- Documenting vital signs daily and reporting any temperature greater than 38° C (100.4° F)
- Providing sterile equipment for vaginal examinations
- Reporting uterine contractions
- Reporting any vaginal discharge or bleeding
- Having the woman remain on bed rest in a lateral position (with bathroom privileges)
- Instructing the woman to document fetal activity (daily kick counts) and report fewer than 10 kicks in a 12-hour period
- Explaining activity restrictions
- Explaining the need to abstain from sexual intercourse and orgasm
- Telling the woman to avoid breast stimulation, which can cause release of oxytocin and initiate uterine contraction
- Assessing psychosocial concerns

DYSTOCIA

Dystocia, also known as *dysfunctional labor*, is a difficult or abnormal labor. It primarily results from one of the following problems (Table 14-3):

Powers: abnormal uterine activity (ineffective uterine contractions)

Passageway: abnormal pelvic size or shape and other conditions that interfere with descent of the presenting part (such as tumors or soft tissue resistance)

Skill 14-1   Testing for the Presence of Amniotic Fluid (Nitrazine Paper Test)

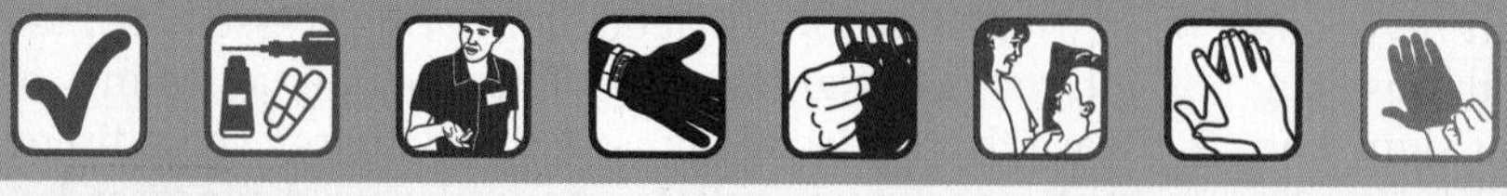

PURPOSE

To determine if "bag of waters" (amniotic sac) is ruptured.

Steps

1. Place piece of Nitrazine paper into fluid from vagina.

2. A blue-green or deep blue color of the Nitrazine paper indicates fluid is alkaline and most likely amniotic fluid.

3. A yellow to yellow-green color of the strip of paper indicates fluid is acidic and is most likely urine.

4. Document and report results, offer and provide peri care, remove gloves, and wash hands.

5. Document presence of bloody show, which may alter accuracy of results.

Table 14-2 Management of Women with Premature Rupture of the Membranes (PROM)

WOMEN WITH PROM	PRETERM FETUS	TERM FETUS
Bed rest	Determination of PROM	Induction of labor if spontaneous labor has not
Hydration	Assessment for prolapsed cord	begun by approximately 12 hours after PROM
Sedation	Observation for infection	Potential for cesarean birth
Antibiotics, if	Administration of corticosteroids, with or without	Expectant management of maternal-fetal infection
needed	delivery in 24-48 hours	Increased chance of asphyxia and respiratory
Reassurance	Delivery when the infant has the best chance for	distress in newborn after birth
	survival (i.e., avoid fetal distress)	
	Have emergency resuscitation equipment available	

Table 14-3 Causes of Dystocia (Dysfunctional Labor)

CAUSE	EXAMPLES
Difficulty with powers	Uterine dysfunction or abnormalities
Difficulty with passageway	Pelvic size and shape, tumors
Difficulty with passenger	Fetal abnormality Excessive size Malpresentation Malposition
Psyche	Maternal anxiety, fatigue

Passenger: abnormal fetal size or presentation (excessive size or less than optimum position)

Psyche: past experiences, culture, preparation, and support system

Dystocia is suspected when the rate of cervical dilation or fetal descent is not progressing normally or uterine contractions are ineffective. A prolonged labor, with potential injury to the fetus, may result. Electronic fetal monitoring (EFM) is used to assess uterine contractions and fetal well-being. Nursing assessment of the intensity, frequency, and duration of contractions is important.

Dystocia can be associated with problems such as maternal dehydration, exhaustion, increased risk of infection, and fetal distress. Change in maternal vital signs, such as elevation of temperature or rise in pulse rate, should be reported. Comfort measures should be implemented by nursing personnel, and the woman and significant other should be kept informed about the progress of labor.

POWERS

Abnormal Uterine Contractions

Dysfunctional labor can result from abnormal uterine contractions that prevent normal progress of cervical dilation, effacement, and descent of the presenting part. It can be further described as being primary (hypertonic dysfunction) or secondary (hypotonic dysfunction).

Hypotonic Dysfunction

Hypotonic uterine dysfunction (secondary uterine inertia) occurs with abnormally slow progress after the labor has been established (Table 14-4). The uterine contractions become weak and inefficient and may even stop. The contractions are fewer than two or three in a 10-minute period and usually are not strong enough to cause the cervix to dilate beyond 4 cm, and the fundus does not feel firm at the height (or acme) of the contraction. Consequently, labor fails to progress. A prolonged labor can occur, which can increase the risk of intrauterine infection, placing both the mother and newborn at risk.

Hypotonic contractions occur as a result of fetopelvic disproportion, fetal malposition, overstretching of the uterus caused by a large newborn, multifetal gestation, or excessive maternal anxiety. The woman with hypotonic contractions can become exhausted and dehydrated. Medical management includes ruling out cephalopelvic disproportion (CPD) by ultrasound. If CPD is not the problem, augmentation by oxytocin is often started. The use of epidural analgesia and other regional anesthesia may reduce the effectiveness of the woman's voluntary pushing efforts. Encouraging position changes and coaching can be helpful.

Hypertonic Uterine Dysfunction

Hypertonic uterine dysfunction refers to a labor with uterine contractions of poor quality that are painful, are out of proportion to their intensity, do not cause cervical dilation or effacement, and are usually uncoordinated and frequent (see Table 14-4). This is more common with a first pregnancy or an anxious woman who has intense pain and lack of labor progression. The latent period of labor is prolonged, which increases her exhaustion and anxiety. Often there is not adequate relaxation of muscle tone between contractions, which causes the woman to complain of constant cramps and results in ischemia or reduced blood flow to the fetus.

Management of hypertonic uterine dysfunction is rest, which is achieved by analgesia to reduce pain and encourage sleep. An intravenous infusion is frequently administered to maintain hydration and electrolyte balance. Often women awaken with normal contractions.

PASSAGEWAY

Abnormal Pelvis Size or Shape

Contractures of the pelvic diameters reduce the capacity of the bony pelvis, including the inlet, midpelvis, outlet, or any combination of these planes.

Table 14-4 Comparison of Hypotonic and Hypertonic Labor

WHEN OCCURS	CONTRACTIONS	IMPLICATIONS	MANAGEMENT
Hypotonic Labor			
Active phase; may occur in latent phase	Infrequent; poor intensity; low resting tone between contractions	Maternal: seldom painful; prolonged labor; PROM; risk of infection; anxiety Fetal: risk of subsequent sepsis	Rule out cephalopelvic disproportion; use intravenous oxytocin to stimulate contractions; perform cesarean birth for abnormal fetal position or large newborn. Nursing interventions: assess contraction pattern; provide support; monitor vital signs; frequently assess fetal status; if considering cesarean birth, instruct mother about procedure.
Hypertonic Labor			
Prolonged latent phase; may occur in active phase	Become more frequent; ineffective; painful; uterus does not relax between contractions	Maternal: exhaustion, discouragement, fatigue, anxiety Fetal: possible distress with decreased placental perfusion	Analgesia for rest; hydration; oxytocin is not administered (discontinue intravenous oxytocin if infusing). Nursing interventions: assess uterine contraction pattern; provide rest (analgesia); provide comfort measures; monitor maternal vital signs; frequently monitor fetal status. Lateral position; administer oxygen by mask.

PROM, premature rupture of membranes.

Pelvic contractures may be caused by congenital malformations, rickets, maternal malnutrition, tumors, and previous pelvic fractures.

Inlet contractures occur when the diagonal conjugate is shortened (less than 11.5 cm [4.5 inches]). Abnormal presentations, such as face and shoulder presentations, increase this problem. Midplane contractures are the most common cause of pelvic dystocia. Fetal descent is arrested (stops), and a cesarean birth is commonly done. Outlet contracture exists when the pubic arch is narrow. If uterine contractions continue when the passageway is obstructed, uterine rupture can occur, placing both the mother and fetus at risk. A common minor obstruction of the passageway is a distended bladder. Catheterization may be needed if the woman cannot void.

Scar tissue on the cervix from previous infections or surgery may not readily yield to labor forces to efface and dilate. A cesarean birth may be indicated when an abnormality of the passageway prolongs or impedes the progress of labor.

PASSENGER

Cephalopelvic Disproportion

Cephalopelvic disproportion (CPD) is a condition in which the presenting part of the fetus (usually the head) is too large to pass through the woman's pelvis. Because of the disproportion, it becomes physically impossible for the fetus to be delivered vaginally, and cesarean birth is necessary. CPD is suspected when the newborn's head does not continue to descend even though the woman is having strong uterine contractions. Excessive fetal size may be associated with diabetes mellitus, multiparity, and genetics (one or both parents of large size). A large newborn (macrosomia) can cause difficulty in birth of the shoulders (shoulder dystocia).

A modified position can aid in delivery (Figure 14-1). Maternal complications that can occur are exhaustion, hemorrhage, and infection. Birth trauma and anoxia are complications for the fetus.

Abnormal Fetal Presentation

A malpresentation refers to any presentation of the fetus other than the vertex presentation, in which the top of the head emerges first. Malpresentation may prolong labor and make it more uncomfortable for the woman.

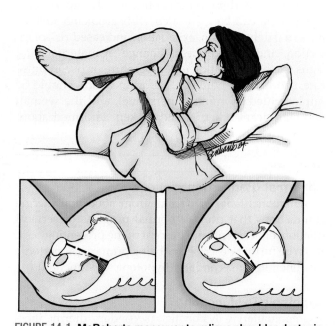

FIGURE 14-1 **McRoberts maneuver to relieve shoulder dystocia.** The woman flexes her thighs sharply against her abdomen to straighten the pelvic curve. A squat position has a similar effect and adds gravity to pushing efforts.

Breech Presentation. Breech presentations are often associated with preterm birth, multiple gestation, congenital anomalies, placenta previa, and multiparity. Breech is the most common example of malpresentation. It occurs in approximately 3% to 4% of all births. During labor, the fetal descent is slow because the breech is a less effective dilating wedge than the fetal head. The buttocks, legs, and feet are softer than the head and therefore exert less pressure on the cervix. Cord prolapse occurs more often during breech birth and increases the risk of birth trauma because the buttocks (presenting part) are smaller than the head and do not fit as tightly into the pelvis. The risk of postpartum hemorrhage is also increased. The three basic types of breech presentation are shown in Figure 14-2. Alternatives to vaginal birth of the fetus in breech presentation are external cephalic version (ECV) or a cesarean birth, in which the fetus is delivered abdominally. The woman should be fully informed of her options and the risks involved in each.

The presence of meconium in the amniotic fluid in breech presentations is not necessarily a sign of fetal distress but results from pressure on the fetal abdominal wall and buttocks. Fetal heart tones are best heard at or above the maternal umbilicus. Forceps are sometimes used to deliver the after-coming fetal head. In a breech delivery, when the lower body is born, the umbilical cord extends above the fetal head and is at risk of compression as the head passes through the bony vaginal canal. Birth of the head must occur quickly to avoid hypoxia. The mechanism of labor in a breech presentation is shown in Figure 14-3.

Face and Brow Presentation. In a face or brow presentation, the diameter of the presenting part is larger than in a vertex or occiput presentation. It is a less effective dilating wedge than the top of the fetal head. The safest means of delivery of the baby in the posterior face position is a cesarean birth. A forceps delivery may be done, but fetal hypoxia and injury are always risks.

Persistent Occiput Posterior Position. Persistent occiput posterior positions occur when the back of the fetal head (the occiput) enters the maternal pelvis and is directed toward the back (posterior) of the maternal pelvis instead of toward the front (anterior). When this position occurs, labor is usually prolonged because, in the process of internal rotation, the head must rotate further. A maternal hands-and-knees position may help the fetus rotate from a posterior to an anterior position (Figure 14-4). A squatting position helps straighten the pelvic curve and aids in rotation. Sometimes the woman is asked to push while lying on her side, which may help the fetus rotate to an anterior position. If the occiput remains posterior, the baby is born with the face upward. The woman usually has a great deal of back discomfort because the baby's head presses against her sacrum during rotation. Sacral counter pressure and back rubs are appreciated by the woman during labor.

External Version

External version is changing the fetal presentation after 37 weeks' gestation, usually from breech or transverse lie to cephalic presentation. Successful external version

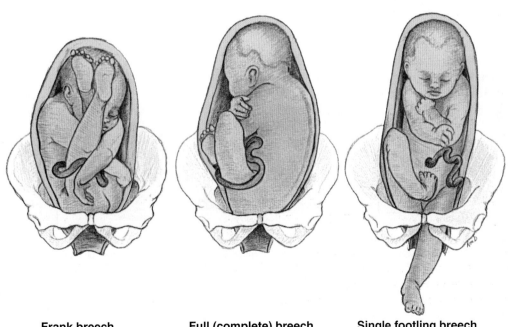

Frank breech   **Full (complete) breech**   **Single footling breech**

FIGURE **14-2** Types of breech presentations.

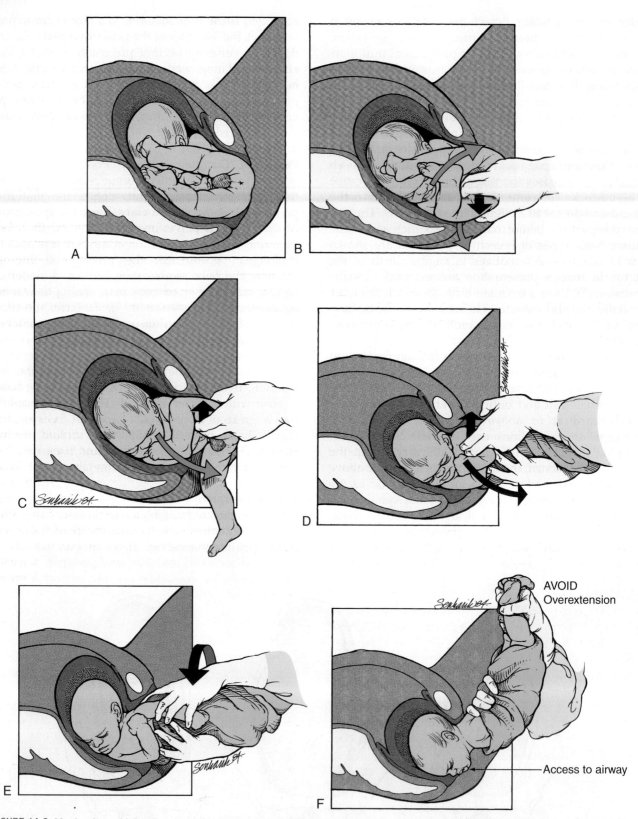

FIGURE 14-3 **Mechanism of labor in a breech presentation. A**, The buttocks reach the perineum. Flexion of the fetal head is maintained. **B**, Traction to the fetal knee enables delivery of the leg. **C**, The fetal pelvis rotates as the second leg is delivered. **D**, As the scapula appears under the symphysis pubis, the arm is delivered. **E**, Gentle rotation of the shoulders facilitates delivery of the other arm. **F**, The fetus is quickly wrapped in a towel for control and slightly elevated. The fetal airway becomes visible at the perineum, and the head is delivered by flexion.

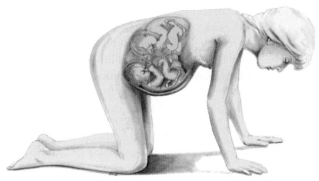

FIGURE 14-4 A hands-and-knees position assists the fetus in rotating from left occiput posterior to left occiput anterior position.

can reduce a woman's chance of having a cesarean birth. The risks of an external version are a **prolapsed umbilical cord** and **abruptio placentae**. Contraindications are uterine malformations, previous cesarean birth, disproportion between fetal size and maternal pelvic size, placenta previa, multifetal gestation, and uteroplacental insufficiency.

Ultrasound guides fetal manipulations during the external version. Most physicians give the woman a tocolytic drug to relax the uterus. After the uterus is relaxed, the physician presses on the abdomen to gently push the breech out of the pelvis and toward the mother's side. The fetal head is pushed downward and to the opposite side. The tocolytic drug is stopped after the version is completed. Fetal heart rate and contractions are monitored, and the woman is taught to report signs of labor that may occur.

Maternal version is usually an emergency procedure that occurs in the delivery room. Most commonly, it is performed during the vaginal birth of twins to change the fetal presentation of the second twin.

CAM Therapy
Complementary and alternative medical (CAM) therapies may play a role in versions. In traditional Chinese medicine, the herb mugwort is used in a therapy, called *moxibustion*. Incense cones of the prepared herb are placed in the outer corner of the fifth toenail (a median point of the body) and allowed to burn near the skin. The heat and odor are believed to increase fetal activity that promotes a breech version (Neri, Airola, Contu, et al., 2004). See Chapter 21 for further discussion of CAM therapies.

PSYCHE
Psychological factors have a strong effect on the progress of labor. The woman's perceived fears of pain, lack of support, embarrassment, or violation of religious rituals can cause the body to respond to the stress in ways that inhibit the progress of labor. Secretions of epinephrine as a response to stress inhibit contractions and divert blood away from the uterus to the skeletal muscle. Tense muscles result in less

effective uterine contractions and a higher perception of pain. Glucose used in the stress response reduces the energy supply available to the labor process. The nursing goal is to help the woman relax by adjusting the environment for maximum comfort and cleanliness, establishing a trusting relationship with the mother and family, guiding the support person, and using pharmacologic and nonpharmacologic methods of pain management.

INDUCTION OF LABOR AND AUGMENTATION

Induction of labor refers to measures to initiate uterine contractions before they spontaneously begin. Labor is usually induced because the benefits of terminating the pregnancy outweigh the benefits of continuing the pregnancy for mother or fetus. Augmentation of labor is the use of an oxytocic drug after spontaneous but ineffective labor has begun. The woman and partner should be fully informed of risks and benefits of these procedures.

REASONS FOR INDUCTION
Induction of labor is often performed because the delay of delivery would place the woman or fetus at significant risk. **Maternal indications** for induction include infection (chorioamnionitis), PROM, and worsening medical disorders (e.g., gestational hypertension, diabetes mellitus type 1, or chronic hypertension). **Fetal indications** include intrauterine growth restriction, postterm newborn, and fetal demise. Elective induction for convenience in planning child care, transportation, and birth attendants is a growing trend. Induction of labor is contraindicated if the mother has active genital herpes, CPD, umbilical cord prolapse, placenta previa, or vertical incision of the uterus from a previous cesarean birth.

METHODS OF INDUCTION
CAM Therapy
CAM therapies (see Chapter 21) for inducing labor have become popular, and admission interviews should include asking the woman whether any practices have been used. Midwives sometimes recommend the use of evening primrose oil (which converts to a prostaglandin compound), black haw, black cohosh, blue cohosh, or red raspberry leaves to induce labor (Tournaire & Theau-Yonneau, 2007). Their value in aiding cervical ripening or enhancing safe labor induction is still under investigation. Castor oil, hot baths, and enemas are not recommended and have no proven value in labor induction. Sexual intercourse is commonly recommended to induce term labor in many cultures. The belief involves the release of oxytocin resulting from breast stimulation, the release of natural prostaglandin from the semen, and the stimulation of uterine contractions that result from female orgasm all

contributing to labor induction. Acupuncture and transcutaneous electrical nerve stimulation (TENS) may stimulate release of natural prostaglandins and oxytocin, but their effectiveness as labor induction techniques is not supported by research data.

Cervical Ripening

Induction of labor will be more successful if the cervix is "ripe," reducing the need for an emergency cesarean birth. Cervical ripening, or maturation, describes a series of biochemical events that result in a soft, pliable cervix. The cervical ripening is evaluated by the Bishop scale (Table 14-5). The American College of Obstetricians and Gynecologists (ACOG) has recommended that a Bishop score of 6 or more is necessary to predict a successful outcome of labor induction (ACOG, 2007). Techniques of cervical ripening include nonpharmacologic and pharmacologic methods.

Nonpharmacologic Methods. Nonpharmacologic methods of cervical ripening include:

Stripping of membranes: The digital separation of the amniotic membranes from the lower uterine segment. The cervix must be dilated enough to allow penetration to reach the membranes. Endogenous prostaglandins are released that stimulate oxytocin production.

Amniotomy: The artificial rupture of the membranes (AROM). Membranes are ruptured by piercing with an amniotic hook. The vertex must be engaged before this procedure is performed to prevent cord prolapse. The fetal heart rate should be monitored after an amniotomy, and the character, odor, and color of the amniotic fluid should be documented.

Mechanical dilators: Dilators can be inserted into the cervix to progressively dilate the cervix and release endogenous prostaglandins. This process is uncomfortable for the woman and has been replaced by hygroscopic dilators.

Hygroscopic dilators: *Laminaria* species, a type of desiccated seaweed; Lamicel, a synthetic dilator containing magnesium sulfate in polyvinyl alcohol; or Dilapan (polyacrylonitrile) is inserted into the cervix, absorbs fluid from surrounding tissues,

and then expands to cause cervical dilation (Gabbe, Niebyl, & Simpson, 2007). The dilator is usually left in place for 6 to 12 hours; the Bishop score is then reevaluated. Nursing responsibilities include documenting the number of dilators inserted, assessing urinary retention, and monitoring fetal heart patterns and uterine contractions.

Pharmacologic Methods. Prostaglandin (PGE$_2$) gel is applied to the cervix before induction to soften and thin (ripen) the cervix. PGE$_2$ gel may be administered through a catheter into the cervical canal or applied to a diaphragm that is placed next to the cervix. Oxytocin induction usually is not started for several hours to avoid uterine hyperstimulation. Side effects of PGE$_2$, which include vomiting, diarrhea, fever, and hyperstimulation of the uterus, are not common but can occur with gel application. The woman may be placed flat or in a modified Trendelenburg position for 30 minutes to 1 hour after gel insertion to prevent leakage. Prostaglandin preparations include dinoprostone (Prepidil, Cervidil) and misoprostol (Cytotec). Misoprostol is a prostaglandin (PGE$_1$) analog approved for use in gastric ulcers and is considered an "off label use" for cervical ripening because it is not FDA approved for this purpose. However, it continues to be used often with special guidelines but is contraindicated for use in women who have had a previous cesarean section due to high risk of uterine hyperstimulation (ACOG, 2006). Uterine contractions and fetal heart rate are monitored for at least 30 minutes after insertion. Women who have asthma, glaucoma, or renal or liver disease may not be candidates for this treatment. Cervical ripening procedures usually reduce the dose of oxytocin needed for induction of labor. Use of these preparations should be in a setting where facilities for emergency cesarean section are immediately available (ACOG, 2007).

Oxytocin Induction and Augmentation

Oxytocin, a hormone normally produced by the posterior pituitary gland, stimulates uterine contractions. Oxytocin (Pitocin) is used to induce the labor process or to augment labor that is progressing slowly because of ineffective uterine contractions.

Table 14-5	Bishop Scale				
SCORE	DILATION (CM)	EFFACEMENT (%)	FETAL STATION	CERVIX	POSITION OF CERVIX
0	0	0-30	−3	Firm	Posterior
1	1-2	40-50	−2	Medium	
2	3-4	60-70	−1	Soft	Anterior
3	5-6	80	+1, +2		

From Bishop, E.H. (1964). Pelvic scoring for elective induction. *Obstetrics and Gynecology, 24,* 266–268. Modification by Brennand, J.E., & Calder, A.A. (1991). Labor and normal delivery: Induction of labor. *Current Opinion in Obstetrics & Gynecology, 3,* 764.
A point may be added to the score for preeclampsia and each prior vaginal delivery. A point may be deducted from the score for a postterm pregnancy, nulliparity, or prolonged ruptured membranes. A high score (8 or 9) is predictive of a successful labor induction because the cervix has ripened, or softened, in preparation for labor. American College of Obstetricians and Gynecologists recommends a score of 6 or above before induction of labor.

Before oxytocin administration is started, a vaginal examination is performed to assess cervical dilation and effacement, fetal presentation and position, and fetal descent. The woman's vital signs are assessed and recorded, and fetal well-being is evaluated. Continuous EFM is started before and is continued during the oxytocin infusion.

Oxytocin has an antidiuretic effect that can decrease urinary output and cause water retention. Maternal water intoxication and fetal hyperbilirubinemia have been associated with prolonged oxytocin infusions. The nurse should be alert for signs of water intoxication, including headache, nausea and vomiting, decreased urinary output, hypertension, tachycardia, and cardiac dysrhythmias. The most common adverse effects of oxytocin administration are uterine hyperstimulation and reduced fetal oxygenation. Hyperstimulation may lead to uteroplacental insufficiency, fetal compromise, uterine rupture, and a very rapid labor with potential uterine or cervical lacerations.

Oxytocin (diluted in an intravenous solution) is administered by a controlled infusion pump. During the oxytocin intravenous infusion, the nurse should report any contractions lasting longer than 90 seconds, intervals between contractions less than 60 seconds, and nonreassuring fetal heart rates. Oxytocin should not be administered without a physician readily available who is capable of performing an emergency cesarean birth. The nursing goals include assessing uterine activity, cervical dilation, and maternal-fetal response. The nurse assesses intake and output to prevent water intoxication. *Oxytocin is discontinued immediately and the primary health care provider notified if uterine hyperstimulation or nonreassuring fetal heart rate occurs.*

The health care provider explains the procedure to the woman and advises her that frequent evaluations will be necessary. Nursing care includes frequent perineal cleansing and linen changes to reduce the introduction of organisms and thus decrease the risk of infection and promote comfort. The side-lying position is recommended to increase placental perfusion. The woman's vital signs should be taken and the external fetal monitor evaluated frequently.

Nipple stimulation may be used to aid stimulation of labor (Chapter 5). Terbutaline should be available to stop labor induction if hyperstimulation of the uterus or adverse fetal responses occur. Oxygen is administered by mask during induction, and the woman is closely monitored. Failure to dilate more than 2 cm in a 4-hour period during active labor may be an indication for cesarean birth.

EPISIOTOMY

Although episiotomies are used when indicated, every effort is made to retain an intact perineum and reduce perineal trauma. An episiotomy is a surgical incision made into the perineum to permit easier passage of the fetus. It is indicated when lacerations of the perineum, vagina, or cervix might occur. It is performed to shorten the second stage of labor, relieve compression on the fetal head, and facilitate breech and forceps births. Episiotomy is not routinely performed but should not be routinely avoided. Two types of episiotomies are (1) the median (midline) episiotomy, which extends from the posterior fourchette of the vagina downward but not to the rectal sphincter; and (2) the mediolateral episiotomy, which is an incision made on an angle to the woman's right or left side (Figure 14-5). An episiotomy is thought to heal more satisfactorily than a laceration. A median episiotomy is considered to be less uncomfortable and heals better than a mediolateral incision. However, a median incision can extend into the rectum. A regional or local block is given before the episiotomy is performed. Ideally, the episiotomy is performed when the fetal head is crowning, just before the birth of the fetus, to reduce the blood loss.

If lacerations of the perineum occur, they are classified in one of four degrees: A **first-degree laceration** extends through the skin and into the mucous membrane. A **second-degree laceration** extends farther, reaching the muscles of the perineal body. In a **third-degree laceration,** the anal sphincter muscles and muscles of the perineum are torn. A **fourth-degree laceration** reaches into the anal sphincter muscles and anterior wall of the rectum.

Measures used (especially by midwives) to enhance perineal stretching are the application of warm compresses, warm oil, and perineal massage. The warm compresses and perineal massage are thought to soften and stretch perineal muscles and may reduce the need for an episiotomy.

Often, after episiotomy repair, an ice bag is applied to the incision to reduce swelling. Other nursing

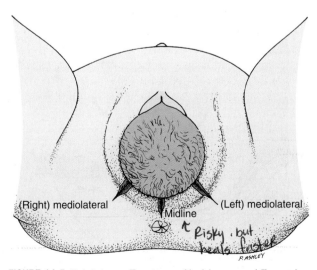

FIGURE 14-5 **Episiotomy**. Two types of incisions are midline and mediolateral.

measures used for an episiotomy are discussed in Chapter 12. Kegel exercises are encouraged after healing to regain muscle tone (see Chapter 12).

ASSISTED VAGINAL DELIVERY

FORCEPS-ASSISTED BIRTH

Forceps are curved metal instruments used by the physician to provide traction to deliver the baby's head, assist the rotation of the head, or both (Figure 14-6). These instruments may be used to deliver preterm newborns to prevent undue pressure from being placed on the fragile fetal skull by continued contractions. They are also used to shorten the second stage of labor when the mother is exhausted and cannot effectively bear down. Sometimes regional or general anesthesia has affected the motor innervation and the mother cannot push effectively. Forceps are also used to assist the descent of the baby as soon as possible when fetal distress occurs. The cervix must be completely dilated and the fetus's head low or visible on the perineum (low forceps delivery) (Box 14-1). Forceps should be applied by a skilled physician only. A Foley catheter is inserted before forceps delivery to prevent bladder injury. The obstetric forceps has a cephalic curve to fit over the fetal head and conforms to the curve of the maternal pelvis. Piper forceps are used for the head in a breech delivery after the body is born. Forceps delivery is no longer in popular use, being replaced by vacuum extraction and elective cesarean section.

Maternal complications of a forceps delivery include lacerations of the birth canal and perineum with increased blood loss. The newborn can have bruising and edema of the scalp, potential cephalhematoma, and intracranial hemorrhage. In a difficult forceps application, temporary or even permanent paralysis of a facial nerve may occur.

Box **14-1**   Criteria for Forceps Delivery
• Membranes ruptured
• Cervix fully dilated
• Fetal head below the ischial spines or on the perineum
• Empty bladder
• Analgesia adequate

The nurse explains the procedure to the woman and helps the woman use breathing techniques to avoid pushing during application of forceps. The health care provider applies traction during a contraction as the woman pushes. After birth, the newborn is assessed for bruising, edema, and other trauma. Bruising and edema in the newborn, called *forceps marks,* resolve without treatment (Figure 14-7). The mother is observed for bleeding, which will be a brighter red than lochia rubra. Cold application to the perineum for the first 12 hours reduces edema and lessens pain. Heat compresses after 12 hours aid in the absorption of edema and hematoma.

VACUUM EXTRACTION

Vacuum extraction is used as an alternative to forceps application. Vacuum extraction involves applying a cup, called a *vacuum extractor,* to the fetal head and withdrawing air from the cup. This creates a vacuum within the cup, which secures it to the fetal head. Traction applied during the uterine contractions assists with the descent of the fetus, and the fetal head is delivered (Figure 14-8). The indications for vacuum extraction are the same as for forceps deliveries.

Side effects of vacuum extraction include edema and bruising to the fetal scalp. Risks to the fetus include cephalhematomas, scalp lacerations, and subdural hematoma. Maternal complications are uncommon. The woman should be informed about the medical procedure. The fetal heart rate should be

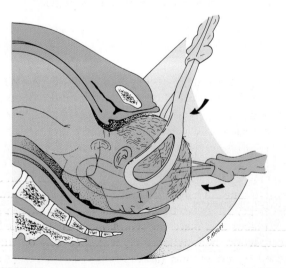

FIGURE 14-6 Application of obstetric forceps (top arrow) and direction of pull during a contraction.

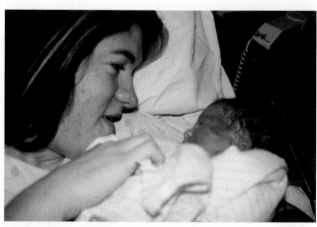

FIGURE 14-7 Note the "forceps mark" on this newborn's face. This bruise will resolve without intervention in a few days.

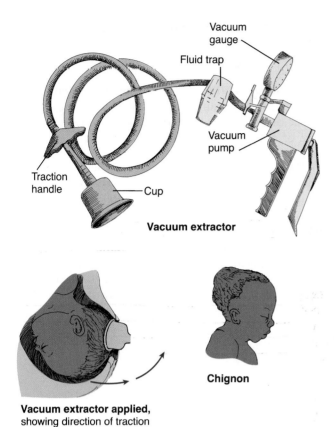

Vacuum extractor

Vacuum extractor applied,
showing direction of traction

Chignon

FIGURE 14-8 Vacuum extractor for assisted vaginal delivery.

monitored. Parents need to be advised that the caput chignon (edema of the fetal scalp) will disappear in approximately 2 or 3 days. Assessment of the newborn includes continued observation for cerebral hemorrhage and injury.

POSTTERM LABOR AND BIRTH

Postterm birth is the birth of a newborn beyond 42 weeks' gestation. The primary maternal risk related to postterm birth is a large newborn, which places the woman at risk for a dysfunctional labor, forceps-assisted birth, lacerations in the vaginal canal, and a potential cesarean delivery. Fetal risks include the possibility of birth trauma, CPD, and hypoxia caused by an aging placenta that begins to deteriorate after 42 weeks' gestation. When placental insufficiency is present, the risk of fetal hypoxia increases.

The management of postterm labor is controversial. Induction of labor is suggested at 42 weeks' gestation. Tests for fetal well-being are performed, including an NST and biophysical profile with ultrasound scanning to assess fetal movements, fetal breathing, and amniotic fluid volume. Amniocentesis may be performed to detect meconium in the amniotic fluid (see Chapter 5). A postmature newborn has a long lean body, long fingernails, and dry, peeling skin (see Chapter 15).

PRECIPITATE LABOR

Precipitate labor is a labor completed in less than 3 hours from the time of the first true labor contraction to the birth of the baby. Because the labor is rapid, maternal and fetal complications can occur. If the uterus has little relaxation between contractions, the intervillous blood flow may be impaired enough to cause fetal hypoxia (lack of oxygen). Also, rapid passage of the fetal head through the birth canal may result in fetal intracranial hemorrhage. The woman may also have cervical, vaginal, or perineal lacerations. Ideally, a physician will be available in the facility to assess the woman and newborn and record the findings. The emergency delivery of the newborn by a nurse is discussed in Chapter 7.

UTERINE RUPTURE

Uterine rupture is rare; however, it represents an emergency condition because it causes severe maternal bleeding and shock. It occurs most often during labor and delivery. When uterine rupture is associated with a previous cesarean birth, the rupture occurs at the site of the previous surgical scar. Aggressive or poorly supervised induction of labor may be responsible for a rupture of the uterus. A prolonged labor with fetopelvic disproportion is another cause.

A clue to a pending rupture is persistent uterine contractions without periods of relaxation. The nurse must report uterine contractions lasting more than 90 seconds. A relaxation period is necessary to maintain fetal oxygenation. Careful EFM monitoring can identify women at risk for rupture. As labor progresses, the woman might have a sharp pain in the suprapubic area. With severe bleeding, symptoms of shock occur. The major complications are maternal hemorrhage and fetal death. Treatment usually consists of an immediate uterine surgery and possible hysterectomy. Blood transfusions may be needed.

HYDRAMNIOS

Hydramnios (also called *polyhydramnios*) is an excessive amount of amniotic fluid, greater than 2 L. When hydramnios is present, congenital anomalies often exist, particularly those of the fetal gastrointestinal tract. It is associated with fetal malformations that affect fetal swallowing and voiding. During pregnancy, the fetus voids in and swallows the amniotic fluid. Any fetal anomaly that upsets this exchange can result in an excessive amount of amniotic fluid. When hydramnios develops, the uterus overdistends. This may cause preterm labor and place the woman at a greater risk for postpartum hemorrhage. Hydramnios can be diagnosed by ultrasound (an amniotic fluid index [AFI] greater than 20) (Gabbe, Niebyl, & Simpson, 2007). Removal of excess amniotic fluid may cause abruptio placentae, as the uterine size is decreased, or the prolapse of the umbilical cord. Psychological support for the mother is an important nursing responsibility. Amniocentesis may be done to avoid a preterm labor caused by an overdistended uterus.

OLIGOHYDRAMNIOS

Oligohydramnios is a decreased amount of amniotic fluid (an AFI less than 5) (Gabbe, Niebyl, & Simpson, 2007). It is associated with fetal renal anomalies and intrauterine growth restriction. Oligohydramnios places the fetus at risk for impaired musculoskeletal development because of the inability to move freely in the uterus and tangling of the long cord around an extremity, or cord compression from twisting or kinking, resulting in fetal distress. Oligohydramnios can be detected by ultrasound, which detects less than 1 cm of fluid in a predetermined pocket or quadrant of the uterus (AFI). During labor, an **amnioinfusion** (a transcervical instillation of warm sterile saline or lactated Ringer's solution into the uterus) may be done if membranes have ruptured to prevent cord compression and relieve the severity of variable decelerations. Fetal monitoring and maintaining a clean, dry bed for the mother are important nursing responsibilities.

PROLAPSED UMBILICAL CORD

Prolapsed umbilical cord occurs when the umbilical cord precedes the fetal presenting part. This condition is more likely to occur when there is a loose fit between the fetal presenting part and the maternal pelvis when the membranes have ruptured. This circumstance leaves room for the cord to slip down (prolapse) (Figure 14-9). The cord can be alongside or ahead of

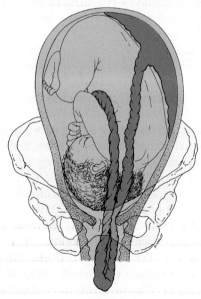

FIGURE 14-9 Prolapsed umbilical cord.

the presenting part. It may be occult (not palpable on vaginal examination), be inside the vagina, or even extend below the vulva. Because compression of the cord between the presenting part and the bony pelvis greatly decreases the flow of oxygen to the fetus, prolapse of the cord can interfere with fetal oxygenation.

Factors that contribute to cord prolapse are (1) rupture of membranes before the fetal head is engaged, carrying a loop of the umbilical cord into the pelvis or vagina; (2) a small fetus; (3) breech presentation; (4) transverse lie; (5) hydramnios; (6) an unusually long cord; and (7) multifetal pregnancy. Signs include prolonged variable decelerations evidenced on the fetal monitor, along with a baseline fetal bradycardia.

Prompt actions must be taken to relieve cord compression and increase fetal oxygenation until help arrives. Nursing interventions include:

- Placing the woman's hips higher than her head by (1) knee-chest position (Figure 14-10), (2) Trendelenburg position, or (3) side-lying position with hips elevated on pillows
- With sterile gloved hand, pushing fetal presenting part away from the cord
- Starting oxygen 8 to 10 L/minute by mask
- Closely monitoring fetal heart rate by EFM
- Preparing for rapid vaginal delivery or cesarean birth

If the cord protrudes, the nurse should apply sterile saline-soaked towels to prevent drying of the cord and to maintain blood flow until the infant is delivered.

AMNIOINFUSION

Amnioinfusion is a procedure during which normal saline or lactated Ringer's solution is instilled into the amniotic cavity through a catheter introduced transcervically into the uterus during labor. It is performed to correct oligohydramnios or reduce thickly stained meconium in the amniotic fluid and to minimize cord compression. An infusion pump should be used so that flow rate is controlled and the amount of infused fluid can be accurately documented. The uterus should be monitored for overdistention and elevated resting tone, which can cause changes in the fetal heart rate. Because the fluid infused will constantly leak out, nursing measures to maintain comfort and dryness should be used. Amnioinfusions with hypertonic solutions are used as a technique of inducing abortions before 20 weeks' gestation (Gabbe, Niebyl, & Simpson, 2007).

MULTIFETAL PREGNANCY

Multifetal pregnancy is the term for two or more fetuses in utero. Types of multifetal pregnancies are discussed in Chapter 3. A positive diagnosis of more than one fetus is made by ultrasound. Preterm labor is common

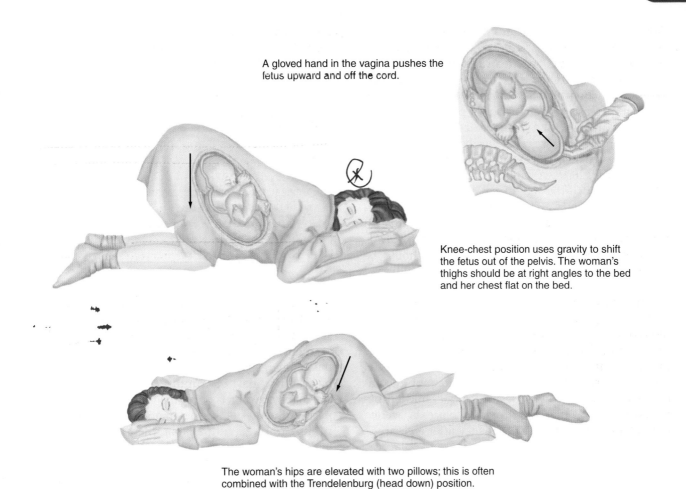

A gloved hand in the vagina pushes the fetus upward and off the cord.

Knee-chest position uses gravity to shift the fetus out of the pelvis. The woman's thighs should be at right angles to the bed and her chest flat on the bed.

The woman's hips are elevated with two pillows; this is often combined with the Trendelenburg (head down) position.

FIGURE 14-10 **Nursing interventions when the umbilical cord prolapses**. Maternal positioning and pushing the fetus away from the cord can relieve pressure on the prolapsed umbilical cord until delivery can take place.

because of an overdistention of the uterus. There is an increased frequency of anemia, hypertension, and hemorrhage. The woman is more likely to hemorrhage because of an overdistention of the uterus; therefore, a multifetal pregnancy poses greater risk than a single fetus.

Twins may be in various positions; one may be breech and the other vertex. The labor may be normal or prolonged. During the birth, the nurse should be prepared to identify each baby at the time it is born. A cesarean birth may be necessary if the cord has prolapsed, if one baby is malpresenting, or if more than two fetuses are present. The nursing care of the woman after the babies are born is the same as for other women, except the nurse is aware of the greater risk for postpartum hemorrhage.

The incidence of multifetal pregnancies has increased because of the popularity of fertility treatments (assisted reproductive technology [ART]) such as in vitro fertilization. Some complications can occur with multifetal pregnancies such as twin-to-twin transfusion syndrome, in which one twin transfuses its blood through a shunt to the other twin. This results in one twin with intrauterine growth restriction and

anemia, whereas the other twin can be larger or have heart failure because of circulatory overload. Another complication involves the death of one twin in utero while the other twin survives. Reabsorption of the tissues of the dead twin can predispose the mother to develop disseminated intravascular coagulation (DIC) (Gabbe, Niebyl, & Simpson, 2007).

Multifetal pregnancy reduction may be necessary when ART results in four or more fetuses, and the survival of all is at risk unless some are selectively aborted. The remaining twins or triplets have a good chance of survival (Gabbe, Niebyl, & Simpson, 2007). Vaginal delivery is advocated for vertex presentation of a twin, but a cesarean is indicated if presentation is not vertex or more than two fetuses are present.

CESAREAN BIRTH

Cesarean birth is a surgical procedure in which the birth is accomplished through an abdominal and uterine incision. The basic purpose of a cesarean birth is to preserve the life or health of the mother and her fetus. The incidence of cesarean births has increased dramatically in the past several years. In 2007, one third (32%)

of all births in the United States were cesarean sections (Menacker & Hamilton, 2010), and vaginal birth after a cesarean birth (VBAC) was at an all-time low of 16.5%. Some reasons cited for the increase include the increased detection of fetal problems from the use of EFM, an increase in the number of pregnancies at an older age, and the high incidence of repeat cesarean births. Complication rates of newborns were higher with cesarean delivery than with VBAC (Kamath, Todd, Glazner, et al., 2009). A national goal of *Healthy People 2020* is to reduce the rate of cesarean births to 15%. ACOG recommends VBAC in a trial of labor after cesarean (TOLAC) with facilities available for cesarean if needed (ACOG, 2010). The risks and benefits of TOLAC as compared to a repeat cesarean section should be discussed and decisions made on an individual basis.

Cesarean Birth on Demand
Part of the increase in the rate of cesarean birth is thought to be due to maternal request for cesarean delivery rather than medical indication for delivery (National Institutes of Health [NIH], 2006). The NIH states that elective cesarean births are not recommended for women who desire several children because the risk of placenta previa or placenta accreta rises with each successive pregnancy after a cesarean birth. Placenta previa may result because the placenta generally cannot attach at the site of a scar and so may attach in a lower segment of the uterus (see Chapter 13). If the placenta does attach at the scar site, it may not release from the site after delivery, resulting in placenta accreta. A goal of *Healthy People 2020* is to reduce cesarean birth on demand and increase normal spontaneous vaginal deliveries that have fewer complications for both mother and infant.

Indications
Four categories are responsible for 75% to 90% indications for cesarean births: dystocia, repeat cesarean, breech, and fetal distress. Other indications for a cesarean birth are active herpes viral infection; prolapsed umbilical cord; medical complications, such as gestational hypertension; placental abnormalities, such as placenta previa and abruptio placentae; and cephalopelvic disproportion (CPD) or fetal anomalies, such as hydrocephaly (Box 14-2).

Surgical Techniques
The skin incisions for a cesarean birth are either transverse (Pfannenstiel's) or vertical; these are not indicative of the type of incision made into the uterus. The transverse incision is made across the lowest part of the abdomen. Because the incision is made just below the pubic hair line, it becomes almost invisible after healing. The major limitation of this incision is that it does not allow extension of the incision if needed. The vertical incision is made between the navel and

Box 14-2   Indications for Cesarean Birth
• Previous cesarean birth with vertical scar
• Failed trial of labor
• Fetal distress
• Uncontrollable third-trimester bleeding
• Placenta previa
• Abruptio placentae
• Cephalopelvic disproportion
• Fetal malpresentation
• Prolapsed cord
• Medical complications of pregnancy, such as maternal heart disorder
• Failure of labor to progress
• Active herpes simplex virus infection
• Postmaturity (with failed induction)

the symphysis pubis. This type of an incision is quicker and is preferred in cases of fetal distress. Uterine incisions are either in the lower segment or in the upper segment of the uterus. The choice of incision affects the woman's opportunity for a subsequent vaginal birth and her risks of a ruptured scar with a subsequent pregnancy. An incision in the body (classic, or upper part) of the uterus is problematic because of potential rupture during a future labor; therefore, a future vaginal birth would be contraindicated. The lower uterine segment incision most commonly used is a transverse incision, although a low vertical incision may be used (Figure 14-11).

Complications and Risks
Cesarean births are not without risks for both mother and fetus. Maternal complications include aspiration, pulmonary embolism, hemorrhage, urinary tract infection, injuries to the bladder or bowel, wound infections, thrombophlebitis, and complications related to anesthesia. Risks to the fetus include preterm birth (if gestational age was not assessed properly), fetal injuries, and respiratory problems resulting from delayed absorption of lung fluids.

Preparation for Cesarean Birth
Because cesarean birth is common, this method should be an integral part of childbirth education classes. Couples need to discuss their specific needs and desires with their physician or nurse-midwife.

Women and their partners have time for psychological preparation when they know that they are going to have a cesarean birth. These women appear to cope with the recovery from surgery better than those who have an unplanned cesarean birth. Women having emergency or unplanned cesarean births have abrupt changes in the expectations for birth, post-birth care, and the care of the newborn at home. The woman may approach surgery exhausted and discouraged with her labor. Time for explanations about the

SKIN INCISION   UTERINE INCISION

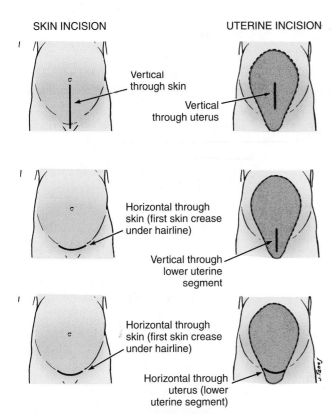

Vertical through skin

Vertical through uterus

Horizontal through skin (first skin crease under hairline)

Vertical through lower uterine segment

Horizontal through skin (first skin crease under hairline)

Horizontal through uterus (lower uterine segment)

FIGURE 14-11 **Various incisions used for cesarean births**. A vertical incision in the skin and the uterus is called a classic incision. A horizontal incision through the lower uterine segment is most favorable for a trial of labor (vaginal birth after cesarean) in the next pregnancy.

procedures for the surgery is often limited. Because procedures for the surgery must be performed quickly, both the woman and her family may have high anxiety levels. These women need adequate psychological support. It is important to explain what is being done and for the nurse to verify that informed consent was obtained.

Nursing Care

Preoperative Care. The preoperative nursing care includes all of the usual procedures for preparing a patient for surgery. The woman receives nothing by mouth to reduce the risk of aspiration. An intravenous infusion through a wide-bore catheter is started. The hair on the skin of the abdomen is considered sterile (Gabbe, Niebyl, & Simpson, 2007). Removal (clipping or shaving) of abdominal hair is only indicated when the hair will interfere with closing and suturing the wound. Routine skin shaving has been shown to predispose the woman to postoperative wound infection. An indwelling Foley catheter is inserted to keep the bladder empty during surgery, which reduces the risk of injury to the bladder when the incisions are made. An antacid is administered intravenously to decrease stomach acids, which could cause pneumonia if the woman should vomit and aspirate during surgery. Laboratory reports are reviewed, including blood type

and cross-match, Rh, complete blood cell count, and urinalysis. Although property and valuables are secured, often the mother wears her eyeglasses to the operating room because she will be awake, and seeing clearly will aid in bonding with her infant (Figure 14-12).

The fetal heart rate is recorded with electronic monitoring until the infant is delivered. Routine preoperative teaching, including coughing, deep breathing, and ambulating postoperatively, is done if time permits (Box 14-3). The use of spinal anesthesia reduces the need for vigorous newborn resuscitation that might be necessary with general anesthesia, which crosses the placental barrier. An infant warmer and resuscitation equipment should be on hand and the pediatrician notified. Preparing the woman for postoperative care expectations is a nursing responsibility. The positive aspects of a cesarean birth should be emphasized and family support offered.

Newborn Care. A nurse from the newborn nursery and a pediatrician are typically present in the operating room to assist in the care of the newborn when delivered. A heated crib and resuscitation equipment are readily available. In most hospitals, the father or partner can be with the mother during the cesarean birth.

After the baby is born, the Apgar score and identification are recorded, the newborn is moved to a radiant warmer to prevent chilling, and the skin temperature probe is applied. The mother and partner are given an opportunity to see, touch, and, depending on the condition of the newborn, hold the newborn.

Postoperative Care. After surgery, the woman is taken to the recovery room. Recovery room care includes observing the firmness of the uterus and the amount of bleeding from the vagina and assessing the abdominal incision. Vital signs are taken every 15 minutes for 1 to 2 hours or until the woman is stable. In addition, the woman receives the usual postoperative care. The woman is given oxytocin intravenously to stimulate the uterus to contract and reduce the blood loss. She is given analgesic medications to promote comfort.

The newborn is brought to the parents as soon as possible to facilitate bonding and attachment. Breastfeeding can be initiated. The woman may be transferred to the postpartum unit after 1 to 2 hours or when her condition is stable. Providing emotional support to the mother and partner after a cesarean birth is essential. Feelings of anxiety, guilt, and inadequacy may prevail. Therapeutic communication helps clear up fears and misunderstandings, and the woman should be encouraged to verbalize her fears and express her anxieties. Special effort to reduce postoperative pain and promote bonding with the newborn is important.

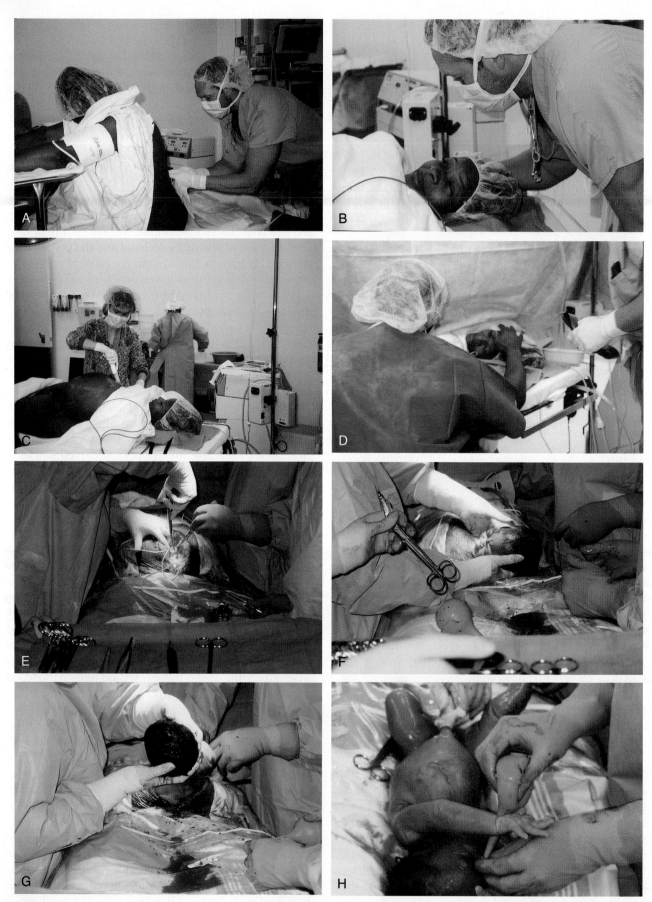

FIGURE 14-12 A cesarean birth. **A**, Spinal anesthesia is administered. **B**, The anesthesiologist reassures the woman. **C**, The nurse cleanses the abdominal skin. **D**, The partner converses with the woman. **E**, An abdominal incision is made. **F**, The newborn's head is lifted out of the uterus. **G**, The newborn's body is lifted out of the uterus. **H**, The newborn is suctioned with a bulb syringe, while the cord is clamped and cut.

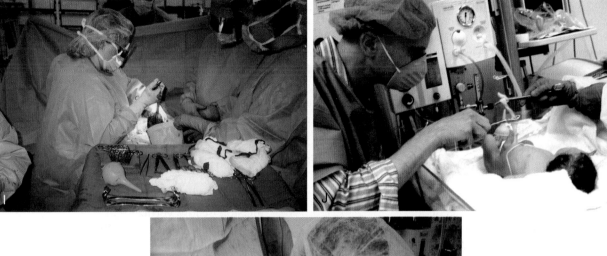

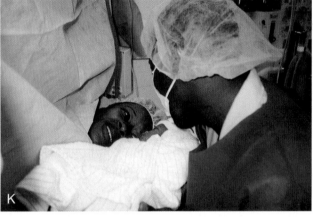

FIGURE 14-12—CONT'D   **I**, The placenta is lifted out of the uterus. **J,** The father cuts the cord above the plastic clamp. **K**, Mother, partner, and newborn get acquainted.

Early ambulation is encouraged to reduce respiratory and circulatory complications. As a rule, the woman with a cesarean birth has less lochial flow, most likely because of the removal of some of the uterine decidua during the surgical procedure. The intravenous infusion may be maintained until the woman is afebrile, has resumption of bowel sounds, and is tolerating fluids. The intravenous infusion often contains oxytocin to keep the uterus well contracted. The indwelling urinary catheter is normally maintained until the intravenous fluids are discontinued. Wound dressings may be removed after the first day.

Analgesic measures for pain at the incision site may be given every 3 to 4 hours, or patient-controlled analgesia (PCA) or epidural narcotics may be prescribed by the physician. Other comfort measures, such as

---

Box 14-3	Nursing Care Summary of the Woman Having Cesarean Birth

BEFORE SURGERY
- Assess when she last had oral intake.
- Explain what to expect with procedure.
- Witness informed consent.
- Monitor intravenous infusion.
- Cleanse abdomen.
- Insert indwelling urinary catheter.
- Administer medications as ordered (antacid and antibiotics).
- Verify blood type, cross-match, and urinalysis reports.

DURING RECOVERY PERIOD
- Start procedures related to postanesthetic period (pulse oximeter, oxygen administration, cardiac monitor).
- Assess fundus for firmness, height, and location per protocol; massage fundus if poorly contracted (boggy).
- Observe vaginal bleeding for color, amount, and consistency (presence of clots).
- Monitor abdominal wound for healing.
- Monitor vital signs every 15 minutes for first hour, every 30 minutes in second hour, then hourly until transfer to postpartum unit.
- Determine urinary output; check catheter and tubing for patency (intake and output).
- Assess for bowel sounds and passage of flatus.
- Change woman's position hourly (if no contraindications).
- Have woman breathe deeply and cough frequently.
- Administer prescribed medication for pain.
- Encourage early ambulation on first day and showering on second day.

position change and splinting the incision with pillows, are demonstrated. Deep breathing and coughing at frequent intervals are encouraged.

Discharge teaching includes information about wound care, personal hygiene, breast care if breastfeeding, bathing, diet, exercise and activity restrictions, sexual activity, contraception, medications, signs of complications, and newborn care. The Newborns' and Mothers' Health Protection Act of 1996 ensures a minimum hospital stay of 96 hours for cesarean births. Aftercare can be enhanced by referral to home care resources. The nurse assesses the need for continued support or counseling and provides a telephone number to call the hospital if needed.

Vaginal Birth After Cesarean

A trial of labor after cesarean (TOLAC) and a vaginal birth after cesarean (VBAC) are recommended by the ACOG for women who have had a previous cesarean birth by low transverse incision (ACOG, 2010). Labor and vaginal birth is not recommended if a previous fundal scar (classic cesarean incision) or evidence of CPD is present. Consent for VBAC should be discussed with the health care provider and the couple based on accepted risk factors. Dystocia, increased maternal age, gestational age over 40 weeks, maternal obesity, preeclampsia and macrosomia may be contraindications for TOLAC.

The labor should occur in a health care facility that is equipped and staffed to conduct a cesarean birth if necessary. Intrapartum care of the woman is essentially the same as for any woman in labor. Close observation of fetal status and uterine contractions is maintained throughout the labor process. The use of cervical ripening with misoprostol (Cytotec) is not recommended, but augmentation with oxytocin can be done with close monitoring. The 2020 ACOG guidelines for VBAC include:

- Previous cesarean birth with transverse uterine incision or low vertical scar
- Documented adequacy of the pelvis
- Availability of the facilities to perform a cesarean birth within 30 minutes
- Provision of EFM
- Availability of intravenous access

Women who have spontaneous labor have a much lower incidence of uterine rupture than women who undergo labor induction. Women who have successful VBACs have lower incidence of infection, less blood loss, and reduced health care costs compared with women who have repeat cesareans.

⭐ Nursing Care Plan 14-1 — Preterm Premature Rupture of the Membranes (PPROM)

Scenario

A woman who is para 0, gravida 1 is admitted to the antepartum unit with possible ruptured membranes. She is at 30 weeks' gestation and has not had any uterine contractions.

Selected Nursing Diagnosis

Risk for infection related to effects of PPROM

Expected Outcomes	Nursing Interventions	Rationales
Woman will be free of infection, as evidenced by: FHR 110-160 beats/minute Maternal temperature 36.1°-37.2° C (97°-99° F) Maternal white blood count <12,000 per mm^3 Absence of foul-smelling vaginal discharge C-reactive protein negative	Determine and record time of PPROM, how much vaginal fluid there was, the color and odor of the fluid, and expected date of delivery (EDD). Assist with sterile speculum examination. Determine FHR and uterine contraction pattern with electronic fetal monitoring.	Provides baseline data. The length of time between rupture of the amniotic membranes and delivery correlates with risk for infection. Color and foul odor can indicate presence of infection. EDD is important in helping to determine whether rupture has occurred prematurely. Confirms rupture by presence of pooling amniotic fluid, Nitrazine paper turning blue, and fern pattern on slide when viewed under a microscope. Also allows for visual inspection of cervix to determine degree of dilation. Identifies nonreassuring FHR patterns so that early intervention can occur. Presence of uterine contractions can be a positive sign if fetus is ≥37 weeks of gestation. However, measures may need to be taken to end contractions if fetus is <37 weeks of gestation. In a term newborn, induction of labor usually will be initiated at 12 hours after rupture if labor has not started.

Nursing Care Plan 14-1   Preterm Premature Rupture of the Membranes (PPROM)—cont'd

Expected Outcomes	Nursing Interventions	Rationales
	Assist with fetal assessment tests if indicated.	Assesses fetal lung maturation and presence of infection. L/S ratio >2:1, prostaglandin positive, and lamellar body count >30,000 units/L are usually indicative of lung maturity. A Gram stain of amniotic fluid can reveal presence of infectious microorganisms.
	Administer glucocorticoids as ordered.	Aids in the maturation of the fetal lungs.
	Assess temperature per protocol and vaginal discharge at least every 4 hours.	Foul-smelling vaginal discharge and maternal fever are indicative of infection and must be reported immediately to the health care provider.
	Review laboratory results.	Elevation of leukocytes, presence of C-reactive protein, and a low amniotic fluid glucose level are indicative of infection.
	Teach patient to wipe perineum from front to back.	Proper peri care reduces the risk of infection.
	Change linens and under pads frequently to keep patient dry.	Moisture is an excellent medium for growth of microorganisms.
	Maintain on bed rest unless fetal presenting part is fully engaged.	Prevents cord prolapse.
	Provide patient with diversional activities.	Eliminates boredom of prolonged bed rest.
	Keep patient informed of fetal condition.	Alleviates anxiety.
	Explain rationales for all treatments.	Information often increases compliance with treatment regimen.
	Provide emotional support.	Anxiety and fear are common reactions to the threat of giving birth to a preterm newborn and to the risk for infection.

Critical Thinking Questions

1. The health care provider tells you to prepare the woman for a vaginal examination to assess for ruptured membranes. What should you have available during the examination?
2. When caring for a woman with PROM, how can you decrease the risk for infection?

FHR, fetal heart rate; *L/S*, lecithin/sphingomyelin.

Get Ready for the NCLEX® Examination!

Key Points

- Preterm labor is the onset of uterine contractions resulting in cervical dilation and effacement between 20 and 37 weeks' gestation. Late preterm labor is between 34 and 36 completed weeks of gestation.
- Management of preterm labor includes assessment of uterine activity and cervical changes, bed rest, hydration, use of tocolytic agents, fetal surveillance, and management to promote fetal lung maturity. Home care management with a HUAM is performed in selected cases.
- PROM occurs when the membranes rupture before the labor has started.
- Dystocia is difficult and often prolonged labor.
- Dystocia is suspected when there is a lack of labor progression in cervical dilation and slow advancement in fetal descent. It is caused by a problem with power (contractions), passenger (fetal position), passageway (small or obstructed pelvic path), or psyche.

- CPD occurs when the fetus is too large to pass through the normal pelvis or the maternal pelvic diameters are too small to allow passage of a normal-size fetus. A cesarean birth may be necessary.
- External version is the turning of the fetal presentation from a breech or transverse lie to cephalic. Ultrasound guides fetal manipulations during the procedure.
- Induction of labor refers to measures to initiate uterine contractions.
- Augmentation of labor is the use of oxytocin drugs to stimulate labor when uterine contractions are ineffective.
- Cervical ripening is performed to soften the cervix before starting an induction of labor. One method is inserting PGE_2 into the cervical canal.
- Amniotomy, or artificial rupture of membranes, usually initiates labor within 12 hours of rupture in the near-term woman with a favorable cervix.

- An episiotomy is a surgical incision made into the perineum to permit easier passage of the fetus.
- Vaginal delivery with forceps or vacuum extraction provides traction to aid in the descent and delivery of the baby's head, to assist the rotation of the head, or both.
- Postterm labor and birth refer to a fetus beyond 42 weeks' gestation.
- Precipitate labor is rapid and lasts less than 3 hours.
- Hydramnios (polyhydramnios) occurs when there is excessive amniotic fluid. It is associated with fetal malformations that affect fetal swallowing and voiding.
- A prolapsed umbilical cord occurs when the cord precedes the fetal presenting part.
- A VBAC is suggested for women who have had a previous cesarean birth by low transverse uterine incision. A trial of labor is recommended, and the woman is closely monitored. VBAC has decreased the incidence of cesarean births.

Additional Learning Resources

SG Go to your Study Guide on pages 499–500 for additional Review Questions for the NCLEX® Examination, Critical Thinking Clinical Situations, and other learning activities to help you master this chapter content.

evolve Go to your Evolve website (http://evolve.elsevier.com/Leifer/maternity) for the following FREE learning resources:
- Animations
- Answer Guidelines for Critical Thinking Questions
- Answers and Rationales for Review Questions for the NCLEX® Examination
- Concept Map Creator
- Glossary with pronunciations in English and Spanish
- Patient Teaching Plans
- Skills Performance Checklists and more!

Online Resources
- www.nlm.nih.gov/exhibition/cesarean/cesarean_1.html
- www.childbirth.org/section/section.html

Review Questions for the NCLEX® Examination

1. A woman experiencing signs and symptoms of preterm labor is admitted to the labor and birth unit. Baseline maternal vital signs are recorded as follows: T 101.5, P 110, R 30, and BP 134/80. These vital signs strongly suggest:
   1. Fetal distress
   2. Amniotic fluid infection
   3. Hypovolemia
   4. Preeclampsia

2. Labor with uterine contractions of poor quality that are painful, out of proportion to their intensity, do not cause cervical dilation or effacement, and are usually uncoordinated and frequent is known as:
   1. Hypotonic uterine dysfunction
   2. Cephalopelvic disproportion
   3. Hypertonic uterine dysfunction
   4. Precipitate labor

3. The most common example of malpresentation is:
   1. Breech presentation
   2. Transverse lie presentation
   3. Shoulder presentation
   4. Face presentation

4. The nonpharmacologic method of cervical ripening that involves rupturing the membranes by piercing with an amniotic hook is called:
   1. Stripping of membranes
   2. Amniotomy
   3. Mechanical dilation
   4. Prostaglandin gel application

5. A woman in the labor and birth unit is undergoing induction with oxytocin (Pitocin). If the nurse notices late decelerations of the fetal heart rate, the first action should be to:
   1. Notify the physician.
   2. Assist the patient into left-side lying position.
   3. Discontinue the oxytocin (Pitocin).
   4. Apply oxygen via nasal cannula.

6. A laceration of the perineum where the anal sphincter muscles and muscles of the perineum are torn is classified as a:
   1. First-degree laceration
   2. Second-degree laceration
   3. Third-degree laceration
   4. Fourth-degree laceration

7. Which clinical manifestation(s) would indicate preterm labor? (*Select all that apply.*)
   1. Thigh pain
   2. Vaginal bleeding
   3. Calf cramping
   4. Low back pain
   5. Nausea

Critical Thinking Questions

1. A woman is 20 years old with her first pregnancy, and her fetus is in persistent occiput posterior position. She is in labor with contractions every 3 to 4 minutes, her membranes are intact, and she is having severe backache with each contraction. If she asks you why she is having such severe back pain during her labor, how would you answer her?

2. A woman began spontaneous labor at 6 AM, and, by 7 PM, she had made no labor progress. Her cervical dilation has not progressed beyond 4 cm. What reasons could you give for her labor not progressing?

The Newborn at Risk: Conditions Associated with Gestational Age and Development

Objectives

1. Define key terms listed.
2. Demonstrate how gestational age is determined.
3. Review the causes of intrauterine growth restriction.
4. Compare and contrast the preterm newborn, the term newborn, and the postterm newborn.
5. Outline the care of the preterm newborn.
6. Explain the factors that predispose the newborn to necrotizing enterocolitis.
7. Describe developmentally supportive care of preterm newborns.
8. Outline the needs of parents who have a preterm newborn.

Key Terms

appropriate for gestational age (AGA) (p. 303)
bronchopulmonary dysplasia (BPD) (brŏng-kō-PŬL-mă-nār-ē dĭs-PLĀ-zhă, p. 314)
intrauterine growth restriction (IUGR) (p. 303)
intraventricular hemorrhage (IVH) (ĭn-tră-věn-TRĬK-ū-lăr HĔM-ŏr-ĭj, p. 315)
kangaroo care (p. 316)
large for gestational age (LGA) (p. 303)
late preterm (p. 303)
necrotizing enterocolitis (NEC) (NĔK-rō-TĪZ-ĭng ěn-tă-rō-kō-LĪ-tĭs, p. 314)

patent ductus arteriosus (PDA) (PĂ-těnt DŬK-tŭs ăr-tē-rē-Ō-sŭs, p. 314)
postterm (p. 303)
preterm (p. 303)
pulse oximeter (ŏk-SĬM-ě-těr, p. 314)
respiratory distress syndrome (RDS) (p. 310)
retinopathy of prematurity (ROP) (rě-tĭ-NŎP-ă-thē, p. 313)
small for gestational age (SGA) (p. 303)

An "at-risk" newborn is one who is susceptible to illness that may be mild to severe resulting from immaturity, physical disorders, or complications during or after birth. By appropriately assessing the gestational age and size, health care providers can make important clinical judgments about the functioning of the body's systems and risk factors facing the newborn. Clinical problems may be quite different in a newborn who is born at 33 weeks' gestation and weighs 1.4 kg (3 lbs) compared with a newborn born at 35 weeks' gestation and weighing the same. Because of these discrepancies, a more precise system of terminology has evolved. The classification of newborns at birth, based on gestational ages and birth weights, is as follows:

Preterm or **premature:** An infant born before the end of 38 weeks' gestation, regardless of weight.
Late preterm: An infant born between 34 weeks' gestation and 37 weeks, regardless of weight.
Term or full term: An infant born between 38 and 42 weeks' gestation, regardless of weight.
Low birth weight: Any newborn who weighs less than 2500 g (5.5 lbs) at birth.

Small for gestational age (SGA): Any newborn whose weight is below the 10th percentile (according to intrauterine growth curve), regardless of gestational age.
Appropriate for gestational age (AGA): Any newborn whose intrauterine growth has been normal (according to intrauterine growth curve) for that length of gestation.
Large for gestational age (LGA): Any newborn whose weight is above the 90th percentile (according to intrauterine growth curve), regardless of gestational age.
Intrauterine growth restriction (IUGR): Failure of the fetus to grow as expected during gestation.
Postterm: A newborn born after 42 weeks' gestation, regardless of weight.

The gestational age can help identify problems to be anticipated. Specific physiologic problems have been linked with specific gestational ages. For example, the preterm infant born before 34 weeks' gestation will potentially face respiratory distress because of immature lungs and lack of surfactant. When the newborn is identified as postterm (postmature), the potential problem is meconium aspiration syndrome as a result of failing placental function.

Improvement in ultrasound and fetal Doppler technology enhances the ability to detect fetal growth restriction, expands the understanding of the pathophysiologic condition, improves the ability to predict certain neonatal outcomes, and enables preparation for the birth of the newborn who may be physiologically compromised. The rate of preterm births increased from 10.2 in 1987 to 12.3 live births in 2003 and accounts for 70% of neonatal morbidity (Giarratano, 2006). The cause of preterm births is thought to be an interaction of genetic factors with environmental factors, such as maternal illness, that increase risk, and therefore prenatal nurses should take a careful family history *prenatally* and teach the woman risk reduction strategies such as proper nutrition, prevention of infection, and management of fatigue (Giarratano, 2006).

GESTATIONAL AGE AND BIRTH WEIGHT

The Ballard scoring system helps determine the newborn's gestational age (Figure 15-1). This system uses growth and maturity criteria, as indicated, by physical and neuromuscular signs. The examiner assigns a score for each characteristic, such as genital development. It is important to remember that newborns can vary in size and weight yet be the same gestational age (Figure 15-2). The clinical course and strategy for management depend on early identification of gestational age.

SMALL-FOR-GESTATIONAL-AGE (SGA) NEWBORN

Factors Contributing to the SGA or IUGR Newborn
Factors that contribute to impaired growth may be caused by maternal, placental, or fetal conditions. The most common factors affecting growth restriction are presented in Table 15-1. SGA newborns may be preterm, term, or postterm.

Two Types of Growth Restriction
Fetal cellular growth occurs by an increase in cell number and an increase in cell size. If some interference with growth occurs early during the critical period of organ development (organogenesis) of the embryo, fewer cells are formed, organs are small, and the organ weight is subnormal. This type of growth impairment is called *symmetric growth restriction* because all parts of the body are small (including the brain). Causes of symmetric IUGR include chronic maternal hypertension, severe malnutrition, intrauterine infection, substance abuse, and anemia. Symmetric IUGR can be noted on ultrasound in the first half of the second trimester. Growth interference that begins later in pregnancy does not affect the total number of cells but their size only. This type of growth restriction is *asymmetric IUGR*. It is most often associated with compromise of uteroplacental blood flow. Causes of

asymmetric IUGR include gestational hypertension, smoking (causing vasoconstriction), maternal drug use (such as cocaine), uncontrolled maternal diabetes, and placental infarcts. The newborn weight is below normal, but length and head circumference are normal. Growth-restricted newborns are at risk for hypoxia, acidosis, and death. Table 15-2 lists problems and risk factors for SGA newborns.

SGA and IUGR newborns are those who are at or below the 10th percentile of weight for the gestational age (Gabbe, Niebyl, & Simpson, 2007). The incidence of SGA newborns is 3% to 10% of all pregnancies. The mortality rate of SGA newborns is higher than that of normal newborns. Prenatal Doppler studies to assess flow abnormalities of fetal or placental vessels and an antenatal biophysical profile should be performed weekly, especially if oligohydramnios is present, because elective delivery may be necessary.

Physical Appearance
On first inspection, many of the SGA newborns show physical characteristics that suggest impaired intrauterine growth. The head might seem large, but its circumference is normal or near normal. The chest and abdominal circumferences are reduced because of decreased subcutaneous fat. The adipose tissue and muscle mass over the cheeks, buttocks, and thighs are diminished. Because the body length is usually normal, the newborns appear thin and long. They often have thin faces, resembling little old people. The skull's sutures are often wide apart as a result of impaired bone growth; thus, the newborn's fontanelles are often large and somewhat sunken.

Behavior
Many SGA newborns are more active than expected for their size. This observation is especially true when comparing them with preterm (AGA) newborns. The cry of an SGA newborn is vigorous and may be impressive in relation to size. The SGA newborn usually has a strong sucking response compared with the weaker sucking response in the preterm newborn. The SGA newborn often eats well and gains weight more quickly than the preterm newborn. The overall impression of vigor and well-being may be misleading. The newborn's wide-eyed, alert facial expression may be caused by chronic hypoxia (lack of oxygen). The SGA newborn is also prone to hypoglycemia because the glycogen stores are often inadequate or depleted. Because of such potential complications, the health care provider needs to observe the SGA newborn closely and intervene as indicated.

Assessment and Management
Because the causes of IUGR are so varied, the care of the SGA newborn must be adapted to meet the specific problems that the newborn demonstrates. These newborns need to be carefully examined for

MATURATIONAL ASSESSMENT OF GESTATIONAL AGE (New Ballard Score)

NAME _____   DATE/TIME OF BIRTH _____   SEX _____

HOSPITAL NO. _____   DATE/TIME OF EXAM _____   BIRTH WEIGHT _____

RACE _____   AGE WHEN EXAMINED _____   LENGTH _____

APGAR SCORE: 1 MINUTE _____ 5 MINUTES _____ 10 MINUTES _____   HEAD CIRC. _____

EXAMINER _____

NEUROMUSCULAR MATURITY

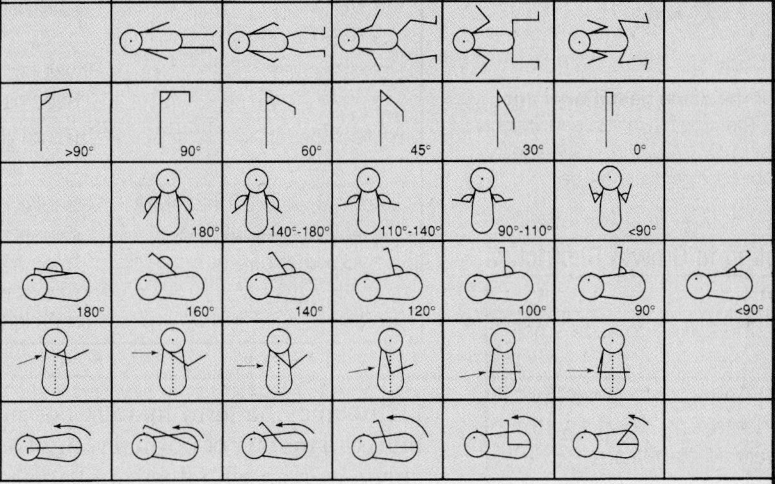

NEUROMUSCULAR MATURITY SIGN	SCORE							RECORD SCORE HERE
	-1	0	1	2	3	4	5	
POSTURE								
SQUARE WINDOW (Wrist)	>90°	90°	60°	45°	30°	0°		
ARM RECOIL		180°	140°-180°	110°-140°	90°-110°	<90°		
POPLITEAL ANGLE	180°	160°	140°	120°	100°	90°	<90°	
SCARF SIGN								
HEEL TO EAR								

TOTAL NEUROMUSCULAR MATURITY SCORE

PHYSICAL MATURITY

PHYSICAL MATURITY SIGN	SCORE							RECORD SCORE HERE
	-1	0	1	2	3	4	5	
SKIN	sticky friable transparent	gelatinous red translucent	smooth pink visible veins	superficial peeling &/or rash, few veins	cracking pale areas rare veins	parchment deep cracking no vessels	leathery cracked wrinkled	
LANUGO	none	sparse	abundant	thinning	bald areas	mostly bald		
PLANTAR SURFACE	heel-toe 40-50 mm:-1 <40 mm:-2	>50 mm no crease	faint red marks	anterior transverse crease only	creases ant. 2/3	creases over entire sole		
BREAST	imperceptible	barely perceptible	flat areola no bud	stippled areola 1-2 mm bud	raised areola 3-4 mm bud	full areola 5-10 mm bud		
EYE/EAR	lids fused loosely: -1 tightly: -2	lids open pinna flat stays folded	sl. curved pinna; soft; slow recoil	well-curved pinna; soft but ready recoil	formed & firm instant recoil	thick cartilage ear stiff		
GENITALS (Male)	scrotum flat, smooth	scrotum empty faint rugae	testes in upper canal rare rugae	testes descending few rugae	testes down good rugae	testes pendulous deep rugae		
GENITALS (Female)	clitoris prominent & labia flat	prominent clitoris & small labia minora	prominent clitoris & enlarging minora	majora & minora equally prominent	majora large minora small	majora cover clitoris & minora		

Reference
Ballard JL, Khoury JC. Wedig K, et al: New Ballard Score, expanded to include extremely premature infants. *J Pediatr* 1991; 119:417-423. Reprinted by permission of Dr Ballard and Mosby · Year Book, Inc.

TOTAL PHYSICAL MATURITY SCORE

SCORE

Neuromuscular _____
Physical _____
Total _____

MATURITY RATING

score	weeks
-10	20
-5	22
0	24
5	26
10	28
15	30
20	32
25	34
30	36
35	38
40	40
45	42
50	44

GESTATIONAL AGE (weeks)

By dates _____
By ultrasound _____
By exam _____

FIGURE 15-1 Ballard scoring system.

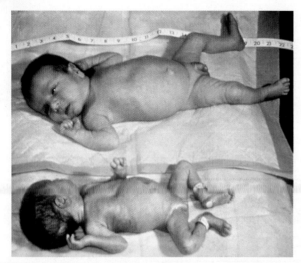

FIGURE 15-2 **Two term newborns of the same gestational age.** These newborns are discordant twins. The variation in size and weight resulted from a malfunction of the placenta. One newborn is average for gestational age, and one newborn is small for gestational age.

Table 15-1	Factors Contributing to Growth Restriction
FACTOR	**EXAMPLES**
Genetics	Small parents more likely to have small newborn
Maternal disease	Complications related to vascular problems, decreasing blood flow to uterus (advanced diabetes, gestational hypertension, kidney disease)
Maternal factors	Smoking, substance abuse
Environmental factors	High altitude, radiographs
Malnutrition	Maternal starvation
Placental factors	Small placenta, placenta previa, decreased placental perfusion
Fetal factors	Congenital infections (rubella, toxoplasmosis, syphilis), multifetal pregnancy, chromosomal abnormalities

Table 15-2	Problems and Risk Factors in Small-for-Gestational-Age Newborns
PROBLEM	**RISK FACTOR**
Hypoxia	Lack of adequate oxygen
Meconium aspiration	Relaxation of anal sphincter with passage of meconium in utero resulting from hypoxia
Hypoglycemia	Poor liver glycogen stores
Hypothermia	Diminished subcutaneous fat and large body surface area
Intraventricular hemorrhage	Fragile blood vessels
Polycythemia	Physiologic response to hypoxia in utero
Hypocalcemia	Calcium depletion caused by birth asphyxia
Maternal factors that cause low birth weight from hypoxia stress	Vascular complications caused by gestational hypertension, advanced diabetes, smoking, poor nutrition, use of drugs

congenital anomalies and monitored for hypoglycemia. Calorie needs are higher for these newborns than for an AGA newborn. Often their care is similar to that of the preterm newborn (Nursing Care Plan 15-1).

Simple measures during prenatal care, such as elimination of cigarette smoking, alcohol, and illicit drugs; improved nutrition; and eradication of genitourinary tract infection would lower the number of infants born with IUGR.

LARGE-FOR-GESTATIONAL-AGE (LGA) NEWBORN

The newborn whose birth weight is at or above the 90th percentile typically weighs 4000 g (8 lbs, 13 oz) or more at birth and is referred to as *LGA*. The LGA

infants may be term infants, postmature, or may be born to a mother of normal weight and health. The diabetic woman who does not have advanced vascular changes is likely to have a large newborn (**macrosomia**) because of high glucose levels that cross the placenta. The large newborn often poses a mechanical problem during delivery and, after a prolonged labor, is usually delivered by cesarean birth. If delivered vaginally, the newborn may incur an injury (e.g., fractured clavicle or central nervous system trauma) during the birth process. LGA newborns are often sluggish, hypotonic, and hypoactive at birth; they may have hypoglycemia or polycythemia. If the newborns have diabetic mothers, they are prone to hypoglycemia; therefore, they need frequent blood glucose level assessments. The newborn of a diabetic mother is discussed in Chapter 16.

POSTTERM NEWBORN

The postterm newborn (postmature) is a newborn born after 42 weeks' gestation. Postterm births occur in about 12% of all pregnancies (Lee, 2008). Many are large. The placenta may not function as well after 40 weeks' gestation because placental insufficiency develops. Because of the progressive degeneration of the placenta, the fetus does not receive adequate oxygen and nutrients. During labor, poor oxygen reserves and limited placental function place the newborn at risk for meconium aspiration. The fetus may use up some of the subcutaneous fat and, when born, will look thin with loose skin. The skin is often cracked and dry, with a parchment-like texture from the decrease in

⭐ Nursing Care Plan 15-1 | Small-for-Gestational-Age Newborn

Scenario

A male newborn is 48 hours old, 38 weeks' gestation, birth weight 1.4 kg (3 lbs) (small for gestational age [SGA]). Physical examination reveals long, thin appearance; scarcity of subcutaneous fat; and sunken abdomen. Apgar scores were 6 and 8 at 1 and 5 minutes, respectively. He is positive for meconium aspiration. His cry is vigorous, and he appears wide-eyed and alert.

Selected Nursing Diagnosis

Impaired gas exchange related to aspiration of meconium

Expected Outcomes	Nursing Interventions	Rationales
Newborn will be free of signs of respiratory distress.	Monitor newborn for signs of respiratory distress. Auscultate breath sounds. Monitor pulse oximetry readings. Suction newborn when necessary to maintain open airway.	In utero, fetal hypoxia causes relaxation of anal sphincter with passage of meconium; newborn inhales meconium in amniotic fluid, which can impair gas exchange. Suctioning maintains open airway.

Selected Nursing Diagnosis

Ineffective thermoregulation related to lack of subcutaneous fat

Expected Outcomes	Nursing Interventions	Rationales
Newborn will maintain normal temperature.	Provide neutral thermal environment. Monitor axillary or skin temperature every 4 hours. Assess for hypoglycemia and observe for respiratory distress syndrome.	Neutral thermal environment aids temperature control. Diminished subcutaneous fat and large body surface area in the SGA newborn predispose him to difficulty in temperature regulation. Glucose stores are used up quickly.

Selected Nursing Diagnosis

Imbalanced nutrition, less than body requirements related to increased metabolic rate

Expected Outcomes	Nursing Interventions	Rationales
Newborn will maintain or gain weight.	Initiate early feeding; monitor, record, and report signs of fatigue or respiratory distress during feeding. Place on right side after feeding to enhance digestion.	SGA newborns are fed frequently; they require more calories per kilogram for growth because of increased metabolic activity and oxygen consumption. Newborns are placed on right side after feeding to facilitate emptying of gastric contents.

Selected Nursing Diagnosis

Risk for injury and *Risk for infection* related to invasive procedures

Expected Outcomes	Nursing Interventions	Rationales
Newborn's tissues will heal promptly.	Because of thin skin, special tape is used to lessen skin injury. Monitor, record, and report skin breakdown.	Invasive procedures will increase risk for tissue injury and infection.

Selected Nursing Diagnosis

Risk for impaired parenting related to mother-newborn separation

Expected Outcomes	Nursing Interventions	Rationales
Parent-newborn bonding will be evidenced by good eye contact. Parent will hold newborn close, frequently touching the baby's body.	Encourage parents to visit the newborn frequently. Refer to baby by his or her given name. Encourage parents to participate in care (feeding and holding).	SGA newborns have prolonged periods of separation from parents. Helps parents see newborn as an individual Encouragement of parents to participate in newborn's care facilitates bonding (parent-newborn attachment).

Critical Thinking Questions

1. A 4-hour-old newborn has vital signs of temperature, 35.8° C (96.4° F); pulse, 120 beats/minute; and respirations, 40 breaths/minute. Color is pink. The mother asks you to bathe the baby so he can room-in with her. Is this a good time to bathe the baby?
2. The physician hands you an SGA newborn immediately after delivery. What should be your priority action?

protective vernix caseosa. The postterm newborn is at risk for hypoxia, meconium aspiration, hypoglycemia, polycythemia, cold stress, and asphyxia. The infant may appear wide-eyed and alert because of chronic intrauterine hypoxia. There is little lanugo or vernix, and the infant has long fingernails. Health care providers should closely monitor all postterm newborns for hypoglycemia, cold stress, and airway obstruction caused by meconium aspiration, regardless of size (Table 15-3).

PRETERM NEWBORN

The most common factor associated with neonatal death is prematurity. The preterm newborn is defined as one who is born at less than 38 weeks' gestation. Preterm births have risen from 9.4% of live births in the United States in 1981 to 12.3% in 2008 (NCHS, 2005). The majority of the increase was in late preterm births, formerly known as "near-term births" (Engel, 2007). Late preterm infants may look more like full-term infants, but they are metabolically and physiologically immature and have needs similar to the more preterm infant. However, a newborn may be born alive much earlier than 34 weeks' gestation and still live, but he or she may be poorly equipped to survive outside of the uterus. Specific organ systems may not be developed enough to function at a level necessary to maintain life and promote growth. The preterm newborn's skin is often wrinkled and delicate and is usually covered with lanugo. The plantar creases on the soles of the feet begin to develop from the toes toward the heel during fetal development, and the term infant has deep creases on the soles of the feet extending from the toes to the heel. In contrast, the preterm has few creases on the sole of the foot (Figure 15-3). The preterm newborn is thin, has little subcutaneous fat, and has prominent fontanelles and suture lines of the skull. Depending on the gestational age, the cry can be very weak, matching the frail appearance, and the body appears limp, with poor muscle tone.

Extremities are in extension rather than flexion, exposing a larger body surface area and increasing the risk of hypothermia (Figure 15-4).

Limitations of the Body System Functionings

The degree of immaturity of each of the preterm newborn's body systems varies with gestational age and determines the potential risks for that newborn.

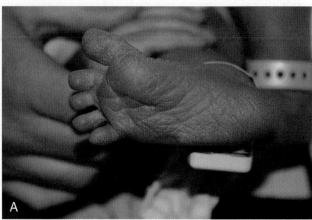

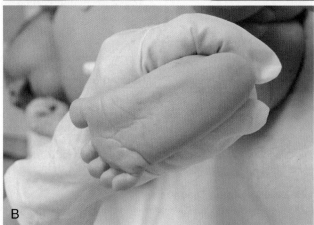

FIGURE 15-3 A, The sole of the foot of a term infant has deep creases extending from toes to heel. **B,** The preterm has few creases on the sole.

Table 15-3   Problems Related to Large-for-Gestational-Age and Postterm Newborns

CAUSE	PROBLEM	NEONATAL RESPONSE	NURSING INTERVENTIONS
Placental degeneration or uteroplacental insufficiency	Chronic hypoxia in utero Fetal distress	Polycythemia Meconium aspiration syndrome Respiratory problems	Monitor intravenous fluid resuscitation. Provide oxygen. Prepare or assist with exchange transfusion if hematocrit is high.
Increased size from high glucose or prolonged gestation Glycogen stores depleted or insulin reserves high	Difficult delivery Cephalopelvic disproportion Insufficient glucose reserves	Birth trauma Clavicle fracture seizures Hypoglycemia at birth (<40 mg/dL in term newborns) Temperature instability	Assess newborn closely for birth injury. Document reflexes. Monitor glucose levels every 2 hours. Provide thermoregulation in incubator care. Prevent cold stress. Provide early feedings.

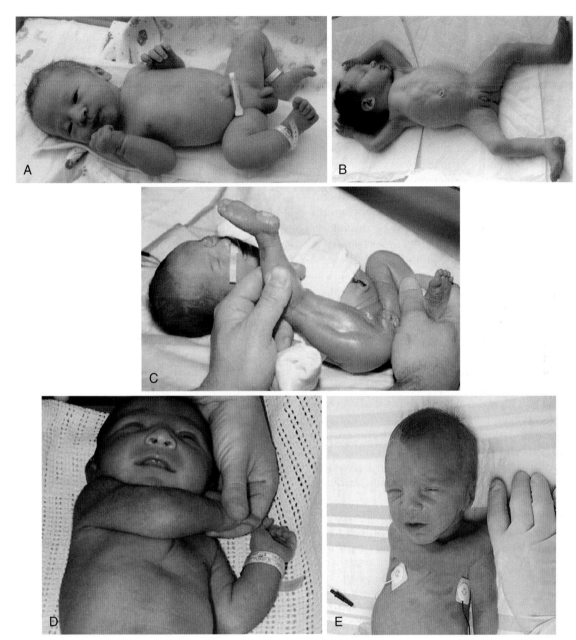

FIGURE 15-4 **A,** The term newborn shows flexion of the arms and legs. Note the acrocyanosis of the hands and feet. **B,** The preterm newborn holds extremities in extension, exposing more of the body surface area to the environment. This factor contributes to the development of cold stress and difficulty with thermoregulation. **C,** Popliteal angle. The knee easily extends so that the toes touch the nose in this preterm newborn (muscle tone prevents the term newborn from extending the knee). Note the thin, transparent skin and open, gaping labia of this preterm newborn. **D,** Scarf sign. In the term newborn, the elbow cannot be drawn past the midline of the body. **E,** Scarf sign in the preterm newborn. The elbow easily passes the midline of the body.

If the hospital does not have an intensive care nursery, and if the newborn requires a great deal of special attention, he or she may be transferred to a regional hospital that has a high-risk intensive care unit for preterm newborns. If it is not possible to transfer the mother before delivery, a transport team may be available to bring the newborn to the regional center after birth. The newborn is given respiratory support as needed, given oxygen, kept warm, and protected from potential sources of infection.

Respiratory System. The newborn's respiratory system is not fully mature until after 35 weeks' gestation. The presence of surfactant in adequate amounts is of primary importance. By 35 weeks' gestation, production of surfactant is usually sufficient to enable the newborn to breathe without a collapse of the alveoli when the newborn exhales. When surfactant is deficient, the lungs' ability to fill easily with air is lessened. On expiration, the alveoli (air sacs) collapse and the exchange of oxygen and carbon dioxide is reduced, resulting in hypoxia, decreased pulmonary blood flow, and depletion of the newborn's energy. Because of surfactant deficiency, respiratory distress often develops in the preterm newborn.

The preterm newborn commonly has irregular breathing patterns, referred to as *periodic breathing*. A danger of periodic breathing in the preterm newborn is prolonged apnea. Apnea is a pause in respirations longer than 20 seconds. Prolonged apnea can cause bradycardia and cyanosis. Weak muscles of the preterm newborn also affect respiratory function; gastroesophageal reflux can cause laryngospasm and apnea, and the gag reflex is weak. The preterm newborn may need respiratory support by intubation and mechanical ventilation. Artificial surfactant is available to be administered to the small preterm newborn.

Newborns who are older than 34 weeks' gestation who have severe respiratory distress may be eligible for extracorporeal membrane oxygenation (ECMO), which serves as an artificial lung outside of the body, allowing time for the lungs to heal. High-frequency ventilators provide smaller volumes of oxygen at a more rapid rate than normal. Very small preterm newborns may be placed on liquid ventilators that recreate the fetal lung environment by pumping an oxygenated liquid solution to the lungs. This type of technology is available in neonatal intensive care facilities and improves survival rates of small preterm newborns. Nitrous oxide therapy is currently under study to replace the invasive ECMO therapy.

Signs of respiratory distress syndrome (RDS) are retractions of the chest wall, **expiratory grunting, nasal flaring,** and changes in the respiratory and heart rates (Figure 15-5). Tiny nasal and respiratory passages are easily occluded by mucous plugs. High concentrations of oxygen, and long-term ventilator therapy, necessary

for initial survival, can result in long-term lung damage (bronchopulmonary dysplasia [BPD]).

Circulatory System. The preterm newborn has a fragile circulatory system and has a tendency toward persistent fetal circulation. A low surfactant level in the lungs of a preterm newborn contributes to hypoxia and low oxygen levels. The transition from fetal circulation to newborn circulation is a direct result of the increase in levels of oxygen because the ductus arteriosus closes in response to high oxygen concentrations. In post-birth hypoxia, it may reopen, causing blood to bypass the lungs and further increasing hypoxia. If pulmonary vascular resistance is high, causing the ductus arteriosus to reopen, more blood will bypass the lungs and further increase hypoxia.

Fluctuations in blood pressure can cause fluctuations in cerebral blood flow, and fragile vessels may rupture, causing intracranial hemorrhage and resulting in long-term neurologic, cognitive, and neuromotor problems. Careful monitoring of the heart rate and rhythm, skin color, blood pressure, and oxygen saturation levels is necessary in the preterm newborn. Although acrocyanosis is normal in all newborns, cyanosis of the body and face is abnormal.

Gastrointestinal System. The preterm newborn is able to take limited nourishment; however, the digestive and absorptive processes are not fully developed and are not fully functional until 36 weeks' gestation. As a result, the preterm newborn is unable to adequately digest some nutrients, such as saturated fats and protein high in casein, because of a decrease in bile salts and pancreatic lipase. In addition, the very preterm newborn may have weak sucking and swallowing reflexes. It is important to remember that the preterm newborn has a limited stomach capacity and

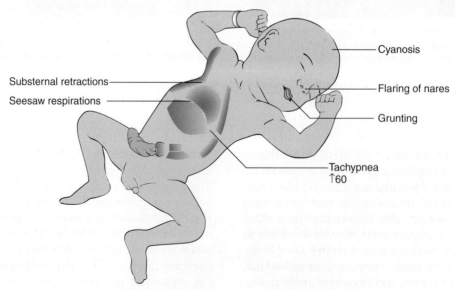

FIGURE 15-5 Signs of respiratory distress in the preterm newborn.

is subject to gastroesophageal reflux and aspiration; therefore, the nurse must be careful in the amount of fluid given, including gastric gavage (tube feeding), to protect the newborn from vomiting and aspiration. Minimal enteral nutrition (MEN) feedings that provide 1 mL/hour may be given until the newborn can tolerate regular tube feedings. Nonnutritive sucking (pacifiers) should be provided when newborns are given a nothing-by-mouth (NPO) order. Skill 15-1 describes the technique of intermittent tube feedings.

Because of delayed stomach emptying and reduced intestinal motility, abdominal distention, rigidity, and failure to absorb liquids can occur. Preterm newborns are prone to hypoxia, and the intestinal cells damaged by hypoxia stop secreting mucus and can be invaded by bacteria, which can be fatal. As a result of the ischemia of the bowel, the newborn becomes predisposed to necrotizing enterocolitis (NEC). Total parenteral nutrition (TPN) may be required.

Increased basal metabolic rate (BMR) requires increased oxygen supply, resulting in fatigue and inability of the newborn to suck.

Liver and Metabolic Function. Because preterm newborns have reduced glycogen, fat, vitamin, and mineral (especially calcium) stores at birth, they are faced with problems of hypoglycemia and hypocalcemia. Some of the clinical signs are twitching, convulsions, and a high-pitched cry. Hypoglycemia in the preterm newborn is evidenced by a blood glucose level of 30 mg/dL or less.

Poor clearance of bilirubin in the liver and reduced fluid intake (small feedings) can inhibit the removal of bilirubin in the intestines. In addition, the preterm newborn is more susceptible to cold stress, which releases free fatty acids. The excess fatty acids compete for albumin-binding sites, which displaces bilirubin. More simply stated, the preterm newborn is at a higher risk for hyperbilirubinemia (see Chapter 16).

With less time in utero, limited amounts of brown fat and glycogen have been stored. This means that when the newborn is stressed by chilling, he or she has an increased need for energy in the form of glucose. The additional need can quickly deplete the newborn's glycogen stores, and hypoglycemia can develop.

Skill 15-1   Gavage Feeding

PURPOSE

To provide nutrition when oral route is ineffective.

Steps

1. Verify correct formula and amount to be administered by gavage.
2. If tube is not in place, verify length of feeding tube. (Measure from the tip of the nose to the base of the ear and then down to point between the xiphoid and umbilicus. Mark tubing with tape.)
3. Give infant pacifier. Insert moistened tube gently via nose or mouth. (Observe for bradycardia, choking, cyanosis which indicates tube is in trachea instead of esophagus.) Securely tape tubing to cheek.
4. Connect the syringe to the feeding tube.
5. Verify placement of tube.
6. Gently pull back on the plunger of the syringe to aspirate stomach contents.
7. Check pH of stomach contents (acidic).
8. Return aspirated contents to stomach.
9. Abnormal or excessive residual stomach contents should be reported before continuing.
10. Connect the barrel of the syringe to the feeding tube, and pinch the tube to prevent air from entering.

11. Pour 1 to 3 mL of sterile water into the syringe to determine tube patency. Pinch tube to prevent air from entering.
12. Pour specified amount of formula or breast milk into the barrel of the syringe.
13. Release pinching of the tube and allow fluid to flow by gravity into the stomach at a rate of approximately 1 mL/minute. Nonnutritive sucking can be provided to the newborn. The newborn should be stimulated by gently touching, stroking, and talking during the procedure.
14. When the prescribed volume is administered, pour 1 to 3 mL sterile water to flush the tube.
15. Pinch the tube, and remove the syringe. A clamp may be applied and the tube placed above the heart level to avoid back-up of milk from the stomach into the tube.
16. Document the residual gastric contents, amount and type of gavage feeding given, and response of the newborn.
17. The newborn is burped and may be propped on the right side after feeding. A rolled blanket can be used to position the infant.

Blood glucose levels of the preterm newborn are closely monitored.

Renal System. The preterm newborn's kidneys are immature, resulting in fluid and electrolyte problems. These newborns have a limited ability to concentrate urine or handle large amounts of fluid. Therefore, the preterm newborn is at risk for fluid retention and overhydration. Excessive bicarbonate losses may cause metabolic acidosis. The preterm newborn has poor drug clearance ability resulting from delayed excretion of the drugs. Because of this, the newborn receiving medications must be closely monitored to avoid toxic side effects.

Radiant warmers and bilirubin lights can cause loss of fluid through the skin. Rapid respiration also causes fluid loss from the lungs. Maintaining fluid and electrolyte balance is a critical challenge.

Behavioral States. Preterm infants may not evidence the same changes in behavioral states as the term infant. The natural reflexes (such as sucking and muscle tone) are weak, and sleep-wake cycles are irregular.

Immune System. The preterm newborn has received limited passive immunity from the mother. Most of the immunity that the fetus receives in utero against a variety of infections from maternal immunoglobulins occurs in the third trimester. Therefore, the preterm newborn has increased susceptibility to infection compared with the term newborn. The skin is fragile, and the many invasive procedures, such as intravenous lines and the use of tape and monitoring devices on the skin, increase the risk of infection. If the mother had group B streptococcal infection during labor, the newborn is at further risk from this infection. To prevent the spread of infection, staff must complete a 2- to 3-minute scrub with a hospital-approved solution before initiating care in the unit, and the use of tape directly on the skin is avoided.

Nurses who have an infection or who recently cared for a patient with an infection should not care for the preterm newborn. Sterilization of supplies and equipment and individual infection control techniques (hand hygiene after handling each newborn and before proceeding to next newborn) must be practiced. In addition, any preterm newborn who is potentially infectious should be immediately isolated from the other newborns.

Management and Nursing Care of the Preterm Newborn

The nurse who cares for the preterm newborn must be skilled in neonatal intensive care procedures, as well as physical and behavioral assessments, and be able to recognize developing complications and intervene accordingly.

Temperature Regulation. The maintenance of a constant neutral thermal environment, discussed in Chapter 10, is essential to the preterm newborn's survival. Term newborns can modify their body temperatures by increasing muscular activity and by adopting a more flexed position that minimizes heat loss; preterm newborns cannot.

The preterm newborn's heat loss is greater than that of a term newborn, and the ability to produce heat is limited. The lack of subcutaneous fat, thin skin, vessels near the surface of the skin, extended extremities (exposing a larger portion of the body surface area to the environment), and scant development of brown fat, along with an immature temperature-regulating center in the brain, result in thermoregulation problems in the preterm newborn. In addition, decreased glucose reserves and hypoxia prevent the increase in metabolism necessary to maintain body warmth.

The preterm newborn is usually placed under a radiant warmer or in an incubator (Figure 15-6). Also, a skin thermometer probe is used to monitor the newborn's skin temperature, which will rise or fall before core temperature. Promptly responding to changes in the skin temperature avoids alterations in the core body temperature.

Skin Care. The preterm newborn is positioned on the back with the head of the mattress slightly elevated, unless contraindicated. While the newborn is in this position, the abdominal contents do not press against the diaphragm and impede breathing. It is important

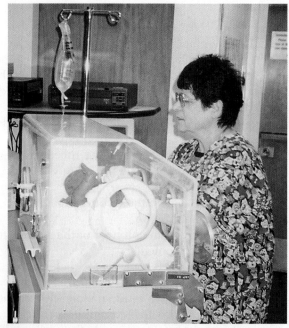

FIGURE 15-6 The nurse cares for a newborn in an isolette, which provides a neutral thermal environment, isolation from outside environment, and supplemental oxygen and humidity if needed.

to position the newborn so that drainage or secretions are not aspirated. Propping the preterm newborn on the side or placing the newborn prone can decrease respiratory effort. The newborn should not be left in one position for long periods because it may be uncomfortable and could potentially cause atelectasis of the lungs. Changing position also prevents breakdown from pressure on the newborn's delicate skin. The use of rolled blankets for support (nesting) and comfort and to relieve pressure on bony prominences is helpful. A rocker bed is used for the very premature newborn in the incubator. A waterbed or sheepskin covered with a cloth diaper or light blanket may also be helpful. Tape can cause skin trauma and should be avoided.

Hydration, Nutrition, and Methods of Feeding.
Providing adequate nutrition and fluids to the preterm newborn is a major challenge to the health care team. Early feedings are extremely important in maintaining normal metabolism and reducing the possibility of hypoglycemia, hyperkalemia, and hyperbilirubinemia.

The preterm newborn has high caloric needs (110 to 130 kcal/kg/day) and requires more whey protein than the term newborn. Many institutions use the mother's breast milk or special preterm formula to meet nutritional requirements. In addition, the preterm newborn may be given supplementary vitamins.

Breastfeeding is possible in small preterm newborns and should be encouraged if the mother has the desire and if the newborn demonstrates an appropriate suck-and-swallow reflex. If the newborn cannot be put to the breast, the mother can pump her breasts (see Chapter 11), and the breast milk can be given to the newborn by gavage (see Skill 15-1). Breast milk provides immunoglobulins A and G, which can protect against some infections such as NEC.

If newborns have a coordinated suck-and-swallow reflex, they may be fed by nipple. The newborn is fed in a semi-sitting position and burped after each half-to-full ounce. To avoid newborn fatigue, the nipple should be soft and the feeding should take no longer than 15 to 20 minutes. The nurse should pay particular attention to the newborn's behavior regarding fatigue and signs of respiratory distress. If the newborn is fed by gavage (nasogastric or orogastric tube), the nurse assesses for gastric residual by aspirating gastric contents; the residual is then readministered. It is important to put the aspirated fluid back in the stomach because the contents contain gastric secretions. Nutritional intake is considered adequate when the newborn gains 20 to 30 g/day. Prolonged gavage feedings may result in nipple aversion, which may prolong adjustment to bottle feeding and delay home discharge.

 Nutrition Considerations

Special Nipple for Bottle Feeding
A "preemie nipple" should be used for bottle feeding preterm newborns to minimize the energy required for sucking.

After feeding, the nurse places the newborn on the right side to decrease the possibility of aspiration and facilitate emptying of the gastric contents.

Fluid Volume. The preterm newborn is monitored for hydration and fluid therapy by accurately calculating the daily weight and intake and output. When the newborn receives intravenous fluids by neonatal infusion pump, hourly monitoring is critical because the preterm newborn is prone to dehydration or fluid overload. Urinary output should be greater than 1 mL/kg/hour. The weight of the dry diaper should be subtracted from the weight of the wet diaper to determine urinary output (1 g = 1 mL). Diapers should be fastened securely on the newborn in a radiant warmer or incubator to prevent evaporation of fluid on the diaper surface, which can result in an inaccurate diaper weight.

 Health Promotion

Signs of Dehydration and Overhydration of Preterm Newborns
SIGNS OF DEHYDRATION
- Urinary output less than 1 mL/kg/hour
- Urine specific gravity more than 1.015
- Weight loss
- Dry mucous membranes
- Poor tissue turgor
- Depressed fontanelle

SIGNS OF OVERHYDRATION
- Urinary output greater than 3 mL/kg/hour
- Urine specific gravity less than 1.001
- Edema
- Increased weight gain
- Rales
- Intake greater than output

COMMON PROBLEMS OF THE COMPROMISED NEWBORN

RETINOPATHY OF PREMATURITY
Prolonged periods of hyperoxygenation (partial pressure of oxygen [PaO$_2$] levels greater than 90 to 100 mm Hg) can be dangerous to the newborn because the condition produces oxygen toxicity. Oxygen toxicity can cause vasoconstriction and leakage in the vessels of the retina, and retinal detachment resulting in retinopathy of prematurity (ROP), previously called **retrolental fibroplasia,** which can lead to loss of vision or blindness. Other problems common to infants weighing less than 1500 g can also cause ROP.

A noninvasive monitoring system, such as transcutaneous oxygen monitor, is a method that uses an electrode to obtain a continuous measurement of PaO$_2$, thereby reducing the frequency of invasive blood sampling. The leads of a pulse oximeter can be attached to the newborn's foot, toe, or hand (Figure 15-7). An alarm sounds with a low perfusion reading. When documenting the saturation level reading, the nurse should note whether the newborn is in room air or receiving supplemental oxygen. The use of the noninvasive pulse oximeter enables the monitoring of oxygen saturation that can avoid hyperoxygenation and resulting damage to the retina. However, very premature infants may require high levels of oxygen for survival and ROP may be a resulting complication. All premature infants who have been treated with oxygen should have follow-up eye exams after discharge. The light on the pulse oximeter lead generates some heat and, therefore, the location of the lead should be rotated each shift to avoid damage to the thin skin of the premature infant.

BRONCHOPULMONARY DYSPLASIA

If the newborn continues to receive supplemental oxygen for a prolonged time, a thickening of the alveolar sacs can develop, with the occurrence of atelectasis and scarring, referred to as bronchopulmonary dysplasia (BPD). This can result in long-term oxygen dependence. Therefore, the concentration of oxygen should be monitored, and the newborn is weaned from supplemental oxygen as soon as weaning is tolerated.

Preterm newborns who have frequent periods of apnea are usually placed on an apnea monitor and are carefully observed. Cutaneous stimulation often restarts their breathing. Suctioning, positioning, and chest physiotherapy aid in maintaining adequate respiratory functioning.

PATENT DUCTUS ARTERIOSUS

Because of the underdeveloped musculature or hypoxia, there may be an incomplete closure of the ductus arteriosus (patent ductus arteriosus [PDA]) in the preterm newborn. When the ductus remains open, left-to-right shunting of the blood in the heart occurs because of the added load placed on the left ventricle of the heart. This results in pulmonary congestion and increased hypoxia.

Administration of a prostaglandin synthesis inhibitor, such as indomethacin, can constrict the ductus arteriosus and cause it to close. The ductus arteriosus may also be closed surgically but not without risks to the newborn. If the PDA is not treated, the newborn is at an even greater risk for complications, including pulmonary edema and heart failure.

NECROTIZING ENTEROCOLITIS

Necrotizing enterocolitis (NEC) is an acute inflammatory process of the bowel. NEC is a multifactorial disorder that involves bowel perfusion, enteric organisms (organisms in the intestine), and nutritional intake. The cause of NEC is not clear, but episodes of asphyxia may reduce the circulation, causing ischemia and necrosis in areas of the bowel. Feeding precedes the onset of the symptoms because milk is a source for the organisms to grow. These organisms then invade the weakened ischemic bowel. Signs of NEC include distention of the abdomen with an increased amount of feeding remaining in the stomach (residual feeding). Diminished or absent bowel sounds, diarrhea, and occult blood in the stools are also signs of NEC. Radiographs reveal a bowel distended with air. Free air in the peritoneum is a sign of bowel perforation and requires immediate intervention.

Management includes discontinuing all oral feedings to give the bowel a rest, nasogastric suction,

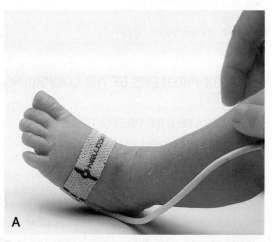 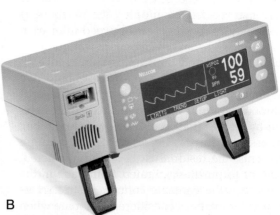

FIGURE 15-7 **Pulse oximeter. A,** A lead with two sensors opposite each other is placed on the toe or foot of the newborn. A red light passes from one sensor, through the vascular bed of the toe or foot, and registers on the sensor on the opposite side. **B,** The oxygen saturation level in the blood is shown on the monitor, which also displays the heart rate. The circle on the foot band indicates the location of the sensor and aids in lining up the sensors for accurate readings. An alarm sounds if saturation is low.

intravenous fluids, and broad-spectrum antibiotics. Frequent measurement of the abdominal girth (for amount of abdominal distention) and abdominal auscultations for bowel sounds are performed. The main indication for surgery is perforation of the bowel, as demonstrated by a radiograph showing free air in the peritoneum. Surgery may be necessary to remove the necrotic areas of the bowel. The newborn with NEC is critically ill.

Breast milk is found to be protective in NEC; therefore, mothers are encouraged to provide breast milk for their newborns in the intensive care unit.

INTRAVENTRICULAR HEMORRHAGE

Intraventricular hemorrhage (IVH) is a common type of intracranial hemorrhage that occurs in infants born less than 32 weeks' gestation. Potential causes include capillary fragility, increased cerebral blood flow, and unstable blood gas levels. Trauma, hypoxia, and asphyxia during the birth process are also implicated in IVH.

Nursing management includes elevating the head of the bed 30 degrees, frequent monitoring of vital signs and blood pressure, and observing for evidence of increasing intracranial pressure such as bulging fontanelles and seizure activity. The outcome depends on the severity and location of the hemorrhage. Gentle handling and a quiet environment are part of the care plan.

PAIN, IRRITABILITY, AND SEDATION

Studies have shown that preterm and term newborns are able to perceive pain. The many necessary invasive procedures performed for newborn survival can produce pain. Evidence-based studies have shown that morphine use in neonates increases positive survival responses (Saniski, 2005; Urso, 2007). The newborn should be assessed for signs of pain, such as intense cry, tightly closed eyes, grimaces, changes in vital signs, and lower oxygen saturation. Pain assessment scales should be posted in the nursery. Nonpharmacologic methods of calming the infant—that is, self-consoling techniques such as providing an enclosed space (nesting or containment), swaddling in a flexed position with one hand near the mouth, nonnutritive sucking (pacifier), soft voice, music, and rocking, including kangaroo care—should be provided (see Chapter 10). Sucrose pacifiers have been found to be an effective pain reliever in neonates (Slater, Cornelissen, Fabrisi, et al., 2010).

Preterm newborns may become irritable when in pain or hyperstimulated by the environment. Numerous caregivers, frequent unpredictable interruptions, the use of nasal catheters, sudden temperature changes, monitor alarms or pagers, and drug sensitivities are other reasons for preterm newborns to demonstrate irritability.

Sedatives do not relieve pain and often reduce the ability to express pain. Sedatives are usually used in the intubated preterm newborn to prevent pneumothorax and other complications when a newborn "fights" the ventilator settings. Patient-triggered ventilation technology can reduce the need for newborn sedation.

Evidence-Based Practice
Signs and Symptoms of Pain in Neonates
- Facial grimace
- Cry
- Increased respiration and heart rate
- Increased movement of extremities
- Increased state of arousal

Evidence-Based Practice
Nonpharmacologic Pain Relief for Neonates
- Reposition newborn (flexed)
- Swaddle
- Rock newborn (vertically)
- Provide kangaroo care
- Give light massage
- Provide sucrose pacifier
- Breastfeed if possible

The organizational phase of brain development starts in the second trimester of pregnancy and continues through the neonatal phase of the preterm infant. Drugs that may be neurotoxic may affect brain growth and organization in the newborn and could result in long-term neurologic deficits. Diazepam is rarely used in the newborn because it increases the risk for kernicterus. Midazolam is a benzodiazepine that has been shown to cause dyskinetic movements and cerebral hypoperfusion that can lead to neurotoxic responses. Chloral hydrate can cause hyperbilirubinemia and has been shown to result in central nervous system depression, arrhythmia, and kidney failure. Morphine has been shown to be safe and effective for infant pain relief. Current assessment tools have been developed to monitor depth of sedation in neonates (see Chapter 10).

The pain scale used in the facility should be posted, and pain scores should be documented as the "fifth vital sign" when vital signs are assessed.

DEVELOPMENTALLY SUPPORTIVE CARE

Developmentally supportive care is the integration of technology with sensitive, family-centered, hands-on nursing care. A developmental care plan can be established to promote growth and development based on the needs and responses of the preterm newborn. Occupational therapists, physical therapists, and speech pathologists can contribute to the preventive care of preterm newborns by providing periodic assessments of the newborn's responses.

Developmental care of the preterm newborn includes protecting his or her quiet sleep state, organizing care interventions to conserve the newborn's energy, and maintaining flexibility of care when the newborn's response indicates a rest is needed. If newborns must be awakened for care, soft whispers and touches can help them make the transition from deep sleep to the wakefulness state.

Parents are kept informed and participate in bonding techniques such as kangaroo care (Skill 15-2; see also Figure 10-4); siblings and grandparents are also recognized and respected. Enabling the face to face (en face) position during caregiver interaction and using mobiles during alert states promote neural development. The newborn's visual field should support developmental tasks when he or she is in the alert phase and restfulness when he or she is in a relaxed or pre-sleep phase. The preterm newborn's eyelid provides little protection to the retina of the eye from light sources in the unit. Isolette covers can protect the

newborn's eyes from direct light and also help provide a circadian rhythm that is important for growth and development and adaptation to home care and healthy sleep cycles. Self-consoling is encouraged by positioning the infant with the hand near the mouth and using pacifiers and nesting (Figure 15-8).

An increase in blood pressure, bradycardia, and agitation is an indicator of pain in nonverbal newborns, and any pain relief medication should be documented. Nurses can assist parents in identifying the cues or signals offered by the newborn that interaction is appropriate and avoiding overstimulation of the newborn by a well-meaning parent who may be trying too hard to obtain a response. The newborn learns to communicate through interactive experiences. Prolonged separation of the preterm newborn from parental care may further predispose the newborn to later developmental delays, including speech development.

Parents of preterm newborns or compromised newborns need teaching, guidance, and emotional support

Skill 15-2   Kangaroo Care

PURPOSE

To maintain skin-to-skin contact to promote warmth and bonding.

Steps

1. Explain the rationale and principles of care to the parents.
2. Provide a comfortable chair and privacy.
3. Have parent wear a gown open in the front, with chest bare.
4. Remove newborn's clothes, except for a clean diaper.
5. Place newborn in a vertical position between the mother's bare breasts.
6. Wrap the parent's gown over the baby.
7. Place a blanket over the newborn.
8. Monitor the newborn's temperature.
9. Document the responses of mother and infant.

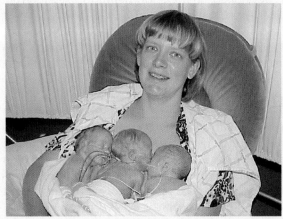

The mother provides kangaroo care for her preterm newborns. Kangaroo care for intubated preterm newborns is also helpful.

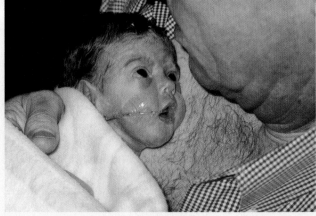

This newborn is responding positively to kangaroo care with the father.

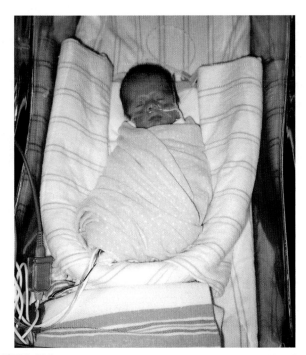

FIGURE 15-8 **Nesting.** An enclosed space bounded by small blanket rolls encircling the preterm newborn provides a calming, supportive environment, also called *containment*. The newborn may or may not be swaddled when placed in nesting.

the care-taking component. Parents should be encouraged to touch, hold, and care for (feed) their newborn. Maintaining touch and participating in care as much as possible are important for parents. Kangaroo care can be given by either parent and helps stabilize the newborn and increase attachment (see Skill 15-2).

COMPLEMENTARY AND ALTERNATIVE MEDICAL THERAPY AND THE PRETERM INFANT

Aromatherapy is the use of scent to alter behavior. An article of clothing with the mother's odor placed near the newborn in the incubator may provide a soothing effect. Research is ongoing concerning the use of peppermint as a respiratory stimulant, chamomile to prompt regular sleep cycles, and special herbs for analgesic properties.

Kangaroo care, or skin-to-skin contact of the newborn on the parent's naked chest, has evidence-based positive effects on newborn oxygenation, thermoregulation, and stabilization of vital signs, in addition to fostering the bonding process.

Music therapy involving soft lullabies can be soothing and has shown a positive influence on nonnutritive sucking.

Massage—gentle touch, with or without stroking—can regulate sleep patterns and reduce motor activity. See Chapter 21 for further discussion of complementary and alternative medical therapy.

HOME CARE

Discharge criteria usually include the newborn's ability to maintain body temperature, cry when hungry, and gain weight. Before discharge, the parents should have the opportunity to care for their newborn with the guidance and support of the nursing staff. Rooming-in can help familiarize the parents with the newborn's nighttime behavior. Feeding techniques, breast pumping, and milk storage are reviewed. Information concerning bathing, diapering, dressing, and wrapping is offered. Bonding behaviors should be reinforced and community resources with telephone numbers and support group referrals given to the parents. Newborn cardiopulmonary resuscitation techniques are reviewed with parents.

Some fragile newborns may require home treatment with oxygen therapy, apnea monitors, tube feedings, or suctioning. The home health nurse is a key link in the interdisciplinary health care team in the discharge and home care of the preterm newborn.

Parents are often anxious about taking home their preterm newborn. The home care nurse must familiarize the parents with the newborn's care. The nurse discusses the newborn's behavioral patterns and

from health care providers. Family members may not be prepared to accept a preterm newborn, and they should be allowed to grieve the loss of their expected normal newborn. They need to work through their emotions and feelings of guilt. They should be encouraged to begin the process of attachment to their newborn, which will take understanding on the part of the nurse. The nurse must offer continued assistance and support to the family and must prepare the family for the newborn's limited ability to respond because of all of the sophisticated medical equipment used in the newborn's care. Also, the nurse should provide explanations to the family concerning the preterm newborn's physical development and remain close to the family on their initial visit. The family should be encouraged to visit the newborn frequently and to call as often as they desire (especially if they live far from the hospital).

It is difficult for some parents to face the realization that they have a preterm newborn who needs special care and accept that they had no control in giving birth to a less than full-term newborn. After the initial attachment, they face the problem of learning about the newborn's special care needs. The two components of the maternal-newborn interaction that are most affected by having the preterm newborn in the high-risk nursery (separated from the mother) are the sensory or touch component and

helps the parents establish realistic expectations about the newborn's catchup development. By 2 years of age, most prematurely born infants catchup to the appropriate developmental level. After discharge, a nursing staff member can extend the hospital interest in the newborn by follow-up telephone calls (see Chapter 18). The social service department may be of help in ensuring that the home environment is satisfactory and that special needs are met.

Get Ready for the NCLEX® Examination!

Key Points

- Accurate assessment of gestational age and size can alert health care providers to specific problems related to prematurity and postmaturity. The Ballard scoring system uses physical and neuromuscular signs as criteria to score maturity.
- SGA newborns usually show physical characteristics that suggest IUGR. They often appear long and thin because adipose tissue and muscle mass over cheeks, buttocks, and thighs are diminished. However, their behavior is impressive in relation to their size. They usually have a strong suck, eat well, and gain weight more quickly than the preterm newborn. The impression of vigor and well-being may be misleading. The wide-eyed, alert facial expression may be caused by chronic hypoxia.
- The LGA newborn is large and may weigh 4000 g (8 lbs, 13 oz) or more at birth. If delivered vaginally, the newborn may incur injury (e.g., shoulder dystocia or fractured clavicle). LGA newborns are often sluggish and hypotonic. Large newborns from non-diabetic mothers are symmetrical and referred to as *LGA*; large newborns from diabetic mothers have hypertrophied organs and fat deposits but the head and length are normal. These infants are called *macrosomic*. Both are large and are prone to birth injury and hypoglycemia.
- The postterm newborn is born after 42 weeks' gestation. The newborn has little lanugo or vernix, and the skin is dry and peeling. These newborns are at risk for hypoxia, meconium aspiration, and asphyxia as a result of placental deterioration.
- The preterm newborn is one born before 38 weeks' gestation. As a result of immature body systems, the preterm newborn may have potential problems, including respiratory distress, hyperbilirubinemia, hypothermia, apnea, infection, and marked insensible water loss.
- Late preterm infants are born after 34 weeks and before 38 weeks of gestation and may look like full-term infants but have needs and problems similar to preterm infants.
- The preterm newborn has a high caloric need and requires more protein than the term newborn. Breast milk has been shown to reduce infections in the preterm newborn. Some preterm newborns do not have a coordinated suck-and-swallow reflex and are fed by gavage.
- NEC is an acute inflammatory process of the bowel. The bowel develops necrotic patches. The necrosis results from hypoxia, ischemia, and bacterial action on weakened bowel tissue after feeding begins. Signs of NEC include distention of the abdomen, diminished or absent bowel sounds, and diarrhea.
- Interventricular hemorrhage, bronchopulmonary dysplasia, and ROP are other conditions that commonly complicate prematurity.
- Parents of at-risk newborns need support from the nurses and other health care providers. The parents must understand the special needs of their newborn. Technical equipment should be explained to them, and they should be encouraged to bond with their newborn, such as by touching and holding the newborn and using kangaroo care.
- Hypoglycemia in the term newborn is manifested by a blood glucose level of 40 mg/dL or less; in the preterm newborn, levels are 30 mg/dL or less.

Additional Learning Resources

SG Go to your Study Guide on pages 501–502 for additional Review Questions for the NCLEX® Examination, Critical Thinking Clinical Situations, and other learning activities to help you master this chapter content.

evolve Go to your Evolve website (http://evolve.elsevier.com/Leifer/maternity) for the following FREE learning resources:
- Animations
- Answer Guidelines for Critical Thinking Questions
- Answers and Rationales for Review Questions for the NCLEX® Examination
- Concept Map Creator
- Glossary with pronunciations in English and Spanish
- Patient Teaching Plans
- Skills Performance Checklists and more!

 Online Resources
- www.childcarseats.org.uk/carrying_safely/premature.htm
- www.mdconsult.com
- www.ntsb.gov/default.htm

Review Questions for the NCLEX® Examination

1. An infant born at 36 weeks' gestation weighing 6.0 pounds would be considered:
   1. Full term
   2. Small for gestational age
   3. Late preterm
   4. Postterm

2. Physical characteristics of the postterm newborn may include: *(Select all that apply.)*
    1. Long fingernails
    2. Loose skin
    3. Cracked, dry skin
    4. Abundant lanugo

3. Retinopathy of prematurity (ROP) is primarily caused by:
    1. Oxygen toxicity
    2. Hypoglycemia
    3. Heat loss
    4. Hyperbilirubinemia

4. The nurse is caring for a newborn diagnosed with thickening of the alveolar sacs with the occurrence of atelectasis and scarring. The newborn's history and physical indicate this diagnosis is the result of the child receiving supplemental oxygen for a prolonged time. The nurse is aware that this complication of prolonged oxygen therapy is:
    1. Necrotizing enterocolitis (NEC)
    2. Patent ductus arteriosus (PDA)
    3. Bronchopulmonary dysplasia (BPD)
    4. Retinopathy of Prematurity (ROP)

5. Which statement made by a student nurse regarding the preterm newborn demonstrates the need for further education?
    1. "Preterm newborns may become irritable when hyperstimulated by the environment."
    2. "Preterm newborns are unable to perceive pain."
    3. "The preterm newborn may be positioned on the back with the head of the mattress slightly elevated."
    4. "The preterm newborn has high caloric needs."

6. Most prematurely born infants catchup to the appropriate developmental level by:
    1. 6 months of age
    2. 12 months of age
    3. 18 months of age
    4. 24 months of age

7. Management of necrotizing enterocolitis (NEC) includes which intervention(s)? *(Select all that apply.)*
    1. Nasogastric suctioning
    2. Frequent measurement of abdominal girth
    3. Decreased number of oral feedings
    4. Administration of intravenous fluids
    5. Administration of corticosteroids

Critical Thinking Questions

1. A woman has just given birth to a preterm newborn, 32 weeks' gestation, weight 1.4 kg (3 lbs). She is anxious and is expressing how she had looked forward to a "normal baby girl." What approach will you take with the woman as you assist her in providing newborn care?

2. A woman gave birth to a 4.4 kg (9 lbs, 11 oz) boy. She had a difficult labor but did deliver vaginally. What patient teaching should you give to the woman?

chapter
16

The Newborn at Risk: Acquired and Congenital Conditions

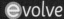

http://evolve.elsevier.com/Leifer/maternity

Objectives

1. Define key terms listed.
2. Discuss the prenatal diagnosis of Down syndrome.
3. Recognize three genetic inborn errors of metabolism.
4. Compare the metabolic disorders hypoglycemia, maple syrup urine disease, hypothyroidism, and phenylketonuria; their effect on the newborn; and the nursing implications.
5. Describe common congenital anomalies.
6. Interpret signs associated with elevated bilirubin in the newborn.
7. Explain the nursing interventions used in phototherapy.
8. Articulate the principles of newborn resuscitation.
9. Outline the common respiratory problems in the newborn.
10. Characterize the effect of maternal diabetes on the newborn.
11. Outline six problems of infants born to mothers with diabetes mellitus.
12. Explain factors responsible for newborn sepsis, and state the nurse's role in reducing the risks.
13. Discuss the nursing assessment that would lead the nurse to suspect newborn sepsis.
14. Identify the defects involved in the tetralogy of Fallot and common manifestations.
15. Compare the alteration of blood flow of cyanotic and noncyanotic congenital heart defects.
16. Explain the pathophysiology of noncyanotic congenital heart defects.
17. Describe care of the newborn who has neonatal abstinence syndrome.

Key Terms

galactosemia (gă-lăk-tō-SĒ-mē-ă, p. 323)
hemolysis (hē-MŎL-ĭ-sĭs, p. 329)
hyperglycemia (hī-pĕr-glī-SĒ-mē-ă, p. 336)
hypoglycemia (hī-pō-glī-SĒ-mē-ă, p. 332)
infants of diabetic mothers (IDMs) (p. 336)
kernicterus (kĕr-NĬK-tĕr-ŭs, p. 329)

macrosomia (măk-rō-SŌ-mē-ă, p. 336)
meconium aspiration syndrome (MAS) (mě-KŌ-nē-ŭm, p. 334)
neonatal sepsis (nē-ō-NĀ-tăl, p. 337)
phenylketonuria (PKU) (fĕn-ŭl-kē-tō-NŪ-rē-ă, p. 322)
phototherapy (p. 330)

Genetics is the scientific study of the transmission of characteristics from parent to child (see Chapters 1 and 3). Genetic defects are common causes of acute and chronic conditions that manifest during fetal life; immediately after birth; or during childhood, adolescence, or adulthood. An understanding of human genetics, including genetic challenges, disorders, and technology, is an integral part of maternity nursing and medical obstetric practice.

Birth defects, abnormalities that are apparent at birth, occur in 3% to 4% of all live births. The rate is even higher if the defects that become evident later in life are counted. An abnormality of structure, function, or metabolism may result in a physical or mental disability, may shorten life, or may be fatal. Box 16-1 shows the system of classification of birth defects. Because these disorders include so many conditions, it is necessary to limit the number discussed in the chapter and to place others in relevant areas of the text (see the index for specific conditions). Defects that are manifested later in life are discussed in pediatric textbooks.

Defects present at birth often involve the skeletal system; limbs may be missing, malformed, or duplicated. Some abnormalities (e.g., congenital hip dysplasia) are more subtle, and the nurse must be alert to detect them. *Inborn errors of metabolism* include a number of inherited diseases that affect body chemistry. There may be an absence or a deficiency of a substance necessary for cell metabolism. The deficient substance is usually an enzyme. Almost any organ of the body may be damaged. Examples of inborn errors of metabolism include cystic fibrosis and phenylketonuria (PKU). In *disorders of the blood*, there is a reduced or missing blood component or an inability of a component to function adequately. Sickle cell disease, thalassemia, and hemophilia fall into this category. *Chromosomal abnormalities* number in the thousands. Most involve some type of mental retardation, and others are incompatible with life. The newborn with Turner's syndrome or Klinefelter's syndrome may have impaired physical growth and sexual development. *Perinatal injuries* have many causes and are seen

Box 16-1   Classification and Examples of Birth Defects

MALFORMATIONS PRESENT AT BIRTH
Structural defects, including:
- Hydrocephalus*
- Spina bifida*
- Congenital heart malformations*
- Cleft lip and palate*
- Clubfoot*
- Developmental hip dysplasia*
- Tracheoesophageal fistula*
- Hypospadias

METABOLIC DEFECTS (BODY CHEMISTRY)
- Cystic fibrosis
- Phenylketonuria (PKU)*
- Galactosemia*
- Maple syrup urine disease*
- Hypothyroidism*
- Tay-Sachs disease
- Family hypercholesterolemia (high cholesterol that often causes early heart attack)

BLOOD DISORDERS
- Sickle cell disease
- Hemophilia
- Thalassemia
- Defects of white blood cells and immune defense

CHROMOSOMAL ABNORMALITIES
Many abnormalities, most involving some combination of mental retardation and physical malformations that range from mild to fatal, including:
- Down syndrome*
- Klinefelter's syndrome
- Turner's syndrome
- Trisomies 13, 18, and 21

PERINATAL INJURY
- Infections*
- Drugs*
- Maternal disorders
- Abnormalities unique to pregnancy (hyperbilirubinemia,* difficult labor or delivery, premature birth)
- Meconium aspiration syndrome*

*Topics discussed in this chapter. More detailed discussions of other conditions can be found in other chapters within this text.

in various forms, the most common of which is premature birth.

As the March of Dimes Foundation (2007) points out, "Few birth defects can be attributed to a single cause. The majority are thought to result from an interplay between environment and heredity, depending on inherited susceptibility, stage of pregnancy, and degree of environmental hazard." Newborns with birth defects may need to remain in the neonatal unit for an extended time for intensive care and treatment. Screening tests are performed prenatally to detect many genetic defects and, in some cases, enable appropriate treatment before or immediately after birth (see Chapter 5).

CHROMOSOMAL DISORDERS

The human body is made up of 23 paired chromosomes, with one pair from the mother and one pair from the father. These chromosomes contain deoxyribonucleic acid (DNA) and other complex proteins. An abnormal chromosome number or arrangement can cause a congenital defect. Sometimes an extra chromosome is present or a chromosome is broken or missing. The resulting imbalance can provide the newborn with too little or too much genetic material. As the embryo grows, the scrambled genetic information may translate into various types of congenital defects.

DOWN SYNDROME

Trisomy 21, also known as **Down syndrome,** is one of the most common chromosomal syndromes, occurring in 1 in 600 to 800 live births (Gabbe, Simpson, & Niebyl, 2007). It affects all races and economic levels equally. Down syndrome often results from having an extra chromosome (usually chromosome 21) and is called trisomy 21 because it was first identified with this chromosome. Occasionally, the extra chromosome 21 is attached to another chromosome in the egg or sperm, which can create a translocation (an alteration in location). The translocation in either parent greatly increases the chances of having another child with Down syndrome. Mothers older than 35 years are at the greatest risk of having a Down syndrome newborn.

The American Academy of Pediatrics recommends screening of all pregnant women for Down syndrome in the first trimester of pregnancy. First trimester screening includes ultrasound assessment of the thickness of the fetal nuchal fold (called *nuchal translucency*). An ultrasound demonstrating absence of the nasal bone (Cicero, Avgidou, Rembouskos, et al., 2006) and a second trimester "quad test" involving blood testing of alpha-fetoprotein (AFP), human chorionic gonadotropin (hCG), unconjugated estriol (UE), and inhibin A (a placental hormone) are additional screening tests for Down syndrome. A low AFP or a high hCG and inhibin A, with a low UE, may indicate a high risk for Down syndrome for the developing fetus. A test of pregnancy-associated plasma protein A (PAPP-A) may also indicate a risk for Down syndrome. Positive tests in the first or second trimester may indicate a need for amniocentesis to confirm the diagnosis.

Characteristics of the Down syndrome newborn are most noted in the craniofacial features (Figure 16-1). The eyes have an upward slant because of an epicanthal fold, speckles known as Brushfield's spots are seen in the iris, the nose is small with a wide nasal bridge, and the ears are low set. The tongue appears large and protrudes from the newborn's mouth, fingers are short and broad, often there is an unusually wide space between the first two toes, and a single

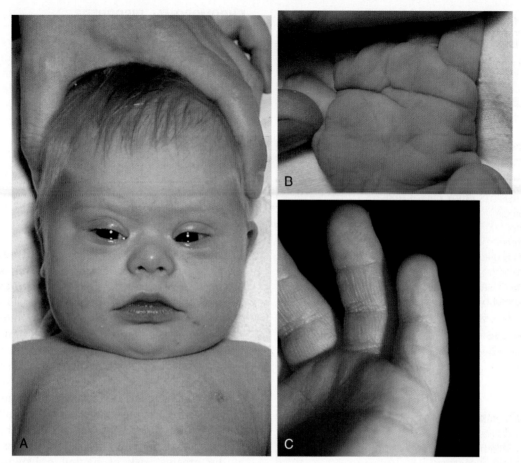

FIGURE 16-1 Down syndrome. A, The typical facial appearance of a newborn with Down syndrome shows the upward slant of the canthal folds of the eyes, protruding tongue, and short, thick neck. **B,** The straight simian crease in the palm of the hand is a typical finding in children with Down syndrome. **C,** The short fifth finger is a typical finding in children with Down syndrome. The tip of the fifth finger does not extend to the distal joint of the adjoining finger.

palmar crease (simian crease) may be present. Relatively common internal anomalies in trisomy 21 newborns include heart defects and duodenal atresia. Mental retardation is exhibited, with the mean IQ of approximately 50 (range: 25 to 70). Females are fertile; however, it is rare for males to be fertile.

At birth, these newborns are usually hypotonic (limp and flaccid) and may have feeding difficulties. They also have increased susceptibility to respiratory tract infections. Parents need guidance in feeding and preventing infections and encouragement to stimulate their newborns developmentally. Children with Down syndrome are usually very affectionate. Parents should be encouraged to join a support group for parents of children with Down syndrome. Developmental disabilities, including mental retardation, are common, with hearing and speech difficulties that complicate efforts at education. Cardiac, orthopedic, and thyroid dysfunction are also common. Alzheimer's disease often develops early in the third decade of life, and an altered immune response increases susceptibility to respiratory and dental infection.

INBORN ERRORS OF METABOLISM

Inborn errors of metabolism do not always manifest symptoms at birth. Screening tests for specific errors of metabolism are required by law in most states. It is important for early identification so that treatment can be started as soon as possible to minimize effects on the newborn.

PHENYLKETONURIA

Phenylketonuria (PKU) is an autosomal recessive inherited inborn error of phenylalanine metabolism that occurs in 1 in 15,000 live births (Trahms, 2008). It is caused by the faulty metabolism of phenylalanine, an amino acid that is essential to life and found in all protein foods. The hepatic enzyme phenylalanine hydrolase, which is required to convert phenylalanine into tyrosine, is missing. As a result, when the newborn ingests protein (found in milk and all protein foods), phenylketones accumulate in the blood and can rise as high as 20 times the normal level. Its byproduct, phenylpyruvic acid, appears in the urine within the first weeks of life. These phenylketones accumulate in the brain and cause irreversible brain damage, resulting in severe mental retardation. Early detection and treatment are essential because by the time the urine test is positive, brain damage has already occurred. The newborn appears normal at birth but begins to show delayed development at approximately 4 to 6 months of age. The newborn may show evidence of failure to thrive or have eczema or other skin conditions. Characteristically, these newborns have an unusual musty odor to their body and in their urine.

A diagnosis is made by the **Guthrie test.** Blood is obtained from a simple heel prick, and a few drops of capillary blood are placed on a filter paper and mailed to the laboratory for screening. It is recommended that the blood be obtained after 48 to 72 hours of life, preferably after ingestion of proteins, to reduce the possibility of false results. All states in the United States require that the test be performed in all newborns before they leave the nursery, but, because of early discharge, the test is often repeated after discharge. The newborn can be tested at home by a public health nurse or at the physician's office or clinic. Confirmation of the diagnosis requires quantitative elevations of phenylalanine compound in both blood and urine. The nurse must stress to the mother the importance of the return visit of the newborn to the physician or clinic for the repeat testing.

Since the development of newborn screening for PKU, several women who had been diagnosed with PKU in the newborn period and then were treated with a phenylalanine-restricted diet have grown up not suffering the damages of untreated PKU. However, newborns born to women with PKU who do not follow the restricted diet during pregnancy have teratogenic effects if high concentrations of phenylalanine are circulating in the mother's blood. Congenital heart defects, microcephaly, and mental retardation are the most commonly seen effects. Therefore, for these women, following dietary restrictions from conception (especially during embryonic development) is critical.

The newborn diagnosed with PKU is fed a special formula (Lofenalac) that has had the phenylalanine reduced or removed. Phenyl-Free is given to children, and Phenex-2 is given to adolescents. The goals of the diet are to provide enough essential proteins to support growth and development while maintaining phenylalanine blood levels between 2 and 10 mg/dL. A phenylalanine level less than 2 mg/dL may result in growth retardation, and a level greater than 10 mg/dL can result in significant brain damage. Levels are monitored throughout childhood.

A dietitian should be consulted for parental guidance and support in maintaining the dietary regimen. This attention is especially needed for the school-age child and the adolescent. The intake of most meat, dairy products, and diet drinks needs to be restricted, and protein intake is restricted to that required for basic growth. The milk substitute can be flavored with a fruit powder or a chocolate substitute, which can increase the child's compliance. Aspartame, a sugar substitute, must be avoided. Genetic counseling is important for future family planning.

GALACTOSEMIA

Galactosemia is an inborn error of metabolism that occurs in 1 in 53,000 live births (Tarini & Freed, 2007). The newborn has a deficiency of the enzyme necessary to convert galactose to glucose, resulting in an increased amount of galactose in the blood (galactosemia), liver, brain, kidney, and urine (galactosuria). An early diagnosis is important so that a milk substitute can be prescribed because galactose is present in milk. Galactosemia can be detected by measuring blood levels of galactose, and screening of all newborns is performed in most states across the United States. Failure to thrive, cataracts, jaundice, cirrhosis of the liver, sepsis, and mental retardation are manifestations of untreated cases. Therapy consists of eliminating galactose from the diet and providing lactose-free formula, such as Nutramigen. Because breast milk contains lactose, breastfeeding must be discontinued. Medications that contain lactose fillers as inactive ingredients also must be avoided. Parents and children often experience frustration and anxiety and must be educated and supported in following this dietary program.

HYPOTHYROIDISM

Congenital hypothyroidism is the result of an inborn error of metabolism caused by a maternal iodine deficiency or the use of antithyroid drugs by the mother. It occurs 1 in 4000 live births (Palma-Sisto, 2004). Thyroxine (T_4) is measured from a drop of blood obtained from heel stick at 2 to 5 days of age. If not treated with thyroid replacement, the infant may develop hypothermia, poor feeding, lethargy, jaundice, and cretinism. The infant has a large protruding tongue, thick lips, and a generally dull appearance.

An important note is that one blood sample can be used to test all three metabolic disorders: PKU, galactosemia, and hypothyroidism. The screening test for hypothyroidism is mandated in all states across the United States and is often performed before discharge from the nursery. Early diagnosis and treatment are essential to maintain normal physical and mental growth and development.

MAPLE SYRUP URINE DISEASE

Maple syrup urine disease is a disorder of amino acid metabolism in which the amino acids leucine, isoleucine, and valine cannot be metabolized because of missing enzymes. Elevated levels of leucine can cause cerebral edema and central nervous system (CNS) symptoms such as seizures. Body fluids have a sweet odor, similar to maple syrup. Some states require routine screening of all newborns for this condition (see Chapter 9). Nursing responsibilities include educating the family concerning strict dietary and exercise limitations throughout the infant's lifetime.

COMMON CONGENITAL ANOMALIES

Although congenital anomalies are generally treated in the pediatric setting, they are usually identified soon after birth. The family of the newborn with the disorder may have been aware of the condition through prenatal testing, or they may be surprised by the birth of a newborn who is not completely normal. The family will need a great deal of support and sensitivity from the health care providers. Some congenital anomalies are noted in Table 16-1. The nursing student is urged to read a pediatric textbook for more detailed information concerning the management of congenital anomalies in the newborn.

COMMON ACQUIRED DISORDERS

HYPERBILIRUBINEMIA (PHYSIOLOGIC JAUNDICE)

Hyperbilirubinemia is defined as an abnormally high level of bilirubin in the blood. This condition occurs when the normal pathways of bilirubin metabolism and excretion in the newborn are altered because of excess products (from normal hemolysis), liver immaturity, delayed feeding (which prevents development of intestinal flora), trauma, or cold stress. An increase in bilirubin also can occur as a result of cephalhematoma, extensive bruising, infections, and acidosis that causes a decrease in liver function. Maternal use of sulfa or salicylates can interfere with conjugation of bilirubin. The result is clinical jaundice (icterus neonatorum), which is seen in approximately 60% of term newborns; it is even more common in preterm newborns, typically occurring after the third day of life. Total serum bilirubin levels greater than 12 mg/dL in the term newborn usually indicate hyperbilirubinemia.

The newborn is born with an excessive amount of red blood cells (RBCs) and, at birth, begins to destroy the RBCs he or she no longer needs. The infant does not need the excess RBCs because he or she is now in an atmosphere of higher oxygen concentration than was available in utero. Bilirubin inside the RBC is released into the bloodstream when the RBC is destroyed. The bilirubin combines with albumin in the blood and is transported to the liver. Under the influence of the enzyme glucuronyl transferase, the bilirubin is conjugated into a water-soluble form and excreted subsequently into the small intestine; most of it is excreted from the body in the feces. Some bilirubin is converted to unconjugated bilirubin, is reabsorbed, and is recirculated back into the blood. The amount of bilirubin in the blood is described in milligrams of bilirubin per deciliter (mg/dL). When the bilirubin accumulates in the blood, it contributes to a condition called *icterus neonatorum,* or physiologic jaundice. The skin and whites of the eyes assume a yellow-orange cast. The higher the bilirubin level the deeper the jaundice. An increase of more than 5 mg/dL in 24 hours or a bilirubin blood level of 12.9 mg/dL or more requires investigation and intervention.

The bilirubin level in newborns typically peaks between 3 and 5 days of age. Therefore, the early discharge of newborns requires follow-up observation within a few days. Conjugation of the bilirubin can be inhibited by a lack of bacteria in the intestines or a low level of glucuronyl transferase enzyme. The immature liver may also be slow to take up the bilirubin that flows to it. For these reasons, the liver may not be able to "clear" the bilirubin from the blood and excrete it from the body at a rapid rate. High levels of bilirubin in the blood can stain the basal nuclei of the brain, causing long-term neurologic problems. This condition is called **kernicterus.**

Because bilirubin conjugated by the liver is excreted by the body via the intestinal tract, the stimulation of meconium stool passage is an important part of the care plan. The initiation of early feedings enhances the passage of meconium and therefore plays an essential role in the management of hyperbilirubinemia. Colostrum, in breast milk, has a natural laxative effect, and therefore breastfeeding at least 10 times a day is recommended for the neonate. Glucose water supplements should be avoided because little bilirubin is excreted by the kidneys and decreased caloric intake is associated with decreased passage of stool, allowing for the reabsorption of bilirubin before it can be excreted. Although there is a factor in human milk that may increase reabsorption of bilirubin from the intestines, this rarely causes a significant rise in serum bilirubin. Some physicians may prefer to feed the infant bottled formula for a 12- to 24-hour period to avoid this small increase. The mother should be encouraged to pump milk from the breast during this short period to enable easy return to breastfeeding.

Assessment and Management of Physiologic Jaundice

All newborns with visible jaundice and all infants under 35 weeks' gestation should have serum bilirubin levels drawn (Rennie, 2010). The visual blanch test is used to help distinguish jaundice from normal skin color. Pressure is applied with a finger over a bony area on the newborn, such as the nose, forehead, or sternum, for several seconds to empty the capillaries in that area. A yellow tinge in the blanched area indicates jaundice. When pressure is released, the capillaries refill. The conjunctivae of the eyes and the buccal mucosa can also be visually assessed to detect jaundice. Assessing for jaundice should be done under natural light

Table **16-1** Common Congenital Anomalies

ANOMALY	TREATMENT AND NURSING CARE
Gastrointestinal	
Cleft Lip and Palate	

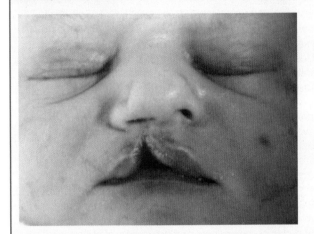

	Degree of cleft determines care.
	Encourage parents to verbalize concerns.
	Determine most effective nipple (soft preemie, lamb's, cleft nipple, rubber-tipped Asepto).
	Feed in upright position to decrease risk of aspiration.
	Feed slowly, burp frequently (tendency to swallow air).
	Cleanse mouth with water after feedings.
	Support parents.
	Refer parents to support group.
	Management is through lip surgery (approximately 10 weeks) and palate repair in stages (approximately 1 year).
	Long-term follow-up, including speech therapy, is necessary.

Failure of fusion of upper lip (may be unilateral or bilateral)
Failure of fusion of hard and soft palate
Defect caused by both genetic and environmental factors

Esophageal Atresia (Failure of Esophagus to Connect with Stomach)

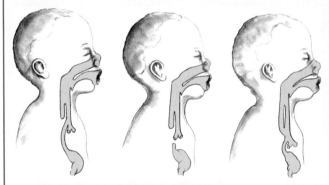

Associated with maternal hydramnios	Withhold feeding until esophageal patency is determined.
Excessive mucous secretions (drooling)	Elevate head of crib to prevent reflux of gastric juices.
Periodic cyanotic episodes and choking	Explain surgical repair to parents.
Abdominal distention after birth	First feeding of all newborns should be supervised by a
Immediate regurgitation of feeding with risk of aspiration	nurse to observe for this anomaly.

Neurologic

Spina Bifida

Occulta	Meningocele	Meningomyelocele
Spinal canal	Spinal cord	Defect in bony canal
Spinal cord	Defect in bony canal	Meninges protrude
Meninges	Meninges protrude	Spinal cord protrudes
Defect in bony canal		

Continued

Table **16-1** Common Congenital Anomalies—cont'd

ANOMALY	TREATMENT AND NURSING CARE
Neurologic	
Spina Bifida—cont'd	
Occulta: Failure of vertebral arch to close (may have a dimple or tuft of hair over lumbosacral region) *Meningocele:* Protrusion of meninges, covered by skin or thin membrane *Meningomyelocele:* Protrusion of both meninges and spinal cord; degree of paralysis depends on location of defect	Prevention includes intake of folic acid in early pregnancy. Protect membrane with sterile cover. Observe sac for leakage of cerebrospinal fluid. Assess sensation and movement of legs. Gently handle newborn; position prone or on side to prevent trauma to sac. Apply sterile dressing and plastic to cover defect to prevent drying. Prevent infection; keep free of contamination by urine and feces; dribbling of urine may affect skin integrity. Measure head circumference to identify early hydrocephalus. Assess for increased intracranial pressure. Long-term treatment includes bowel and bladder control management with prevention of urinary tract infections, management of paralysis with prevention of orthopedic and skin complications, and prevention of obesity. Watch for latex allergy; 73% of children with spina bifida are sensitive to latex and must be cared for in a latex-free environment.
Hydrocephalus 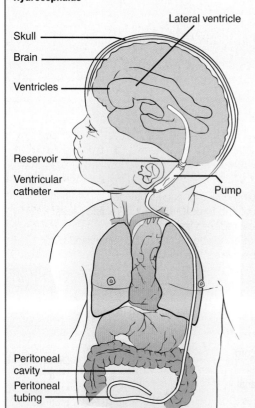	
Excessive accumulation of spinal fluid in ventricles of brain; head enlarged and fontanelles bulging Setting-sun sign common (whites of eyes visible above iris)	Reposition head frequently to prevent pressure sores (newborn often cannot move heavy head). Measure head circumference daily. Assess for signs of increased intracranial pressure such as vomiting and shrill cry. Surgery is performed to place shunt with pump device (directed from ventricle to peritoneal cavity [ventriculoperitoneal shunt]).

Labels on figure: Skull, Brain, Ventricles, Lateral ventricle, Reservoir, Ventricular catheter, Pump, Peritoneal cavity, Peritoneal tubing

| Table 16-1 | Common Congenital Anomalies—cont'd |

ANOMALY	TREATMENT AND NURSING CARE

Musculoskeletal

Developmental Dysplasia of the Hip

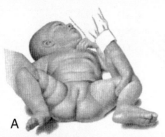

A

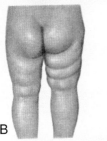

B

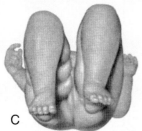

C

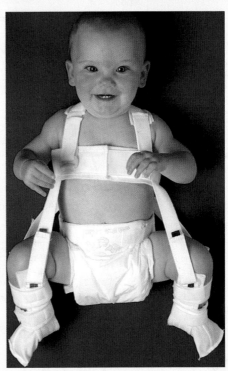

Pavlik harness

Femoral head and hip improperly aligned

May be genetic or involve extended position of hip in utero, such as a breech position, resulting in an unstable hip

Early signs of dislocation include limitation of abduction (A), asymmetry of skin folds (B), and shortening of femur (C)

Signs and symptoms include limited abduction of the hip, asymmetry of the gluteal folds, extra thigh fold, and a positive Barlow and Ortolani test.

X-ray studies are not reliable until bone formation is more complete.

Treatment may be use of Pavlik harness to maintain hip flexion.

Traction and spica cast may be required.

Clubfoot

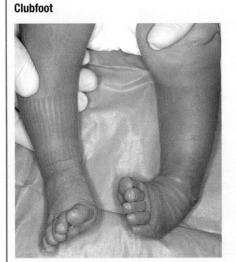

Talipes equinovarus: an abnormal twisting of the foot out of normal alignment

Early treatment is essential before ossification of bone is complete.

Exercise and casting are the treatments of choice soon after birth.

Continued

Table **16-1**   Common Congenital Anomalies—cont'd

ANOMALY	TREATMENT AND NURSING CARE

Cardiac (Heart Defects)*

Normal heart and blood flow

Atrial septal defect

Ventriculoseptal defect

Patent ductus arteriosus

Coarctation of aorta

Tetralogy of Fallot

Patent Ductus Arteriosus

Noncyanotic heart defect

Failure of the ductus arteriosus, connecting the pulmonary artery and the aorta, to close after birth

Cyanosis does not occur because blood recirculates to the lung and is fully oxygenated when it flows to general circulation

Heart defects may or may not be identified immediately.

Newborn with heart defect may exhibit murmurs, abnormal heart rate or rhythm, breathlessness, and fatigue while feeding.

Surgery may be postponed until newborn is physiologically stable.

Tetralogy of Fallot

Cyanotic heart defect

Involves four characteristic defects: a ventricular septal defect, aorta positioned over the ventricular septal defect, stenosis of the pulmonary valve, and hypertrophy of the left ventricle

Cyanosis results from venous blood from the right ventricle flowing through the septal defect and directly into the overriding aorta; blood flow to the lungs is decreased because of the narrowed pulmonary valve; cyanosis occurs because unoxygenated blood reaches the general circulation

Monitor closely; observe for respiratory difficulties, cyanosis, tachycardia, tachypnea, diaphoresis.

Conserve newborn's energy to reduce workload on heart.

Gavage feedings or oral feedings with special nipple may be given.

Elevate newborn's head and shoulders to improve respirations and reduce cardiac workload.

Prevent infection.

Place in knee-chest position for respiratory distress during "tet" attack.

Management includes corrective surgery.

LA, left aorta; *LV*, left ventricle; *RA*, right aorta; *RV*, right ventricle.
*For other common congenital heart defects, students should consult their pediatric textbooks.

because reflections of wall color can influence the appearance of skin color (Skill 16-1). The cephalocaudal (head-to-toe) pattern of circulation results in a head-to-toe progression of jaundice in the newborn so that jaundice affecting the head and upper body may be a reflection of a lower serum bilirubin level than in infants who evidence jaundice of the chest and lower body. Serum bilirubin levels are taken whenever the jaundice levels appear before 24 hours of age. A bilirubin threshold table is available as a guideline in the management of infants with hyperbilirubinemia (Rennie, 2010).

Noninvasive Methods of Bilirubin Measurement
The trauma, cost, and inconvenience of obtaining a blood sample for serum bilirubin levels can be saved by measuring the transcutaneous bilirubin (TcB). Hand-held electronic devices such as the BiliCheck (Respironics) measure TcB levels. TcB monitoring is a screening tool. Those infants with TcB bilirubin levels above 14.6 mg/dL should have serum bilirubin levels drawn and referred for further follow-up.

HYPERBILIRUBINEMIA (PATHOLOGIC JAUNDICE)
A major cause of hyperbilirubinemia is hemolytic disease, in which there is an excessive breakdown of RBCs of the newborn as a result of maternal antibodies passing through the placenta to the fetus in the uterus. Isoimmune hemolytic disease, also known as **erythroblastosis fetalis,** occurs when an Rh-negative mother is pregnant with an Rh-positive fetus and transplacental passage of maternal antibodies occurs. When maternal antibodies enter the fetal circulation, they destroy the fetal RBCs. The fetal system responds by increasing the RBC production with a marked increase in immature RBCs (erythroblasts). A high level of maternal antibodies may have developed during a previous pregnancy, abortion, amniocentesis, or abruptio placentae. A previous blood transfusion with

Rh-positive blood would also cause the development of maternal antibodies. At birth, the newborn with hemolytic disease caused by Rh incompatibility has a positive direct Coombs' test, which reveals the presence of antibody-coated (sensitized) Rh-positive RBCs in the newborn. The indirect Coombs' test measures the amount of Rh-positive antibodies in the mother's blood. If the mother prophylactically receives $Rh_o(D)$ immune globulin (RhoGAM), maternal development of antibodies to Rh-positive blood greatly decreases (Figure 16-2). Pathologic jaundice, such as that caused by Rh incompatibility, is evident *before* the third day of life because the hemolysis begins before birth.

 Did You Know?

Pathologic Jaundice

In pathologic jaundice of erythroblastosis (Rh hemolytic disease), jaundice is evident **before** the third day of life. Jaundice that is first evident **after** the third day of life is usually caused by physiologic icterus neonatorum.

ABO incompatibility may also cause pathologic jaundice. Mothers with type O blood are most likely to be involved; however, the hemolysis (destruction of RBCs) is much less than with Rh incompatibility. Pathologic jaundice also can result from infection, hypothyroidism, and biliary atresia.

Management of the Jaundiced Newborn
The goals of management are prompt identification of newborns who are at risk for jaundice (based on the woman's Rh history and antibody levels) and prompt treatment to prevent the development of kernicterus, a staining of the basal nuclei of the brain that results in toxicity to the CNS. Newborn hyperbilirubinemia is considered pathologic if clinical jaundice is evident within the first 24 hours of life, the clinical jaundice persists for more than 14 days, serum bilirubin level

Skill 16-1   Detecting Jaundice in the Newborn

PURPOSE
To determine whether a blood test for bilirubin level is indicated.

Steps
1. Place the newborn in a well-lighted area.
2. With one finger, press the area of the skin at the bridge of the nose near the forehead to cause blanching of the skin.
3. Observe the skin and subcutaneous tissue for yellowish color as the skin is blanched.
4. Blanch areas of the body at the sternum and below. As the degree of jaundice increases, the yellow-orange color will be observable in the torso and lower extremities as well as the face.
5. Document findings.
6. Report abnormal findings.

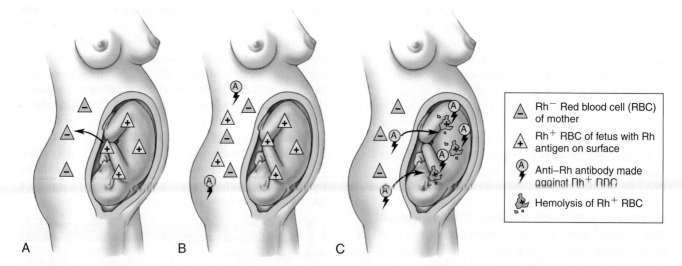

△ ⎯	Rh⁻ Red blood cell (RBC) of mother
△ +	Rh⁺ RBC of fetus with Rh antigen on surface
Ⓐ	Anti–Rh antibody made against Rh⁺ RBC
🦂	Hemolysis of Rh⁺ RBC

FIGURE 16-2 Maternal sensitization producing erythroblastosis in newborn. A, During the first pregnancy the mother is sensitized to the Rh-positive (*Rh⁺*) antigen from the fetus. **B,** The mother produces Rh antibodies to the Rh antigen to which she was exposed. **C,** During a second pregnancy, these Rh-positive antibodies cross the placenta to the fetus and destroy the fetal Rh-positive blood cells. *Rh⁻*, Rh negative.

rises more than 5 mg/dL/day, or the total bilirubin level is greater than 12 mg/dL.

Clinical signs associated with the development of kernicterus include temperature instability, poor feeding, decreased muscle tone, poor Moro's reflex, lethargy, high-pitched cry, rigidity, irritability, opisthotonos position (arched back), seizures, upward gaze, dark urine, and light stools. In preterm newborns, apnea and seizures may also occur.

Phototherapy. Management includes phototherapy as the primary treatment of choice for an infant with serum bilirubin levels above 12 mg/dL (Figure 16-3). Exposing the newborn to high-intensity light in the blue light spectrum decreases bilirubin levels by converting unconjugated bilirubin into isomers, called *photobilirubin*, which is transported to the liver, where it combines with bile and is excreted in the feces (without conjugation by the liver). Some light-oxidized bilirubin is also excreted in the urine. It is important for frequent feedings to continue to facilitate the excretion process. Phototherapy can be provided by a bank of green or fluorescent blue lights placed above an incubator, a fiberoptic blanket attached to a halogen light source wrapped around the body of the infant, or a fiberoptic mattress attached to a halogen light source placed under the infant (Figure 16-4). The newborn receiving standard phototherapy will have his or her eyes covered by a shield or mask to prevent potential retinal damage caused by the lights (Figure 16-5). The eye patches are removed, and the newborn is removed from the incubator during feeding and short parental visits. It is also recommended that the newborn's genital area be shielded to protect the testicles and ovaries. Surgical masks can be used like a "bikini" diaper to

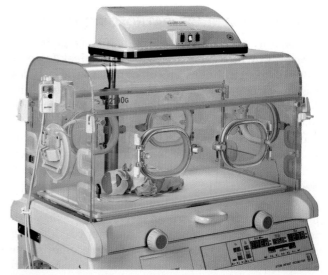

FIGURE 16-3 Phototherapy. The neoBLUE provides a high-intensity, narrow band of blue light that helps break down excess bilirubin. A flip of a switch allows change from conventional to intense phototherapy treatment. Note: In the clinical setting, the infant would be diapered only, not fully clothed.

provide protection. Repeat bilirubin measurements should be taken q6-12 hours and then again 12 hours after phototherapy is stopped (Rennie, 2010).

Frequent stools occur with rapid decrease in bilirubin and can lead to perineal excoriation; thus, careful and frequent cleansing of the newborn's skin is essential. Ointment should not be used because it could cause a burn to the skin during the phototherapy. The newborn should be assessed for dehydration and the intake and output accurately monitored. The newborn's temperature is monitored frequently, and the newborn's position is changed a minimum of every 2 hours.

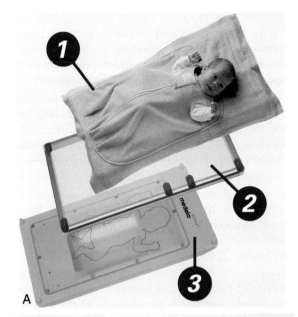

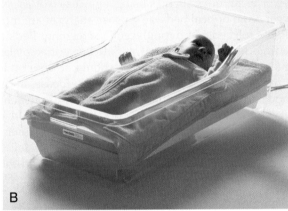

FIGURE 16-4 **Phototherapy BiliBed. A,** Newborn lies on a transparent film over a blue light source. **B,** Romper blanket in which the newborn is wrapped has a light, porous fabric on the anterior and posterior surfaces. Newborn's eyes do not need covering, and newborn can room with the mother during therapy.

Advantages of using a fiberoptic blanket or mattress method of phototherapy are that the eyes do not have to be covered, the newborn is accessible for care and interaction, and fluid and weight loss are usually not problems.

If the newborn is to receive phototherapy using home equipment, parents are taught how to assess the baby and use the equipment (see Chapter 18). Breastfeeding may continue, and the infant should not be given additional fluids routinely (Rennie, 2010).

Exchange Transfusion. Treatment by blood exchange transfusions may be indicated if the bilirubin level is greater than 25 mg/dL within 6 hours of phototherapy (Rennie, 2010).

An exchange transfusion is accomplished by alternately removing a small amount (5 to 10 mL) of the newborn's blood from the umbilical vessels and replacing it with 5 to 10 mL of donor blood. A maximum of 500 mL of donor blood is transfused, and the technique results in an approximately 75% exchange of the newborn's total blood volume.

The newborn's blood is Rh positive. Because antibodies are present in the newborn's blood against the Rh-positive factor, transfusing Rh-positive donor blood to the newborn will cause the antibodies to destroy the new blood cells and result in an increased bilirubin level. For this reason, Rh-negative blood is used for the exchange transfusion. The Rh-positive antibodies will not destroy Rh-negative blood cells, and the bilirubin levels will not increase. The life cycle of all RBCs is approximately 180 days. Therefore, after 180 days, the Rh-positive antibodies are no longer active in the newborn's blood and the Rh-negative blood cells are no longer present. The newborn will produce his or her own RBCs, reverting to the Rh-positive blood type the newborn was born with.

During the procedure, the newborn's vital signs are monitored, infection control measures are maintained, and the newborn is closely observed for transfusion reactions (hypocalcemia), such as jitteriness, convulsions, and edema or signs of fluid volume overload. Research is ongoing to develop a safe drug that will prevent the development of elevated blood bilirubin levels.

Administration of RhoGAM. Prevention of erythroblastosis by administering RhoGAM to the mother is routine. An intramuscular injection is given to the Rh-negative mother within 72 hours of delivery of an Rh-positive newborn, provided she has not been previously sensitized. Also, RhoGAM is usually given to the Rh-negative pregnant woman at 28 weeks' gestation. Rh-negative women need to have RhoGAM when they have had an abortion, after an amniocentesis, or when they have bleeding during pregnancy. Fetal blood may leak into the mother's circulation at these times and

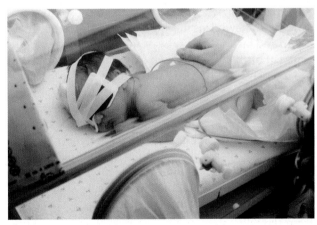

FIGURE 16-5 This newborn is in an incubator receiving phototherapy; note the eyes covered for protection. The mother provides gentle touch and massage. The newborn's position is changed frequently to expose all areas to the light.

Box **16-2**   Rh Sensitization

- The potential for sensitization occurs when an Rh-negative woman and an Rh-positive man conceive a fetus that is Rh positive.
- If the woman becomes sensitized, her body will produce antibodies to her fetus's Rh-positive blood.
- Tests used to detect antibody formation or sensitization are (1) an indirect Coombs' test on the mother's blood to measure the amount of Rh-positive antibodies and (2) a direct Coombs' test on the baby's blood to detect antibody-coated Rh-positive red blood cells.
- Rh₀(D) immune globulin (RhoGAM) is given at 28 weeks' gestation (prenatally) to reduce the potential fetal Rh-positive cell antibody development in the Rh-negative mother's bloodstream.
- RhoGAM should be administered after each amniocentesis, abortion, or ectopic pregnancy and within 72 hours or less after birth of an Rh-positive newborn.
- Phototherapy is the treatment of choice for newborns who develop hyperbilirubinemia.

stimulate antibody production (Box 16-2). Rophylac, approved by the FDA in 2004, is used in many facilities in place of RhoGAM. Rophylac is derived from human plasma and has never contained thimerosal (mercury). It can be administered IM or IV but cannot be administered at the same time as administration of other vaccines.

HYPOGLYCEMIA

Blood glucose levels decrease during the first 2 hours of life to approximately 50 mg/dL and then start to rise and stabilize. Hypoglycemia (*hypo* refers to below, and *glycemia* refers to sugar in the blood) is usually based on two consecutively low values on blood samples taken 30 minutes apart. Plasma glucose levels of less than 40 mg/dL indicate hypoglycemia and are considered abnormal. Blood glucose less than 25 mg/dL is usually treated with intravenous glucose solutions. The brain requires a constant supply of glucose, and therefore hypoglycemia must be treated promptly.

Preterm newborns may not have enough stored glycogen and fat and so may be prone to develop hypoglycemia at birth. Preterm newborns who are admitted to the intensive care nursery may be too sick to swallow formula and often require gavage or parenteral feedings to supply their need for 110 to 130 kcal/kg/day. Newborns born to diabetic mothers are at risk of hypoglycemia when insulin levels of the newborn remain high and glucose levels supplied by the placenta decrease. In fetal life, insulin is secreted by the fetal pancreas in response to the maternal glucose that crosses the placenta (see Chapter 4). After birth, the newborn has to stabilize glucose levels. Transient hypoglycemia most often occurs during the first 24 hours after birth, but it may be delayed for up to 72 hours. Any newborn who experiences stress at birth, such as asphyxia or cold stress, quickly uses up available glucose stores and may be predisposed to develop hypoglycemia. Maternal epidural anesthesia may alter glucose homeostasis in the fetus and also predispose the newborn to develop hypoglycemia at birth.

The most common signs of hypoglycemia are lethargy, hypotonia, jitteriness, poor feeding, tachypnea, apnea, sweating, shrill cry, low temperature, and seizures (Box 16-3). The newborn often demonstrates a combination of these signs. Careful control of environmental body temperature, establishment of early feedings, and aggressive blood screening minimize the occurrence of hypoglycemia. Testing may be performed by a bedside glucose capillary heel stick (Figure 16-6). For guaranteed accuracy of glucose determination (Chemstick), the alcohol should be allowed to dry before the skin is punctured, and the first drop of blood should be wiped away with sterile gauze before placing a blood drop in the test strip. Newer techniques such as using a glucose oxidase analyzer or an optical bedside glucose analyzer are more reliable for bedside hypoglycemia screening. Bedside readings less than 40 mg/dL should be verified by laboratory analysis. Blood samples should be kept on ice to prevent RBCs from metabolizing glucose in the blood sample, and samples should be sent to the clinical laboratory promptly. Blood sampling should be performed before feedings. Feeding glucose water is not recommended because it raises glucose levels, which results in elevated insulin production and then a drop in glucose levels. Breast milk or formula sustains blood glucose levels for a longer time.

RESPIRATORY DISORDERS

The respiratory system plays a critical role in successful adaptation to extrauterine life. At birth, interruption of the fetoplacental circulation requires the newborn to achieve effective gas exchange immediately. Maturation of the respiratory system in utero is essential for extrauterine life. Pulmonary surfactant is an antiatelectasis factor located in the alveolar lining layer, which provides a low surface tension to the

Box **16-3**   Signs of Hypoglycemia

- Poor feeding
- Jitteriness or tremors
- Tachypnea
- Cyanosis
- Lethargy
- Hypotonia (possible weak swallowing reflex)
- Irritability
- Temperature instability
- Apnea
- Seizures and coma

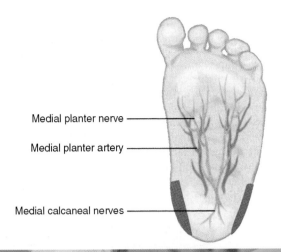

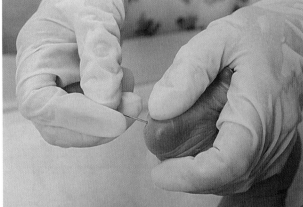

FIGURE 16-6 The shaded areas at the side of the heel are used for heel sticks in newborns to avoid the nerves, blood vessels, and bony areas. Warming the heel before puncture will promote better blood flow.

tissues that prevents collapse of the alveoli during expiration.

Common respiratory disorders that manifest during the beginning of extrauterine life include respiratory distress syndrome, meconium aspiration syndrome (MAS), transient tachypnea of the newborn, persistent pulmonary hypertension of the newborn, and sepsis.

RESPIRATORY DISTRESS SYNDROME

Respiratory distress syndrome (RDS), also known as hyaline membrane disease, is a major cause of newborn morbidity and death. Impaired or delayed surfactant appears to play a key role in this condition, and it often occurs in preterm infants. Hypoxemia occurs and causes metabolic acidosis, and both contribute to pulmonary vasoconstriction. The newborn then has decreased ability to exchange oxygen and carbon dioxide necessary for perfusion of oxygenated blood to vital organs and for removal of metabolic waste products.

Newborns with RDS are typically seen initially with a combination of tachypnea, nasal flaring, subcostal and intercostal retractions, cyanosis, and expiratory grunting. Retractions occur as the result of the soft rib cage being drawn in on inspiration. The expiratory grunt results from partial closure of the glottis during an expiration, which is a means of trapping alveolar air. Clinical signs of the disorder often occur within 1 hour of birth. Signs of respiratory distress in the newborn are illustrated in Figure 16-7. Principles of newborn resuscitation are reviewed in Table 16-2.

Prevention and Treatment

Essential preventive measures for RDS include avoiding preterm birth (from either elective cesarean birth or premature labor). If preterm delivery is necessary, the administration of corticosteroids to the mother before birth stimulates fetal lung production of surfactant. After birth, the severity of RDS may be lessened by administration of surfactants by trachea using strict sterile technique. Nursing responsibilities include:

- Weighing the newborn to ensure the proper dosage is administered.
- Deep suctioning before the procedure to ensure the medication will not be mixed with thick mucus. Suctioning is not performed for 2 hours after the procedure to avoid removing the instilled liquid.
- Administering appropriate sedatives as prescribed.
- Assisting with chest x-ray examinations as needed.
- Positioning the newborn during procedure. Positioning required is often head down, turned in specific directions, and held in place for 30 seconds after each dose is administered. A respiratory therapist should be available.
- Monitoring the newborn's vital signs and status. Bradycardia, decreased oxygen saturation, and poor general color may indicate a pause in the procedure is necessary.
- Monitoring oxygen saturation, vital signs, signs of respiratory distress, and signs of cerebral hemorrhage after the procedure.

Assisted ventilation is given with high-speed jet ventilation or a high-frequency oscillation ventilator (HFOV), which delivers small volumes of gas at high frequencies and limits development of high airway pressure. An intermittent positive pressure ventilation (IPPV), a continuous positive airway pressure (CPAP), high-frequency extracorporeal membrane oxygenation (ECMO), or nitric oxide inhalation is also used. Careful assessment and parenteral nutritional support are essential. Documenting an accurate intake and output is essential.

⚠ Safety Alert

Signs of Respiratory Distress in Neonates

- Pale, mottled skin color
- Tachypnea and periods of apnea
- Retractions on inspiration (substernal or intercostal)
- Flared nares on inspiration
- Expiratory grunt
- Decreased response to stimuli

Observation of Retractions

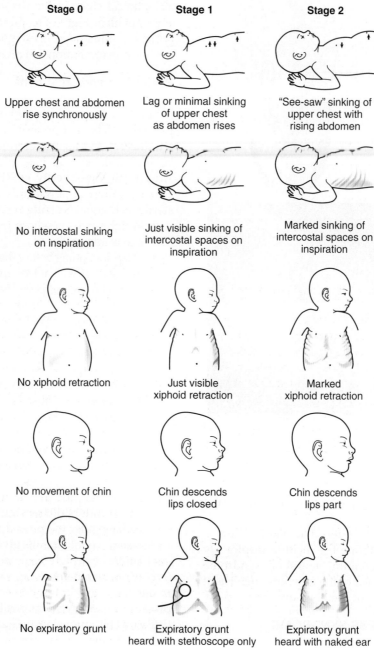

Stage 0	Stage 1	Stage 2
Upper chest and abdomen rise synchronously	Lag or minimal sinking of upper chest as abdomen rises	"See-saw" sinking of upper chest with rising abdomen
No intercostal sinking on inspiration	Just visible sinking of intercostal spaces on inspiration	Marked sinking of intercostal spaces on inspiration
No xiphoid retraction	Just visible xiphoid retraction	Marked xiphoid retraction
No movement of chin	Chin descends lips closed	Chin descends lips part
No expiratory grunt	Expiratory grunt heard with stethoscope only	Expiratory grunt heard with naked ear

FIGURE 16-7 **Assessment of respiratory distress.** The Silverman-Andersen index is used to score the newborn's degree of respiratory difficulty. The score for individual criteria matches the grade, with a total maximum score of 10, indicating severe distress.

MECONIUM ASPIRATION SYNDROME

The fetal physical response to asphyxia in utero is increased intestinal peristalsis, relaxation of the anal sphincter, and the passage of meconium into the amniotic fluid. When the fetus experiences hypoxia, gasping movements can draw meconium into the fetal airways. Interestingly, the passage and subsequent aspiration of meconium are rarely seen before 34 weeks' gestation. Meconium aspiration syndrome (MAS) primarily affects postterm newborns and those who have had a prolonged labor and intrauterine asphyxia. The presence of thick (particulate or pea soup–like) amniotic fluid increases the risk for MAS. The key to management of MAS is its prevention and, using the skilled team approach, immediate routine upper airway suctioning at birth as soon as the head is delivered to the perineum. After birth, tracheal suctioning should be performed when the Apgar score is low and must be completed before using positive pressure ventilation.

When meconium is aspirated, obstruction of the newborn's airways can occur. Obstruction of the large or upper airways results in an acute hypoxic emergency.

Table 16-2	Steps in Newborn Resuscitation
INTERVENTION	**RATIONALE AND NURSING RESPONSIBILITY**
Place infant in head down position.	Avoids aspiration of oropharyngeal secretions.
Suction.	Suctioning nose and mouth establishes a patent airway.
Rub infant's back.	Provides noninvasive respiratory stimulation.
Provide positive pressure puffs of inflation at 40-60 breaths/ minute with infant's head in neutral (sniff) position.	Sniff position opens the airway (avoid hyperextension of the neck).
Intubate.	Have resuscitation equipment and medications on hand. In delivery room, may be given by umbilical vein. • Epinephrine • Sodium bicarbonate • Intravenous dextrose 10% • Naloxone (Narcan) • Normal saline (intravenous) • Lactated Ringer's solution (intravenous) • Dopamine

Presence of meconium in the lungs produces a ball-valve action, in which air is allowed in but cannot escape on expiration. This problem results in overdistention of alveoli, which leads to alveolar rupture, pulmonary air leaks, chemical inflammation (pneumonitis), and atelectasis (incomplete expansion of lungs). With air leaks, pneumothorax often occurs. These newborns can have extreme acidosis from cardiac shunting and decreased perfusion, and extreme hypoxia may result, even with 100% oxygen concentration and ventilatory assistance. Clinical signs of MAS include the skin, nails, and umbilical cord stained a yellowish green; tachypnea; retractions; generalized cyanosis; and metabolic acidosis.

Prophylactic surfactant therapy may be indicated, and chest physiotherapy is usually prescribed. Fortunately, the use of amnioinfusion (the infusion of sterile saline into the uterine cavity to dilute the meconium-stained fluid) during labor has reduced the severity of MAS (see Chapter 7). The nurse should be alert to and report abnormal fetal heart rates and meconium in the vaginal discharge of women in labor, and they should prepare for the prevention and management of meconium aspiration.

PERSISTENT PULMONARY HYPERTENSION OF THE NEWBORN

Persistent pulmonary hypertension of the newborn (PPHN) refers to the combination of pulmonary hypertension and persistence of right-to-left shunting. Blood bypasses the lungs by flowing through the foramen ovale or ductus arteriosus. PPHN may be present either as a single entity or as the main component of MAS, pneumonia, sepsis, or diaphragmatic hernia. PPHN is also known as **persistent fetal circulation.** Actually, any process that interferes with the transition from fetal to extrauterine circulation may precipitate PPHN. Maternal use of aspirin, nonsteroidal antiinflammatory drugs, or general hypoxia is implicated as a contributory factor.

When there is a sustained elevation of pulmonary vascular resistance after birth, the transition to extrauterine circulation is hindered. When right-to-left shunting occurs, hypoxemia results and progresses to hypoxia and metabolic acidosis, which cause a worsening of pulmonary vasoconstriction. ECMO may be used. Incubators, ECMO, parenteral nutrition, and minimum external stimulation have achieved positive results in the treatment of PPHN.

TRANSIENT TACHYPNEA OF THE NEWBORN

Transient tachypnea of the newborn (TTN) is seen more often in newborns delivered by cesarean birth, probably because of insufficient thoracic squeeze resulting in retained fetal lung fluid, and in large infants of diabetic mothers (IDMs). Shortly after birth, a transient elevation in respiratory rate occurs in an effort to get rid of amniotic fluid in the newborn's lungs. Newborns breathing room air will show expiratory grunting, nasal flaring, and mild cyanosis. Respirations may reach 100 to 140 breaths/minute. It is a self-limiting disorder resulting from a slight lack of surfactant or a delayed reabsorption of fetal lung fluid. The newborn is given oxygen, respiratory support, parenteral nutrition, and intravenous fluids because the infant is placed on NPO (nothing by mouth) status when respiratory rates are increased. Improvement is often seen within 48 hours (Figure 16-8).

INFANTS OF DIABETIC MOTHERS

Maternal diabetes is a problem for the mother and the newborn (see Chapter 13). The effect of diabetes on pregnancy depends on the type of diabetes and how well it is controlled. Newborns of mothers with long-term diabetes may have a deficiency of nutrients as a result of decreased blood flow reaching the fetus. Hypertension, which occurs more often in diabetic

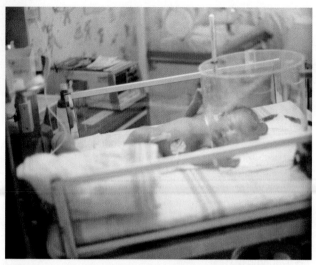

FIGURE 16-8 Oxygen is administered by an oxygen hood. The newborn is accessible for treatment without interrupting oxygen supply.

mothers compared with other women, can further compromise the uteroplacental blood flow and can cause fetal growth restriction and even death.

A high maternal glucose level can result in a large fetus (macrosomia) for the gestational age and an increased risk for problems at birth. The most common congenital defects associated with uncontrolled hyperglycemia throughout pregnancy include congenital heart defects, tracheoesophageal fistulas, and CNS anomalies. Close observation in the first few days of life is essential. Infants of diabetic mothers (IDMs) have an increased risk of RDS compared with healthy newborns because high levels of insulin appear to interfere with the production of surfactant in the lungs. Another complication for the IDMs is an increased risk for hypoglycemia after birth. After birth, the maternal glucose is no longer available; however, the newborn's pancreas continues to produce an increased amount of insulin (overproduction of insulin), and hypoglycemia results. For this reason, early and frequent heel sticks are performed to assess the newborn's blood glucose level. A Chemstick determination of less than 40 mg/dL indicates hypoglycemia in a term newborn. *Levels less than 30 mg/dL indicate hypoglycemia in the preterm newborn.* Early feedings or intravenous therapy is administered to maintain normal glucose levels. If hypoglycemia is left untreated, seizures, brain damage, and death can occur. See Box 16-3 on p. 332 for signs of hypoglycemia.

Polycythemia (hematocrit level greater than 65%) may be a problem with IDMs because these newborns often produce more erythrocytes than normal because of poor oxygenation during fetal life. Polycythemia often results in *hyperbilirubinemia* as the excessive RBCs break down after birth. *Hypocalcemia* may be a problem in response to a long and difficult birth process, and the large-for-gestational-age (LGA) newborn may exhibit tremors. Polycythemia from intrauterine hypoxia,

combined with an immature liver, can predispose the LGA newborn to hyperbilirubinemia. IDM babies may have immature lungs and insufficient surfactant at birth and so are susceptible to *respiratory distress.* Administration of surfactant by endotracheal tube is often necessary. Birth defects may occur if the mother had uncontrolled diabetes mellitus during pregnancy.

IDMs can vary in their appearance. The newborn may be small for gestational age if he or she experiences growth restriction in utero because of poor diabetic control and maternal vascular involvement. Macrosomia (large newborn) is the result of maternal hyperglycemia in which elevated maternal levels of amino acids and fatty acids, along with hyperglycemia, cross the placenta. The resulting accelerated protein synthesis and fat stores produce the typical macrosomia newborn, with a round, puffy face and characteristic cushingoid appearance from increased subcutaneous fat. The macrosomic infant differs from the typical LGA infant who is symmetric in appearance and does not have excess fatty deposits and (hypertrophy) enlarged organs (Figure 16-9).

The risk of birth trauma resulting from macrosomia, including cephalhematoma, paralysis of the facial nerve (seventh cranial nerve), fracture of the clavicle, brachial plexus paralysis, and Erb-Duchenne (upper right arm) paralysis, is increased.

Nursing Management

The onset of hypoglycemia in IDMs is rapid because insulin production remains high when the glucose supplied by the mother is suddenly cut off. Hourly glucose checks should be done, and a level below 40 mg/dL should be reported. Early feedings with formula or breast milk or an infusion of 10% dextrose in water may be required. Once the glucose level is stable for 24 hours, the normal feeding regimen may be resumed. The infant is assessed for signs of respiratory

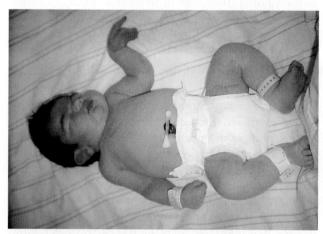

FIGURE 16-9 **A newborn with macrosomia caused by maternal diabetes mellitus during pregnancy.** This newborn weighed 5 kg (11 lbs) at birth. Newborns with macrosomia often have respiratory and other problems.

distress, hyperbilirubinemia, birth trauma, and anomalies. Education of the mother concerning diabetes control and self-care is essential.

NEONATAL SEPSIS

Neonatal sepsis refers to a systemic infection from bacteria in the bloodstream that occurs during the first month after birth. Newborns lack immunoglobulin M, which protects against bacteria, because that immunoglobulin does not cross the placenta from the mother to the fetus. The positive diagnosis of the infection is based on clinical symptoms and positive blood culture. The infection is usually polymicrobial (i.e., caused by more than one pathogen). Organisms responsible for neonatal infection include *Staphylococcus aureus, Staphylococcus epidermidis, Escherichia coli, Haemophilus influenzae,* and group B streptococci (GBS). Infection can result from transplacental passage of organisms, pathogens ascending from the vagina, cutaneous transmission as the fetus passes through the birth canal, environmental contamination after birth, and health care–associated transmission after birth from health care providers or invasive procedures performed in the nursery. Because of the newborn's limited immunity and inability to localize infection, it can spread rapidly into the bloodstream, and generalized sepsis can occur.

The infected newborn may demonstrate nonspecific signs, including poor feeding, vomiting, diarrhea, and lethargy; later, the newborn may show cyanosis, jaundice, and hypothermia. Because of the immaturity of the thermoregulatory center in the brain, the newborn commonly has low body temperature with an infection; however, newborns may also demonstrate temperature instability and fever. As sepsis becomes more severe, respiratory difficulty and septic shock may follow (Nursing Care Plan 16-1).

Prevention of Neonatal Sepsis

Prevention of neonatal sepsis starts prenatally with maternal screening for sexually transmitted infections (STIs). Sterile technique during delivery and aseptic technique, maintaining strict standard precautions during all hospital care, are essential in preventing neonatal sepsis. Mothers with positive cultures for GBS prenatally and during labor and delivery are treated with prophylactic antibiotic therapy to reduce the risk of neonatal sepsis. Genital lesions such as herpes require elective cesarean birth to prevent the newborn from being exposed to the virus. The prophylactic antibiotic treatment of the eyes of all newborns and appropriate umbilical cord care also help prevent neonatal sepsis. Laboratory reports are monitored. A white blood cell (WBC) count of $30,000/mm^3$ may be normal in the first 24 hours of life in a term newborn. A low neutrophil and high immature WBC level may indicate infection. Antibiotics such as ampicillin or gentamicin or a cephalosporin may be prescribed for 7 to 14 days. Placing the newborn in an incubator provides isolation from others and allows close observation. Home care for long-term antibiotic therapy can be initiated.

Management of the newborn includes cultures of blood, urine, stool, spinal fluid, and, in some cases, any intravenous lines. Cultures are also taken from an area with suspicious drainage, such as the eyes or umbilical stump. Nurses play a crucial role in providing education for preventive strategies and in helping families cope with their high-risk newborn.

NEWBORN WITH EFFECTS OF MATERNAL SUBSTANCE ABUSE

The woman who abuses drugs, alcohol, or other substances can deliver a newborn with varied physical and neurobehavioral manifestations. In addition, newborns may have neonatal abstinence syndrome (formerly referred to as *narcotic withdrawal*) after birth (Box 16-4). The substance-abusing mother is at risk of malnutrition, resulting in an infant who is small for gestational age, or the newborn may have congenital anomalies if the drug was taken in early pregnancy and crossed the placental barrier. The use of cocaine during pregnancy is associated with the development of abruptio placentae (Table 16-3). When drug use by the mother is suspected, a urine specimen may be collected from the infant for analysis (Skill 16-2 on p. 340). A pediatric urine collection bag may also be applied to a newborn to assess accurate intake and output when indicated.

THE NURSE AND THE FAMILY OF THE NEWBORN AT RISK

The birth of a newborn who has an anomaly, infection, or other problem is a crisis for the family. A grief reaction may occur for the loss of the anticipated "perfect baby." Parent-newborn attachment may be interrupted by incubators, intravenous lines, and ventilators. Parents may blame themselves, and self-esteem may plunge. Parents need support; recognition of the problem; and a clear explanation of the problem, treatment, and anticipated prognosis. The nurse's role is to provide support by helping the parents recognize the reality of the problem, establish trust in the health care provider, dispel misconceptions, and mobilize family support systems. The nurse must realize that some parents, although they are grateful for the expert care given to their newborn in the neonatal intensive care unit, may be jealous that the nurse is able to care for their infant and they cannot. Feelings of inferiority may influence the nurse-parent rapport. It is important to help the parents participate in the care of their newborn while providing positive support

Scenario

A 1-day-old female newborn has an axillary temperature of 39.7° C (103.4° F). She had apnea during the first 4 hours of life and demonstrates some lethargy. Maternal history reveals premature rupture of membranes (PROMs) 18 hours before birth. Her physician orders a chest radiograph, complete blood cell count, and cultures from a large pustule on her chest area and from the umbilical cord.

Selected Nursing Diagnosis

Risk for infection related to events before, during, or after birth

Expected Outcomes	Nursing Interventions	Rationales
Causative organism(s) will be identified and treated, and disease process will resolve.	Assess for risks of infection and initiate appropriate isolation and infection control management.	Newborn's defense mechanisms are immature and overwhelmed. Maternal source of infection must be identified to prevent reinfection.
	Monitor vital signs continuously by mechanical means.	Ongoing assessment indicates early changes, making adjustment of treatment possible.
	Calculate and administer medications at the proper route, rate, time, and dose.	
	Calculate and administer electrolyte replacements.	Electrolytes are lost in the presence of sepsis.
Newborn will be protected from exposure to pathogens from hospital environment, staff, or visitors.	Clean and sterilize all equipment to be used. Change tubing, lines, or humidifiers according to facility's protocol.	Cross-contamination is minimized and controlled.
	Monitor visitors for signs of illness.	Protects health of newborn by preventing exposure to pathogens.
Newborn will be free from signs of infection.	Inspect umbilical cord stump for signs of infection.	An open wound is a potential site of infection.
	Note on newborn record if mother has history of a condition that may increase potential for newborn sepsis.	Enables planning for detection or treatment of infection.
	Assess for signs of infection such as poor feeding, poor muscle tone, pallor, increased temperature.	Temperature may be subnormal in newborn sepsis. The nurse must be alert for other signs of infection.

Selected Nursing Diagnosis

Imbalanced nutrition, less than body requirements related to poor feeding or intolerance

Expected Outcomes	Nursing Interventions	Rationales
Nutritional needs will be met and maintained.	Assess for weight loss, vomiting or diarrhea, poor sucking ability, large residual if feeding by gavage.	Caloric loss through vomiting and diarrhea or poor intake will cause weight loss.
	Initiate oral feedings as soon as possible with breast milk if appropriate.	Breast milk contains natural immunoglobulins and offers some passive immunity from mother.

Selected Nursing Diagnosis

Deficient knowledge related to infection control

Expected Outcomes	Nursing Interventions	Rationales
Parents and support system will be taught effective infection control measures.	Provide videos on infection control and supervise handwashing.	Demonstrations and videos increase understanding of techniques. Written information can be referred to when at home.
	Furnish parents with booklets, brochures, informative articles, and up-to-date references from Internet.	
Parents will state effective measures to prevent infection and manage minor illness.	Instruct mother to use clean bottle and nipple for each feeding and not store leftover formula.	Microorganisms can move from a contaminated nipple into bottle. Proper storage and use of formula preparations can prevent spoilage.
	Teach mother to consult health care provider before medicating newborn.	Use of aspirin has been linked to development of Reye's syndrome. Safe dosage of medications for neonates differs from that for adults. Neonate is at risk for toxic responses.

Critical Thinking Question

1. A 1-day-old newborn has been diagnosed as having sepsis. He is increasingly lethargic and has a poor sucking reflex and decreased oral intake. What are the priority nursing interventions?

Box 16-4	Signs Typical of Neonatal Abstinence Syndrome

RESPIRATORY DISTRESS
- Stuffy nose
- Tachypnea
- Flaring of nares
- Retractions
- Apnea

GASTROINTESTINAL DYSFUNCTION
- Diarrhea
- Vomiting
- Frantic sucking
- Poor feeder

CENTRAL NERVOUS SYSTEM
- Shrill, high-pitched cry
- Irritability
- Hypertonicity
- Tremors
- Short sleep cycles
- Occasional seizures

OTHER
- Sweating
- Fever
- Sneezing
- Yawning
- Mottled color
- Abrasions of elbows and knees

and encouragement. The nurse can use strategies to maintain parent-infant attachment whenever possible. The nurse should observe the stages of grief as parents deal with the reality (denial, anger, depression, bargaining, and acceptance) and help them toward reorganization that maintains family cohesiveness and communication. Contact with the multidisciplinary team should be maintained and community resources assessed.

DISCHARGE PLANNING AND HOME CARE

Discharge planning for the compromised newborn begins as soon as the disorder is identified. Questions about the mother's situation and home environment include: Who makes up the immediate family? Does the mother have others to provide support and care for her and the newborn? Is there access to a telephone for emergencies? Are finances available to cover necessary newborn therapy? Is a social services referral indicated?

Successful discharge and home care of the newborn with a health problem often require a multidisciplinary approach. The newborn may be transferred back from the neonatal intensive care unit to the community hospital before discharge to the home, and this transfer requires interfacility communication. Long-term care may be planned for those newborns

Table 16-3	Maternal Substance Abuse and the Newborn	
PROBLEM	**SYMPTOMS**	**INTERVENTION**
Fetal alcohol syndrome (FAS): the most serious of a range of disorders caused by maternal alcohol consumption during pregnancy. Fetal alcohol spectrum disorders are a range of effects that include fetal alcohol effects (FAE), alcohol-related neurodevelopmental disorders (ARNDs), and alcohol-related birth defects (ARBDs).	Diagnosis may be confirmed by identifying fatty acid ethyl esters (FAEEs) in the meconium of the newborn. Symptoms include failure to thrive (FTT), feeding problems, CNS dysfunctions, hypotonia, speech and behavior problems, and mental retardation.	Provide quiet environment, swaddling, nutritional support, and referral for developmental monitoring.
Drug-dependent newborns: history of the mother ingesting illicit drugs during pregnancy	At birth, the newborn may manifest IUGR, jaundice (heroin and cocaine contribute to early liver maturity in the fetus and rarely show jaundice). Behavioral abnormalities and withdrawal symptoms are common.	Nursing interventions include snug swaddling, with hand near the mouth; monitoring intake and output; offering a pacifier; vertical rocking when infant is irritable; protecting skin from excoriation with the use of sheepskin or mittens; and maintaining a quiet, dimly lit environment.
Infants of tobacco-dependent mothers	Nicotine reduces the oxygen-carrying power of hemoglobin, resulting in intrauterine hypoxia and growth restriction. IUGR is common. Vasoconstriction caused by nicotine can result in placental insufficiency and prematurity with decreased Apgar scores at birth. Nicotine toxicity, including tachycardia, irritability, and poor feeding, is common.	Nurses must be alert to these signs and monitor the newborn closely.

Data from Moore, C., Jones, J., Levis, D., & Buchi, K. (2003). Prevalence of fatty acid ethyl esters in meconium specimens. *Clinical Chemistry, 49(1),* 133–136; Goren, J., Klein, J., & Koren, G. (2006). Drugs of abuse testing in meconium. *Clinica Chimica Acta, 366(1),* 101–111; and Plate, C., Alder, S., Jones, M., Jones, F., & Christiansen, R. (2006). Testing for fetal exposure to illicit drugs using umblical cord tissue vs meconium. *Journal of Perinatology, 26(1),* 11–14.
CNS, central nervous system; *IUGR,* intrauterine growth restriction.

Skill 16-2 Applying a Urine Collection Bag to a Newborn

PURPOSE
To obtain a specimen for clinical laboratory assessment.

Steps
1. Prepare newborn: place in supine position and remove diaper.
2. Wash genitalia, perineum, and surrounding area; dry thoroughly. (The urine collection bag is usually a single-use, clear plastic bag with self-adhering material around the opening at the point of attachment. Adhesive will not stick to moist or oily skin, which may cause leakage of urine.)

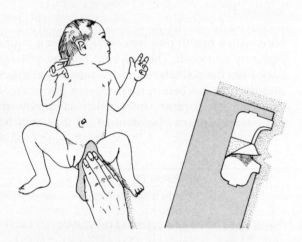

3. Remove the paper covering on the adhesive tabs of the collector bag.
4. In female newborns, fold bag in half and apply smoothly over the perineum (above the rectum), extending the tabs to the side.

For Girls

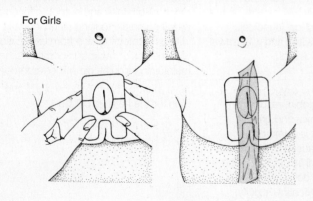

5. For the male newborn, place the penis and scrotum inside the bag before removing the tabs. Apply the posterior adhesive tabs to the perineum (above the rectum), not to the scrotum.

For Boys

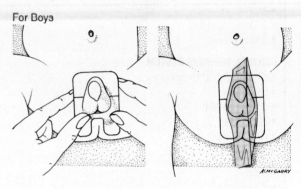

6. Apply the anterior adhesive tab to cover genitalia. Make sure there are no wrinkles. Wrinkles allow openings for urine to leak out of the bag and stool to enter.
7. Carefully and loosely, replace diaper. Diaper can be cut; pull the bag through the slit. This allows bag to be visible.
8. Check frequently for urine. The urine can be aspirated with a syringe or drained from the bag.

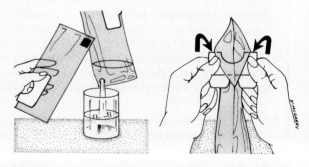

9. For small newborns, a cotton ball can be placed inside collection bag and urine aspirated from it with a syringe.
10. Remove collection bag, and pour urine into sterile container; label and send to laboratory.
11. Clean genitalia and observe for irritation where adhesive tabs were attached. Apply clean diaper.
12. Document in medical record that the labeled urine specimen was sent to the laboratory, and record output.

with congenital malformations and some congenital infections.

Discharge of the newborn to the home setting requires parental competence. Parents must learn normal newborn care and specific information relating to their infant's medical condition. Allowing the family members to handle equipment and care for their newborn under supervision of the staff nurse helps them develop self-confidence, which is particularly important if special equipment is needed when the newborn is discharged. Follow-up care by the nurse practitioner or the pediatrician is essential. Parents must be reassured that they can call the appropriate nursing staff (high-risk nursery staff), telephone help lines (see Chapter 18), hospital or community clinics, private agencies with home care services, or other community resources when they have questions about their newborn's care.

Get Ready for the NCLEX® Examination!

Key Points

- An abnormal gene can cause a birth defect of body structure, function, or metabolism. Birth defects can also result from environmental factors. Identifying the gene involved in the defect is the first step toward developing the specific treatments.
- Inherited inborn errors of metabolism include PKU, galactosemia, and congenital hypothyroidism. The same (heel stick) blood sample can be used to test for all three of these metabolic disorders in the newborn.
- PKU is an inborn error of metabolism in which the newborn cannot process an amino acid called phenylalanine; if untreated, it can result in severe mental retardation.
- In galactosemia, the newborn has a deficiency in the enzyme galactose, resulting in the inability to convert galactose to glucose.
- Congenital hypothyroidism can result from a maternal iodine deficiency or use of antithyroid drugs by the mother during pregnancy.
- The defects involved in tetralogy of Fallot include ventricular septal defect, pulmonary stenosis, hypertrophy of the left ventricle, and an overriding aorta. Cyanosis occurs. The defect is surgically corrected.
- Noncyanotic heart defects result from the blood recirculating to the lungs.
- Hyperbilirubinemia is an abnormally high level of bilirubin in the newborn's blood. Elevated bilirubin levels can cause kernicterus, which results in mental retardation.
- Standard phototherapy is the exposure of the newborn to high-intensity light. Phototherapy helps break down and excrete elevated bilirubin in the blood. Precautions are taken during phototherapy, such as shielding the newborn's eyes for protection. Other methods of phototherapy, such as using a fiberoptic blanket, do not require covering the newborn's eyes.
- The respiratory system plays a critical role in successful adaptation to extrauterine life. Common respiratory disorders occurring after birth include RDS, MAS, PPHN, and TTN.
- Blood glucose levels less than 40 mg/dL indicate hypoglycemia in term newborns. IDMs are at risk for hypoglycemia because of high insulin production and sudden cutoff of mother's glucose supply at birth. Glucose is essential for normal brain functioning.
- Newborns of diabetic mothers are at risk for respiratory distress, congenital anomalies, hypoglycemia, polycythemia, hyperbilirubinemia, and respiratory distress.
- Neonatal sepsis is an infection occurring during the first month after birth. Bacteria are found primarily in the newborn's blood.
- The newborn with special problems, such as congenital anomalies, requires interdisciplinary care, communication with the parents, identification of needs, care and support groups for parents, and follow-up care. The nurse is often the facilitator for this team communication and is the key health care provider to give the family emotional support.
- Nursing care for newborns with neonatal abstinence syndrome includes decreasing stimuli such as noise, lights, and handling. The nurse should be nonjudgmental toward the mother and encourage her in newborn attachment and newborn care.
- Maternal nicotine intake during pregnancy causes vasoconstriction, resulting in fetal hypoxia that affects fetal development.
- Fetal alcohol spectrum disorders include FAS, caused by maternal ingestion of alcohol during pregnancy and manifested by newborn neurodevelopmental delays. Diagnosis may be confirmed by examination of fetal meconium.

Additional Learning Resources

SG Go to your Study Guide on pages 503–504 for additional Review Questions for the NCLEX® Examination, Critical Thinking Clinical Situations, and other learning activities to help you master this chapter content.

evolve Go to your Evolve website (http://evolve.elsevier.com/Leifer/maternity) for the following FREE learning resources:
- Animations
- Answer Guidelines for Critical Thinking Questions
- Answers and Rationales for Review Questions for the NCLEX® Examination
- Concept Map Creator
- Glossary with pronunciations in English and Spanish
- Patient Teaching Plans
- Skills Performance Checklists and more!

Online Resources
- www.aap.org/policy/hyperb.htm
- www.cleftline.org
- www.marchofdimes.com
- www.medem.com
- www.sbaa.org/html/sbaa_facts2.html

Review Questions for the NCLEX® Examination

1. A newborn baby is diagnosed with Turner's syndrome, which is considered a(n).
    1. Disorder of the blood
    2. Perinatal injury
    3. Inborn error of metabolism
    4. Chromosomal abnormality

2. Down syndrome is also known as:
    1. Trisomy 13
    2. Trisomy 15
    3. Trisomy 18
    4. Trisomy 21

3. Characteristically, a newborn with phenylketonuria has a(n):
    1. Deficiency of the enzyme necessary to convert galactose to glucose
    2. Sweet odor in body fluids
    3. Large protruding tongue
    4. Unusual musty odor to his or her urine

4. The nurse caring for a newborn with a serum bilirubin level of 14 mg/dL is aware that the primary treatment of choice is:
    1. Phototherapy
    2. Exchange transfusion
    3. Intravenous therapy
    4. Gavage feedings

5. A newborn infant diagnosed with hypoglycemia requires treatment with intravenous glucose. The nurse is aware that in order to require this treatment the infant's blood glucose must have been:
    1. Less than 40 mg/dL
    2. Between 40 and 50 mg/dL
    3. Above 50 mg/dL
    4. Between 70 and 100 mg/dL

6. Which disorder would be categorized as a malformation present at birth?
    1. Spina bifida
    2. Cystic fibrosis
    3. Hemophilia
    4. Meconium aspiration syndrome

7. Infants of diabetic mothers (IDMs) have an increased risk of which disorder(s)? *(Select all that apply.)*
    1. Respiratory distress syndrome
    2. Hypoglycemia
    3. Polycythemia
    4. Macrosomia
    5. Cephalhematoma

Critical Thinking Questions

1. A 3-day-old newborn has been placed in an incubator to treat hyperbilirubinemia. The mother states she doesn't understand why the baby is jaundiced because she is not Rh negative. What is the best response of the nurse?

2. A mother asks the nurse why the PKU blood screening test can't be performed at birth instead of waiting until the time of discharge. What is the best response of the nurse?

Postpartum Complications

Objectives

1. Define key terms listed.
2. Summarize major causes of postpartum hemorrhage.
3. Identify nursing interventions in the care of the woman with postpartum hemorrhage.
4. Describe the dangers that deep vein thrombosis presents.
5. Explain the nursing care of a woman who has a thromboembolism.

6. List four common sites for puerperal infection.
7. Describe predisposing factors for infections of the reproductive system.
8. Discuss the nursing care of a woman who has an infected episiotomy.
9. Compare postpartum blues with postpartum psychosis.

Key Terms

endometritis (ĕn-dō-mĕ -TRĪ-tĭs, p. 350)
mastitis (măs-TĪ-tĭs, p. 351)
parametritis (păr-ămĕ -TRĪ-tĭs, p. 350)
placenta accreta (plăSĒ N-tă ăKRĒ-tă, p. 345)
postpartum hemorrhage (HĔ M-ŏr-ĭj, p. 343)
puerperal fever (pū-Ĕ R-pĕ r-ăl, p. 350)

pulmonary embolism (PŬL-mō-nărē Ĕ M-bō-lĭz-ŭm, p. 349)
REEDA (p. 350)
subinvolution (sŭb-ĭn-vō-LŪ-shŭn, p. 345)
thrombophlebitis (thrŏm-bō-flĕ BĪ-tŭs, p. 349)
uterine atony (Ū-tĕ r-ĭn ĂT-ŏnē, p. 344)

Shortened inpatient (postpartum) stays are common in maternity care. Women are often discharged after childbirth before clinical signs of puerperal infection and other postpartum disorders are evident. Consequently, hospital-based nurses are challenged to perform a risk assessment and attempt to recognize subtle signs of complications that may require a delay in discharge. Before discharge, the nurse teaches preventive measures to avoid common postpartum complications.

Many problems can occur during the postpartum period, but most problems fall into the following five categories:

- Hemorrhage *greater than 500mL vaginally*
- Thromboembolic disorders
- Subinvolution of the uterus
- Infections
- Depression

POSTPARTUM HEMORRHAGE: OVERVIEW

Postpartum hemorrhage is the most common cause of excessive bleeding during the childbearing cycle. Postpartum hemorrhage is traditionally defined as loss of more than 500 mL of blood after an uncomplicated vaginal birth or 1000 mL after a cesarean birth. Excessive blood loss after a *complicated* birth, such as placenta previa (see Chapter 13) or accreta placenta, is discussed later in this chapter. Because most women have 1 to 2 L of increased blood volume during pregnancy, they can tolerate this amount of blood loss. Postpartum hemorrhage can occur early (in the first 24 hours) or late (between 24 hours and 6 weeks after birth). The greatest danger, however, is in the first 24 hours because of the large venous area exposed after placental separation from the uterine wall (Box 17-1).

The most common causes of **early postpartum hemorrhage** are uterine atony and laceration. **Late postpartum hemorrhage** (secondary postpartum hemorrhage) is caused by retained placental fragments or subinvolution. Coagulation defects and infection can also result in postpartum hemorrhage (Simpson, 2010). Women at greatest risk for postpartum hemorrhage include those who have labor induction or augmentation, multiple fetuses (twins, etc.), macrosomia, preeclampsia, operative deliveries, and chorioamnionitis.

The body responds to hypovolemia (reduced blood volume) with increased heart and respiratory rates. These reactions increase the oxygen content of circulating erythrocytes (red blood cells). A decrease in blood volume causes the woman's skin and mucous membranes to become pale, cold, and moist (clammy). As the blood loss continues, blood flow to the brain decreases and the woman becomes restless, confused, anxious, and lethargic. A collaborative effort by the health care team is necessary to provide prompt care.

Box 17-1 | Risk Factors for Postpartum Hemorrhage

- Uterine atony
- Overdistention of the uterus
- Multifetal gestation
- Hydramnios
- Fetal macrosomia
- Oxytocin induction or augmentation
- Lacerations
- Bladder distention
- Disseminated intravascular coagulation
- Retained placental fragments

The management for hypovolemic shock (reduced blood volume) resulting from postpartum hemorrhage includes:

- Recognizing the specific cause (where the blood is coming from)
- Stopping the blood loss
- Starting intravenous fluids to maintain circulating volume
- Monitoring vital signs
- Providing oxygen to increase saturation of red blood cells (with a pulse oximeter used to assess blood oxygen saturation)
- Inserting an indwelling (Foley) catheter to assess kidney function and urinary output

EARLY POSTPARTUM HEMORRHAGE

UTERINE ATONY

Uterine atony (hypotonic uterus) is the inability of the myometrium muscle (middle muscle, which has interlacing "figure eight" fibers) of the uterus to contract and stay contracted around the open blood vessels. Without this contraction, the vessels at the placental implantation site cannot close and begin to heal. Uterine atony is the most common cause of early postpartum hemorrhage and occurs during the first hours after birth.

Mechanical factors that contribute to the inability of muscles to contract include retained placental fragments or large blood clots. Extreme uterine distention (e.g., multifetal gestations, hydramnios) can cause uterine atony. Overstretching may cause a lack of efficiency of the smooth muscle cells to contract. A full bladder can also prevent the uterus from contracting (Figure 17-1).

Metabolic factors may contribute to uterine atony. Muscle exhaustion can occur from lactic acid buildup (derived from prolonged muscle activity and the breakdown of glycogen). Because calcium is an important regulator of smooth muscle tone, hypocalcemia may be implicated in some cases of uterine atony.

Drugs have important effects on postpartum uterine tone. Magnesium sulfate administered to prevent seizures or as a tocolytic agent may result in uterine atony by impairing calcium-mediated properties

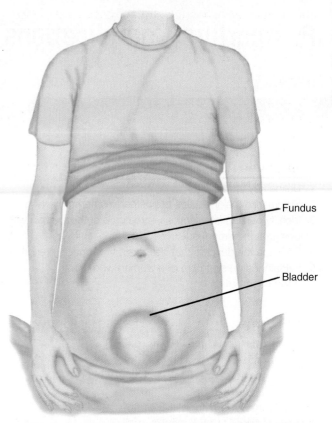

FIGURE 17-1 A distended bladder pushes the uterus upward and usually to one side of the abdomen. The fundus may be boggy or firm. If not emptied, a distended bladder can result in uterine atony and hemorrhage because it interferes with the normal contraction of the uterus.

within the cells. In addition, calcium channel blockers, such as nifedipine, used in preterm uterine contractions may also inhibit postpartum uterine contractions.

[!] Safety Alert

Signs of Hemorrhage

In a postpartum patient, a narrowing of the pulse pressure (the difference between the systolic and diastolic blood pressure) may be a sign of compensated hemorrhage and an early sign of a serious problem.

TRAUMA AND LACERATIONS

Trauma includes vaginal, cervical, or perineal lacerations. Postpartum hemorrhage can occur as a result of extension of the perineal incisions (and incisions during a cesarean birth). All lacerations should be promptly sutured. Large perineal lacerations can occur in difficult or precipitate deliveries, in primigravidas with large newborns (more than 4.1 kg [9 lbs]), and in deliveries requiring instrument assistance such as forceps or a vacuum extractor.

Lacerations are suspected when excessive bleeding occurs and the uterine fundus is firmly contracted. Bleeding from

severe preclampsia w/ enduced labor = ↑ early post-partum hemorrhage

the vagina is usually bright red, compared with lochia, which is dark red and not profuse or continuous. Signs of shock may occur.

RETAINED PLACENTA

Hemorrhage may occur if pieces of the placenta remain in the uterus. This prevents the uterus from contracting effectively and can result in either early or late hemorrhage. Careful examination of the placenta after delivery is essential. Oxytocics are administered to expel the fragments of the placenta but may not be sufficient to expel all of the fragments, so dilation and evacuation (D&E) may be necessary. Placenta accreta is the term used for a placenta that adheres to the uterine wall. Profuse bleeding may result, and a hysterectomy may be required.

HEMATOMA

Hematoma (collection of blood within the tissues) may result from injury to blood vessels in the perineum or in the vagina. Soft tissues in other areas may be involved, which are typically seen as a bulging, bluish mass. Hematomas containing 250 to 500 mL of blood may develop rapidly. A hematoma may form in the upper portion of the vagina or may occur upward into the broad ligament, which can result in massive hemorrhage.

Perineal pain, rather than noticeable bleeding, is a distinguishing characteristic of a hematoma, and the uterus remains firm but the blood pressure decreases. The woman may not be able to void because of pressure on the urethra, or she may feel the urge to defecate because of pressure on the rectum. A hematoma can cause severe pain and may require a surgical incision to remove the clot. Small vulvar hematomas may be treated with the application of ice packs or alternate hot and cold applications.

LATE POSTPARTUM HEMORRHAGE

Late postpartum hemorrhage can occur 1 to 2 weeks after delivery and is typically due to subinvolution (failure of the uterus to return to pre-pregnant size). The site of placental implantation is the last to heal and regenerate after delivery. A vascular area, retained placental fragments, or infection may be the cause of late postpartum hemorrhage. The clinic nurse should be alert to symptoms that include a fundal height higher than expected postpartum (after 10 days it should be difficult to palpate because it should be well into the pelvis) and persistent lochia rubra. Infection may be suspected if a foul odor to the lochia is noted. Treatment may include administration of methylergonovine (Methergine), oxytocin, or prostaglandins to contract the uterus, antimicrobials if infection is present, or D&E if retained placental fragments are suspected.

SUBINVOLUTION

Subinvolution of the uterus occurs when the uterus fails to return to its nonpregnant size; instead, it remains enlarged and still has a lochial discharge. Subinvolution may result from a small retained placental fragment or mild endometritis. Ultrasound can be used to identify retained placental fragments. Excessively vigorous massage of the uterus may contribute to this problem. Long-term loss of blood from subinvolution results in anemia, lack of energy, and exhaustion. Conservative treatment consists of the administration of methylergonovine orally or intramuscularly. Methylergonovine may be contraindicated in hypertensive women. D&E may be needed to remove retained placental fragments.

COAGULATION PATHOLOGY
DISSEMINATED INTRAVASCULAR COAGULATION

Disseminated intravascular coagulation (DIC) is a condition in which clotting and anticoagulation stimulation occur at the same time. The release of thromboplastin uses up available fibrinogen and platelets, which results in profuse bleeding and intravascular clotting. The key to successful management of DIC is treatment of the causative event. It often is a secondary condition associated with abruptio placentae, gestational hypertension, missed abortion, or fetal death in utero. DIC is discussed in more detail in Chapter 13.

DIC is suspected when the usual measures to stimulate uterine contractions fail to stop vaginal bleeding. Signs of DIC include oozing from an intravenous insertion site, petechiae, ecchymosis, oliguria, and restlessness. In pregnancy and the early postpartum period, shock is considered a late sign of DIC because the increased blood volume during pregnancy delays evidence of the serious blood loss. However, a decreasing pulse pressure (the difference between systolic and diastolic blood pressure) with continued bleeding may indicate a serious problem and should be promptly reported to the health care provider. Recombinant activated factor VIIa given intravenously can reverse symptoms of DIC (Karrie, 2006).

VON WILLEBRAND'S DISEASE

Von Willebrand's disease is an inherited disorder characterized by a decrease in plasma factor VIII, which is essential for proper platelet function. The woman may have a history of easy bruising, frequent nosebleeds, and heavy menses. There is typically a normal increase in plasma factor VIII during pregnancy, so symptoms can be masked. Hemorrhage from von Willebrand's disease is treated with the administration of cryoprecipitate to raise factor VIII levels.

Ⓧ uterine atony, laceration.

ANAPHYLACTOID SYNDROME OF PREGNANCY (AMNIOTIC FLUID EMBOLISM)

Amniotic fluid embolism, currently known as *anaphylactoid syndrome of pregnancy*, is due to the unanticipated entrance of amniotic fluid into maternal circulation, which triggers the release of mediators (such as bradykinin, cytokines, prostaglandins, leukotrienes, thromboxane, and others) that causes pulmonary artery vasospasm and hypoxia. The hypoxia results in myocardial (heart muscle) damage that can cause maternal left-sided heart failure.

Nursing interventions include recognizing symptoms such as acute dyspnea, hypotension, and possibly seizures; providing oxygen for the woman; preparing blood work for laboratory coagulation studies; providing emotional support for the family; and assisting in the transfer of the patient to the intensive care unit (ICU). This condition appears without warning, and the morbidity and mortality rate is high.

INTERVENTIONS FOR HEMORRHAGE

PREVENTION OF HEMORRHAGE

Postpartum hemorrhage caused by uterine atony after a vaginal birth can be greatly reduced by prophylactic administration of uterotonic drugs (oxytocin) after the delivery of the placenta. An intravenous solution of oxytocin may be started to contract the uterus. Early clamping of the umbilical cord and assisted delivery of the placenta may also prevent uterine atony and postpartum hemorrhage. The placenta should be carefully examined to determine that it is intact. Massage of the uterine fundus can aid in uterine muscle contraction. Observation and prevention of bladder distention is an important postpartum nursing responsibility (see Figure 17-1).

NURSING ASSESSMENT AND MANAGEMENT OF POSTPARTUM HEMORRHAGE

Prompt assessment and management can minimize blood loss. Essential nursing interventions are shown in Box 17-2 and Nursing Care Plan 17-1. In the first 24 hours after delivery, the nurse should be alert to the signs and symptoms of uterine atony and postpartum hemorrhage, which include a soft, boggy uterine fundus, a fundus that quickly loses firmness after massage, a fundus that is not midline or above the level of the umbilicus, excessive lochia, or excessive clots. The nurse should report signs of shock, including tachycardia and low blood pressure.

The first nursing action with uterine atony should be to massage the uterus until firm and to express clots that may have accumulated in the uterus. One hand should be placed above the symphysis pubis to support the lower uterine segment while the fundus is gently but firmly massaged in a circular motion

| Box 17-2 | Essential Nursing Interventions for Postpartum Hemorrhage |

- Uterine massage (avoid potential uterine inversion)
- Maintenance of large-bore intravenous catheters
- Administration of intravenous fluids (e.g., rapid volume expanders, blood products)
- Blood samples for hemoglobin, hematocrit, type and cross-match, coagulation profile (prothrombin time [PT], partial thromboplastin time [PTT], platelet count, fibrin level, arterial blood gases)
- Foley catheter (to maintain accurate measurement of output)
- Pulse oximeter use and saturation level monitoring
- Administration of oxygen (per protocol)
- Elevation of legs to a 20- to 30-degree angle to increase venous return
- Avoidance of Trendelenburg position (unless ordered) because it may interfere with cardiac and respiratory function
- Explanation of procedures to the woman (why they are necessary)
- Emotional support for the woman and her family
- Blood loss assessment (weigh perineal pads)
- Surveillance of vital signs

(Skill 17-1). It is critical not to try to express clots until the uterus is firmly contracted. Pushing on an uncontracted uterus can invert the uterus and cause a massive hemorrhage. If the uterus does not stay contracted, the health care provider may order an intravenous infusion of dilute oxytocin, which usually will increase muscle tone and control bleeding. Methylergonovine may be given intramuscularly if bleeding continues. This drug has side effects of elevating blood pressure; therefore, it should not be given to a woman who is hypertensive. If uterine massage and administration of oxytocin and other medications are not effective, it may be necessary to return the woman to a birthing room to stop the bleeding. A physician may attempt bimanual compression by placing one hand in the vagina with the other pushing against the fundus through the abdominal wall or surgical intervention may be needed.

An accurate assessment of blood loss is important. Blood loss can be assessed by weighing the perineal pad (1 g = 1 mL, subtracting weight of dry pad from saturated pad). If possible, a gram scale should be kept in the postpartum unit and used to measure blood loss. Vital signs should be assessed at least every 15 minutes until stabilized, and the woman should be assessed for signs of hypovolemic shock. Accurate assessment of intake and output is necessary. Urinary output should be at least 30 mL/hour.

Other measures include observing for a full bladder. A full bladder pushes on the uterus and can keep the uterus from contracting; catheterization may be

Nursing Care Plan 17-1   **The Woman with Postpartum Hemorrhage**

Scenario

A recently delivered woman is admitted to the postpartum unit. She appears anxious and frightened, and her lochia has saturated three perineal pads in the last hour.

Selected Nursing Diagnosis

Ineffective tissue perfusion related to excessive blood loss from uterine atony or birth injury

Expected Outcomes	Nursing Interventions	Rationales
Patient's blood pressure and pulse will be within 10% of her baseline values when she was admitted.	Identify whether woman has added risk factors for postpartum hemorrhage.	Women who have risk factors should be assessed more often than those who do not.
Patient will be free of signs or symptoms of hypovolemic shock.	Observe fundus for height, firmness, and position.	The fundus must be firm to compress bleeding vessels at the placenta site.
Patient will void as needed.	Palpate abdomen above symphysis to detect distended bladder.	Bladder distention interferes with uterine contractions and causes the fundus to be high and displaced to one side.
	Assess lochia for color, quantity, and clots. Count pads and degree of saturation (weigh pads for greater accuracy).	Most blood lost after birth is visible rather than concealed. Observing lochia provides an estimate of actual blood loss.
	Check blood pressure, pulse, and respiratory rates per hospital protocol.	A rising pulse rate is often a first sign of inadequate blood volume. A rising pulse and falling blood pressure can also occur.
	Observe for less obvious signs of bleeding: constant trickle of bright red blood with a firm fundus; severe, poorly relieved pain, especially if accompanied by changes in the vital signs or signs and symptoms of shock.	Most postpartum hemorrhage is caused by uterine atony, which often produces dramatic blood loss. However, blood loss from a laceration or hematoma can be significant, even though it is less obvious.
	Observe for other signs and symptoms of hypovolemic shock.	Excessive blood loss can result in hypovolemic shock.
	If signs of hemorrhage are noted, take appropriate actions according to the probable cause for hemorrhage:	Hemorrhage can cause death of a new mother if not promptly corrected.
	Uterine atony: Massage uterus until firm—do not overmassage; expel blood from uterine cavity when uterus is firm; have breastfeeding woman nurse newborn; notify registered nurse or health care provider for orders and medication if uterus does not become firm and stay firm.	Most minor episodes of uterine atony are easily corrected with fundal massage and newborn suckling. If the uterus does not remain firm, the health care provider examines the woman to identify and correct cause of bleeding. Oxytocin (Pitocin) infusions are often ordered to contract the uterus. Other drugs, such as methylergonovine (Methergine) or prostaglandin, may be needed. Excessive massage of uterus can tire it, possibly resulting in the inability to contract.
	Lacerations: Notify registered nurse or health care provider to examine woman.	Trauma such as laceration or hematoma may require repair by health care provider.
	Hematomas on the vulva: Place cold pack on the area.	Small hematomas on the vulva can be limited by cold applications because they reduce blood flow to areas; cold applications also numb area and make woman more comfortable.

Selected Nursing Diagnosis

Fear related to powerlessness

Expected Outcomes	Nursing Interventions	Rationales
Patient will be able to cope with the unexpected complications.	Identify woman's reaction to unexpected complications and correct misconceptions and exaggerations of fact or myth.	Supplying factual information reduces fear. Identifying reaction establishes basis for intervention.

Continued

Nursing Care Plan 17-1	The Woman with Postpartum Hemorrhage—cont'd	
Expected Outcomes	**Nursing Interventions**	**Rationales**
Anxiety will be at a manageable level.	Be calm and reassuring when in contact with the woman. Encourage woman to verbalize her fears and perceptions. Stay with the woman and her partner.	Anxiety can be transferred by voice or body language. Helps establish a basis for patient teaching and identification of fears. Having a professional presence promotes a feeling of security.

Critical Thinking Questions

1. A patient delivered a healthy 4.4 kg (9 lbs, 11 oz) baby 2 hours ago. The woman's fundus is at the level of her umbilicus; lochia rubra is moderate; and vital signs are blood pressure, 88/46 mm Hg; pulse, 110 beats/minute; and respirations, 28 breaths/minute. What should you assess before calling the health care provider?
2. A woman delivered her fourth child this morning. Her husband comes to the nurses' station and tells the nurse that his wife changed her perineal pad 10 minutes ago and it is already saturated. You assess the woman and find that the uterus is boggy. What nursing actions should you take?

Skill 17-1 Assessment of Uterine Fundus Postpartum

PURPOSE

To assess and maintain uterine tone postpartum.

Steps

1. Place one hand just above the symphysis pubis and exert gentle pressure.

2. Cup the other hand around the uterine fundus.
3. If the uterus does not feel firm, lightly massage it with the hands in the same position.

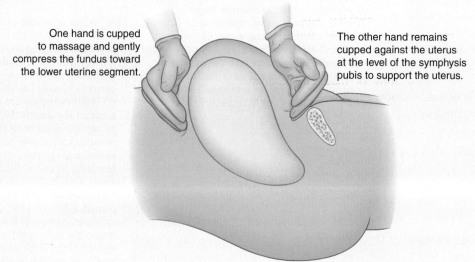

One hand is cupped to massage and gently compress the fundus toward the lower uterine segment.

The other hand remains cupped against the uterus at the level of the symphysis pubis to support the uterus.

necessary. The woman should be assessed for respiratory distress from decreasing blood volume. Oxygen is administered by mask and the woman positioned supine to allow adequate blood flow to her brain and other vital organs.

In planning continuing care, the nurse must remember that the woman will be exhausted after birth, and with additional bleeding, she will feel even more exhausted. The nurse should explain the importance of frequent assessments. Nursing assessments need to be planned so that they can be performed as quickly as possible, allowing the woman time to rest between assessments. Guidelines for managing postpartum hemorrhage can be accessed online (AWHONN, 2006) and sample approaches to managing care can be accessed online at www.cmqcc.org

THROMBOPHLEBITIS AND THROMBOEMBOLISM

Thrombophlebitis is inflammation of the inner blood vessel wall with a blood clot attached to that wall. When the blood clot tears away and moves into the circulation, it is called an *embolus*. If the embolus lands in the lung, it is called a *pulmonary embolus*—a common postpartum complication. Thrombophlebitis can be superficial and involve saphenous or surface veins, or it may be deep (deep vein thrombosis [DVT]) and involve the deep venous system from the foot to the iliofemoral region.

All postpartum women are at high risk for thrombophlebitis because of the normal hypercoagulability of the blood at delivery that prevents hemorrhage, venous stasis from pressure of the gravid uterus, and inactivity (Box 17-3).

Assessment

The nurse, in a routine postpartum assessment, may be the first person to identify signs of thromboembolic disorders. The nurse may note subjective signs of pain when she palpates the calves of the legs for heat and tenderness. Pain in the calf when the foot is passively dorsiflexed is called a positive **Homans' sign.** However, DVT can be present despite a negative Homans' sign. Comparison of pulses in both extremities may reveal decreased blood flow to the affected area. Serial measurements of the affected extremity will reveal an increased diameter (edema and swelling) caused by venous inflammation. Leg pain that extends above the knee may indicate DVT. Fever and chills may occur. Computed tomography or magnetic resonance angiography is helpful to show the presence of a thrombus, and ultrasound or duplex scanning may be used.

Nursing Care

Management for superficial venous thrombosis includes rest, antiembolism stockings, analgesics for comfort, and elevation of the leg. The nurse should

Box **17-3**   Risk Factors for Thrombophlebitis

- Cesarean birth
- Varicose veins
- Inactivity
- Diabetes mellitus
- Smoking
- Obesity
- History of thrombophlebitis
- Prolonged standing or sitting
- Prolonged time in stirrups for delivery
- Parity greater than three
- Maternal age older than 35 years

instruct the woman about the importance of frequent ambulation to prevent this disorder.

Patient Teaching
Measures to Prevent Thrombophlebitis
- Avoid prolonged standing or sitting.
- Elevate legs when sitting.
- Avoid crossing legs (will reduce circulation and encourage venous stasis).
- Exercise to improve circulation (e.g., walking).
- Maintain 2500 mL (2.5 quarts) fluid intake per day.
- Prevent dehydration, which encourages sluggish circulation.
- Stop smoking (a known risk factor).

If the woman is diagnosed with DVT, anticoagulation therapy is started with intravenous heparin administered by continuous intravenous infusion. Doses of heparin are adjusted according to coagulation studies (partial thromboplastin time [PTT]). While the woman is receiving heparin therapy, her platelet count must be monitored closely because of the potential for developing heparin-induced antiplatelet antibodies. The heparin antidote protamine sulfate should be readily available.

Measures to prevent thrombophlebitis should be part of every teaching plan throughout pregnancy and postpartum. Early ambulation, avoidance of prolonged sitting and crossing of legs, elevation of legs when possible, and adequate hydration are important preventive measures.

PULMONARY EMBOLISM

Pulmonary embolism is reported as one of the three leading causes of maternal death, along with hemorrhage and gestational hypertension, and is a feared complication of DVT. It occurs when fragments of a blood clot dislodge and are carried to the pulmonary artery or one of its branches. The embolism can occlude the vessel and obstruct the flow of blood into the lungs. If the pulmonary circulation is severely compromised, death may occur in minutes. An embolectomy (surgical removal of the embolus) may be required.

Signs and symptoms of pulmonary embolism include chills, hypotension, dyspnea, and chest pain. Other signs are tachypnea and apprehension. Immediate medical and nursing interventions include raising the head of the bed to facilitate breathing and administering oxygen by mask. Critical care nursing is necessary, and the woman will be transferred to the ICU.

POSTPARTUM (PUERPERAL) INFECTION

Associated Risk Factors

The uterus and cervix are open after delivery of the fetus and are exposed through the vagina to the external environment. Exposed blood vessels are well supplied, and wounds from lacerations or incisions may be present; therefore, the risk of microorganisms entering the reproductive tract and extending into the blood and other parts of the body is high, which could result in life-threatening septicemia.

Normal physiologic changes that occur during pregnancy increase the risk of infection. During labor, amniotic fluid, blood, and lochia, which are alkaline, decrease the acidity of the vagina; therefore, the vaginal environment encourages the growth of pathogens. Many small lacerations (some microscopic) occur in the endometrium, cervix, and vagina, which allow pathogens to enter the tissues. Infections do not occur in most women, partly because of the presence of granulocytes in the lochia and endometrium, which aid in preventing infection. The most effective method of preventing infection is scrupulous aseptic technique and proper handwashing and gloving during labor, birth, and postpartum care.

A cesarean birth is a major predisposing factor and poses a greater risk than a vaginal birth. This is because of the trauma to tissues during surgery and the fact that many of these women have other risks, such as prolonged labor. When premature rupture of membranes occurs, organisms from the vagina are more likely to ascend into the uterine cavity and increase the risk of infection. Each vaginal examination increases the risk of pathogens entering the vagina and, in effect, being pushed into the cervix. As the area of placental attachment heals, necrotic tissue develops, which provides an ideal medium for bacterial growth. Poor perineal hygiene permits an increase in pathogens entering the vagina. If the woman has a large blood loss or has anemia, she is at increased risk for a postpartum infection because her ability to fight the infection is low.

Postpartum infection (puerperal sepsis) still accounts for significant rates of postpartum maternal morbidity and mortality. Postpartum infections fall into two broad categories. The first covers reproductive system infections (puerperal infection or **puerperal fever**), which are bacterial infections that arise in the genital tract after delivery. The second category includes nonreproductive system infections that arise in sites other than the genital tract and influence maternal morbidity during the postpartum recovery phase. These infections, which include mastitis and urinary tract infections, are indirectly related to the physiologic features of pregnancy, labor, birth, and lactation. A woman is considered to have a puerperal infection if she has a fever of 38° C (100.4° F) or higher after the first 24 hours following delivery and the fever is maintained at least 2 days within the first 10 days postpartum.

Safety Alert

Signs and Symptoms of Postpartum (Puerperal) Infection
- Fever, tachycardia, chills (temperature greater than 38° C [100.4° F])
- Uterine tenderness
- Localized reddened, warm, and tender area
- Purulent wound drainage
- Lochia: appearance varies, depending on causative organism; may be normal, profuse, scant, foul smelling
- Uterine subinvolution (uterus boggy, soft fundus, location higher than normal)
- Malaise

ENDOMETRITIS

Endometritis (also called *metritis*) is the most common postpartum infection. It is an infection of the endometrial lining, decidua, and adjacent myometrium of the uterus. Symptoms begin on the second to fifth day postpartum. This condition affects approximately 1% to 3% of women delivering vaginally and 10% to 15% of those delivering by cesarean birth. Endometritis, if untreated, can quickly progress to **parametritis** (infection spread by lymphatics through the uterine wall to the broad ligament or the entire pelvis) and can spread, causing peritonitis (infection of the peritoneum) and possibly a pelvic abscess.

Signs and Symptoms
The major clinical findings include:
- Onset usually 24 hours after delivery
- Uterine tenderness and enlargement
- Foul odor or purulent lochia that may increase or decrease in amount
- Malaise, fatigue, tachycardia
- Temperature elevation

Assessment and Nursing Care
Blood cultures may reveal the organism involved, and intravenous antibiotics are prescribed. Supportive care includes rest and pain relief. Vital signs and lochia are monitored. Mothers may need to be encouraged to maintain mother-newborn interaction.

WOUND INFECTION
Wound infections are common in women with a history of chorioamnionitis, intraamniotic infection, hemorrhage, underlying medical problems such as diabetes mellitus, and obesity. Multiple vaginal examinations also increase the risk of infection. The most common sites are the perineum, where episiotomies and lacerations are located, and the cesarean surgical incision.

Assessment and Management
REEDA is an acronym for *R*edness, *E*dema, *E*cchymosis, *D*ischarge, and *A*pproximation and is useful in assessing wounds. Cultures are performed to identify the

offending organisms. Episiotomy infection may result in a wound breakdown and stool incontinence, which can further contaminate the site. Drainage of the area, irrigation, and occasionally debridement are necessary. The wound may be packed with sterile gauze, and pain management is offered before dressing changes. Extended hospitalization or hospital readmission may be needed. Frequent perineal hygiene and perineal pad changes are important.

Necrotizing fasciitis is a serious complication of wound infections; women with diabetes mellitus are at highest risk. Symptoms include a blue discoloration and numbness of the wound edges. Aggressive treatment is required because the condition is life threatening. Wound debridement may require follow-up with plastic reconstructive surgery. Patients with chorioamnionitis and endometritis are at risk for septic shock. Symptoms include restlessness, disorientation, and hypovolemia. Acute respiratory distress syndrome (ARDS) or DIC may develop as life-threatening complications. High-level intensive care is required for survival.

URINARY TRACT INFECTION

Urinary tract infection can occur after birth from hypotonia of the bladder, urinary stasis, birth trauma, catheterization, frequent vaginal examinations, or epidural anesthesia. During birth, the bladder and urethra can be traumatized by pressure from the descending fetus. After birth, a hypotonic bladder and urethra can increase both urinary stasis and urinary retention.

Dysuria, frequency, urgency, and low-grade fever may be the presenting symptoms on the first or second postpartum day. Occasionally, fever is the only presenting sign. Pyelonephritis may be accompanied by costovertebral angle tenderness, chills, fever, malaise, hematuria, and nausea and vomiting (Box 17-4).

Cystitis is often treated on an outpatient basis with oral antibiotic therapy. Nursing intervention includes taking vital signs every 4 hours and encouraging increased fluid intake to dilute the bacterial count and flush the infection from the bladder. Acidification of urine inhibits multiplication of bacteria; therefore,

Box **17-4**	**Signs and Symptoms of Postpartum Urinary Tract Infection**

- Cystitis (inflammation of urinary bladder)
- Pyelonephritis (inflammation of kidney)
- Urinary urgency
- Urinary frequency
- Suprapubic pain
- Dysuria
- Hematuria (not always present)
- Fever, chills
- Costovertebral angle tenderness
- Leukocytosis
- Nausea and vomiting

cranberry juice may be recommended. The nurse reviews perineal hygiene and ensures the woman recognizes the need to wipe the perineum from the front to back and to wear cotton underclothing. Antispasmodic or urinary analgesic agents, such as phenazopyridine hydrochloride (Pyridium), may be prescribed to relieve bladder discomfort.

MASTITIS

Mastitis (infection of breasts) usually occurs approximately 2 to 3 weeks after birth and may occur as early as the seventh postpartum day. The infection involves the interlobular connective tissue, usually involving one breast.

Predisposing factors include milk stasis (from a blocked duct), nipple trauma (cracked or fissured nipples), and poor breastfeeding technique. Therefore, the nurse should ensure that the baby is positioned correctly and properly latches onto the nipple, including both the nipple and areola, and that the mother is releasing the baby's grasp on the nipple before removing the baby from the breast (see Chapter 11). Other causes of mastitis are inadequate handwashing between handling perineal pads and then the breasts.

The woman's chief symptoms are a painful or tender localized hard mass and reddened area, usually of one breast (Figure 17-2). She also may have enlarged glands in the axilla on the affected side. Fever, chills, and malaise may accompany the infection and, if untreated, may progress into an abscess.

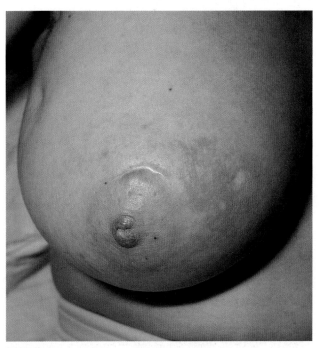

FIGURE 17-2 Mastitis is an infection that usually occurs 2 to 3 weeks' postpartum in the breastfeeding woman. Bacteria usually enter the breasts through small cracks in the nipples. Breast engorgement and milk stasis increase the risk for mastitis.

Nursing Care

With early administration of antibiotics, mastitis usually resolves within 24 to 48 hours, and abscess formation is not common. In many cases, the mother can continue to breastfeed from both breasts. With vigorous sucking, it is thought that the newborn can empty the breast better than a breast pump or manual expression. To prevent stasis of milk, the breasts must be completely emptied at each feeding. This can be done every 1½ to 2 hours to make the mother more comfortable and prevent stasis. The woman is encouraged to wear a well-supporting, properly fitted brassiere. To relieve discomfort, she can take analgesics or use ice or warm packs (whichever feels better). Moist heat promotes comfort and increases circulation. Occasionally, temporary lactation failure may occur in that breast, and the woman may become frustrated and depressed. Weaning during an episode of mastitis can cause an engorgement and stasis that can result in the development of an abscess. To prevent mastitis, the woman should be taught breast hygiene, how to prevent breast engorgement, adequate breast support, proper hand hygiene, and breastfeeding techniques (see Chapter 11).

 Patient Teaching

Self-Care for Mastitis

- Wash hands thoroughly before breastfeeding.
- Maintain breast cleanliness with frequent breast pad change.
- Expose nipples to air.
- Correct newborn latch-on and removal from breast.
- Encourage the newborn to empty the breast because milk provides a medium for bacterial growth.
- Frequently breastfeed to encourage milk flow.
- If an area of the breast is distended or tender, breastfeed from the uninfected side first at each feeding (to initiate let-down reflex in the affected breast).
- Massage distended area as the newborn nurses.
- Report redness and fever.
- Apply ice packs or moist heat to relieve discomfort.

GESTATIONAL DIABETES

Pregnancy is considered to be a "stress test" for glucose homeostasis mechanisms. Therefore, women who develop gestational diabetes during pregnancy can be considered to have "failed that test" and may be at risk for developing type 2 diabetes later in life. ACOG recommends that women who developed gestational diabetes during pregnancy be checked 6 to 12 weeks postpartum and monitored for 5 to 10 years after delivery (Callaghan, 2010). The nurse should provide the mother with patient education materials concerning diabetes mellitus before discharge and refer for follow-up care.

POSTPARTUM SEXUAL DYSFUNCTION

Sexual activity usually decreases in the third trimester of pregnancy but often returns to "normal" by 6 months postpartum. However, sexual activity may be delayed for up to a year in some women who experience trauma during delivery (Katz, 2010). Women who experience a prolonged labor, difficult delivery, episiotomies, or perineal lacerations may develop urinary incontinence that can delay the return to normal sexuality. A decreased hormonal level during breastfeeding may also result in painful intercourse. A distorted body self-image, supported by the media that portray women who regain their pre-pregnant shape within weeks after delivery can also delay the return to pre-pregnant vitality and sexual activity. Of course, sleep deprivation, anxiety, and infant needs can cause stress on relationships that can impact sexual activity. Nurses should provide anticipatory guidance and discuss sexual issues as part of postpartum education. A PLISSIT model to discuss sexual concerns with new parents is available for guidance. The PLISSIT model is an acronym for *Permission* (permission to discuss the problem without feeling they are abnormal); *Limited Information* (concerning causes of the problem); *Specific Suggestions* (techniques to cope); and *Intensive Therapy* (referral to psychologist if other methods fail; the PLISSIT model is merely a framework for intervention to address concerns about a topic many patients are embarrassed to discuss openly) (Katz, 2010).

POSTPARTUM BLUES AND DEPRESSION

Postpartum blues, postpartum depression, and postpartum psychosis are not part of a continuum of the same disorder. The symptoms may be similar, but the conditions are different (Gabbe, Niebyl, & Simpson, 2007).

POSTPARTUM BLUES

Postpartum blues is a transient state of weepiness, mood changes, anxiety, and irritability that occurs in 50% to 80% of women after birth and rarely lasts more than 10 to 14 days. It may be a transient response to rapid role changes and tasks that occur after delivery combined with sleep disruptions. There are no established social, economic, or personality factors that place a woman at risk, and there is no established correlation with changes in hormone levels (Driscoll, 2008). The woman may complain of being overwhelmed and unable to cope and may be oversensitive with periods of unexplained tearfulness. Increased rest, anticipatory guidance, empathy, reassurance, support, and assistance are the treatments of choice.

POSTPARTUM DEPRESSION

The causes of postpartum depression may include an interaction between biochemical, genetic, and psychosocial factors. The signs of postpartum depression include general signs of depression such as weight

usually for the 1st few days

↳ don't interact w/the baby.

loss, sleeplessness, and ambivalence toward the new-born and her family. Postpartum depression occurs in approximately 7% to 50% of new mothers and may have long-term effects on mother-newborn interaction (Callister, Beckstrand, & Corbett, 2010). However, many cases of postpartum depression go unrecognized and untreated. Some women do not seek care due to lack of access, lack of time, stigma associated with depression, and child care issues.

Symptoms of postpartum depression may be evident before hospital discharge, and patients at risk should be scheduled for follow-up visits before the traditional 6-week postpartum visit. Women at high risk for postpartum depression have risk factors such as:

- Unstable or abusive family environment
- History of previous depressive episode
- History of limited support system
- Low self-esteem
- Dissatisfaction with education, economics, or choice of partner
- Dissatisfaction with the gender of the newborn

Women may evidence anxiety, sleeplessness, feelings of guilt, agitation, feelings of worthlessness, and have difficulty concentrating and making decisions. Depression may not be the first sign. Nurses should be sensitive to the different ways women perceive, display, and report symptoms of depression. Screening strategies and education of parents concerning signs and symptoms should start in the postpartum unit. Culturally sensitive postpartum care provides the woman with the opportunity to discuss the birth, future plans, and support systems.

The Edinburgh Postnatal Depression Scale (EPDS) is a 10-question survey that can identify women at high risk of depression (Beck, 2008). Treatment includes supportive counseling and medication with selective serotonin reuptake inhibitors or tricyclic antidepressants. Symptoms may last up to a year; untreated women may progress to psychosis and suicide.

POSTPARTUM PSYCHOSIS

The symptoms of postpartum psychosis are similar to those of other psychoses. Early signs of depression may be evident, or it may start abruptly within a few

Suicidal / harming the neonate

days after childbirth. Confusion, restlessness, anxiety, and suicidal thoughts may occur, and delusional thoughts may be expressed. The woman and her newborn are at risk for their safety. Psychiatric supervision is necessary, and antipsychotic medications may be prescribed.

The Nurse's Role

A combination of factors may be involved in the cause or predisposition to postpartum depression, and nurses can play a key role in providing appropriate support and referral for the mother, based on assessments and data collection during care. Screening strategies should start in the postpartum unit. Nurses must be sensitive to the different ways women perceive, explain, and report symptoms of depression. Culturally appropriate postpartum care that encourages expressions of feelings, validating the mother's emotions, addressing personal conflicts, and reinforcing personal power and autonomy may be helpful if the mother finds her view of motherhood in conflict with what she believes society expects of her. If a new mother perceives herself as lacking social support in her new role, referral to social agencies or couples therapy may be helpful. Postpartum support groups and screening tools are available in some communities and online (Beck, 2008).

Not every new mother feels competent to manage the role, plans motherhood at that particular time in her life, or has a realistic view of her new responsibilities. A woman's culture, experiences, and coping strategies influence her adjustment to becoming a mother. Helping a new mother resolve these issues and referring her for appropriate guidance can help prevent or alleviate postpartum depression (Douglas, Pierce, Rosenkoetter, Callister, Hattar-Pallara, et al., 2009). Telling a new mother what her newborn needs and how she should respond to newborn cues may not help the depressed mother develop the feelings of competence or confidence that she needs. The nurse must listen to the woman's concerns, respect the woman's knowledge, and help her use her own strengths and resources to meet her challenges.

Get Ready for the NCLEX® Examination!

Key Points

- Postpartum hemorrhage is blood loss exceeding 500 mL in a vaginal delivery and 1000 mL in a cesarean birth. Hemorrhage may occur early or late in the postpartum period. Leading causes of early postpartum hemorrhage are uterine atony, lacerations, and retained placental

- fragments. The leading cause of delayed hemorrhage is subinvolution of the uterus, which may result from retained tissue fragments.
- Thromboembolic disorders can complicate the postpartum period. Changes in the blood coagulation system during the postpartum period place the woman at

risk for thromboembolic conditions such as superficial venous thrombophlebitis and DVT. A life-threatening complication is pulmonary embolism, which requires immediate intensive care.

- Pulmonary embolism, although not common, is reported as a major cause of maternal death. It occurs when fragments of a blood clot dislodge, are carried to a pulmonary artery, and block the flow of blood into the lungs.
- Puerperal infections involving the reproductive system account for many complications in the postpartum period.
- Two common postpartum infections are mastitis and urinary tract infection.
- Postpartum blues is commonly observed and is a transient experience of mood changes, weepiness, and anxiety.
- Understanding factors that may contribute to postpartum depression can aid in developing a care plan.
- Postpartum depression has more intense and long-lasting symptoms of depression that interfere with caring for the newborn and maintaining family relations. The assistance of a psychiatrist can help the woman develop effective coping strategies.

Additional Learning Resources

SG Go to your Study Guide on pages 505–506 for additional Review Questions for the NCLEX® Examination, Critical Thinking Clinical Situations, and other learning activities to help you master this chapter content.

⊖volve Go to your Evolve website (http://evolve.elsevier.com/Leifer/maternity) for the following FREE learning resources:

- Animations
- Answer Guidelines for Critical Thinking Questions
- Answers and Rationales for Review Questions for the NCLEX® Examination
- Concept Map Creator
- Glossary with pronunciations in English and Spanish
- Patient Teaching Plans
- Skills Performance Checklists and more!

Online Resources
- www.awhonn.org
- www.babycenter.com/pregnancy/pregcomplications/index
- www.cmqcc.org
- www.depressionafterdelivery.com
- www.nlm.nih.gov/medlinePlus/postpartumdepression.html
- www.postpartum.net
- www.postpartumsupport.com
- www.postpartumstress.com
- www.4woman.gov/faq/postpartum.htm

Review Questions for the NCLEX® Examination

1. Postpartum hemorrhage is traditionally defined as the loss of more than 500 mL after an uncomplicated vaginal birth or:
   1. 600 mL after a cesarean birth
   2. 800 mL after a cesarean birth
   3. 1000 mL after a cesarean birth
   4. 1200 mL after a cesarean birth

2. When performing a morning assessment on a 1-day postpartum mother, the nurse notes excessive bright red vaginal bleeding with uterine fundus firmly contracted. The nurse suspects:
   1. Hematoma
   2. Placenta accreta
   3. Disseminated intravascular coagulation
   4. Lacerations

3. The first action with uterine atony should be to:
   1. Assess for bladder distention.
   2. Massage the uterus until firm.
   3. Express clots.
   4. Administer oxytocin intravenously.

4. The physician has ordered an accurate assessment of blood loss on a postpartum patient. When subtracting the weight of a dry perineal pad from a saturated pad the nurse notes a weight of 7 g. This blood loss would be recorded on the liquid section of the output record as:
   1. 7 g
   2. 7 mL
   3. 0.07 kg
   4. 3.5 cc

5. It is suspected that a woman on the postpartum unit has a deep vein thrombosis. The nurse can expect the possibility of which diagnostic test(s) to be ordered to confirm this diagnosis? (Select all that apply.)
   1. Computed tomography
   2. Magnetic resonance angiography
   3. Ultrasound
   4. X-ray

6. What are the most common cause(s) of early postpartum hemorrhage? (Select all that apply.)
   1. Retained placental fragments
   2. Subinvolution
   3. Uterine atony
   4. Laceration
   5. Infection

7. What are the three leading causes of maternal death? (Select all that apply.)
   1. Pulmonary embolism
   2. Endometritis
   3. Hemorrhage
   4. Gestational hypertension
   5. Necrotizing fasciitis

Critical Thinking Questions

1. A married woman, age 36 years, had twins. She had prolonged labor but delivered vaginally. Two hours after the delivery, she began bleeding excessively. What do you think is the potential cause of the excessive bleeding? What nursing action must you immediately consider?

2. A woman has extreme perineal pain 1 hour after birth. The physician performed a midline episiotomy before the delivery of her daughter, and the nurse applied an ice pack to her perineum. You are assigned to the woman's care. What nursing interventions will you provide?

The Pregnant Adolescent and Maternity Nursing in the Community

Objectives

1. Define key terms listed.
2. Review the phases of adolescent development.
3. Discuss the impact of pregnancy on the development of the adolescent.
4. Examine the influence of pregnancy on adolescent fathers.
5. Discuss the impact of unplanned adolescent pregnancy on achieving the tasks of pregnancy.
6. Explain the risks related to childbearing in adolescents.
7. Outline the health education needs of the adolescent.
8. Recognize two major risks for newborns of adolescent mothers.
9. Name three specific sexually transmitted infections that are increased in the adolescent population.
10. List reasons for the high rate of contraceptive failure in adolescents.
11. List the principles involved in counseling adolescents.
12. Discuss community approaches to pregnancy prevention in adolescents.
13. Explain three ways to offer continuity of follow-up care to families who are discharged early from the hospital after childbirth.
14. Describe a prenatal home visit.
15. Outline postpartum teaching that may be provided in the home.
16. Identify two high-risk newborn conditions that may be followed at home.
17. Discuss legal liability and home care.
18. Review the nurse's role in home care of new mothers and newborns.
19. Review and discuss the *Healthy People 2020* objectives related to maternal-infant care.

Key Terms

adolescence (p. 355)
advice telephone lines (p. 365)
hotlines (p. 367)

pelvic inflammatory disease (PID) (p. 362)
warm lines (p. 367)

THE ADOLESCENT AS OBSTETRIC PATIENT

Adolescent pregnancy continues to be a social, economic, and health concern in the United States and worldwide. Rates of adolescent pregnancies, abortions, and live births are significantly higher in the United States than in most other developed countries. Clearly, nursing professionals must be aware of all aspects of teen pregnancy. They must be familiar with developmental tasks of adolescents and recognize that teen pregnancy comes at a time when the developmental tasks of adolescents are incomplete. The adolescent is not prepared psychologically or economically for parenthood; thus, both the adolescent (mother or father) and the child are at high risk. This chapter explores the physiologic and psychosocial aspects of pregnancy regarding the adolescent and society, risk factors and outcomes of pregnancy, parenting, and sexually transmitted infections (STIs).

ADOLESCENT DEVELOPMENT

Adolescence is the period of transition from childhood to adulthood. It involves change, and adolescents often feel a sense of stress and anxiety throughout this period (Table 18-1). Nurses must understand the types of physical and psychological changes that face the adolescent and the sources of frustration they meet in society. Although specific ages are assigned to young or early adolescents (10 to 13 years), middle adolescents (14 to 16 years), and late adolescents (17 to 20 years), passage of these periods is smooth for some and stormy for others, and some adolescents never complete all aspects of the journey.

Table 18-1 Social Influences of the Community on Adolescent Behavior

TASK WITHIN THE COMMUNITY	INFLUENCE	RESULTS
Change from elementary school to middle school and high school with new organization of classes.	Changes from core home room classes to independent classes with different teachers are representative of leaving the family concept of elementary school to independent concept of middle school and high school.	The community reinforces the decreasing role of family values and controls and increases self-control and self-responsibility. Selection of classes and friends in this new setting is crucial to positive developmental outcome.
Respond to economic pressure and job availability for funds.	Teens need money for fad foods, stylish clothes, and dates and look for sources of income.	In the United States, laws concerning the number of hours young adolescents can work after school keep focus on school; decreased school attendance leads to increased risk behaviors.
Teens must develop their own sense of self as it relates to their own sexuality in order to prevent interpreting the public availability of condoms and other barrier control methods of contraception as permission to believe that it is OK to have sex if they use them and that they are safe from unintended pregnancy.	The devices available in public places do not come with detailed instructions on use. Often the teen will be embarrassed to ask questions.	Providing contraceptive devices without appropriate teaching on proper use leads to ineffective birth control, sexually transmitted infections, and unplanned pregnancy.

The adolescent is confronted by developmental tasks, which vary slightly in different cultures. Tasks and issues that are especially significant during adolescence have been described by many researchers. Major tasks for the adolescent include developing:

- An identity
- Autonomy and independence
- Intimacy in a relationship
- Comfort with one's own sexuality
- A sense of achievement

EARLY ADOLESCENCE: AGES 10 TO 13 YEARS

Early adolescence is a period of rapid growth and development. The physical changes involve all body systems but especially the cardiovascular, musculoskeletal, and reproductive systems. The adolescent's self-image is affected as he or she attempts to incorporate both physical and psychological changes. These young adolescents have questions about menstruation, breast development, testicular and penis size, and wet dreams. They wonder whether they are normal and compare themselves with their peers. During early adolescence, exploratory sexual behavior may occur with friends of the same or opposite sex.

During this phase, thinking remains concrete, and the young teenager lacks the capacity for abstract thinking or introspection. The early adolescent has a rich fantasy life. Peer acceptance and conformity are important to the adolescent and may result in parental-adolescent conflict.

MIDDLE ADOLESCENCE: AGES 14 TO 16 YEARS

Physiologic growth and development of secondary sexual characteristics may be completed during this period. Middle adolescents focus on making their appearance as attractive as possible. At this time, in an effort to adjust to body changes, adolescents experiment with new images. They use peers to share experiences and try out new roles. Adolescents in this age group have the ability to think more abstractly and may begin to realize the limits of their potential. For those in disadvantaged situations, a feeling of hopelessness may begin. The middle adolescent may become increasingly self-centered and feel invincible. While testing the limits of power, teens may engage in high-risk behaviors. Experiments with drugs, alcohol, and sex are avenues for rebellion. This can be a period of great turmoil for the family as the adolescent struggles for independence and challenges family values and expectations. During this time, adolescents would like to be treated as adults; however, their behavior fluctuates. They may or may not recognize that risk-taking behaviors can bring negative consequences.

LATE ADOLESCENCE: AGES 17 TO 20 YEARS

Late adolescence is characterized by the ability to maintain stable, reciprocal relationships. The family becomes more important; however, independence from parents is a major part of the developmental task. By late adolescence, many teens have more realistic images of themselves and are more secure about their appearance.

Sexual identity is usually firmly established during late adolescence. Problem solving is used to view consequences of behavior, and plans are more future-oriented. Ideally, the late adolescent will have developed an ability to solve problems, assess many aspects of life situations, and delay immediate gratification. It is important for them to understand the impact of their choices on their future. For example, they need to think through the consequences of not using birth control;

recognize that using contraception will prevent pregnancy; and be aware that unprotected sex can lead to illness, which may involve discomfort or be life threatening.

ADOLESCENT PREGNANCY

INFLUENCES ON SEXUAL BEHAVIOR

The meaning of sexuality to adolescents is influenced by communication and visual images. Adolescents' communication with their parents may be open or limited. Teenagers may avoid conversations about sexuality with their parents because they perceive that their parents send negative messages (admonitions) about sex, resulting in feelings of ambivalence, guilt, and fear for the teen. Some parents live vicariously through their teens and may send messages that actually encourage risk-taking behaviors.

Televisions and computers and the Internet in the home create an environment in which the adolescent can observe sexual activity and form opinions about sexuality. Some adolescents confuse what is portrayed by the media as moral standards or publicly acceptable standards of behavior.

Schools may or may not include sex education in the curriculum. The impact of learning about sexuality in school and from parents, peers, and the media has been studied, and broad well-prepared programs introduced early can have a positive impact. We do know that the outcomes of active sexual behavior are often an unplanned pregnancy and STIs. Health care providers must make use of every opportunity to counsel adolescents about their sexual behavior.

Health Promotion

Preventing Teen Pregnancy

Approaches include providing:
- Anticipatory guidance
- School education programs
- Improved access to health care and counseling
- Use of emergency contraceptives as appropriate
- Ready access to nurse or physicians
- Choice of positive group membership (e.g., Scouts)
- Choices and ability to be autonomous

According to comments made by teenagers, risk-taking behaviors with uncertain outcomes are enjoyable, the consequences do not seem that great, and "everybody else is doing it—why shouldn't I?" Some adolescents are known to brag about their sexual experiences. An adolescent boy may not want to be stigmatized as being the only virgin in his group, and, as a result, sexually inexperienced adolescents conform to their peers. In other words, many adolescent boys and girls become sexually active not because of sexual desire, but because of the need to belong to the group (Table 18-2).

Table 18-2	Psychosocial Tasks that Influence Sexual Activity, Pregnancy, and Parenting in Adolescents		
PSYCHOSOCIAL TASK	**INFLUENCES**	**RESULTS**
Develops sense of identity	Influenced by friends, media, and parents, young adolescents are interested in experimenting, whereas older adolescents are interested in commitment.	Dysfunctional, absent, or strict family may increase rebellious response, negative self-image, and risk-taking behaviors.
Is egocentric and self-centered	Does not think of others or effect of behavior on newborn or responsibility of parental role.	Self-centered behavior contributes to failed relationships. Adolescent may not respond to needs of newborn, resulting in safety concerns.
Seeks independence from family	Values of peers become more important than values of parents; late adolescent selects role models, rejects parents' rules, and develops own personal values.	Young teens respond to peer pressure; this may influence need to "belong" and influence sexual behavior; Scouts, sports, and church groups provide positive role models.
Develops emotional intimacy	Develops role models, heroes, close friends of same and, later, opposite sex.	Teen may misinterpret intimacy as sexual relationships and may be disappointed that early sexual relationships are not always related to intimacy or commitment.
Develops sexual identity	Accepts puberty and develops relationships.	Sexual abuse and peer pressure can influence early sexual activity and positive sexual identity; early sexual activity is correlated with poor school performance at all socioeconomic levels.
Develops sense of career and future	Choice of future depends on exposure and opportunities available.	Use of contraceptives is higher in adolescents with career goals.
Develops sense of morality	Operational thought begins in middle adolescence, and personal code of ethics emerges.	Knowledge does not consistently control behavior. Proper role models are helpful guides to adolescents.

PREVENTION OF ADOLESCENT PREGNANCY

In 1996, the U.S. Congress authorized Title V, Section 110 of the Social Security Act, providing funding to administer abstinence-only sex education in school programs and omitting content related to contraception, abortion, and safer sex. Sex education in the schools remains a controversial topic, and there is little agreement about specific content to be taught. Some schools teach abstinence-only programs, and some teach abstinence along with safe sex practices and STI prevention. In one study, abstinence-only programs did not delay intercourse, improve birth control, or decrease pregnancy rates (Oski, 2010). The effective prevention of teen pregnancies and STIs may need to involve theory-based education as well as behavior control (Jemmott, Jemmott, & Fong, 2010). The U.S. teen pregnancy rate for 15 to 17 year olds fell from 77.1 per 1000 in 1990 to 44.4 per 1000 in 2002. Sixty percent of adolescents today are using some form of contraceptive compared to 46% in 1991, and nearly half of the 15 to 19 year olds in the United States report having at least one sexual experience. Eighty percent of teen pregnancies are unplanned, and, although this is a decline since the 1980s and 1990s, it still indicates a need for teen education and counseling (Oski, 2010).

The National Campaign to Prevent Teen Pregnancy is an organization that has a goal of reducing the rate of teen pregnancy by one third between 2006 and 2015. Teen pregnancy in the United States cost taxpayers $9.1 billion in 2004, with a $1 billion cost in Texas alone and a $12 million cost in Vermont. This organization distributes user-friendly educational materials for practitioners, policy makers, and advocates. Parents may not realize the impact they have in preventing teen pregnancy over their child's teen peers. The organization also distributes a curriculum-based pamphlet for educational programs and offers tips for parents in how to intervene and prevent teen pregnancy.

The overwhelming consensus is that adolescent pregnancy is a serious problem. As the adolescent matures, parents have less influence on behavior, and peers have more. Peer pressure controls many behaviors. The desire to please peers, the feeling of invincibility, and the belief that "everyone is looking at me" contribute to participation in high-risk behaviors. The occurrence of sexual abuse and date rape contribute to pregnancy in the adolescent (Box 18-1). Pregnancy prevention programs in schools and the media should assist teens in focusing on their future education and career goals and provide information concerning birth control and STI prevention.

CONFIDENTIALITY AND THE ADOLESCENT

Confidentiality laws differ in various states, meaning that some adolescents may not have access to confidential counseling and contraceptive advice. If the health

---

| Box 18-1 | Date Rape Prevention Teaching Guidelines |

- Do not get into a vehicle with someone you have just met.
- When you begin to date someone, go on a double date, participate in group activities, or meet in public places.
- When meeting in public places, provide your own transportation to avoid being alone in a car with an acquaintance.
- Never be alone in a private residence, hotel room, or secluded place with someone you barely know.
- Request to drive separately when invited to a party; you can leave immediately if you feel uncomfortable.
- Do not accept beverages at parties or from a stranger unless you observe them being prepared.
- Keep beverages within sight at all times and hold at waist level or above. Dispose of any beverage left unattended.
- Before dates, tell someone where you are going and when you expect to return.
- Plan ahead what you would do if your date tried to force or started intimidating you to have sex.
- Program your cell phone to call 911 with an easy dialing code. When out alone on a date, keep your cell phone on and easily accessible.
- Trust your instincts and leave whenever you feel uncomfortable.

For more information, see National Dating Abuse Helpline, www.ndvh.org/press/article.php?id5110, and http://loveisrespect.org/.

care worker cannot ensure confidentiality, some teens will not seek health care. Adolescents are at greater risk for complications than adults because they are the least likely to seek early health care.

All 50 states have enacted legislation that entitles adolescents to consent to treatment with confidentiality for "medically emancipated conditions." Although the law varies from state to state (see Online Resources), the list of medically emancipated conditions generally refers to contraception, pregnancy, pregnancy-related care, STIs, substance abuse, and sexual assault. The Health Insurance Portability and Accountability Act (HIPAA) ensures patient privacy in all adult cases. All 50 states allow confidential STI testing of adolescents.

PREGNANCY AND THE ADOLESCENT

Menstruation is a sign of a girl's transition into womanhood and fertility and is celebrated in many cultures. However, in the United States, it is often viewed as a nuisance, stressful, and sometimes uncomfortable. Many young women opt to take medications to reduce the number of menstrual periods from the natural 12 times a year to 1 or 3 times a year. This may prevent unplanned pregnancies but these methods do not protect against STI infection.

Because teens may not receive accurate information elsewhere, parents must be open to discussing sexuality with their adolescent children, and the community must have input to educational programs through organizations such as the parent-teacher associations

(PTAs). Providing education and accessible care can have a positive impact on preventing adolescent pregnancy and helping teens understand their own emotional and physical feelings. Nurses can use creative ways to incorporate sexuality information into regular clinic visits. Sexuality should be discussed in the context of relationship issues, rather than dos and don'ts of safe practice. The American Cancer Society recommends that regular Pap smears should begin about 3 years after sexual activity, and the test should be integrated into the health education plan. The impact of pregnancy on the adolescent is discussed in Table 18-3.

TERMINATION OF EDUCATION

Teenage pregnancy remains the main cause of dropping out of school for adolescent girls. Sexual activity is often associated with poor school performance. The level of formal education is an important predictor of job advancement and earning potential. Adolescent girls who have not completed high school are more likely to be unemployed or employed in entry-level jobs, and lack job security. Generally, in addition to holding low-paying jobs, they may have no health care benefits for themselves and their children.

ADOLESCENT FATHERS

It is estimated that 1 in 15 boys fathers a child while he is a teenager. In general, the adolescent father faces sociologic and psychological risks. Many adolescent couples do not plan to marry; however, if the adolescent boy is from a rural area or a specific cultural group, marriage is more likely. Some adolescent fathers, even without marriage, may be involved in the adolescent girl's pregnancy and child rearing.

Adolescent fathers tend to achieve less formal education than older fathers, and they enter the labor force earlier and with less education. The stresses of pregnancy on the male adolescent come from several sources. He is likely to face a negative reaction from his own family and from the girl's family. The young girl's parents may refuse to let him see their daughter, which often makes him feel isolated, alone, and unable to give her support. His future career may be threatened by early marriage or quitting school to support the pregnant girl and new child. Also, his relationship with his peers is altered.

The lack of responsibility shown by some adolescent fathers is a reflection of cultural and community attitudes. Sometimes an adolescent's ability to impregnate may be viewed, among peers, with a sense of pride and as a sign of manhood.

As part of counseling, the nurse should assess the young man's stressors, his support system, and his plans for involvement in the pregnancy. If the father is involved in the pregnancy, the young mother may feel less alone and may be better able to discuss her future plans. The young father should be welcomed in the prenatal sessions.

A sizable number of fathers are 6 or more years older than the adolescent mother. Some younger girls are more likely to have much older sexual partners. Older sex partners may be supportive of the pregnant adolescent before the delivery, but their relationship

Table 18-3	Developmental and Physiologic Impact of Pregnancy on the Adolescent	
FACTOR	**RISK**	**EFFECT**
Age at which pregnancy occurs	At menarche, the first menstrual cycles are irregular and anovulatory.	"Natural" methods of birth control are ineffective in young adolescents.
	Young adolescents have immature vascular development in the uterus.	Condition may lead to gestational hypertension and fetal perfusion problems that result in poor pregnancy outcome, such as prematurity and low birth weight.
	Long bone growth is incomplete until 2 years after menses start.	Pregnancy before long bone growth is complete can cause early closure of epiphysis because of increase in estrogen.
	Pelvis does not reach adult size and dimensions until 3 years after menarche.	A small pelvis increases problems during labor and delivery and increases need for cesarean birth.
Nutritional intake	Dietary intake often contains "empty" calories and consists of fad diets; eating disorders may be present; dieting to control weight and meet media definition of a beautiful body is common.	Inadequate nutrition, especially in early months of pregnancy, results in negative pregnancy outcome and birth defects. Poor nutrition can result in gestational hypertension, low-birth-weight newborn, and prematurity.
Sexual activity	Multiple partners or unprotected sex can result in sexually transmitted infections (STIs).	STIs increase risk to fetus and newborn.
Limited access to health care	Adolescent may fear revealing pregnancy to parents.	Delayed prenatal care can result in problems for mother and fetus.

Studies have shown that pregnancy in late adolescence accompanied by good prenatal care is not as high risk for physiologic problems as in early and middle adolescence. A multidisciplinary approach is essential because teen pregnancy is a complex problem.

with the mother and newborn may weaken over time. Before delivery, many unwed fathers may plan to contribute to the support of the mother and newborn, but during delivery, most adolescent girls select their mothers as their support person.

NURSING CARE OF THE PREGNANT ADOLESCENT

ANTEPARTUM CARE OF ADOLESCENTS

During the first prenatal visit, the teen should be welcomed and praised for seeking prenatal care. Knowledge of the adolescent's individual needs, cultural preferences, and developmental level is essential in planning effective prenatal care and education (Table 18-4). Teaching techniques most effective for adolescents include orienting care protocols to current needs and using visual aids and simple language. Immature communication skills may prevent the teen from expressing herself and asking questions about the pregnancy. Pregnant adolescents should be screened for STIs and substance abuse and offered detailed, mutually developed nutritional plans. Eating foods rich in calcium and vitamin D, regular exercise and muscle activity is necessary for bone health in the adolescent as well as fetal development during pregnancy. A support person who accompanies the adolescent to the clinic should be actively involved in the prenatal education. Community resources and agencies for additional information and counseling should be provided.

CARE OF THE ADOLESCENT DURING LABOR AND DELIVERY

The adolescent is often modest and may not tolerate pain well. Breathing and relaxation and concentration techniques require patience that many teens lack. Pain control and adequate coaching are essential, especially if a support person is not present. Suggestions to an adolescent support person must be given in a clear, concrete, detailed manner and involve specific directions and activities. The nurse must carefully explain to the adolescent in labor what is being done and what can be expected in order to prevent fear from developing and establish a trusting patient-nurse relationship.

CARE OF THE POSTPARTUM ADOLESCENT

The adolescent may have inadequate coping skills to manage the transition to parenthood and parenting responsibilities. She may feel overwhelmed. Issues of child care, finances, schooling, and family dynamics need to be addressed. Encouragement, support, instruction, and an opportunity to practice perineal self-care and care of the newborn should be provided. The nurse can help adolescent parents integrate the newborn into their lives and offer them resources in the community for follow-up care. Grandparents who take over the complete care of the newborn may interfere with the teen's development of parent-newborn attachment and adversely affect the teen's self-image and future parenting skills. Grandparents can be encouraged to help with household tasks and offer positive suggestions and guidance that enable the teen parent to develop coping and parenting skills.

ADOLESCENT PARENTING

The transition to parenthood is not easy for adolescents. Often they still have unmet needs in their own phase of development. Acceptance of the role of parenting, including the responsibility of newborn care and their changed self-image, now sets them apart from their peers. Often they feel excluded from desirable "fun"

Table 18-4	Nursing Care and the Effect of Adolescence on the Tasks of an Unplanned Pregnancy		
STAGE OF PREGNANCY	**TASK**	**ADOLESCENT RESPONSE**	**NURSING INTERVENTIONS**
First trimester	Confirmation of pregnancy	Fear of telling may result in delayed confirmation, hidden pregnancy, and delayed prenatal care.	Educate concerning signs and symptoms of pregnancy so as not to confuse with other conditions. Discuss options concerning pregnancy and the plan for the baby. Discuss health behaviors required for healthy fetus.
Second trimester	Focus on newborn as real	Family chaos may result when parents and father and friends see reality of pregnancy; adolescent may try to maintain control by dieting and continuing to conceal pregnancy. Egocentric phase may prevent full focus on baby as being real.	Preserve adolescent image in clothes needed during pregnancy. Discuss disclosure to parents and friends. Discuss prenatal needs; show attractive pictures of fetus at various gestational ages.
Third trimester	Preparation for newborn and birth process	Adolescent focuses on ending experience but may fear labor; may not wish to bond or consider needs of newborn.	Initiate discussion of child care; tour facility and refer to community agencies as needed; provide education regarding birth process.

activities characteristic of others their age because they are prematurely forced into the adult role.

Parenting programs available for adolescent mothers may be limited or nonexistent in the community. Adolescent mothers may also find they have little social and financial support. Many adolescent girls welcome the assistance of newborn care offered by their mothers, aunts, or grandmothers. In some cultures, a designated member of the family may accept the complete responsibility of rearing the child.

Many adolescent mothers tend to have repeated pregnancies that are closely spaced, which increases the risks to their health, continued education, and economic future. These factors create family instability and further impair good parenting. If the couple marries as teenagers, divorce tends to be more common.

Characteristic adolescent mother child-rearing practices have been identified, including insensitivity to newborn behavioral cues (e.g., crying, soiling diaper), pattern of limited nonverbal interaction, lack of knowledge of child development, preference for aggressive behavior and physical punishment, and limited learning in their home environment. Adolescent mothers tend to be at risk for non-nurturing behaviors, particularly in areas of inappropriate expectations. They may expect too much of their children because of limited knowledge of child developmental tasks. Adolescents often characterize their newborns as being "fussy." This description may relate to lack of knowledge that newborn crying is expected behavior. These findings suggest a need for parenting classes for high school students.

Nurses must understand that the adolescent faces many hardships of living in two worlds—adolescence and motherhood. Appointment schedules need to be flexible, or follow-up care may not be sought. Support groups and child care resources may be needed so the adolescent can finish school and participate in some adolescent-type activities. Referral to agencies or professionals to help the adolescent develop coping skills and adapt to the parenting role may be necessary to develop a plan for a more positive future.

URINARY TRACT INFECTIONS AND SEXUALLY TRANSMITTED INFECTIONS IN ADOLESCENTS

URINARY TRACT INFECTIONS

Urinary tract infections (UTIs) in sexually active young women must be differentiated from STIs. Periurethral bacteria ascend into the bladder, especially after sexual intercourse. Spermicidal coated condoms can alter vaginal flora allowing colonization of bacteria that increases the risk for UTIs. Voiding after sexual intercourse is encouraged. Signs and symptoms of UTIs include:

- Suprapubic pain
- Urgency and frequency

- Hematuria
- Back pain

The drugs used to treat the adolescent with a UTI include nitrofurantoin or trimethoprim and sulfamethoxazole (TMP-SMX), which replaces amoxicillin as the drug of choice for a 3- or 7-day course. Nursing care and teaching include encouraging a glass of cranberry juice every day, which prevents *Escherichia coli* from colonizing the wall of the bladder and probiotics to maintain a normal protective flora.

There are usually no vaginal signs and symptoms (e.g., vaginal discharge) with a UTI. Generally speaking, urinary signs and symptoms *without* vaginal discharge often means a diagnosis of UTI, whereas urinary signs and symptoms *with* vaginal discharge often result in the diagnosis of an STI (Robbins & Shew, 2010).

SEXUALLY TRANSMITTED INFECTIONS

Unprotected sexual behavior among teens can have two major consequences: pregnancy and STIs. The Centers for Disease Control and Prevention (CDC) state that people younger than 25 years account for half of new STIs in the United States (Oski, 2010). It is estimated that 46.8% of U.S. high school students have had sexual intercourse with 14% having had multiple partners (Ventura, Abma, Mosher, & Henshaw, 2008).

Adolescents often do not seek health care because of limited access, preference for nonpharmacologic birth control methods, involvement with multiple partners, fear of lack of confidentiality, lack of knowledge about free programs, and other personal preferences. Attention to these factors is essential to reduce the alarming STI incidence among adolescents. The role of a nurse as a health care provider is to use all opportunities to increase adolescents' understanding of the relationship of their lifestyle to their health, including STIs.

Adolescent girls are biologically more susceptible than adult women to STIs because of epithelium that is present on the cervix (Kliegman, Behrman, Jenson, & Stanton, 2007) and the typical risk-taking behaviors common in this age group. Because young teens are concrete thinkers, they often do not seriously consider long-term effects of their actions. STIs are discussed in more detail in Chapter 20.

DIAGNOSTIC TESTS

A pelvic examination may be required to obtain specimens for testing. Nucleic acid amplification tests (NAATs) are highly sensitive tests for *Chlamydia* and *Neisseria gonorrhoeae* and use urine samples for testing. A DNA probe for the diagnosis of vaginitis and bacterial vaginosis, candidiasis, and trichomoniasis is also available. Other tests are available that use first-void urine specimens in male patients and a vaginal fluid specimen in female patients.

Teen Pelvic Examination

- Use a slender speculum.
- Provide privacy.
- Provide chaperone or support person.
- Use specially trained team with assault kit and support person if needed.
- Maintain confidentiality.
- Fully inform adolescent of any legal requirements (a teen who is voluntarily sexually active needs confidentiality, whereas a teen who is being sexually abused needs protection).

TREATMENT REGIMENS

Single-dose therapy is available for chlamydia, gonorrhea, and trichomoniasis, and follow-up care is advised. Quinolones are not recommended for treatment of gonorrhea infections in Hawaii, Asia, and the Pacific and are contraindicated in persons younger than 18 years (see Chapter 20). Bacterial vaginosis can be treated by intravaginal metronidazole gel or an oral metronidazole pill for 7 days. It is recommended that the teen abstain from alcohol during treatment and avoid latex barrier contraceptives if intravaginal (oil-based) gel is used. Vulvovaginal candidiasis can also be treated with a single-dose tablet of fluconazole.

Pelvic inflammatory disease (PID) is a common complication of STIs in adolescents and can increase risk for ectopic pregnancy, infertility, and chronic pelvic pain later in life. PID is an infection of the upper genital tract, endometrium, fallopian tubes, and adjacent structures, usually from organisms present in the lower genital tract (vagina). Broad-spectrum antibiotics are the treatment of choice.

PREVENTION OF STIs

Teaching developmentally appropriate, positive health behaviors, and "safer sex" practices such as proper condom use and effective communication techniques is an important strategy for STI prevention. Risk assessment and preventive screening are essential for sexually active teens.

CONTRACEPTION AND ADOLESCENTS

Adolescents who are sexually active often do not use contraceptives correctly. There may be an increase in the use of condoms among adolescents; however, their use is not consistent. Many adolescents believe that preparing for sexual intercourse by having contraceptives available interferes with the spontaneity and romance of the moment. Many teenagers think that they are not vulnerable to pregnancy (i.e., they will not become pregnant). Others, because of confusion or misinformation about the physiology of their bodies, do not understand the risk of pregnancy. Many

girls are afraid that they will be considered "bad girls" if they use contraception because that means they have planned for sexual intercourse. Many adolescents are not aware that withdrawal at the beginning of ejaculation is not an effective birth control technique because the pre-ejaculate fluid contains sperm.

Adolescent boys are known to carry condoms in their wallets merely as a symbol. However, body heat can decrease effectiveness of the spermicide contained within the condom. Many boys say they do not use condoms because it can decrease their pleasure. Other adolescents say that they do not use contraceptives because they do not anticipate having intercourse.

Other factors contributing to the use or disuse of contraceptives include availability, cost, and confidentiality. In a large study (Guttmacher Institute, 2006) found that many students may be unaware of their rights to confidentiality for certain health problems (Box 18-2).

In counseling adolescents about contraception, the nurse must consider the adolescent's maturity level, moral and religious beliefs, motivation to avoid pregnancy, frequency of intercourse, regularity of menses, and knowledge of risks of contracting STIs, including human immunodeficiency virus (HIV) or acquired immunodeficiency syndrome (AIDS). Adolescents need education about all contraceptive methods, including abstinence. The method chosen should reflect the teenager's lifestyle. Outcomes of active sexual behavior must be emphasized. Emergency contraception is available within a 5-day window of unprotected sexual intercourse and is effective (Glasier, Cameron, Fine, et al., 2010). Contraception is discussed in detail in Chapter 19.

| Box 18-2 | Legal Issues of Adolescent Care |

In the United States, state laws give the minor some rights to give consent without parents' knowledge. The treatment of sexually transmitted infections (STIs) is addressed by special health statutes in some states, and this may extend to the treatment of drug abuse and mental health problems. Providing contraceptives to teens without parental consent is still a legal issue in some states, as is the right of a minor to seek abortion without parental consent. Minors may be exempt from parental consent in the following conditions:

- Emancipated minor status: If the adolescent lives away from home, is married, or is in the military service, treatment can be provided.
- Emergencies: If the delay required for parental consent would jeopardize the minor's life, treatment can proceed.
- Low risk: In some cases of low-risk treatment, documentation by the health care provider that informed consent was obtained and the teen appeared mature may be sufficient.

A mandatory report to the state is required when:

- Child abuse (including rape) is involved or suspected.
- Danger to the minor is evident (requires appropriate referral for protection).

ELECTIVE ABORTION

Many adolescent pregnancies are terminated by elective abortion, which is not an easy decision for most teenagers. Many adolescents are aware of conflicting religious and moral views about abortion, and some view having a baby as exciting without understanding the responsibilities involved. Many adolescents do not know where to seek services or various options such as adoption; they may lack transportation to facilities or the financial means to pay for services available. The parents of the adolescent often intervene in the decision to carry the pregnancy to term or to seek termination of the pregnancy. Adolescents may be in denial about their pregnancy or not tell their parents for fear of violence or loss of support. The delay in discussing their pregnancy may limit the options available. Professional counseling is essential to avoid serious psychological consequences in later life. Effective, early contraceptive education can prevent the need for abortion in adolescents. Abortions are discussed in detail in Chapter 13.

PRENATAL PROGRAMS AVAILABLE TO ADOLESCENTS

Three types of programs that offer prenatal care to adolescents are clinic programs, private medical services, and school-based programs. The choice of program depends on the program's accessibility and the financial circumstances of the adolescent and her family. Private practice care is provided by physicians in a single or group practice or associated with managed health care organizations. Until the Health Care Reform Act of 2010, these services were usually available only to people who were covered by a medical insurance plan or who could afford to pay. For families without insurance or financial resources, an option is medical assistance paid by Medicaid benefits or through federal programs. The community nurse may act as a resource by providing the family with a list of health care practitioners who accept Medicaid patients. Principles of teaching the adolescent are reviewed in Box 18-3.

Nurses can provide or refer young parents to education or counseling programs designed for adolescents. School-based and community clinics and school curricula can help adolescents delay pregnancy or assist them in understanding basic child care. Sex education and guidance to prevent repeated pregnancies can be provided during well-child clinic visits.

Adolescent pregnancy and parenting issues are complex and challenge nurses to search for effective approaches to reduce or alleviate the problems (Box 18-4). Some high schools offer "reality experiences" with computerized dolls that help teens role play and understand parental responsibilities. Interventions

---

Box 18-3 **Principles of an Effective Adolescent Interview and Teaching Session**

- Establish rapport.
- Assure patient of confidentiality.
- Fully inform.
- Provide privacy.
- Be nonjudgmental.
- Respect maturity of adolescent.
- Provide open communication lines.
- Use open-ended questions.
- Give opportunity for adolescent to express concerns.
- Recognize positive success and achievements of teen.
- Allow sufficient time for interview.
- Use native language of adolescent or an interpreter.
- Provide follow-up or referral as needed.
- Provide anticipatory guidance.
- Provide contraceptive, drug, and alcohol information.
- Discuss high-risk behavior.
- Let the adolescent make final choices and decisions.

that promote positive choices, nurturing attitudes, and self-esteem among adolescents should be a goal of the nurse (Table 18-5).

COMMUNITY RESPONSIBILITY

The National Campaign to Prevent Teen Pregnancy, initiated in 1996, is a private, nonprofit organization made up of a broad spectrum of religious, political, social, human services, health, and academic organizations. The Association of Women's Health, Obstetric and Neonatal Nurses (AWHONN) is one of the professional organizations that joined this group and has made a commitment to focus on prevention of adolescent pregnancy. In its first year, the national campaign allocated money to fund better evaluation of adolescent pregnancy programs and offered some incentive grants for communities. In addition, the national campaign has a task force to review the incidence of adolescent pregnancy and another task force to review the research on the effectiveness of pregnancy prevention programs.

Thus far, the campaign has found that adolescent pregnancy is a multifaceted problem with no easy answers. The best approach in local areas is strong, community-wide involvement with a variety of programs directed at multiple causes of the problem. The national campaign's task force has identified the following critical characteristics of successful programs:
- Involvement of adolescents in planning the programs
- Role models from the same cultural and racial backgrounds
- Long-term and intensive programs
- Focus on adolescent needs and providing confidentiality
- Nonjudgmental counselors who understand the developing adolescent

Box 18-4 **The Nurse as an Adolescent Counselor**

1. Nurses who counsel adolescents must consider special factors when planning their educational programs:
   - Adolescents may know little about their own anatomy.
   - Adolescents may understand little about the physiology of menstruation and conception.
   - Adolescents are risk takers.
   - Adolescents feel "it can't happen to me."
   - Adolescents often do not ask about contraception because they expect that adults will tell them not to be sexually active and think they are "bad."
   - Adolescents need secrecy and will not discuss their sexual activity unless they feel their discussion will be held confidential.
   - Adolescents may be noncompliant in taking daily medication (pills).
2. The nurse who counsels adolescents should use audiovisual materials such as samples, pictures, and anatomic models. The adolescent should help in selecting the method of contraception to be used and should have a backup if a problem arises. Condoms should be used to prevent STIs, even if other methods of pregnancy prevention are selected.
3. The nurse should counsel the adolescent in a private setting to ensure confidentiality and answer all questions completely. Role-playing and referral to a female nurse practitioner rather than a male physician may be acceptable to some female adolescents who require follow-up care.
4. The nurse should provide referral sources and discuss options available with the teen who is pregnant.
5. The nurse can involve the community in accepting responsibility for meeting the needs of adolescents and reducing adolescent pregnancy and its associated problems by:
   - Encouraging business groups or organizations to "adopt a school" and help plan educational programs
   - Involving the community in fund-raising for educational programs and teen centers
   - Including teens as leaders in planning and implementing programs
   - Targeting high-risk populations, especially in shopping malls
6. Community programs developed should include:
   - Community health clinics for teens
   - Teen hotlines
   - Prevention of school dropout
   - Job opportunity and training
   - Sex education and sexually transmitted infection prevention
   - Parenting classes
   - Peer counseling
   - Activities for teens in a safe environment

Table 18-5 **Coping with Teen Problems**

TEEN CONCERN	NURSING INTERVENTIONS
Need for acknowledgment of sexuality	Initiate discussions.
Fear of parental knowledge	Provide confidentiality.
Fear of unknown	Provide factual information.
Ambivalence	Inform of positive effects of contraception.
Lack of funds	Refer for community assistance or Medicaid coverage.
Contraceptive use failure	Discuss backup plans; educate regarding technique.
Noncompliance	Encourage counseling before deciding to discontinue; provide telephone numbers of help lines and hotlines.
Need for peer acceptance	Use group teaching and discussion.

OVERVIEW OF ISSUES IN OBSTETRICAL HOME CARE

In response to efforts at containing health care costs, consumer demand for participation in their own care, and the availability of new technologies, options concerning health care delivery continue to be developed. A dramatic increase has occurred in both antepartum and postpartum maternal-newborn home care. Both low-risk and high-risk women and newborns, if they meet certain criteria, are able to be monitored or treated at home, whereas previously they would have been kept in the hospital.

Essential teaching and patient or caregiver competencies must be achieved and documented before hospital discharge of a high-risk patient. For postpartum care, these include cord and circumcision care, use of a bulb syringe, maternal perineal hygiene, diet, breast care and breastfeeding, exercise, rest, and follow-up care. Written instructions are included because often the excitement of the moment decreases retention of the information given. In 1996, the Newborns' and Mothers' Health Protection Act was signed into law and guaranteed a 48-hour hospital stay for normal births and a 96-hour stay after cesarean birth. Many states mandate home care follow-up for women discharged in less than 48 hours.

HOME CARE SETTINGS

Community health nurses have long been providers of maternity and pediatric home care. Traditionally, professional nursing care has been delivered in the home by community health nurses within a public health system or by visiting nurse agencies. The goals of community health nursing have always included **health promotion** and **disease prevention.** The movement toward patient-managed high-technology care, both prenatal and postpartum, in the home setting continues to rise. Advances in portable machines and wireless technology allow care in the home that in the past could be given in the hospital only. Wireless Internet provides the nurse with access to patient information and the orders of the health care provider. The goals of home care services are to fill the gap made by the brief hospital stay, coordinate multidisciplinary care, and make appropriate referrals. Home care can take place in the patient's own home, short- or long-term care facilities, foster care, or hospice care. Telephones, hand-held computers, Internet and e-mail, and videoconferencing are also available and part of the home health care scenario.

PROTOCOLS AND TOOLS

Maternal-newborn professional organizations have developed tools, such as a critical pathway, to delineate a time frame for all significant tasks to be accomplished during a hospital stay (see Chapter 1). Emphasis is placed on identifying learning needs and skills most essential in the peripartum period and in providing supportive newborn care. Written material is given to the women to aid in the teaching and learning process. Help or advice telephone lines are used for extended home care, but this method relies on the family to initiate the telephone contact and usually deals with immediate concerns. E-mail is a method of communication between the family and the health care provider or nurse via the electronic medical record (EMR). Many managed care organizations send health care publications to their members' homes, offering timely tips on health care. Some hospitals have a maternal-newborn outpatient clinic to replace or supplement a home visit program. Nursing protocols for postpartum home care are available from the AWHONN and are used as guidelines for assessing families.

The nurse assists in teaching, caregiving, and preparing the woman and her family for discharge. The nurse also collaborates with the woman in planning the extended care in the home and counsels and provides referrals as needed.

LEGAL ISSUES

The provision of home care services is not without risk of legal liability. Two types of legal liability that can be faced by home care agencies and nursing staff are **professional negligence** and **violation of state licensing laws.** The nurse can be involved in a lawsuit for professional negligence when a patient is injured or dies, and it is alleged that the nurse or other home health care team member's conduct was the direct, or proximate, cause of the injury or death. The nurse must have a thorough understanding of the nurse practice act related to his or her level of expertise and be careful to work within those guidelines, referring the patients as needed. Counseling and advice must be objective and have a sound rationale. Community health nurses need to have maternal-child nursing knowledge and skills, teaching skills, the ability to work with a multidisciplinary team, use high technology, and communicate effectively. Telephone counseling is also a type of home care. Telephone techniques require special triage competence. Open-ended questions reveal information necessary to determine whether a problem is serious and requires immediate medical care or not serious and can benefit from telephone advice and reassurance. Written protocols and guidelines are usually provided.

To reduce the risks of legal liability, **consent forms** and **documentation** are extremely important. Health care interventions must be established on a sound scientific basis and backed up by evidence-based practice. In the home, the nurse must act as a member of the interdisciplinary health care team and maintain close communication with the team members to ensure that proper patient care is provided. AWHONN has identified the knowledge and skills necessary for competent nursing practice in providing perinatal care in the home setting. Clinical protocols and pathways for home care have been designed, and adherence is reviewed by accrediting agencies such as The Joint Commission (TJC).

ALTERNATIVE HEALTH CARE PRACTICES

The nurse in the home care setting can best observe the use or abuse of home remedies, the impact of cultural practices and alternative health care practices on the pregnant or postpartum woman, and their effect on the outcome of pregnancy. See Chapter 21 for a detailed discussion of alternative health care practices.

HOME PREGNANCY TESTS

Home pregnancy tests are sold over the counter in most drugstores at a reasonable cost, and the nurse is often asked about their reliability. If the test result is positive, the mother should be encouraged to seek early prenatal care. The positive pregnancy test does not confirm a uterine pregnancy but merely confirms presence of human chorionic gonadotropin (hCG) in the urine. Other conditions requiring immediate care, such as ectopic pregnancy or hydatidiform mole, could cause a positive pregnancy test.

PRENATAL HOME VISITS

Home care during pregnancy usually includes a discussion of:

- Physiologic and psychological changes
- Compliance with prenatal visits
- Use of monitors or other special instructions
- Common discomforts of pregnancy

Self-care for common discomforts of pregnancy, including good body mechanics and other preventive care, is reviewed by the nurse with the pregnant woman in the home. The nurse also reviews the use of home monitors and kick counts for prenatal women. The home setting is the ideal place to review home safety and medicines in the woman's medicine cabinet that should be avoided during pregnancy or while breastfeeding.

PRENATAL CARE FOR LOW-RISK PREGNANCIES

Home care can be beneficial to a pregnant woman, especially if the woman is having difficulty accessing health care. There may be a lack of locally available health care facilities, problems with transportation to the facility, or difficulty with available appointment times because of family responsibilities or employment hours. The nurse can help identify and remove barriers that are keeping the woman from attending the prenatal clinic appointments.

The nurse conducts typical prenatal health assessments and interventions. He or she takes a health history and performs screening procedures typically conducted in the office or clinic, including vital signs, urine screen, weight, fundal height, dietary intake, hygiene, and physical activity. Depending on the gestational age, the nurse listens to fetal heart rate and discusses fetal activity with the woman. The nurse discusses the use of phone contact as an option for continuity of care. He or she also mentions available social support services. Documentation of all assessments made by the nurse is essential.

Throughout the home visit, the nurse takes the opportunity to teach self-care, including changes that may indicate a potential health problem. Health education is aimed at reducing poor health habits, such as smoking. The nurse provides anticipatory guidance to help the family plan for changes that must be made after the birth of the newborn, such as identification of an available support person. The nurse can assist the parents in preparing for newborn needs (e.g., crib). The extended family should be involved in the planning, and the nurse should be culturally sensitive.

PRENATAL CARE FOR HIGH-RISK PREGNANCIES

In high-risk pregnancies, limited activity is commonly prescribed to prevent preterm delivery and to provide time for the fetus to develop in utero. Home care allows a more normal environment while minimizing family disruption and allows the woman to have greater control while continuing to receive safe, supervised health care. The nurse discusses the importance of rest and asks whether any barriers, such as caring for other children or family members, will keep the woman from carrying out the prescribed treatment.

A woman who is at risk for preterm delivery may be discharged from the hospital to be monitored at home. Home fetal assessments include kick counts. Although three kicks per hour is average, if there are fewer than 10 movements in 12 hours, the woman should contact her health care provider (Gabbe, Simpson, & Niebyl, 2007). Kick counts provide reassurance of fetal life, assist in bonding, and help the mother take responsibility for fetal surveillance. Some monitoring devices can transmit information by phone to a central unit at the hospital, where it can be evaluated by the expert health care provider. The home nurse may also review techniques for monitoring glucose levels when indicated and reinforce responses to the test results.

Set standards and criteria must be met for women to be eligible for home care in a high-risk pregnancy. Standard protocols for the home care of high-risk pregnancies have been developed by the American College of Obstetricians and Gynecologists (ACOG).

Education concerning signs and symptoms of preterm labor, the use of the monitor, and the importance of communication with the advice nurse by phone is reinforced with each home visit. The nurse reviews the woman's ability to cope with her home environment and responsibilities, assesses her compliance, and documents an individualized care plan for each patient visit made.

POSTPARTUM HOME VISITS

POSTPARTUM CARE FOR LOW-RISK MOTHERS

Postpartum home visits are an extension of the hospital or agency service. The decision to extend home visits beyond one or two times depends on the family's needs. The mother is assessed to determine whether her recovery is proceeding normally and whether any complications exist. The newborn is assessed for normal and potentially abnormal clinical findings (e.g., jaundice). Referrals are made as needed.

Documentation is extremely important and includes recording the assessment findings, interventions, and teaching provided. Documentation serves as a legal record of the visit and also justifies reimbursement or payment for the services.

Early discharge from the hospital setting places a special responsibility on the home care nurse concerning the mother's health and the baby's progress. Promoting bonding between parents and child, observing the parent's ability to care for the child and recognize cues regarding needs, and assessing flexibility of care are important activities that should be documented (Figure 18-1). Kangaroo care (i.e., skin-to-skin contact) should be encouraged (see Skill 15-2). This can be done with preterm and term newborns.

Readiness for learning does not always occur in the first days of the postpartum hospital experience. The nurse reviews warm lines, which are telephone numbers that can be used to answer questions that may arise, and hotlines, which are telephone numbers that can be called 24 hours a day in case an emergency arises.

The nurse answers questions concerning common postpartum discomforts (such as episiotomy sutures, constipation, cramping, lochia, and resumption of sexual activity) and discusses complaints or problems (such as urinary burning). Optimum rest periods, the use of a support person, and psychological status (postpartum blues) are discussed. The nurse also reviews family planning issues. The family picture is more readily available to the home care nurse who actually sees the home situation, and he or she can be a valuable link with the maternity staff for follow-up care and referral. Adaptation to the new roles of parenthood can be best evaluated by the use of open-ended questions such as, "What is it like being a new father?"

Postpartum home care goals include assessing, teaching, counseling, and referral (Box 18-5). Documentation of the information provided in the hospital can aid the home care nurse in deciding which areas of teaching need coverage or reinforcement for the individual patient and family. The postpartum visit is a short-term plan in normal situations. Further follow-up is usually initiated by the mother by using a telephone warm line or hotline for advice.

The postpartum home care nurse usually prepares content for the visit, plans the travel and directions

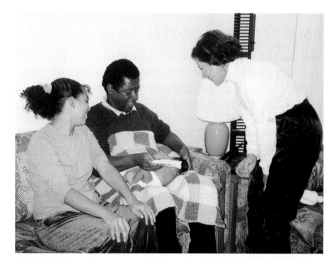

FIGURE 18-1 A father learns how to dress a newborn under the guidance of a home health nurse.

Box 18-5   Guidelines for Postpartum Home Visit

PRE-VISIT PREPARATION
- Inform family about the purpose of the visit.
- Establish a convenient time for the visit. Confirm address and route to family home.
- Obtain written consent for skilled nursing services to be provided.
- Obtain a physician's order for procedures such as blood tests.
- Review all appropriate information for mother and newborn (e.g., hospital discharge summaries, referral forms).
- Identify appropriate community resources and teaching material to meet needs.

IN-HOME INTERVENTIONS
- Introduce self and establish purpose of postpartum follow-up visit.
- Establish trusting relationship by brief period of social interaction.
- Obtain complete health history for both mother and newborn.
- Perform complete physical assessment for mother, including vital signs, breast examination, fundal height, lochia, and episiotomy or abdominal incision.
- Perform complete physical assessment for the newborn, including vital signs, weight, hydration, and bowel and bladder functions.

- Throughout visit, collect data to assess emotional adjustments of individual family members to newborn and lifestyle changes.
- Perform procedures or treatments, such as a phenylketonuria (PKU) blood test, ordered for newborn.
- Assess the safety of the home environment, including the newborn's sleeping arrangements.
- Assess mother's ability to provide care, including emergency care and cardiopulmonary resuscitation.
- Provide teaching regarding previously identified problems.
- Refer family to appropriate community resources, such as warm lines and support groups.
- Develop plans for subsequent visits if authorized.

IN-HOME END OF VISIT
- Summarize the main points of the visit with the parents.
- Provide information about reaching the nurse or agency if needed before the next scheduled visit.

POST-VISIT ACTIVITIES
- Document the visit thoroughly to serve as a legal record of the visit and to allow third-party reimbursement.
- Communicate with appropriate care providers as needed.

(ensuring her own safety in unfamiliar neighborhoods is important), consults with the office or hospital staff, and reports findings to the health care provider. Postpartum parenting classes are available in some communities to discuss postpartum self-care, exercises, newborn care, bonding, and parenting issues (Figure 18-2). Videos are available at community libraries, and newsletters are often part of a hospital's follow-up care program. The Internet has become an avenue for information, but the nurse needs to assist parents in assessing the reliability of the source or website.

HOME CARE FOR LOW-RISK NEWBORNS

During the routine newborn follow-up visit at home, the nurse observes and demonstrates, as needed, newborn positioning, carrying, home facilities, household safety, and the condition of the newborn's cord and circumcision areas. Information concerning growth and development, anticipated safety needs, immunizations, and follow-up care is discussed. Bonding between parent and child is a major goal. The nurse also reviews newborn feeding technique, including formula preparation or breastfeeding. A lactation consultant can be contacted if needed.

HOME CARE FOR HIGH-RISK NEWBORNS

Apnea monitoring and **phototherapy** are the most common monitoring procedures performed at home for high-risk newborns (see Chapter 16).

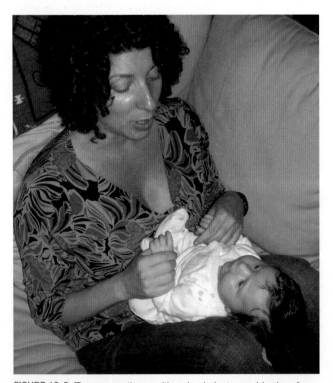

FIGURE 18-2 The new mother positions her baby to provide close face-to-face interaction to promote bonding.

Jaundice

Because newborns are especially at risk for dehydration and jaundice, which may not be manifested before discharge, most pediatricians recommend that early newborn discharge include follow-up home visits within at least 48 hours after birth. Assessments of degree of jaundice, normal stool patterns, newborn behavior, and maternal-newborn interaction can be critical for the newborn's well-being. Some agencies have standing orders to obtain blood for specific reasons; therefore, if the newborn appears jaundiced, a heel stick for bilirubin levels may be performed.

If the bilirubin level is elevated, the newborn can receive phototherapy at home. The parents are taught how to assess the newborn and how to use the equipment. A fiberoptic phototherapy blanket (BiliBlanket) is effective and easy to use (Figure 18-3). During phototherapy, bilirubin in the skin absorbs the light and changes into water-soluble products, which can be excreted in the bile and urine, thereby lowering the elevated serum bilirubin level and decreasing the potential for neurologic damage. Hyperbilirubinemia and phototherapy are discussed in Chapter 16.

Respiratory Problems

Newborns with suspected respiratory problems may be sent home with oxygen or an apnea monitor. The home health nurse must assess the use of the equipment and parent competencies in cardiopulmonary resuscitation (CPR) for the newborn. Strategies to prevent overprotection are important.

BREASTFEEDING

Healthy People 2020 set a goal to increase to at least 82% the number of women who begin breastfeeding by the time of discharge from the hospital, exclusively breastfeed for at least 6 months, and continue breastfeeding for 1 year. The goals also include increasing "baby friendly hospitals" and workplace accommodations for breastfeeding. The World Health Organization (WHO) recommends breastfeeding to 1 year of age and encourages breastfeeding until age 2. Breast milk provides a specifically tailored combination of proteins, carbohydrates, and fats for the newborn. In addition, breast milk provides immunologic protection against infection and may decrease the incidence of chronic illnesses later in life. Breastfeeding also facilitates early maternal-newborn attachment. The nurse can assist the mother in breastfeeding techniques and refer to community sources for continued support and guidance. Breastfeeding techniques are discussed in Chapter 11.

Breastfeeding education and intervention home visit programs are available to provide in-home support for mothers and newborns who are thought to be at high risk for breastfeeding failure. One or two home visits often enable mothers and newborns to

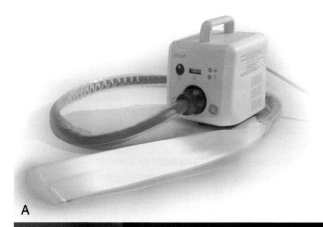

and others stay with friends or live in the garage of extended family. Homeless women often have difficulty accessing care, receive care from different health care providers at different sites, and have incomplete medical records. Follow-up is difficult. Before discharging a mother with her newborn infant, it is essential to determine that she has a place to go and has a way of obtaining help for herself or her newborn. The nurse can be a key link in facilitating referrals to outreach programs, support services, counseling, shelters, and follow-up medical care.

Much of the homeless population in the United States results from domestic violence or single-parent poverty. The parent and newborn health problems involved with homelessness include malnutrition, respiratory and nutritional disorders, lack of preventive care, and development or continuation of high-risk behaviors (such as use of drugs or alcohol and prostitution) or mental illness, to survive in the streets. The benefits offered in the Health Care Reform Act of 2010 have not yet been evaluated, and some actions do not take effect until the year 2014. Often the nurse's first contact with a pregnant homeless woman is late in her pregnancy unless a serious complication developed that caused the woman to go to a public health care facility for care.

Nursing intervention includes getting involved with the community leaders and legislators, speaking out, identifying women at risk, providing support and referrals to existing community resources, educating for self-care, and documenting the woman's inability to obtain care as evidence of a community problem. Free or low-cost child health care is available, and nurses should be aware of how to refer families to these agencies.

Affordable child care is a challenging issue, and any nurse in the home or community setting should inquire about facilities used. Women who try to work and support themselves need to have child care for their preschool children. National goals for *Healthy People 2020* include national accreditation of childcare

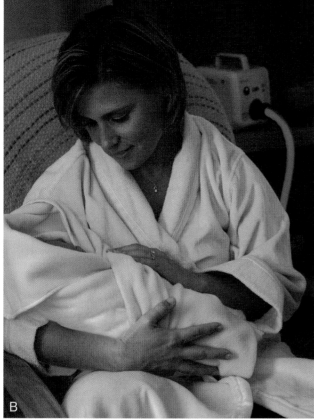

FIGURE 18-3 BiliBlanket plus high output phototherapy system. A, A pad of woven fibers is used to transport light from a source to the newborn. This fiberoptic pad is wrapped directly around the newborn's skin to bathe the skin in light. **B,** The newborn can then be diapered, clothed, held, and nursed during treatment at home. Eye protection is not necessary.

breastfeed with success. In many communities, the home health nurse can call on a lactation specialist to assist in initiating the breastfeeding process (Figure 18-4).

THE HOMELESS MOTHER AND NEWBORN

Homelessness is defined as a lack of a permanent home and is not limited to women who must live on the street. Some women live in single-room hotels,

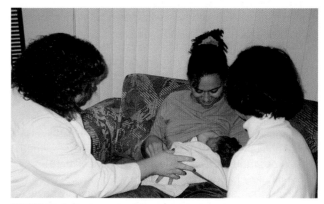

FIGURE 18-4 The home health nurse and a lactation specialist help the mother develop good breastfeeding techniques.

facilities with background checks for all workers and interventions in the community to prevent teen pregnancy.

COSTS OF EARLY DISCHARGE AND HOME CARE

The potential reduction in the cost of hospital care is a positive benefit of early discharge programs. It is argued that the true cost of early discharge and services compared with the longer hospitalization stay has not been thoroughly analyzed. Post-discharge services, such as follow-up visits by maternal and newborn health care providers, have not always been included in these data. Consequently, although hospital costs have decreased, total costs for the care of the mother and newborn are unknown. Continued research is necessary.

HEALTHY PEOPLE 2020

The origins and purpose of the *Healthy People* program are discussed in Chapter 1. Goals of *Healthy People 2020* focus on health promotion and illness prevention rather than disease specific objectives seen in *Healthy People 2010*. Many *Healthy People 2010* objectives have been retained in *Healthy People 2020*, and several new objectives have been added that are related specifically to adolescents and maternal-infant care. These include:
- Improving the health of women, infants, and children by:
  - Providing genetic counseling and education about nutrition and weight maintenance
  - Increasing access to preconception and pregnancy care
  - Providing pregnancy planning and prevention
  - Increasing baby-friendly hospitals
  - Increasing to 82% of mothers who exclusive breastfeeding for 6 months and increasing workplace accommodations for breastfeeding
- Improving the health development and safety of adolescents by:
  - Reducing STI infections
  - Reducing delinquency, violence, and teen pregnancy
- Using genomics to support health and early intervention
- Using health information technology to improve communication

A comprehensive and detailed listing of the goals can be found on the *Healthy People* website in the Online Resources at the end of the chapter.

Get Ready for the NCLEX® Examination!

Key Points

- Adolescence is a period from the beginning of puberty to maturity. Early adolescence is 10 to 13 years of age, middle adolescence is 14 to 16 years of age, and late adolescence is 17 to 20 years of age. Specific developmental and psychologic behaviors are characteristic of each phase.
- Specific tasks of adolescence include developing an identity, autonomy and independence, intimacy, comfort with one's own sexuality, and sense of achievement.
- Peer values become more important to adolescents than parents' values, and risk-taking behavior is seen as a way of conforming to peer groups.
- Increased sexual activity is associated with poor school performance.
- The adolescent father is likely to face negative reactions from his own family and from the pregnant girl's family. His future career may be threatened by early marriage or quitting school to support the pregnant girl and new child. Also, his relationship with his peers can be altered.
- Accepting the new role of parenting includes accepting responsibility of newborn care, developing a self-image that differs from that of their peers, and being excluded from desirable "fun" activities. Pregnant teens are prematurely forced into the adult role.
- The newborns of adolescent parents commonly have major risks such as preterm birth and low birth weight.

Factors that influence these newborn risks are low socioeconomic status, inadequate prenatal care, poor weight gain, inadequate nutrition, and smoking.
- Many adolescents are involved in risk-taking behaviors, which include taking drugs and alcohol; smoking; and becoming sexually active and participating in unprotected sex with multiple partners.
- Among adolescents the incidence of STIs is high, especially gonorrhea, chlamydia, genital herpes, genital warts, and HIV infection.
- Preventing teen pregnancy and STIs may need to involve both theory-based education as well as behavior control.
- Periurethral bacteria can ascend into the bladder after sexual intercourse and cause urinary tract infection.
- Community health nurses have long been providers of maternal-newborn home care. Their emphasis has been on health promotion and disease prevention. The more recent movement is for patient-managed, high-technology health care in the home setting.
- Home care services are not without risk of legal liability. Two types of legal liability face home care professionals: professional negligence and violation of state licensing laws. Consent forms for nursing care and documentation of all nursing interventions are essential.

- Home care visits during the prenatal period can help women with high-risk pregnancies monitor themselves at home.
- Home care programs for postpartum follow-up care are offered by hospitals, childbirth centers, public health agencies, private physicians, and independent entrepreneurs.
- The variety of postpartum follow-up services includes early discharge classes, hospital outpatient clinics, telephone follow-up, warm lines, hotlines, home visit follow-up, and support groups.
- Postpartum home visits include assessments of the mother and newborn. Questions are answered, and teaching is reinforced. The nurse can refer the family to community resources as needed.
- The most common special equipment for home health care of high-risk newborns is for apnea monitoring and phototherapy.
- The home health nurse is part of an interdisciplinary team and coordinates care with other health care providers, maintaining communication.
- *Healthy People 2020* proposes many goals related to maternal-infant care that can be achieved by nurses in the community and patient education.

Additional Learning Resources

SG Go to your Study Guide on pages 507–508 for additional Review Questions for the NCLEX® Examination, Critical Thinking Clinical Situations, and other learning activities to help you master this chapter content.

 Go to your Evolve website (http://evolve.elsevier.com/Leifer/maternity) for the following FREE learning resources:

- Animations
- Answer Guidelines for Critical Thinking Questions
- Answers and Rationales for Review Questions for the NCLEX® Examination
- Concept Map Creator
- Glossary with pronunciations in English and Spanish
- Patient Teaching Plans
- Skills Performance Checklists and more!

Online Resources
- www.arhp.org
- www.asrm.org
- www.bestbonesforever.gov/whatsbest/calcium/index.cfm
- www.cdc.gov/nchs/fastats/teenbrth.htm
- www.dol.gov/ebsa/newsroom/fsnmhafs.html
- www.guttmacher.org/pubs/FB_sexEd2006.html
- www.healthypeople.gov/hp2020
- www.law.cornell.edu/Topics/table_Emancipation.htm
- www.teenpregnancy.org/resources/data/pdf/STBYST06.pdf

Review Questions for the NCLEX® Examination

1. Sexual identity is usually firmly established during:
   1. Early adolescence
   2. Middle adolescence
   3. Late adolescence
   4. Early adulthood

2. Early adolescence is a period:
   1. Of rapid growth and development
   2. When development of secondary sexual characteristics may be completed
   3. When problem solving is used to view consequences of behavior
   4. When teens are more secure about their appearance

3. Many adolescent boys and girls become sexually active because of:
   1. Sexual desire
   2. A need to belong to the group
   3. A need for physical intimacy
   4. A desire to have a child

4. A clinic nurse is providing education to a female patient. When instructing the patient, the nurse includes that the American Cancer Society recommends that regular Pap smears should begin:
   1. Immediately following menarche
   2. After the first sexual experience
   3. At 16 years of age
   4. About 3 years after sexual activity

5. Development of which characteristic(s) would be included in the major tasks for the adolescent? *(Select all that apply.)*
   1. Trust
   2. Identity
   3. Intimacy
   4. Independence
   5. Career satisfaction

6. All 50 states have enacted legislation that entitles adolescents to consent to treatment with confidentiality for "medically emancipated conditions." Which condition(s) generally would be characterized as medically emancipated? *(Select all that apply.)*
   1. Pregnancy
   2. Sexually transmitted infections
   3. Substance abuse
   4. Contraception
   5. Sexual assault

Critical Thinking Questions

1. A 16-year-old adolescent, whom you met in an ambulatory clinic, has been menstruating regularly for approximately 2 years. She appears anxious and tells you that she has not menstruated for 2 months. What questions would you ask to help her identify the potential problem?

2. After discharge from the hospital, a newborn became jaundiced. Bilirubin was found to be elevated, and fiberoptic phototherapy was prescribed with a BiliBlanket. Explain to the mother how the BiliBlanket reduces the bilirubin.

3. Review the *Healthy People 2020* proposed goals. Select one and discuss how the nurse can help achieve that goal.

chapter

19

Family Planning and Infertility

evolve

http://evolve.elsevier.com/Leifer/maternity

Objectives

1. Define key terms listed.
2. Identify factors that influence the woman's choice of contraceptive method.
3. Discuss five types of contraception.
4. Explain how the male condom should be used to be most effective.
5. Describe a method of contraception that reduces the risk of sexually transmitted infections.
6. List advantages and disadvantages of five types of contraception.
7. Explain male sterilization.
8. Explain female sterilization.
9. Discuss the role of the nurse in caring for patients with contraceptive or fertility problems.
10. Describe a therapy to facilitate pregnancy.
11. Review factors that contribute to infertility.
12. Describe four types of treatment protocols in the management of infertility.

Ⓧ test!

Key Terms

assisted reproductive technology (ART) (p. 385)
basal body temperature (BBT) (p. 373)
Billings method (p. 373)
calendar method (p. 374)
cervical cap (p. 376)
cervical mucus method (p. 373)
chemical predictor test (p. 374)
coitus interruptus (KŌ-ĭ-tŭs ĭn-tĕ-RŬP-tŭs, p. 381)
contraception (p. 372)
diaphragm (DĪ-ă-frăm, p. 376)
ELLA (p. 381)
female condom (p. 376)
fertility (p. 383)
infertility (p. 383)

intrauterine device (IUD) (ĭn-tră-Ū-tĕ-rĭn, p. 378)
male condom (p. 375)
mittelschmerz (MĬT-ĕl-shmĕrtz, p. 374)
oral contraceptives (OCs) (p. 378)
Plan B (p. 380)
spermicides (SPĔR-mă-sīdz, p. 374)
spinnbarkeit (SPĬN-băr-kīt, p. 373)
sterilization (stĕr-ĭ-lĭ-ZĀ-shŭn, p. 381)
symptothermal method (sĭmp-tō-THĔR-măl, p. 374)
therapeutic insemination (thĕr-ă-PŪ-tĭk ĭn-sĕm-ĭ-NĀ-shŭn, p. 386)
tubal ligation (TŪ-băl lĭ-GĀ-shŭn, p. 382)
vasectomy (vă-SĔK-tō-mē, p. 382)

FAMILY PLANNING

Family planning involves personal, social, economic, religious, and cultural decisions about planning a pregnancy. For many, it will mean seeking ways to prevent or postpone pregnancy. For others, it will mean seeking infertility treatment or assisted reproductive technology. Today, couples choosing contraception must be informed about the prevention of unintended pregnancy and protection against sexually transmitted infections (STIs). This chapter discusses methods to prevent pregnancy and ways to achieve pregnancy.

REVERSIBLE CONTRACEPTION

Two goals of *Healthy People 2020* are to reduce the percentage of unintended pregnancy to less than 30% and reduce contraceptive failures to less than 7% (U.S. Department of Health and Human Services, 2010). To aid in achieving these goals, the nurse can guide couples to select reliable methods of birth control and educate them about proper use of methods, back-up techniques, and emergency contraception available. The main objective for couples using contraception is to prevent unintended pregnancy. Some contraceptive methods also reduce the risk of STIs. Decisions about contraception should be made voluntarily, with full knowledge of advantages and disadvantages, effectiveness, side effects, contraindications, and long-term effects for each technique. Many personal, cultural, religious, and cost factors influence the contraceptive choice. In addition, different methods of contraception may be appropriate at different times according to the couple's changing needs (Figure 19-1).

The nurse should document the contraception information discussed with the patient and partner, including the benefits, risks, alternatives, questions asked and answered, and discussion concerning the techniques required to safely and appropriately use the various products (Box 19-1).

Selecting which contraceptive method to use is a highly personal decision. Factors to consider include:
- Cost in using the method (insurance coverage)
- Effectiveness of method in preventing pregnancy
- Availability of method
- Partner's support and willingness to cooperate
- Safety of the method
- Protection against STIs
- Convenience
- Desirability or personal preference
- Personal motivation and compliance
- Religious and moral factors
- Medical problems such as blood clotting disorders or cancer

NATURAL METHODS
Abstinence
Abstinence has become associated with saying "no," but it can be viewed from another perspective. Abstinence can include saying "yes" to other satisfying sexual activities. Touching and communication are forms of affection. Holding hands, kissing, massage, and activities such as dancing or going to movies all fit along the sexual continuum.

Abstinence acts as a contraceptive by eliminating the possibility of sperm entering the woman's vagina. It is completely effective in preventing pregnancy and is a means to avoid STIs. This method has been integrated into many human immunodeficiency virus (HIV) prevention educational programs. Abstinence is receiving more emphasis in some educational programs for teenagers; however, whether more adolescents are using it is debatable (see Chapter 18).

The rhythm method of contraception (abstinence during the woman's fertile period) requires understanding of the menstrual cycle and fertility awareness.

Fertility Awareness
Fertility awareness is the understanding that a woman is fertile at ovulation, which occurs approximately 14 days before the next menstrual period. This method is not effective for women who have irregular menstrual cycles. Time of ovulation can be confirmed by assessing:
- **Basal body temperature (BBT)**: The woman takes her temperature with a special thermometer every morning before getting out of bed. The BBT will increase very slightly at ovulation and remain increased until menstruation or pregnancy occurs. Many factors, such as use of a heated waterbed, use of alcohol, fatigue, and infection, affect the BBT and may cause inaccurate interpretation of the reading.
- **Cervical mucus method** (also known as the **Billings method** or ovulation method): After ovulation, the cervical mucus becomes thick and sticky and can be stretched between the fingers (a sign known as **spinnbarkeit**) which is essential for sperm motility (Figure 19-2). After ovulation, the mucus is cloudy and forms a mucous plug that obstructs sperm flow. If the vaginal mucus is mixed with semen or contraceptive foams or an infection is present, the result may be inaccurate (Torske, 2010).

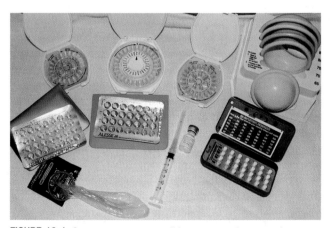

FIGURE 19-1 Some common reversible contraceptives: condom, diaphragm, oral contraceptives, and parenteral contraception.

Box 19-1   Key Points About Contraceptives

- Abstinence is the single most effective means of preventing pregnancy.
- Compliance in taking a daily pill is essential for effective oral birth control.
- Teenagers are less likely to be compliant.
- Using two methods at once (e.g., diaphragm with a spermicidal barrier or a condom with spermicidal barrier) dramatically lowers the risk of accidental pregnancy, provided they are used consistently.
- Condoms can help protect against infections (e.g., sexually transmitted infections).
- Oral contraceptives (OCs) may ease menstrual discomforts.
- The cost of contraceptives (e.g., monthly cost of OCs) may impose financial problems.
- Sterilization must be considered permanent.

and calculation of her fertile period. Intercourse is then avoided during the fertile period. The calendar method is based on the assumption that ovulation occurs approximately 14 days before the onset of the next menstrual period and the knowledge that the sperm is viable for 48 to 120 hours (5 days) and the ovum is viable for 24 hours. The calendar method is not a very reliable birth control technique because it requires cooperation and compliance by both partners in keeping records of the menstrual cycle and abstaining when appropriate and also understanding of various factors that may affect ovulation.

MECHANICAL BARRIER METHODS

Barrier methods are chemicals or devices that provide a barrier or block that prevents either the transport of sperm to the cervix or the implantation of the fertilized ovum. Spermicides (agents that kill sperm) should be deeply inserted into the vagina 1 hour before coitus. Spermicides are rarely effective when used alone and should be used with a diaphragm or condom. Chemical barriers that contain nonoxynol-9 have been shown to protect against *Neisseria gonorrhoeae*, chlamydial infection, and HIV, but frequent use can cause genital lesions and actually increase the risk for HIV infection (Hatcher, Trussell, & Nelson, 2008). Barrier methods include the male and female condom, diaphragm, intrauterine device, and cervical cap.

Vaginal Spermicides

Vaginal spermicides immobilize and destroy sperm and neutralize vaginal secretions. Many products contain nonoxynol-9, which is the active agent that destroys sperm. However, viruses and some other pathogens are less susceptible to spermicidal destruction. For this reason, spermicides cannot be relied on to provide complete protection from STIs. Spermicides are available as creams, foam, jellies, film, and suppositories that are inserted into the vagina 1 hour before intercourse. Correct placement of the spermicide and correct timing of insertion are important for contraceptive success. The spermicide applicator should be used with the foam gels and cream to reach the cervix. Suppositories need time (30 minutes) for dispersion. Spermicidal products become activated rapidly when exposed to body warmth in the vagina; therefore, they are short-acting and become inactive an hour after insertion. Also important to remember is that an application of the spermicide provides protection for one sexual intercourse ejaculation only. Typical failure rate of vaginal spermicides is approximately 6%. Some women who use spermicides develop a reaction to nonoxynol-9 and develop vaginal lesions, which can increase the risk for some STIs. Insertion may be messy, and the spermicide may leak out of the vagina after intercourse. Spermicides are relatively low cost and are safe.

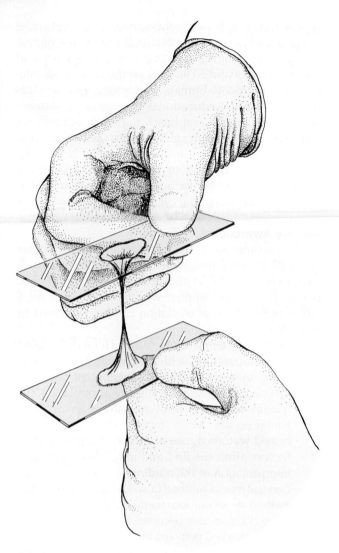

FIGURE 19-2 **Spinnbarkeit.** Cervical mucus changes under the influence of estrogen and progesterone during the menstrual cycle. The stretching ability of cervical mucus is greatest at the time of ovulation.

Some women may feel uncomfortable touching their genitalia and mucous discharge.

- Symptothermal method: This method combines the BBT with the cervical mucus stretching test and also self-recognition of physical or psychological symptoms of ovulation, which can include mittelschmerz (abdominal pain at ovulation) and pelvic fullness and tenderness.
- Chemical predictor test: A test kit that can be purchased over the counter has a chemically treated strip that will turn a specific color when it comes in contact with fluid that contains high luteal hormone levels. (There is a surge of luteal hormone 12 to 24 hours before ovulation.) Some test kits are available that are based on presence of estrogen and luteinizing hormone in the urine.
- **Rhythm method,** also known as the calendar method: This method is based on a calendar documentation of the woman's menstrual cycles

Male Condom

The male condom, a flexible sheath worn over the penis, is an inexpensive, accessible, and effective means of contraception when used properly and consistently (Skill 19-1). Condoms cover the penis and prevent sperm from entering the vagina. This method has an additional advantage of reducing the spread of STIs. Condoms are small, lightweight, and disposable; have almost no side effects; and require no medical examination. However, they may reduce the spontaneity of the sexual act.

Skill 19-1   How to Use a Male Condom Effectively*

PURPOSE

To learn to use a male condom for contraception.

Steps

1. Use a new condom each time you have intercourse.
2. Check the expiration date on packages, because condoms deteriorate over time.
3. Apply the condom before you have any contact with the woman's vagina, because there are sperm in the secretions before you ejaculate.
4. Squeeze the air from the tip when placing the condom over the end of your penis. Leave a half inch of space at the tip to allow sperm to collect and to prevent breakage.

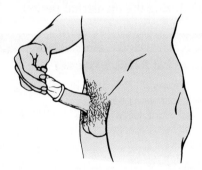

5. Hold the tip while you unroll the condom over the erect penis.

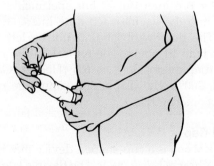

6. Do not use petroleum jelly, grease, or oil as lubricants because they can cause the condom to burst. Instead, use a water-soluble lubricant such as K-Y Jelly.
7. HOLD on to the condom at the base of the penis to prevent spillage as you withdraw from the vagina.

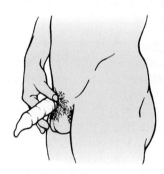

8. Remove the condom carefully to be sure that no semen spills from it.
9. Place the condom in the trash or in some safe disposal.

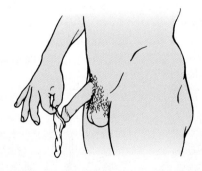

↳ Sperm usually dies when it's exposed to air.

---

*Proper use increases effectiveness. The failure rate is 3% with proper use and can be decreased to 2% or less by properly using spermicide with the condom (Hatcher, Trussell, & Nelson, 2008). The effectiveness of condoms is largely determined by their correct and consistent use.

Four basic features that differ among condoms are material, shape, lubricants, and spermicides. Most condoms are made of latex rubber and can cause allergic reactions. The functional difference in condom shape is the presence or absence of the sperm reservoir tip. Some condoms are rippled or have roughened surfaces to increase vaginal stimulation. A wet jelly or dry powder lubricates some condoms. Prolonged storage in hot humid climates or contact with vaginal antifungal creams, suntan oil, or oil-based lubricants, such as petroleum jelly, will cause latex to break down, and the condom may be ineffective.

Condoms made of polyurethane are thinner and stronger than those made from latex, provide less constricting fit, are more resistant to deterioration, and may enhance sensitivity. Unlike latex, condoms made of polyurethane are compatible with oil-based lubricants. Acceptance has been increasing because they afford protection against many STIs. Natural skin condoms (made from lamb's intestines) also may be used by men who are allergic to latex; however, they do not provide protection from STIs.

Female Condom

The female condom (or vaginal pouch) is a thick, lubricated, polyurethane sheath, 7 inches long, with a flexible ring at each end. The inner ring, at the closed end of the condom, serves as the means of insertion and covers the cervix like a diaphragm. The second ring of the device remains outside, thus covering part of the perineum and protecting the labia during intercourse (Figure 19-3). It may be inserted up to 8 hours before intercourse. It is approved for over-the-counter purchase and is intended for one-time use. It should not be used with a male condom. It is stronger than latex, is less likely to tear, and offers protection against various pathogens. The typical failure rate is 21% in the first year. The woman should wash her hands with soap and water before inserting the condom.

Diaphragm

The diaphragm is a latex or rubber dome-shaped cup surrounded by a spring or coil that fits snugly over the cervix. Spermicidal cream or gel is placed into the dome and around the rim; it is then inserted over the cervix by hand or with a plastic introducer (Skill 19-2). The diaphragm prevents passage of sperm into the cervix. The woman must be fitted with a diaphragm by a health care provider, at which time she is given instructions in its use. It should be rechecked for correct size after each term birth and if a woman gains or loses 4.5 kg (10 lbs) or more. Except for an allergic response to the diaphragm or spermicide, there are no known side effects from a well-fitted device.

If a woman is uncomfortable manipulating her genitalia to insert the diaphragm, check for its placement, and remove it, then this method may be an unsatisfactory choice. In addition, if the woman has a history of toxic shock syndrome (TSS) (see Chapter 20) or a history of frequent urinary tract infections, she should not use the diaphragm or other barrier methods. A diaphragm can put pressure on the urethra, which may interfere with complete emptying of the bladder. Leaving the diaphragm in place for prolonged periods can increase the risk for TSS. For this reason, it should not be used during the menstrual period.

> **Patient Teaching**
>
> **Danger Signs of Toxic Shock Syndrome**
> - Sudden high fever 38.9° C (102° F)
> - Sunburn-like rash with peeling
> - Aching muscles and joints
> - Dizziness, faintness, weakness
> - Hypotension
> - Signs of shock

The diaphragm holds the spermicide in place against the cervix for the 6 hours it takes to destroy the sperm. The diaphragm can be inserted up to 4 hours before intercourse, but spermicide must be inserted into the vagina each time intercourse is repeated. The diaphragm should not be left in place for more than 24 hours. The typical failure rate with using a diaphragm alone is 6% (Hacker, Gambone, & Hobel, 2009). The diaphragm cannot be relied on to protect against STIs.

Cervical Cap

The cervical cap is a cup-shaped device that is similar to the diaphragm but smaller. The flexible latex or rubber cup fits over the cervix and remains in place by suction. Cervical cap sizes are limited; therefore, it is not possible to fit all women properly.

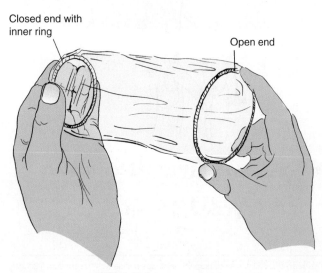

Closed end with inner ring

Open end

FIGURE 19-3 Female condom.

Skill 19-2   How to Use a Diaphragm Effectively

PURPOSE

To learn to use a diaphragm for contraception.

Steps

1. A diaphragm can be inserted up to 4 hours before intercourse. Skill of insertion and removal increases with practice.
2. Perform hand hygiene.
3. Apply spermicidal cream or gel inside at center and around the rim of the diaphragm. This aids the insertion and offers a more complete seal.

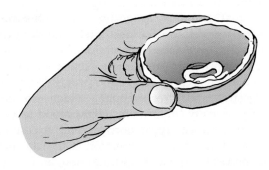

4. Hold diaphragm between your thumb and fingers and compress diaphragm. Use fingers of other hand to spread the labia (lips of vagina).

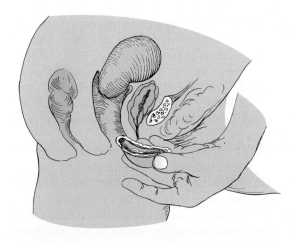

5. Insert diaphragm into vagina with spermicide toward the cervix. Squatting or placing one foot on a chair makes insertion (and removal) easier.
6. Insert diaphragm into vagina. Direct it inward and downward behind and below the cervix.
7. Tuck the front of the rim of diaphragm behind the pubic bone.

8. Feel your cervix through the center of the diaphragm.

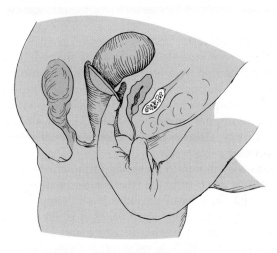

9. Leave diaphragm in place at least 6 hours after intercourse.
10. To remove diaphragm, assume squatting position and bear down. Hook a finger over the top rim to break suction and pull diaphragm down and out.

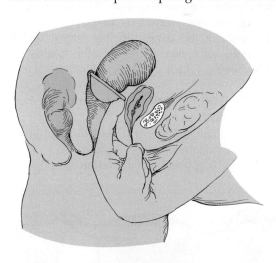

11. Wash diaphragm with mild soap and dry well after each use and store according to manufacturer's recommendations. (Scented talc or baby powder can weaken the rubber and therefore should not be applied to the diaphragm.)
12. Inspect the diaphragm occasionally for small holes by holding it up to light. If a light is seen, the diaphragm must be replaced.

The cervical cap fitting should be checked yearly, after childbirth, and after vaginal or uterine surgery. The insertion and instructions for use and removal of the cap are similar to those for the diaphragm. The cervical cap can remain in place for 24 to 48 hours.

Some women who have had abnormal Papanicolaou (Pap) test results, cannot be fitted properly with the cap sizes, have a history of TSS, have vaginal or cervical infections, or find it difficult to insert or remove the device are not candidates for using the cervical cap.

Intrauterine Device

An intrauterine device (IUD) is a small, T-shaped, flexible device inserted by a health care provider into the uterine cavity through the cervix to provide continuous pregnancy prevention (Figure 19-4). More popular than the traditional copper IUD (ParaGard), a smaller progestin-only IUD is also available for long-term contraception.

Mirena, a levonorgestrel-releasing intrauterine system (LNG-IUS), is an effective IUD that is inserted during an office visit by a health care provider. It is a T-shaped IUD that releases its hormone for 5 years; it is effective in controlling abnormal uterine bleeding and can cause amenorrhea. This IUD is most often prescribed for women who have had at least one term pregnancy.

IUDs are not recommended for women who have multiple sexual partners and are at risk for STIs because they provide no protection against STIs. Contraindications for IUDs are listed in Box 19-2.

Teaching the woman about an IUD is important. After insertion, the woman is instructed to check for the presence of strings. If she cannot feel the strings (tail), she should notify her health care provider.

HORMONAL CONTRACEPTIVES

Oral Contraceptives

Oral contraceptives (OCs) (birth control pills) are the most popular hormonal contraception. OCs prevent pregnancy by suppressing ovulation through the

| Box 19-2 | **Contraindications for Intrauterine Device Insertion** |

- Liver disease
- Copper allergy (for copper intrauterine device)
- Breast cancer (for Mirena)
- Immunodeficiency disorders
- Immunosuppressive therapy
- Uterine abnormality
- Pelvic infection or disorder
- Undiagnosed vaginal bleeding

combined actions of synthetic estrogen and progestin. In addition, the hormones thicken the cervical mucus and alter the decidua of the uterus to prevent implantation. If taken as directed, OCs have an effectiveness rate of 99% (Oats & Abraham, 2010). For women who cannot take estrogen, a minipill is available that contains progestin only. This pill thickens the cervical mucus and alters the decidua of the uterus to prevent implantation, but it is less effective in suppressing ovulation. Newer combination OCs contain second-generation progestins, such as desogestrel and drospirenone, which do not reduce high-density lipoprotein (HDL) blood levels, but they do reduce dysmenorrhea and excessive blood loss. Low-dose combination OCs do not increase the risk of myocardial infarction, and some may improve acne as a side effect (Oats & Abraham, 2010).

Although highly effective, OCs may produce side effects ranging from nausea and breakthrough bleeding to thrombus formation. Side effects may be either estrogen or progestin related. At least three regular ovulatory cycles should be evidenced before adolescents initiate OC use. After a term delivery, OCs can be started approximately 3 weeks postpartum to decrease thromboembolic risk. Combination OCs reduce the volume of breast milk and should not be started before lactation is well established.

The World Health Organization (WHO), in consultation with international clinicians, has developed comprehensive guidelines for the safe use of OCs and listed more than 120 chronic diseases that pose a health risk for OC use (see Online Resources). Some contraindications for taking OCs are listed in Box 19-3. Combination OCs result in lighter menstrual flow and decreased cramping (decreased dysmenorrhea).

Women who choose OCs as their method of birth control should be fully advised of the risks and benefits. OCs also have some noncontraceptive benefits, listed in Box 19-4. It is important to advise the woman to notify the health care provider if certain warning signs appear.

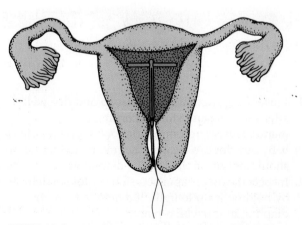

FIGURE 19-4 Intrauterine device (IUD) inside the uterine cavity.

Box **19-3**	Some Contraindications to Oral Contraceptive Use

- Vascular pathologic condition
- Thromboembolism or pulmonary embolism
- Stroke, atherosclerosis, heart failure, or hypertension
- Valvular heart disease
- Uncontrolled hypertension
- Breast cancer within 5 years
- Diabetes with neuropathy
- Retinopathy, liver disease
- Smoking
- Age older than 35 years
- Pregnancy
- Migraines with aura

Box **19-4**	Potential Benefits and Risks of Oral Contraceptives

BENEFITS
- Very effective if taken correctly
- Benefit to regular menstrual cycle: reduces cramping, menstrual blood loss, and associated anemia
- Does not affect fertility (3 months average for becoming pregnant after cessation)
- Fewer side effects with low estrogen content
- May reduce risk of ovarian and endometrial cancer by as much as 50%
- Decreased risk for:
  - Benign breast disease
  - Ovarian cysts
  - Pelvic inflammatory disease
  - Toxic shock syndrome
- Improves:
  - Endometriosis
  - Premenstrual syndrome
  - Dysmenorrhea
  - Acne
  - Menopause management

RISKS
- No protection against sexually transmitted infections (STIs)
- Can affect carbohydrate metabolism and insulin levels
- Worsens conditions affected by fluid retention, such as migraine, asthma, epilepsy, and kidney or heart disease
- Increased risks of:
  - Thrombosis
  - Breast tenderness or pain
  - Scant or missed periods
  - Stroke (especially in smokers and women older than 35 years)
  - Nausea
  - Headaches
- May be contraindicated in women with specific chronic illnesses
- Decreased effectiveness with some medications such as antibiotics

Safety Alert

Warning Signs During Oral Contraceptive Use

When taking oral contraceptives (OCs), women should notify the health care provider if they:
- Develop a breast lump
- Become depressed
- Become jaundiced
- Have abdominal pain
- Have severe leg pain (calf or thigh)
- Have severe headaches or dizziness
- Have weakness or numbness
- Have vision loss or blurred vision
- Have speech problems
- Have chest pain, cough, or shortness of breath

Teaching the proper use of OCs can increase their effectiveness. The combination OCs are purchased in packets of 21 or 28 tablets. With a packet of 28 tablets, 7 tablets are made of a noncontraceptive substance (e.g., sugar pills), and women take a pill every day. With the 21-day packet, the woman takes one pill every day for 3 weeks, then stops for a week, during which time menses (usually light bleeding) occurs. It is important to take the pill at the same time each day to keep the blood hormone levels stable. Experts in reproductive health now recommend that healthy, nonsmoking women older than 40 years with no cardiovascular problems continue to take OCs until menopause.

Some pill packs, such as Loestrin 24 FE and Yaz, use 24 hormone pills and 4 inert (hormone-free) pills only. Mircette pill packs follow the traditional 21 estrogen-progestin tablets with 5 tablets of low-dose estrogen and two inert pills only. A shorter time without hormones decreases the chance of ovulation and pregnancy. A contraceptive is also available that provides a menstrual period just once a year.

Missed doses require appropriate responses. OCs may interact with other medications; therefore, the woman should consult her health care provider about prescribed drugs (e.g., antibiotics, rifampin, and griseofulvin) that may decrease the effectiveness of OCs (Hacker, Gambone, & Hobel, 2009).

Patient Teaching

What to Do When Oral Contraceptive Pills Are Missed

- Oral contraceptive pills should be taken at the same time every day for the prescribed time.
- If one pill is missed, take it as soon as you remember it.
- If you miss two or more pills in succession in the first 2 weeks of the cycle, take two pills for the next 2 days and use a backup method of contraception until the end of the cycle.
- If you are using a 28-day pack and you miss any of the 7-day "blank" pills without hormones, throw out the pills you missed and keep taking one pill a day until the pack is empty. You do not need a backup method in this situation.
- If three pills are missed, throw away the pack. Start a new pack of pills on the first day of menstrual flow.

Research has shown that there are no specific health benefits to monthly menstruation. An extended-therapy OC (e.g., Seasonale) has been approved by the U.S. Food and Drug Administration (FDA). The contraceptive contains levonorgestrel and ethinyl estradiol and is taken daily for 84 days, followed by 1 week of placebo to allow menstruation to occur. This pattern reduces menstruation to four times per year.

In May 2007, the FDA approved a contraceptive called Lybrel (a name meant to invoke thoughts of liberty), which is designed to suppress monthly bleeding indefinitely. Lybrel contains 90 mg of levonorgestrel and 20 mg ethenyl estradiol and is taken continuously 365 days a year. Wyeth Laboratories markets the pill in the United States.

Follow-up care is important for a woman taking OCs. She should have a yearly pelvic examination, Pap smear, breast examination, and blood pressure measurement.

Hormonal Skin Patch

The hormonal contraceptive transdermal patch, Ortho Evra, contains norelgestromin (NGMN) and ethinyl estradiol. The patch is applied to the dry skin of the buttock, abdomen, upper arm, or torso. (It should not be applied to the breast or waist area, where it is subject to friction from clothing or accessories.) The first patch is applied the first day of the menstrual period. The patch is worn 1 week, then replaced on a different part of the body. A new patch is applied on the same day each week for 3 weeks; the patch is not applied during the fourth week, and menstruation occurs.

The advantages of the skin patch include maintaining a consistent level of hormones in the blood, avoiding liver metabolism of the drug (because the drug is not absorbed by the gastrointestinal tract), and avoiding the risk of forgetting to take a daily pill. The patch should not be placed on a skin rash or lesion. Women who weigh more than 90 kg (198 lbs) may require special counseling because the pregnancy protection may not be reliable. If the patch loosens and cannot be reapplied with brief pressure, that patch should be discarded and a new one applied. Occluding the top of the patch by taping it to the skin can adversely alter its effectiveness. Baby oil or a cotton ball can be used to clean away minor stains that may occur around the patch. If a skin patch remains off for more than 24 hours during the 3 weeks it should be in place, a new patch should be applied on a new cycle schedule and backup contraception used for at least 1 week.

The patch was recently removed from the U.S. market because of some risk of higher than expected exposure levels to the hormone. It was returned to the market with new FDA approval and a warning that absorption of high levels of hormones increases risk of complications. Studies are continuing.

Vaginal Ring

The NuvaRing (etonogestrel and ethinyl estradiol ring) is a flexible silicone ring that is inserted into the vagina for 3 weeks and removed for 1 week to allow for menstruation to occur. Steady levels of the low-dose hormone are achieved, with leukorrhea (increased white vaginal discharge) and vaginal infections being the most common side effects. Other side effects are similar to those of OCs, with fewer gastrointestinal and liver problems because it does not pass through the gastrointestinal tract. Fertility returns rapidly after the ring is discontinued.

Implantable Contraceptives

Implanon, a single silicone rod implant that uses etonogestrel, is inserted subdermally and provides contraception for up to 3 years. This rod has recently been approved in the United States by the FDA. The rod can be removed in the outpatient clinic under local anesthesia.

Injectable Contraceptives

Depo-medroxyprogesterone acetate (DMPA) suspension (Depo-Provera), a long-acting, injectable progestin, has been approved for contraceptive use in the United States. It alters the cervical mucus so that it becomes hostile to sperm, which impairs ovulation and implantation. A single injection is given every 3 months. It can be used in women with sickle cell disease and those taking anticonvulsants or rifampin. A pregnancy test is performed before the first injection. Side effects are similar to those of subcutaneous implants: menstrual spotting, headache, and weight gain. Women should be advised to take additional calcium and to exercise to minimize the risk of osteoporosis. Research shows that teens in the active phase of bone development who use DMPA recover bone density after stopping the drug, so being a teenager is not a contraindication for use, but the use in teenagers for longer than a 2-year period is not recommended. The injection site should not be massaged to avoid altering absorption rate. Contraceptive effects may last up to 1 year after injection. Postpartum women who are breastfeeding should start treatment at 6 weeks after lactation is firmly established. If the woman is not breastfeeding, she may start treatment at 5 days' postpartum with progestin only contraceptives (ACOG, 2007).

EMERGENCY CONTRACEPTION

There are three types of emergency oral contraception regimes available in the United States (ACOG, 2010):

1. A combined estrogen/progestin pill that requires two doses 12 hours apart taken up to 72 hours after unprotected sexual intercourse.
2. A progestin-only pill or a generic form, "Next Choice," which is the most popular "Plan B"

Pre-ejaculation = ↑ risk of pregnancy

1 pill/1 step regimen taken up to 72 hours after unprotected sexual intercourse (approved by the FDA in 2009).

3. Antiprogestin pill known as "ELLA," which contains mifepristone or ulipristal acetate that can be taken up to 5 days after unprotected sexual intercourse (approved by the FDA in 2010).

Emergency contraceptives are thought to work by delaying ovulation or impairing ovulation or the luteal function that supports fertilization and therefore will not be effective after fertilization and implantation has occurred.

The side effects of high-dose estrogens include nausea, vomiting, breast tenderness, and menstrual irregularities. An antiemetic is often recommended when these products are used.

Emergency contraception is available over the counter in most states to women over 17 years of age. Each state has "hotlines" on the Internet, most supported by Planned Parenthood for advice and education, or the woman may call 1-888-665-2528 for information. The insertion of a copper IUD within 5 days of unprotected midcycle coitus also may be an effective emergency contraceptive for the woman who desires long-term contraception.

ADVERSE EFFECTS OF ORAL CONTRACEPTIVES

Oral contraceptives may interact with other medications such as fluoroquinolones, anticonvulsants, asthmatic drugs, tricyclic antidepressants, and some CAM therapies. The physician should be consulted whenever medications are prescribed and an accurate history provided. Oral contraceptives may decrease milk production and should not be taken before lactation is established at 6 weeks' postpartum. Adverse responses should be reported and the woman counseled to use the acronym *ACHES* to be alert to adverse effects. Mood changes, depression, or jaundice should also be reported.

Memory Jogger

ACHES

Symptoms to report when taking OCs:
Abdominal pain
Chest discomfort
Headaches
Eye problems
Severe leg cramps

ONGOING RESEARCH

Research is ongoing concerning the use of chemical means of contraception (inserting a chemical into the fallopian tubes) and the development of contraceptive vaccines. Other methods of contraception are under investigation in the United States and other countries.

Information concerning postcoital contraception can be obtained from the Office of Population Research.

LEAST EFFECTIVE METHODS OF CONTRACEPTION

COITUS INTERRUPTUS (WITHDRAWAL)

Coitus interruptus prevents pregnancy when the man withdraws his penis from the woman's vagina before he ejaculates. This action prevents sperm from being deposited in the vaginal orifice. However, it requires control by the man and may be unsatisfying for both partners. In addition, he may misjudge the timing and withdraw too late because the fluid that escapes from the penis before ejaculation contains sperm. It also is possible for sperm to be deposited on the skin near the vulva and still enter the vagina, possibly resulting in pregnancy. Coitus interruptus is not a reliable method of birth control.

POSTCOITAL DOUCHE

The postcoital douche is a very unreliable method of contraception. Because sperm are known to appear in the cervical mucus within a few seconds after ejaculation, they can reach the fallopian tube within a short time. Once the sperm reaches the fallopian tube, pregnancy can result, and douching will not prevent it.

BREASTFEEDING

Lactation (breastfeeding) should not be recommended as a reliable form of contraception. Breastfeeding inhibits ovulation because prolactin alters ovarian response to hormones and the return of menses. The frequency (at least 10 to 12 times per day), intensity, and duration of breastfeeding may maintain the status for 4 to 6 months, and then prolactin decreases and ovulation returns. The woman should be cautioned that pregnancy can occur before menstruation returns. Some types of OCs have no known adverse effect on the milk or the newborn once lactation has been established.

PERMANENT CONTRACEPTION

LEGAL ASPECTS

Surgical sterilization is used to permanently prevent any future pregnancy. Male and female sterilization procedures are relatively simple to perform. Informed consent is required by law before any voluntary permanent sterilization is performed. A partner's consent may not be required by law, but the patient is advised to discuss the plan with his or her partner. Both the man and woman should be counseled, and the decision for sterilization must be made after a thorough discussion of the risks, benefits, and alternatives. In addition, the couple should be informed that there is no absolute guarantee that the procedure will prevent pregnancy; however, the failure rate is very low.

The informed consent form must be signed before any medication is administered before surgery. Informed consent should be in the patient's native language and at a reading level he or she can understand. It should include risks, benefits, alternatives, and a statement that the procedure is permanent and may be irreversible. Some states require a 30-day waiting period between signing consent and the surgery. Sterilization of minors or mentally incompetent women requires a court-appointed team of professionals for consent.

MALE STERILIZATION

Male sterilization, vasectomy, is achieved by an in-office "no scalpel" technique or an outpatient minor surgical procedure (Dassow & Bennett, 2006). A 3-cm incision is made over the vas deferens on each side of the scrotum, usually with the patient under local anesthesia (Figure 19-5). The vas deferens, which carry sperm to the ejaculatory ducts, are isolated, severed, and occluded. The man is advised to apply ice to reduce pain and swelling and to use a scrotal support for approximately a week. He must be informed that it takes approximately 6 weeks and up to 36 ejaculations to clear the remaining sperm from the vas deferens. The couple is advised to use another method of contraception for that time. The man is asked to bring semen samples to assess sperm count. Side effects of a vasectomy are immediate discomfort and a potential hematoma. Vasectomies can be reversed with the use of microsurgery, and fertility can be restored in 30% to 60% of the men, but declines over time (Hatcher, Trussell, & Nelson, 2008). Vasectomy has no effect on sexual performance.

FEMALE STERILIZATION

One type of female sterilization, tubal ligation, is relatively simple and very effective. A variety of approaches to this type of procedure is available. The surgery can be performed on an outpatient or inpatient basis with local or regional anesthesia, and in the postpartum or an interval period. Proper counseling and informed consent are mandatory before the voluntary procedure. The woman must fully understand that tubal sterilization is considered permanent. Sterilization reversals can be attempted, but the success depends on the type of procedure performed.

A minilaparotomy uses a suprapubic or subumbilical incision. The tubes are isolated and then may be crushed, ligated, or electrocoagulated. The tubes may be banded (rings) or plugged (Figure 19-6). For reversibility, microsurgical techniques are used; the greater the amount of tubal destruction, the less opportunity for successful reversal. The transcervical occlusion procedure introduces fibrosing elements into the fallopian tubes hysteroscopically (Hacker, Gambone, & Hobel, 2009). An Essure coil promotes tissue growth in each fallopian tube, leading to complete occlusion within 3 months after insertion (Simon, 2006). It is the first nonsurgical (no incision) permanent sterilization available to women; it is safe for use with magnetic resonance imaging (MRI) and is not detectable by security gate metal detectors (Simon, 2006).

Complications of female sterilization include coagulation burns on the intestines, infection, hemorrhage, and adverse anesthesia effects. Tubal ligation does not protect against STIs and does not affect menstruation or sexual performance.

NURSING RESPONSIBILITIES

The nursing responsibilities and interventions in permanent reproductive sterilization involve listening to the patient's concerns; verifying information concerning benefits, risks, and alternatives; and providing emotional support. Referral to community resources, social service agencies, and so forth should be done as indicated. The nurse should discuss preoperative preparation, postoperative home care, and signs and symptoms that require return to the health care

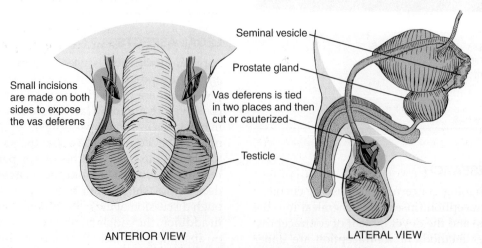

Small incisions are made on both sides to expose the vas deferens

Seminal vesicle

Prostate gland

Vas deferens is tied in two places and then cut or cauterized

Testicle

ANTERIOR VIEW　　　　LATERAL VIEW

FIGURE 19-5 **Vasectomy.** The sperm duct is cut and tied.

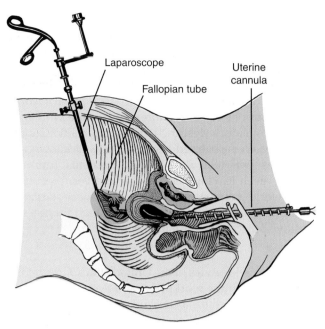

FIGURE 19-6 **Tubal ligation.** The fallopian tubes are cut and tied.

Box 19-5   Sterilization Documentation

The nurse should document that the following occurred:
- Patient gave informed consent, which included benefits, risks, and alternatives to permanent sterilization.
- Discussion was in the patient's native language.
- Patient is older than 21 years.
- Mandatory waiting period was discussed. Some states may require up to 30 days after consent before the procedure can be performed.
- Preoperative and postoperative self-care was discussed.
- Written material was given to the couple.
- Follow-up appointment was scheduled.

---

provider. The patient should be informed that sterilization does not offer STI protection. Sterilization also does not affect sexual functioning. Detailed documentation concerning patient teaching and preparation is essential (Box 19-5).

INFERTILITY AND THERAPIES TO FACILITATE PREGNANCY

DEFINITIONS OF FERTILITY AND INFERTILITY

Fertility is defined as the capacity to conceive or reproduce. The definition of infertility has changed with changing lifestyles. In 2008, the Practice Committee of the American Society of Reproductive Medicine (ASRM) defined infertility as a failure to achieve a successful pregnancy after 12 months or more of unprotected sexual intercourse. Earlier evaluation and treatment may be justified, based upon medical history or physical findings and is warranted after a 6-month period for women over age 35 (ASRM, 2008). The term

subfertility is used when both partners have a factor present that reduces fertility. The term *sterility* refers to a partner who has an irreversible factor that prevents fertility, such as a hysterectomy. Different types of infertility problems encountered in the infertility clinic are as follows:

- **Primary infertility:** The couple is unable to conceive at all after at least 1 year of unprotected sexual intercourse.
- **Secondary infertility:** After one successful pregnancy, the couple is unable to conceive a second time.
- **Unsuccessful pregnancies:** Couples conceive but repeatedly lose the fetus before it is viable.
- **Single infertility:** A single woman desires pregnancy without a male partner (e.g., same-sex marriages, unattached woman, or sudden widowhood).

Each of these women can receive help from an infertility clinic; however, their needs differ and the nurse must be sensitive and supportive (Box 19-6). The woman seeking fertility services may have occlusion of the fallopian tubes or removal of the fallopian tubes. In the past, she would have been declared sterile and advised to adjust to a childless marriage. Today, with advanced reproductive technologies available, having a baby for some of these women becomes a possibility. Some couples, after extensive counseling and education in a fertility clinic, may decide not to have children, and their decision should be supported. Only some health care plans cover fertility services.

CULTURAL AND RELIGIOUS CONSIDERATIONS

In many cultures, fertility (or the lack thereof) is considered strictly a female problem. It may be closely linked to the woman's social status. The stigma of infertility can lead to divorce and rejection from family and society. Choosing treatment for infertility may go against the couple's cultural norms, particularly if the man must be treated to achieve pregnancy.

Religious norms influence what tests and treatments a couple is willing to pursue. Surrogate parenting, in vitro fertilization, or other techniques may not be acceptable in terms of the couple's personal or

---

Box 19-6   Self-Help Fertility Aids

- Recognize signs of ovulation, and time intercourse one to three times during that period.
- Avoid altering pH of vagina with douches or scented inserts.
- Use male-superior position during intercourse.
- Remain lying flat after intercourse for 1 hour, with hips elevated to encourage retention of sperm.
- Maintain adequate nutrition.
- Minimize stress and anxiety.
- Avoid lubricants that can be spermicidal.

religious beliefs. Conflict can arise if a potentially successful therapy is acceptable to one member of the couple but not to the other.

FACTORS RELATED TO FERTILITY

Before a specific method for treating infertility is selected, factors contributing to fertility must be explored with the couple. These factors include coital frequency, age, smoking, exercise and weight loss, diet, stress, medical conditions, use of drugs, and exposure to chemicals.

COITAL FREQUENCY

Unprotected intercourse more than three times a week offers the best opportunity for conception to occur, whereas daily intercourse may result in decreased volume of ejaculate and a low sperm count. Planning intercourse around the time of ovulation is essential because the ova can be fertilized only within 24 hours after ovulation. Because the sperm live for 48 to 120 hours after ejaculation, sexual intercourse immediately before ovulation contributes to successful fertilization. Only water-soluble lubricants should be used because others may have spermicidal properties.

AGE

Coital frequency often decreases as marriage length increases, and, as the woman ages, medical conditions that interfere with pregnancy may develop. The woman older than 35 years has a decreased chance of successful conception. The increasing age of the man may decrease conception rates, but firm research data have not been collected concerning this factor. Donor fertilization of a young woman with an older man's sperm has been successful.

SMOKING

In vitro studies have been conducted regarding the effect of nicotine on ovulation. Cigarette smoking increases the peristalsis within the fallopian tubes, causing the ovum to pass more quickly. This may increase the risk of ectopic pregnancy. Heavy cigarette smoking has been associated with poor pregnancy outcomes and may play a role in impaired fertility. Research is ongoing, and anti-smoking education is offered at most schools, by managed care organizations, and in the media.

EXERCISE AND WEIGHT LOSS

Heavy exercise has been associated with menstrual irregularity, and excessive weight loss can cause amenorrhea. However, continued research is required for definitive information regarding the relation of male and female exercise and weight loss to fertility. High scrotal temperatures from frequent sauna or hot tub use or tight nylon underpants can decrease male sperm production.

DIET

A deficiency in vitamin B_{12} has been linked to infertility in some studies. A low-calorie, strict vegetarian diet has a possible relation to altering the luteal phase and the release of gonadotropins. Hypercarotenemia may also play a role in altering ovarian function (Morin, 2010). Both obesity and anorexia place the woman at risk for ovulatory dysfunction and infertility. Continued research is required because it is well known that the fetus will take its required nutrients from the mother, even leaving her without reserves. Women in third-world countries suffering from near-starvation conditions do become pregnant, although the rates of positive outcome require further study.

STRESS

With today's lifestyles in the United States, stress exists in the home, in the workplace, and even in the recreation arenas. Much has been said about the couple who decides to adopt and then "relaxes" and goes on to have a successful conception. Infertile women may be expected to have high stress and anxiety levels concerning their inability to conceive. However, studies have not shown definitive proof that stress is a significant cause of infertility. Because women who seek treatment for infertility may be anxious or stressed, and some religious groups require successful pregnancy and heirs for the marriage to continue, marital discord may also be present in couples seeking fertility treatment. Listening to the couple and providing an interdisciplinary referral to clergy, a social worker, or support groups are helpful. Open communication and the development of a true partnership between the couple and the staff are essential.

MEDICAL CONDITIONS

Pelvic adhesions and a history of previous pelvic inflammatory disease (PID) or endometriosis may affect fertility. Other abdominal surgeries can influence tubal patency. Abnormalities of the reproductive tract in the woman or her partner and immunologic and endocrine disorders can also alter fertility and may require treatment before infertility therapy is initiated.

USE OF DRUGS AND CHEMICALS

The use of recreational drugs has been associated with increased infertility relating to tubal function in women and sperm concentration in men. Repeated workplace exposure to chemicals, such as nitrous oxide and soil fumigants, has been suspected as a result of some studies. Prescribed and over-the-counter drugs, such as antihistamines, can reduce vaginal lubrication. Some antihypertensives impair male erection, barbiturates can inhibit hormone release, and nonsteroidal antiinflammatory drugs can inhibit ovulation. Occupational Safety and Health Administration (OSHA) guidelines in the workplace require disclosure of toxic chemicals the worker may be exposed to because the exposures may be risk factors for infertility or birth defects. A database is kept at the Reproductive Toxicology Center (REPROTOX), and websites can be accessed to address specific questions.

MALE INFERTILITY

Male infertility plays a role in about half of all cases. A defect in the transport system of the sperm (such as orchitis or varicocele), a defect in sperm production (such as a hormonal deficiency), or the inability to deposit sperm into the woman (such as erection problem or hypospadias) contributes to male infertility. The use of tobacco, alcohol, and illicit drugs can also contribute to male infertility. Use of over-the-counter or prescription drugs such as sulfasalazine, spironolactone, calcium channel blockers, allopurinol, nitrofurantoin, and cimetidine can inhibit sperm production; diuretics can result in ejaculatory problems; and steroids can reduce sperm production or contribute to erectile dysfunction. Lead and pesticide exposure can also reduce sperm count.

Fertility tests for the male partner include semen and sperm analysis, transrectal ultrasound, hormonal profile, post-ejaculatory urinalysis to test for retrograde ejaculation, vasograph, genetic testing, and a postcoital test of sperm count.

Treatment of Male Infertility

Autoimmune antibodies against sperm can be stimulated by genital infection or trauma. Treatment of male infertility involving erectile dysfunction can include drugs such as sildenafil (Viagra) or vardenafil (Levitra), injectable or mechanical aids to erection, or ART procedures. To increase sperm count, men should be instructed to wear loose-fitting underwear; to avoid saunas, smoking, St. John's wort, and anabolic steroids; and to eat a healthy diet.

INFERTILITY MANAGEMENT PROGRAMS

In a good infertility management program, the factors that contribute to infertility are discussed and dealt with before specific interventions are implemented. A nurturing but value-free environment must be created for couples who may be aggressively and impatiently seeking fertility treatment and who may suddenly decide to abandon efforts. Acceptance and support of their values and decisions are essential. The couple must be empowered to make the decisions on the basis of their own needs and values and to change those decisions without an expression of disappointment by the fertility clinic staff.

Before infertility treatment is initiated, diagnostic tests may be performed to help in selecting the best treatment protocol. They include physical examination; tests for tubal function, tubal patency, ovulation, and hormonal levels; BBT records; a transvaginal ultrasound; an endometrial biopsy; and ferning capacity of the cervical mucus.

Evaluation of the couple identifies whether therapy can increase their chance to conceive. The initial evaluation involves education and preparation of the couple, which empower them to make informed choices and control the evaluation and fertilization procedures. The couple's psychosocial and marital health should be considered in determining the best approach to infertility management. A multidisciplinary approach to the management of infertility involves the endocrinologist, urologist, psychologist, gynecologist, and nurse.

ASSISTED REPRODUCTIVE TECHNOLOGY

Legal and Ethical Factors in Assisted Reproduction

Noncoital reproduction brings with it many legal and ethical problems that must be dealt with. In most cases, assisted reproductive technology (ART) is used to assist infertile couples. However, this technique can also be used by a married couple to avoid known genetic anomalies carried by one or both partners. Sperm or egg donors and surrogates involve third parties, and their emotional bonds and legal rights must be considered. Homosexual couples or single parents can create a child through the donation of eggs or sperm or surrogacy, and a changed family structure evolves.

Parental rights are a legal challenge. It is now possible for a child to have five parents: a sperm donor, an egg donor, a gestational surrogate, and the two parents who will rear the child. The right to bear a child is protected by the U.S. Constitution; the government cannot usually interfere. The nontraditional family is therefore entitled to constitutional protection.

Cloning one's lost child is not yet a possibility. The fate of a frozen embryo when the parents divorce has been challenged in court. The sale of frozen embryos also is increasingly challenged in our legal system. However, federally funded research on fetal tissue and stem cells can control future research and development. State laws can also prevent funding of private research. The problems of insurance coverage and access to care are also highly debated issues related to ART.

Assisted Reproductive Technology Procedures

Extraordinary progress has been made in ART toward the treatment of infertility. In vitro fertilization, gamete intrafallopian transfer (GIFT), and in vitro fertilization–embryo transfer (IVF-ET) are techniques that bypass many of the natural means to conception. Each of these procedures begins with ovulation induction to permit retrieval of ova to improve the chance of a successful pregnancy. Maternal risks include multiple births, prematurity, preeclampsia, cesarean birth, ectopic pregnancies, pelvic organ infection or damage, and ovarian hyperstimulation syndrome (OHSS). Fetal risks include prematurity, chromosomal anomalies, and other problems (Scoccia, 2006).

Ovulation Induction

Medications to induce ovulation may be given to the woman who does not ovulate or ovulates irregularly (Table 19-1). Medications are also prescribed to provide multiple ova if the woman plans to have in vitro fertilization, GIFT, tubal embryo transfer (TET), or IVF-ET. Clomiphene citrate is the drug most commonly given to stimulate ovulation. OHSS is not uncommon when ovarian enlargement and follicular cysts are present. More than one ovum may be released and fertilized, making twins and triplets more common. Dosage and responses must be closely monitored. Other medications have been developed to combat specific factors known to inhibit ovulation (see Table 19-1).

Ovulation induction typically involves three types of medications:

- Selective estrogen receptor modulators (SERMs) (e.g., clomiphene)
- Aromatase inhibitors (AIs) (e.g., anastrozole [Arimidex] and letrozole [Femara])
- Injectable gonadotropins (e.g., menotropins [Repronex, Menopur] and urofollitropin [Bravelle])

There is a small window of time that is appropriate to administer an ovulatory stimulant, and hormone measurements are used as a guide. OHSS is a serious complication if the drug is given at an inappropriate time in the menstrual cycle. Gonadotropin-releasing hormones (GnRHs) are used to prevent ovulation and control ovarian hyperstimulation.

Surgical Procedures

In men, correction of a varicocele may improve sperm quality and quantity. Laser surgery may be used to correct adhesions, or microsurgery technique can be used. In women, transcervical balloon tuboplasty may be used to unblock the woman's fallopian tubes without using more invasive procedures such as laparoscopy or laparotomy. In this procedure, a thin catheter is threaded through the uterus into the fallopian tube, and the balloon is inflated to clear the blockage.

Therapeutic Insemination

Therapeutic insemination (a technique formerly referred to as **artificial insemination**) is the instillation of ova or sperm into the uterus to aid conception. Either the partner's semen or a donor's semen may be used. Donor semen may be used if the partner carries a genetic defect or if a woman wants to have a child without a relationship with a male partner. Intrauterine insemination can be performed, allowing the sperm to bypass cervical mucus and decreasing some immunologic problems. Donors are screened to reduce the risk of transmitting genetic defects and STIs. Tests determine whether the donor is in good general health, determine the blood type and Rh factor, and screen for STIs. Donor sperm and donor ova may be frozen and held for 6 months before use to reduce the risk of infections not realized at the initial screening.

In Vitro Fertilization. In vitro fertilization is a technique that involves bypassing blocked or absent fallopian tubes. In a surgical procedure, ova are removed by laparoscope and mixed with prepared sperm from the woman's partner or donor. Approximately 2 days later, up to four embryos are returned to the uterus. In vitro fertilization may or may not be successful. Not all ova are successfully fertilized by this technique, and embryos that are transferred to the woman's uterus may not implant.

Gamete Intrafallopian Transfer. Hormones are given to stimulate ovulation, and ova are collected laparoscopically. The woman has to have at least one normal,

Table 19-1 Drugs Used to Assist Ovulation

DRUG	ACTION
Clomiphene citrate (Clomid)	Stimulates hypothalamus to secrete GnRH that results in LH and FSH secretions, which stimulate maturity and release of ova Side effects include hot flashes and vision changes
Human menopause gonadotropin (hMG) (menotropins [Pergonal, Humegon, Repronex, Menopur], urofollitropin [Bravelle, Fertinex])	Daily injections are required, and serum estradiol levels are measured to avoid ovarian hyperstimulation syndrome
Bromocriptine (Parlodel)	Lowers prolactin levels that may impair FSH and LH action on the ovaries Must be discontinued when ovulation occurs
Zoladex; Lupron	GnRH agonists are used for endometriosis-related infertility
Recombinant LH	FDA approved in 2004 for follicular stimulation
Aromatase inhibitors	Inhibit the conversion of androgen into estrogen

[handwritten: ℞ have to be fully aware before starting it]

FDA, Food and Drug Administration; *FSH,* follicle-stimulating hormone; *GnRH,* gonadotropin-releasing hormone; *LH,* luteinizing hormone.

patent fallopian tube. After a 3- to 7-day abstinence period, the male sperm is collected and prepared, and both the sperm and ova are placed into the ampullary portion of the fallopian tube, allowing fertilization in vivo at the site where it naturally occurs. A transcervical route for GIFT by hysteroscopy is in the research and development stage.

Indications for GIFT include unexplained infertility, pelvic endometriosis, male factor infertility, adhesions, failure of previous cycles of artificial insemination (either by partner or donor), cervical factors, and immunologic causes. Zygote intrafallopian transfer (ZIFT) involves the transfer at the zygote state. Donor embryos or surrogate mothers are also popular approaches to infertility treatment.

Intracytoplasmic Sperm Injection. When the male cannot ejaculate sperm, a microsurgical sperm aspiration can retrieve sperm from the epididymis via the testes. The sperm is then used to fertilize ova by intercytoplasmic sperm injection and the fertilized ova are implanted in the uterus.

COMPLEMENTARY AND ALTERNATIVE MEDICAL THERAPY FOR INFERTILITY

Some couples prefer to use complementary and alternative medical (CAM) therapy before or during use of prescribed assisted reproductive technology (ART). The National Institutes of Health defines CAM therapy as a group of diverse medical and health care systems, practices, and products that are not presently considered to be part of conventional medicine. *Complementary medicine* is used together with conventional medicine, and *alternative medicine* is used in place of conventional medicine (NIH, 2009). Integrative medicine combines treatments from conventional medicine and CAM for which there is some high quality evidence of safety and effectiveness (NIH, 2009).

Acupuncture for the male is thought to increase sperm counts and, for the female, it is thought to enhance success of ART by improving ovarian and uterine blood flow, improving the endometrial environment and relieving stress and uterine motility, thereby improving embryo implantation. Ginseng and astragalus are herbs used to increase sperm motility. Studies are underway using repeated low frequency electroacupuncture to inhibit the action of ovarian sympathetic nerves and influence ovulation (Bennington, 2010). Ayurveda and relaxation techniques provide a mind-body balance and avoidance of stress that positively affects ovulation, fertility, and pregnancy. Aromatherapy can enhance relaxation, and massage both relaxes and increases blood flow as well as reduces stress hormones, all of which can enhance fertility. See Chapter 21 for a detailed discussion of CAM therapy.

Biologic supplements, such as folic acid and iron supplements, are known to have a positive effect on a positive pregnancy outcome. Antioxidants that prevent stress, vitamin E, selenium, vitamin A, and coenzyme Q are all thought to support pregnancy. Women should be cautioned not to consume over-the-counter individual supplements without consulting the health care provider. If a substance has a U.S. Pharmacopeia verification symbol, it has been evaluated for content and manufacturing practices (Bennington, 2010).

ROLE OF THE NURSE IN CONTRACEPTION AND INFERTILITY

In the United States, the woman most often chooses the type of contraception to use. Information is often obtained from friends or the media—television, newspapers, and magazine advertisements. The risk of incomplete, inaccurate, or misinterpreted information results in improperly selected or improperly used techniques that fail and result in an unintended pregnancy.

Couples should obtain contraceptive information from qualified health professionals. It is therefore the responsibility of the health professional to educate the consumer in the community. Opportunities for education occur in the school nurse's office, at parent-teacher meetings, and at physicians' offices and clinics. Every postpartum woman should receive instruction concerning family planning before discharge. The nurse's role is to assess contraceptive knowledge, attitudes and plans for pregnancies, the need for family planning, and the preferred methods, and counsel the woman and her partner to help them choose the method best for them, taking into consideration religious beliefs, cultural values, and personal needs. The nurse must feel comfortable discussing contraception and conception and help the woman and her partner express their personal needs and concerns.

The couple's needs and preferences should be the focus of counseling and education. The nurse can help the couple understand the information concerning ART. Information regarding surrogate mothers and adoption should also be provided and appropriate referrals made. Infertility treatments are expensive, can be frustrating, and are intrusive in the private lives of the couple. Guilt and shame may enter the relationship, and couples often feel a loss of control. The nurse can act as an educator, an advocate, and a counselor, offering the couple a sense of control and acceptance.

Get Ready for the NCLEX® Examination!

Key Points

- Family planning involves personal, social, and cultural considerations. For many, it means seeking ways to prevent pregnancy; for others, it means finding ways to achieve pregnancy.
- Abstinence has become associated with saying "no," but it can be viewed as saying "yes" to other satisfying sexual activities, such as touching, kissing, and communication.
- Fertility awareness is also known as natural family planning. Periodic abstinence requires cooperation of both partners and an understanding of how to identify fertile days.
- Contraceptive failure is related to noncompliance, lack of cooperation in the partner's attitude toward consistent use, and, most important, misinformation or lack of information about how to use the technique selected.
- Barrier methods include the male and female condoms, diaphragm, IUD, and cervical cap, all of which prevent the transport of sperm into the vagina.
- Vaginal spermicides are available in foams, gels, creams, and suppositories, which are inserted into the vagina before sexual intercourse. Their action is to destroy sperm or alter vaginal secretions and immobilize sperm. They are short acting and are often used with another contraceptive method.
- Hormonal contraceptives include OCs, hormone injections, the vaginal ring, and the skin patch. They inhibit ovulation and also make the cervical mucus unfavorable for sperm penetration.
- Combination OCs are available at lower doses that have fewer side effects. Use of synthetic progesterone can decrease bloating and avoid increased appetite.
- Oral contraceptives are available in formulas that support monthly menstruation, limit menstruation to four times a year, and suppress menstruation completely.
- IUDs are inserted into the uterus to provide continuous pregnancy protection, but they do not protect the woman from STIs.
- Surgical sterilization offers permanent contraception. A tubal ligation can be performed on the woman, and a vasectomy can be performed on the man. Although surgery to reverse sterilization is possible, it is expensive and may not be successful.
- Emergency contraception is available as a combination of estrogen and progestin, progestin only (Plan B), or an antiprogestin tablet (ELLA) taken shortly after unprotected sex. An insertion of a copper IUD within 5 days after unprotected sex is also an effective emergency contraception technique for women who prefer long-term contraception.
- Therapies to facilitate pregnancy or increase the couple's chance to conceive include ovulation induction by medications and therapeutic insemination by the partner's or donor's sperm. In vitro fertilization is a surgical procedure of inserting embryos into the woman's uterus. The GIFT procedure involves the direct placement of both gametes into the ampullary portion of the fallopian tubes.

Additional Learning Resources

SG Go to your Study Guide on pages 509–510 for additional Review Questions for the NCLEX® Examination, Critical Thinking Clinical Situations, and other learning activities to help you master this chapter content.

evolve Go to your Evolve website (http://evolve.elsevier.com/Leifer/maternity) for the following FREE learning resources:

- Animations
- Answer Guidelines for Critical Thinking Questions
- Answers and Rationales for Review Questions for the NCLEX® Examination
- Concept Map Creator
- Glossary with pronunciations in English and Spanish
- Patient Teaching Plans
- Skills Performance Checklists and more!

 Online Resources
- www.asrm.org
- www.cdc.gov/reproductivehealth/art.htm
- www.knowmycycle.com
- www.managingcontraception.com
- www.mayoclinic.com/health/infertility/DS00310/DSECTION=8
- www.nlm.nih.gov/medlinePlus/birthcontrol.html
- www.not-2-late.com
- http://opr.princeton.edu
- www.plannedparenthood.org/birthcontrol-pregnancy/birthcontrol.htm
- www.thefemalepatient.com/pdf/supplementcontocsintr40.pdf
- www.who.int

Review Questions for the NCLEX® Examination

1. The calendar method of contraception is based on the assumption that:

   1. Luteal hormone surges 12 to 24 hours after ovulation.
   2. Ovulation occurs approximately 14 days before the onset of the next menstrual period.
   3. Basal body temperature decreases slightly at ovulation.
   4. Cervical mucus becomes cloudy and sticky before ovulation.

2. Following a term delivery, a postpartum patient who is breastfeeding asks the health care provider how soon she can begin using oral contraceptives. The health care provider should reply:

   1. "You may begin to use oral contraceptives immediately."
   2. "You must wait until the end of the 6 week postpartum period."
   3. "You can start using oral contraceptives approximately 4 weeks' postpartum."
   4. "You must wait until your menstrual period begins to start using oral contraceptives."

3. When providing information regarding the use of the hormonal skin patch, the nurse should include the following: *(Select all that apply.)*

　1. The patch is worn for 4 weeks then replaced on a different part of the body.
　2. The patch is applied to dry skin of the buttock, abdomen, upper arm, or torso.
　3. The initial application of the patch is the first day of the menstrual period.
　4. Occluding the patch by taping it to the skin can adversely alter its effectiveness.

4. Which patient should not use Depo-Provera?

　1. Woman with sickle cell disease
　2. Adolescent
　3. 2-week postpartum, breastfeeding mother
　4. Woman taking anticonvulsant medications

5. Primary infertility is diagnosed when:

　1. A single woman desires pregnancy without a male partner.
　2. Couples conceive but repeatedly lose the fetus before it is viable.
　3. After one successful pregnancy, the couple is unable to conceive a second time.
　4. The couple is unable to conceive at all after at least 1 year of unprotected sexual intercourse.

6. A technique that involves bypassing blocked or absent fallopian tubes is called:

　1. Transcervical balloon tuboplasty
　2. Gamete intrafallopian transfer
　3. In vitro fertilization
　4. Intracytoplasmic sperm injection

7. When providing information to a patient at a family planning clinic, the nurse should include which instruction(s)? *(Select all that apply.)*

　1. Spermicides are highly effective forms of birth control.
　2. Abstinence is completely effective in preventing pregnancy.
　3. The diaphragm should not be left in place for more than 24 hours.
　4. IUDs are not recommended for women who have multiple sexual partners.
　5. Oral contraceptives may interact with other medications.

Critical Thinking Questions

1. A woman, married for 6 months, does not want to become pregnant for 2 years so that she can establish her career. She is interested in using an IUD. What advice would you give her about using this method?

2. A woman states that she is sexually active. The physician prescribed an OC for her. What advice would you give her about taking OCs? What advice would you give her about protection against STIs?

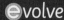
Objectives

1. Define key terms listed.
2. Describe toxic shock syndrome, list four of its symptoms and prevention measures.
3. Describe premenstrual syndrome, and list potential ways to reduce it.
4. Identify potential causes of dysmenorrhea, and explain how it can be relieved.
5. Explain the physiologic factor that initiates menopause.
6. State two screening techniques for early detection of breast cancer.
7. Explain the technique of breast self-examination.
8. Describe two options in the management of breast cancer.
9. Define endometriosis, and state one typical symptom.
10. Describe the transmission, treatment, and prevention of common sexually transmitted infections.
11. Explain methods to prevent transmission of infections acquired through blood and body fluids.
12. Discuss the prevention of human papillomavirus infections.

Key Terms

amenorrhea (ə-men″o-re′ə, p. 393)
climacteric (klī-MĂK-tĕr-ĭk, p. 393)
dysmenorrhea (dĭs-mĕn-ō-RĒ-ă, p. 392)
dyspareunia (dĭs-pă-ROO-nē-ă, p. 399)
endometriosis (ĕn-dō-mē-trē-Ō-sĭs, p. 398)
leiomyomas (lī-ō-mī-Ō-măs, p. 393)
menopause (MĔN-ō-păwz, p. 393)
menorrhagia (mĕn-ō-RĀ-jă, p. 393)
metrorrhagia (mĕ-trō-RĀ-jă, p. 393)
oligomenorrhea (ol′~ĭ-go-men″o-re′ə, p.393)
osteoporosis (ŏs-tē-ō-pŏ-RŌ-sĭs, p. 394)

Papanicolaou (Pap) test (păp″ə-nĭ′ko-la′oō, p. 395)
pelvic inflammatory disease (PID) (PĔL-vĭk ĭn-FLĂM-ă-tō-rē, p. 399)
polymenorrhea (pol′e-men″o-re′ə, p. 393)
premenstrual dysphoric disorder (PMDD) (prē-MĔN-strŭl, p. 392)
premenstrual syndrome (PMS) (p. 392)
sexually transmitted infections (STIs) (p. 400)
stress incontinence (p. 394)
toxic shock syndrome (TSS) (p. 391)

WOMEN'S HEALTH CARE

® Test!!

Today, women from all ethnic backgrounds choose to be active participants in their health care and therefore need information about their bodies, health promotion, self-care techniques, and choices concerning treatment options.

Culturally competent communication is the key to empowering the woman to feel confident about her ability to care for herself and her family. In some cultures, women ask questions when they want to know something related to their health; in other cultures, women wait to be told what to do (see Chapters 1 and 7). To be an effective teacher about health behaviors, the nurse must understand the patient's cultural needs, experiences, and individual goals. The nurse offers support, knowledge, and caring behaviors that help the woman cope with screening tests or problems.

Some goals of *Healthy People 2020* relate to women's health, including curbing the rise in breast cancer,

increasing the number of women over the age of 40 who have mammograms, reducing the number of deaths from cervical cancer, increasing the number of women over the age of 18 who have Papanicolaou (Pap) tests, reducing the occurrence of vertebral fractures in older women with osteoporosis, and reducing the occurrence of sexually transmitted infections (STIs [formerly known as sexually transmitted diseases, or STDs]). Achievement of these goals requires preventive care, screening, and increased accessibility to health care.

Women are assertive health care consumers. As women age, the intergenerational phase (caring for young children and older parents) influences their health care needs. As a woman's life expectancy increases, living with disabilities or long-term illness presents financial, psychological, and physical strains that affect their health care needs.

Lifestyle management, adaptation to multiple roles, and self-care play a large role in women's health care, especially in the areas of health promotion and illness prevention. The perinatal experience is often the first encounter with a health care provider that is maintained on a long-term basis as the new mother assumes the caregiving role for her child.

The older woman presents a unique challenge to nurses and health care providers. Older women may be single, live alone, have below-poverty income, and be without caregivers. The nurse must be aware of normal physiologic changes associated with aging when assessing the older woman. Although normal physiologic changes cannot be modified, associated decline in the ability to function depends on lifestyle choices and the individual's ability to adapt to change. Aerobic and resistance exercise programs are popular, and exercise programs for the older woman can be individualized for best results.

The majority of health care delivery for women is based in a location other than the acute care hospital facility. This chapter provides an overview of the more common health care problems of women in the community.

SMOKING AND HEALTH

Newborns and children who live in an environment where parents smoke are at increased risk for respiratory problems, including sudden infant death syndrome (SIDS) and asthma. Smoking during pregnancy places the woman at risk for preterm delivery or places the fetus at risk for intrauterine growth restriction. Counseling, public health campaigns, and smoking cessation programs have been implemented, and these are some of the continued goals of *Healthy People 2020*.

Stress is often associated with smoking, and stress management programs may be an important part of any smoking cessation program. An understanding of addictive behavior, motivation for change, and behavioral strategies to accomplish smoking cessation is important to the success of any program. A sample interview concerning smoking assessment, intervention, and self-help is shown in Table 20-1.

TOXIC SHOCK SYNDROME

Toxic shock syndrome (TSS), a multisystem infection that results from the response of the body to toxins produced by *Staphylococcus aureus* and group A streptococci, is potentially fatal. The toxin produced alters capillary permeability, which allows intravascular fluid to leak from the blood vessels, resulting in hypovolemia, hypotension, and shock. The toxin also causes direct tissue damage to organs and precipitates serious defects in blood coagulation.

Table 20-1	Tobacco Cessation Teaching Plan	
Ask About Tobacco Use and Exposure		
Risks to self and fetus or newborn include increased risk for cancer, lung disease, strokes, heart disease, stomach ulcers, preterm labor, low-birth-weight newborns, sudden infant death syndrome, learning problems, more colds, and ear infections.		
Benefits to mother and fetus or newborn include living an average of 20-25 years longer, better health, more money, food tastes better, better chance of normal birth weight, fewer health problems at birth, fewer respiratory illnesses, and fewer allergies.		
Ask Whether Patient Wants to Quit		
No	**Yes**	**Exposure Only**
Continue telling about risks of smoking and benefits of quitting at every prenatal visit.	Help patient develop a plan to quit smoking.	Help the patient's partner quit smoking in the same way, and also teach about nicotine replacement products,* such as nicotine gum and patches or medications such as bupropion.
Join smoking cessation programs. Stop "cold turkey" (choose a date and time then never smoke again). Smoke at fixed intervals (only smoke at set times and make the times progressively further and further apart). Change smoking behaviors (take shorter puffs or smoke less of each cigarette). Change routines (e.g., if patient is used to smoking while reading the newspaper after breakfast, suggest reading the newspaper while eating and then going for a walk after breakfast).		Do not let anyone smoke inside of the house. Stay away from smoky areas. Spend more time with friends who do not smoke.
Find Out Whether Patient Has Attempted to Stop Smoking in the Past		
No	**Yes**	
Arrange follow-up. Suggest that the patient join smoking cessation groups, attend counseling sessions, make office visits, make phone calls, or choose someone to help stick to the plan.	Explain that it often takes seven attempts before successfully quitting. Ask what got in the way of success when he or she last tried to quit. Help develop a plan to avoid the same problems that interfered with the previous attempt at quitting.	

*Nicotine-replacement products have not been proven to have fewer health risks than regular tobacco.

Certain factors increase the risk for the toxin to gain entry into the bloodstream. These include the use of high-absorbency tampons during menstruation and barrier methods of contraception (diaphragm or cervical cap), both of which can trap and hold bacteria if left in place for more than 48 hours.

Early diagnosis and treatment are important in preventing a fatal outcome. Symptoms include a sudden spiking fever and flulike symptoms (headache, muscle aches, vomiting, diarrhea, and sore throat), hypotension, generalized rash resembling sunburn, and skin peeling from the palms of the hands and soles of the feet 1 to 2 weeks after the onset of the illness. Laboratory findings usually reveal elevated blood urea nitrogen (BUN) and creatinine levels and low platelet count. Prevention includes changing tampons every 4 hours, using peri pads rather than tampons during sleep, not using diaphragms or cervical caps during menstruation, and washing the hands before and after inserting anything into the vagina. Hospitalization and intensive care may be required if TSS occurs.

PREMENSTRUAL SYNDROMES

Premenstrual syndrome (PMS), also known as **ovarian cycle syndrome,** is defined as the presence of physical, psychological, or behavioral symptoms that regularly recur with the luteal phase of the menstrual cycle, significantly disappear during the remainder of the cycle, and completely disappear the week after the menstrual period. Approximately 5% to 10% of menstruating women experience PMS that interferes with activities of daily living. The symptoms that occur between ovulation and the onset of menses include weight gain, bloating, irritability, loss of concentration, headaches, constipation, acne, breast tenderness, anger, fatigue, and feelings of being out of control that may interfere with work or school.

Premenstrual dysphoric disorder (PMDD) is a more severe type of PMS that involves irritability, dysphoria, mood swings, fatigue, appetite changes, and a sense of being overwhelmed (American Psychiatric Association, 2000). A woman's personal diary can confirm symptoms recurring during the specific phase of the ovarian cycle. The psychological symptoms are usually the result of a decreased ability to cope with psychological stressors rather than the appearance of new emotional distress. For this reason, psychotherapy may help the woman cope with or resolve problems that are aggravated by PMS. Medical treatment often includes drugs that inhibit ovulation. Pyridoxine (vitamin B_6) is thought to be helpful, although its use is not validated by research. Excess dosages of vitamin B_6 (more than 1000 mg/day) may result in peripheral nerve toxicity. Calcium and multivitamins with vitamin E may be advised by some obstetricians. Diuretics may be helpful when water retention is a problem. Selective serotonin reuptake inhibitors (SSRIs), such as fluoxetine (Prozac) and sertraline (Zoloft), have been shown to be effective in decreasing psychological symptoms. Gonadotropin-releasing hormone (GnRH) agonists do not show strong evidence of efficacy in the comprehensive treatment of PMS symptoms. Diet modifications include eating a well-balanced diet and avoiding a high salt intake to prevent water retention. Reducing caffeine intake to reduce breast tenderness and consuming low-fat, high-complex carbohydrates to increase brain serotonin synthesis help decrease nervousness, frustration, irritability, and agitation that the woman may be experiencing.

Management includes self-care measures directed toward developing a healthy behavior. The nurse can suggest stress management such as relaxation techniques and aerobic exercise, especially during the luteal phase of the cycle. Exercise has been found to increase blood levels of beta-endorphin (an opiate-like substance produced in the body). Complementary and alternative medicine (CAM) approaches to care include yoga, massage therapy, and herbs such as black cohosh, ginger, and chaste tree fruit (see Chapter 21).

DYSMENORRHEA

Dysmenorrhea refers to painful menstrual cramps that occur during or before the onset of menstruation and disappear by the end of menses. Dysmenorrhea is classified as primary or secondary. Primary dysmenorrhea is caused by prostaglandins, which are produced by the uterus in higher concentrations during menses. This increases uterine contractility and decreases uterine artery blood flow, resulting in painful ischemia, which is known to cause the sensation of cramps. Treatment of primary dysmenorrhea includes oral contraceptives (which block ovulation) and prostaglandin inhibitors (such as ibuprofen and aspirin). Self-care measures such as exercise, rest, heat, and proper nutrition help some women. Biofeedback has also been used with some success.

Secondary dysmenorrhea is associated with a pathologic condition of the reproductive tract. The symptoms appear after menstruation has been established. Some causes are endometriosis, pelvic inflammatory disease, and ovarian cysts. Some nutritionists suggest that vitamin E, a mild prostaglandin inhibitor, may decrease uterine discomfort. Warmth helps by promoting increased blood flow. Drinking hot herbal tea or sitting in a warm bath is soothing. Massage can soothe aching back muscles and promote relaxation, and daily exercise can ease the cramps.

MENSTRUAL IRREGULARITIES (DYSFUNCTIONAL BLEEDING)

Menstruation relies on a balance of several hormonal events that involve the hypothalamic, pituitary, ovarian, and uterine function that results in sloughing of the endometrium when pregnancy does not occur. Dysfunctional bleeding includes:

- **Menorrhagia**: More than 80 mL of blood is lost or menstruation lasts more than 7 days.
- **Polymenorrhea**: Menstruation occurs regularly in less than 21-day cycles (more frequent than normal).
- **Oligomenorrhea**: Menstruation occurs in cycles of more than 35 days.
- **Metrorrhagia**: Menstruation occurs at irregular and frequent intervals.
- *Menometrorrhagia:* Prolonged or excessive bleeding occurring at frequent intervals.
- *Postmenopausal vaginal bleeding:* Occurs at least 1 year after cessation of spontaneous menstruation.
- **Amenorrhea**: The absence of menstrual bleeding (primary, before regular menses is established, or secondary, after regular menses has been established).

Bleeding can be anovulatory, which is most common at the beginning or the end of reproductive life. There is no ovum, corpus luteum, or progestin to prepare uterine lining. Bleeding can also be ovulatory, which usually occurs at the height of the reproductive life cycle. It is associated with prolonged progesterone secretion or prostaglandin release. Risk factors include, age, obesity, excessive exercise, and high stress or medical condition such as polycystic ovarian syndrome (Ayers & Montgomery, 2009).

The form of management depends on the cause of the bleeding and should be investigated by the health care provider. The treatment of anovulatory bleeding includes combination oral contraceptives, and the treatment of ovulatory bleeding includes NSAIDs taken 1-2 days before menses to decrease prostaglandin production. OCs may also be used. Lysteda (tranexamic acid) has been approved by the FDA as a non-hormonal treatment for menorrhagia. It works by reducing clot breakdown in the uterus. It should not be used with oral contraceptives (USFDA, 2010). Surgical removal of polyps may be performed to diagnose endometrial hyperplasia.

LEIOMYOMAS

Uterine fibroids, also known as leiomyomas or myomas, are benign uterine tumors that develop during the woman's reproductive years. They are estrogen-dependent and progress to cancer in about 0.5% of patients diagnosed with fibroids. The majority of women with fibroids are diagnosed at the time of pelvic examination and may receive confirmation with a pelvic ultrasound. Detectable fibroids manifest as a pelvic mass, excessive menstrual bleeding, or both. In some women, the excessive bleeding leads to iron deficiency anemia. Small tumors are often undetectable and present no symptoms. Diagnosis can be confirmed with ultrasound, in most cases.

Although it is commonly believed that all fibroids grow larger during pregnancy, some fibroid tumors increase in size, whereas others actually regress. Women who have fibroids and become pregnant are subject to certain risks, including antepartum bleeding, dystocia from interference with the efficiency of uterine contractions, potential cesarean birth, and early pregnancy loss. There also appears to be an increased risk of preterm labor. Although specific risks exist, most pregnancy outcomes are quite favorable. Therefore, women with fibroids should not be discouraged from becoming pregnant.

Hormonal management includes the use of oral contraceptives (as an off-label use) or GnRH analogs, such as Lupron (Leuprolide), Synarel (Nafarelin acetate), and Zoladex (Goserelin acetate) to treat endometriosis and decrease the size of fibroids prior to surgery (Flowers, 2008).

The removal of the fibroid or myoma that impinges on or interferes with the endometrial cavity reduces the risk of pregnancy loss. Treatment options include a nonsurgical uterine fibroid embolization, magnetic resonance imaging (MRI)–guided focused ultrasound embolization, or a surgical myomectomy. For women with heavy or prolonged menstrual bleeding, a hysterectomy may be performed.

MENOPAUSE

Menopause occurs when a woman's menstrual periods have ceased for 1 year. The climacteric (change of life) refers to the physiologic and psychological alterations that occur around the time of menopause. Pregnancy can occur during the climacteric period. Psychological responses are affected by the woman's expectations, marital and financial stability, family views, and social or ethnic cultural values. The changes in women's health care enable women to cope more effectively, form new goals and priorities for this new phase, and enjoy a productive life.

Physical changes are a result of lowered estrogen levels. The average age of menopause in the United States is 51.5 years (Cedars & Evans, 2008). The uterine endometrium and myometrium atrophy, as do the cervical glands. The vaginal mucosa becomes smooth and thin, and the rugae disappear, leading to loss of elasticity. Sexual intercourse may be painful, but this can be overcome by using water-soluble lubricating gels. The woman may have hot flashes and feel a burning

Box 20-1 Contraindications to Menopausal Estrogen Treatment

- Pregnancy or possible pregnancy
- Unexplained vaginal bleeding
- Active or chronic impaired liver function
- Breast cancer
- Endometrial cancer, except in certain circumstances
- Recent vascular thrombosis (with or without emboli)

sensation in the face and chest, followed by perspiration. The woman may also notice chills, palpitations, dizziness, and tingling of the skin resulting from vasomotor instability.

A woman's view of menopause as a normal life transition or as a medical condition that requires treatment will determine management strategies. Decreasing estrogen does increase the risk for osteoporosis or increased cholesterol levels. Treatment options include exercise, a high-fiber diet that is rich in antioxidants, and calcium and magnesium supplements. Hormone replacement therapy (HRT) is acceptable for short-term treatment in younger women but not long-term treatment in older women (NAMS, 2008) (Box 20-1). CAM therapy includes yam root, which contains a natural progesterone-like substance; ginseng; soy products that contain phytoestrogens; black cohosh (thought to reduce luteinizing hormone); and vitamin E (see Chapter 21).

PELVIC FLOOR DYSFUNCTION

Pelvic floor dysfunction occurs when the supporting structures to pelvic organs are damaged or weakened. The damage may be the result of childbirth injury. Two classifications of pelvic floor dysfunction, which may occur at the same time, are vaginal wall prolapse (which includes cystocele, enterocele, and rectocele) and uterine prolapse. A **cystocele** occurs when the upper vaginal wall becomes weakened and unable to support the bladder, causing a downward displacement of the bladder. Stress incontinence (loss of urine) may result and is particularly noticeable when the woman coughs or sneezes. An **enterocele** occurs when the upper posterior vagina is weakened, allowing a loop of bowel to herniate downward between the uterus and rectum. A **rectocele** occurs when the posterior vaginal wall becomes weakened. When the woman strains to defecate, the feces are pushed against the wall instead of toward the rectum. Digital pressure against the posterior vaginal wall may facilitate defecation.

A **uterine prolapse** occurs when the supporting structures (ligaments) of the uterus and vagina are weakened, causing the uterus to protrude through the vagina. The woman feels pelvic pressure, fatigue, and backache. Uterine prolapse may occur in a woman who has had several vaginal births or large newborns born vaginally.

Treatment and Nursing Care

Age, physical condition, and sexual activity are considered in the medical management of pelvic floor relaxations. The vaginal wall(s) may be repaired, or a vaginal hysterectomy may be done. A pessary support device can be used if the woman is unable or chooses not to have surgery. Kegel exercises can help strengthen the pubococcygeal muscle—the major support for the urethra, vagina, and rectum (see Chapter 5). A diet high in fiber and adequate fluids can soften the stools and make it easier to defecate.

OSTEOPOROSIS

Osteoporosis is a degenerative musculoskeletal disorder in which a decrease in bone density results in an increased porosity in bone, making the person more vulnerable to fractures. The North American Menopause Society (NAMS) defines *osteoporosis* as a bone-mineral density score under 2.5 or presence of fragility fractures. In the United States, 1.3 million fractures occur yearly as a result of osteoporosis. Women at greatest risk are of Asian descent or small-boned, fair-skinned white women of Northern European descent. Other risk factors are family history, early menopause, a sedentary lifestyle, and inadequate calcium intake. Caffeine, alcohol, smoking, and long-term use of steroids also contribute to the decrease in bony skeletal mass.

Prevention of osteoporosis is the primary goal of care. Preventive measures should begin during youth. Women are advised to maintain an adequate calcium intake. Young women should have at least 1200 mg calcium per day, and postmenopausal women should take 1500 mg per day. Vitamin D, 400 to 800 units, should be taken to aid in calcium absorption. Calcium supplementation is most efficient when single doses do not exceed 500 mg and when it is taken with meals. Medications can be used, such as calcitonin (nasal spray), with nasal irritation as the major side effect, and alendronate (Fosamax), which is effective but has side effects such as esophageal irritation and gastric discomfort. To reduce the side effects of esophageal irritation, the drug must be taken on awakening, with a minimum of 8 oz of water, followed by staying in an upright position for 30 minutes. Although there is some evidence that estrogen replacement therapy increases bone density and reduces fractures, the risks involved with HRT must be weighed against the benefits. Low impact exercises are advised. Raloxifene (Evista), a selective estrogen receptor modifier (SERM) may be prescribed to prevent bone loss, Teriparatide (Forteo), an injectable parathyroid hormone is approved for menopausal women with high risk for fractures, for a 2-year period of therapy (NAMS, 2008).

The woman's height should be measured at each annual checkup because loss of height is often an early

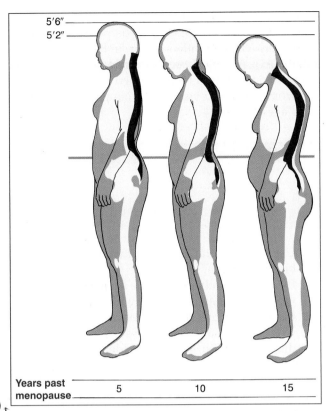

FIGURE 20-1 With progression of osteoporosis, the vertebral column collapses as a result of loss of bone mass, causing loss of height and back pain. Dowager's hump refers to the curvature of the upper back.

sign of compressed vertebrae caused by decreasing bone mass (Figure 20-1). A dowager's hump (cervical lordosis with dorsal kyphosis) occurs when the vertebrae can no longer support the upper body in an upright position. Treatment recommendations include educating the woman concerning healthy nutrition, calcium and vitamin D intake, regular exercise, and fall prevention. Follow-up concerning compliance and repeat bone density studies are recommended at 1-2 years after start of treatment or 5 years after initial testing (Bonnick, 2010). Further information can be found at www.nof.org.

BENIGN BREAST DISORDERS

The breast undergoes regular cyclic changes in response to hormonal stimulation. Each month, in rhythm with the ovulatory cycle of the ovaries and uterus, the breasts become engorged with fluid and the woman may have sensations of tenderness, lumpiness, or discomfort. Mastodynia (pain in the breasts) is common and usually lasts for 3 or 4 days before the onset of menses. In fibrocystic breast disease, a mobile, localized cyst may form that can be diagnosed and treated by needle aspiration. A fibroadenoma is a movable, well-defined solid breast mass that is nontender. Surgical removal may be indicated. A nonpalpable solitary nodule discovered by mammogram may be an interductal papilloma. Excision is the treatment of

choice. These conditions are most often benign but require follow-up and referral to a health care provider.

SCREENING TESTS FOR CANCER DETECTION

PAPANICOLAOU TEST

In most cases, changes occur in cells of the cervix before cervical cancer develops. The Papanicolaou (Pap) test (a screening device) is useful for detecting precancerous and cancerous cells that may be shed by the cervix. Regular Pap test screening detects early changes and enables early treatment, thereby increasing survival rates for cervical cancer. The U.S. Food and Drug Administration (FDA)–approved PapNet testing is an advanced method of computer technology that automatically detects and displays abnormal cells on a high-resolution color monitor for interpretation and diagnosis.

Health education concerning the need for regular Pap tests as part of routine health care and emotional support for women who have a positive Pap test result are nursing responsibilities. Gardasil is the first human papillomavirus (HPV) vaccine approved by the FDA. It is almost 100% effective in preventing HPV type 6, 11, 16, and 18 and associated precancerous lesions. It is indicated for women 9 to 26 years of age as a regular part of routine immunization programs. Annual PAP tests are recommended to start at age 21 and repeated every 2 years between 21 and 29 years of age unless pathology is seen. Women over 30 years of age with three consecutive negative PAP tests can lengthen the interval to every 3 years. Women with cervical cancer should be screened annually for 20 years after treatment. Screening is not necessary for women who have had elective cesarean sections or women over age 70 with 3 consecutive negative screenings (ACOG, 2009).

VULVAR SELF-EXAMINATION

During the pelvic examination, the nurse or health care provider can educate the woman about her vulva. Self-examination of the vulva, like breast self-examination, permits early detection of abnormalities, with possible early treatment and cure. The vulvar self-examination should be performed monthly, especially for all sexually active women. Vulvar self-examination is composed of visual inspection and palpation of the female external genitalia. Any abnormalities (discharge, irritation, or growths observed) should be reported to the health care provider. A good light and mirror are needed for the examination.

BREAST SELF-EXAMINATION

Women have been encouraged to perform a breast self-examination (BSE) every month. If the woman becomes knowledgeable about her breasts by performing a regular self-examination, she often is able to detect an abnormality earlier or recognize that the finding is normal and has not changed for years. The BSE should begin during adolescence. Some health care providers feel mammography alone is sufficient because many BSEs result in false-positive interpretations (Chiarelli, Majpruz, Brown, et al., 2009).

The nurse or health care provider should teach the woman how to perform a BSE during a routine physical examination. BSE should be performed approximately 1 week after each menstrual period, when the breasts are usually not tender or swollen. After menopause, the BSE should be performed on the same day each month so that it becomes routine (Skill 20-1). A clinical breast examination by a health care provider should be performed every 1 to 3 years for women ages 40 years and younger and annually after age 40 years.

Skill 20-1   Breast Self-Examination

PURPOSE
To learn how the breasts feel and detect any changes.

Note: Perform breast self-examination (BSE) monthly, approximately 1 week after the menstrual period, when breasts are not tender or swollen from hormonal changes. This is an ideal time to feel breasts for consistency in breast tissue. Perform BSE the same day each month so it becomes routine (you will be less likely to forget to do it).

Steps
1. Lie down.
2. Flatten your breast by placing a pillow under your shoulder on the side being examined.
3. Put one hand behind your head.
4. Use finger pads of your three middle fingers to feel for lumps or thickening.

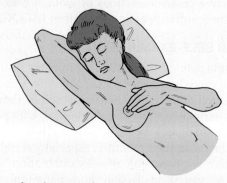

5. Press firmly enough to distinguish different breast textures.
6. Move around the breast in a set way. (You can choose the circle movement, the up-and-down line, or the wedge movement.)

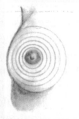 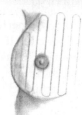 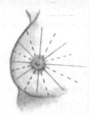

7. Use the same way each time to remember how the breast feels.
8. Examine the other breast the same way. Compare what you feel in one breast with the other.
9. Inspect your breasts while looking in the mirror with your hands at your sides. Look for noticeable dimpling of skin, swelling, reddening, asymmetry, or changes in the nipple.
10. You may want to palpate your breasts while taking a shower, when the skin is wet and lumps may be easier to feel. Your soapy hands will glide over the wet skin, making it easy to check how your breast feels.

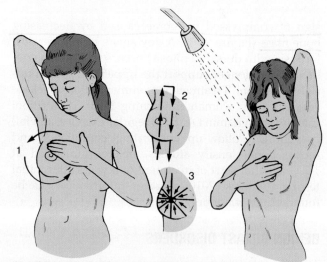

11. Report any changes, such as lumps, dimpling, thickening of skin, or nipple discharge.

MAMMOGRAPHY

A **mammogram** is a soft-tissue radiographic image of the breast taken without the injection of a contrast medium. It can detect lesions in the breast before they can be felt and is an effective screening tool for breast cancer. Currently, the American Cancer Society suggests that all women age 40 years and older have an annual mammogram. The National Cancer Institute recommends mammograms every 1 to 2 years for women ages 40 to 49 years and annually for all women ages 50 years and older. The National Cancer Advisory Board also suggests that women at high risk for breast cancer should ask their physicians about beginning mammography before the age of 40 years. The digital mammography technique has reduced the occurrence of false-positive readings (Buzek, 2010).

One national goal for *Healthy People 2010* related to women's health was met in the year 2010: access to mammograms for women ages 50 years and older. Mammography is a useful tool, but it cannot replace BSE and clinical examination; both are needed. Up to 10% of early-stage breast cancers are first detected by clinical examination, not by mammogram. Transillumination, thermography, and ultrasound can aid in detecting cancerous lesions in dense breast tissue.

☀ BREAST CANCER

RISK FACTORS

Each year an estimated 1 in 8 women is diagnosed with breast cancer in the United States. Two inherited genes linked to breast cancer have been identified: *BRCA-1*, located on chromosome 17, and *BRCA-2*, located on chromosome 13. It is thought that as many as 30% of women given the diagnosis of cancer before 45 years of age may be carriers of the *BRCA-1* gene. Other risk factors include age greater than 50 years, family history of premenopausal breast cancer, use of alcohol, smoking, high-fat diet, high caffeine intake, early menarche, late menopause, and nulligravid status. Studies concerning genetic links to breast and gynecologic cancer are ongoing.

Although genetic testing for the risk of breast cancer was intended to enhance informed decision making and influence self-care, often the early knowledge that a genetic mutation is present with a high risk for developing breast cancer sometime during the life cycle may result only in increased anxiety and depression that may decrease quality of life.

Inflammatory breast cancer (IBC) is a rare type of cancer that is very aggressive and occurs in younger women and many African American women. A rapidly appearing red, inflamed breast tissue typically occurs rather than the traditional breast lump. Breast conservation therapy is not an option for this type of breast cancer at this time (Morris, 2010).

Treatment and Nursing Care

Surgical Procedures. When the woman is told that she has breast cancer, important decisions must be made regarding the type of surgery available or whether she has other options. Conservative breast surgery in early disease combined with radiation or adjuvant chemotherapy improves survival rates comparable to those for radical mastectomy (Box 20-2). Today, less emphasis is placed on radical procedures. Mastectomy rates from 1997 to 2003 decreased from 45% to 31% but then increased to 43% in 2006, even though the outcomes were not shown to be better than lumpectomy or radiation (Katipamula, Degnim, Hoskin, et al., 2009; Morrow & Harris, 2009). The most common surgical procedures are:

- **Lumpectomy:** Removal of a tumor from the breast. This is considered conservative treatment, and the excision is performed without major cosmetic deformity. Some axillary lymph nodes are often removed to rule out spread of the disease. Radiotherapy may or may not be prescribed.
- **Simple mastectomy:** Removal of the entire breast. Axillary dissection is omitted, although some lymph nodes may be removed to rule out the spread of the disease.
- **Modified radical mastectomy:** Removal of breast tissue, axillary nodes, and some chest muscles. The pectoralis major muscles are preserved. This procedure is recommended when a large primary lesion is found in a relatively small breast.
- **Radical mastectomy:** Removal of the entire breast, including the axillary nodes and the pectoral muscles. It is rarely performed today.

The nurse should encourage the woman to verbalize her feelings and express her fears. The loss of a body part and fear of pain, disability, and death can be overwhelming. Education concerning the diagnosis and treatment options is a nursing responsibility.

Adjuvant Therapy. Adjuvant therapy is additional therapy after the surgical procedures. Some tumors are estrogen-receptor positive, meaning that their growth is stimulated by estrogen; therefore, estrogen-blocking drugs are administered, such as tamoxifen, which blocks estrogen by binding with it. The side effects of tamoxifen vary, but the most

---

Box 20-2 | **Breast Surgery Options**

- **Lumpectomy:** Removing the tumor mass and a narrow margin of normal tissue surrounding it.
- **Simple mastectomy:** Removing the tumor, nipple, and areola and removing axillary lymph nodes for staging purposes.
- **Modified radical mastectomy:** Removing breast tissue, axillary nodes, and some chest muscles, while preserving the pectoralis major muscles.
- **Radical mastectomy:** Removing all breast tissue, pectoral muscles, and axillary nodes; less common.

Box 20-3 Discharge Planning After Breast Surgery

- Assist the woman in understanding her diagnosis, therapy, and long-term prognosis.
- Encourage the woman to participate in her recovery program.
- Teach the woman to recognize complications that may occur.
- Advise the woman about planned exercises, activities, and follow-up care.
- Encourage the woman to attend Reach to Recovery group discussions.

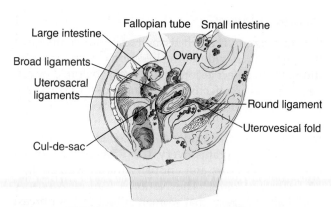

FIGURE 20-2 Common sites of endometriosis.

common are hot flashes, leg cramps, bladder problems, nausea, and anorexia. Raloxifene is a similar drug, which may have fewer side effects. Initial treatment may interfere with nutrition due to nausea and vomiting or loss of appetite, but patients should be warned that antioxidant supplements may reduce the effectiveness of chemotherapy or radiation treatment. Megadoses of vitamins are not recommended. The American Cancer Association guidelines include the use of plant sources of vitamins with limited supplements, limiting high-fat foods and daily physical activity. Green tea is a natural antioxidant, soy contains isoflavones that can mimic estrogens and are a source of protein and fish-oil, omega-3 fatty acids from 3 oz of fish twice a week are helpful suggestions (Blackwell & Burns, 2010). Statin drugs have been prescribed to reduce cholesterol and prevent heart attacks, but now some studies show that statin drugs may be useful in reducing the risk of cancer and increasing the response to chemotherapy (Elmore & Li, 2010).

Discharge teaching and follow-up care are important (Box 20-3). Women who take aspirin 2-5 days per week after breast surgery may reduce complications (Holmes, Chen, Li, Hertzmark, Spiegelman, & Hankinson, 2010). Most women benefit from information about support groups, such as Reach to Recovery and Encore. Someone from Reach to Recovery who has had breast cancer surgery may visit the woman before she leaves the hospital. The visitor will explain the importance of rehabilitation, such as arm exercises, and encourage the patient to join a support group of women who have had breast cancer surgery.

ENDOMETRIOSIS

Endometriosis is the presence of endometrial tissue implanted predominantly in extrauterine sites (ovaries, fallopian tubes, cul-de-sac, uterine ligaments, and other areas in the reproductive tract; Figure 20-2). Endometrial cells contain glands and stroma, which respond to the cyclic hormonal stimulation in the same way that the uterine endometrium does. As the lesions build up and slough off during the menstrual cycles,

they often cause pelvic pain, pressure, and inflammation to the adjacent organs. This results in an inflammatory response, causing adhesions to form. The exact cause of endometriosis is poorly understood. Proposed causative factors include retrograde menstrual flow that transplants endometrial tissue outside of the uterus, hereditary tendency, and possible immunologic defect.

Management varies with the severity of the pain, extent of the disease, desire for children, patient age, and threat to the gastrointestinal or urinary tract. NSAIDs provide pain relief for some women. Continuous OC therapy for 6 to 12 months may suppress endometrial growth. Surgical intervention is often needed for severe symptoms. For women who want to retain their reproductive capacity, laser therapy or surgery with careful removal of all endometrial tissue is an option.

Other interventions include teaching nonpharmacologic measures to relieve pain, such as frequent rest periods, application of heat to the lower abdomen, moderate exercise, and a well-balanced diet. Suppressing endocrine production to limit lesion growth and medically induced menopause can be used to treat this condition. The nurse should advise the woman about potential side effects of GnRH agonists, which may cause hot flashes, vaginal dryness, mood swings, bone loss, and irregular bleeding. Nafarelin acetate (Synarel [a GnRH agonist]) is used as a nasal spray, or leuprolide acetate (Lupron depot, a time-release injection) may be given. Recent studies provide evidence that the use of aromatase inhibitors along with combination oral contraceptives or progestin effectively treats pelvic pain that is resistant to other therapies in both premenopausal and postmenopausal women.

DOUCHING

Douching is placing a liquid into the vagina for cleanliness, odor control, or comfort. It is estimated that 32% of women douche regularly. There are no evidence-based benefits of douching, but the risks are great. Douching alters the vaginal flora predisposing the development of bacterial vaginosis, which can be a risk to a normal pregnancy or cause pelvic inflammatory disease (PID). Douching may increase the risk for ectopic pregnancy and susceptibility to HIV and STI pathogens. The risks of douching should be discussed with women, especially those considering pregnancy (Cottrell, 2010).

PELVIC INFLAMMATORY DISEASE

Pelvic inflammatory disease (PID) is an infection of the upper genital tract involving a tubal infection (salpingitis). Although many organisms have been found to cause PID, *Chlamydia trachomatis* and *Neisseria gonorrhoeae* are most common, and infectious organisms can ascend from the vagina to the cervix and upper genital tract. Early onset of sexual activity and multiple sexual partners increase the risk for PID. PID may also place the woman at risk for infertility, ectopic pregnancies, pelvic abscess, and adhesions.

Minimal criteria established for diagnosis and treatment include pelvic pain; adnexal tenderness; cervical motion tenderness, which often causes dyspareunia (painful intercourse); fever; and purulent vaginal discharge. Positive ultrasound and elevated erythrocyte sedimentation rate (ESR) further confirm diagnosis. The use of a home test for vaginal pH can determine the need for early intervention for vaginitis. A decrease in vaginal acidity allows pathogens to invade and can result in PID (Wysocki, 2010).

Women with serious infection may require hospital care and intravenous therapy with cefotetan or doxycycline hyclate (Vibramycin). Outpatient treatment with levofloxacin and metronidazole for 14 days has had high success rates. The sexual partner should also be seen by a health care provider and treated as indicated. Follow-up care is important. Health education concerning safer sexual practices and prevention of repeated PID is imperative.

VIOLENCE AGAINST WOMEN

Violence against women is a widespread problem. It is known by a variety of names, such as domestic violence, intimate partner violence, spouse abuse, wife battering, and marital rape. Battering is the single most common source of injury to women. Each year, 3 million to 4 million women in the United States are battered by men with whom they live. Battering is often associated with rape. Violence may start or become worse during pregnancy, and the abdomen is often the target for battery.

Violence comes in many forms. Because physical assault is the easiest to measure, it is the type of abuse most discussed. However, emotional abuse, characterized by intimidation and assault on self-esteem, is receiving more attention than in the past. Abuse may be physical, emotional, sexual, social, or financial and involves one individual exercising power and control over another in the relationship.

Often the abuser does not perceive his violent behavior as a problem and denies responsibility for the violence by blaming the woman. Although many abusive men have alcohol or other substance abuse problems, many also batter women when they are sober. It is important to remember that violence against women is deliberate, can be severe, and generally is repeated. Often the abusive episode is followed by apologies and a kind, loving "honeymoon" period. However, the cycle typically repeats.

Assessment, such as observing bruises and injuries, is an important nursing intervention. These women may wait for someone to ask them about their injuries because they are too ashamed to volunteer the information (Nursing Care Plan 20-1). The nurse can help gather sufficient information in a nonthreatening, nonjudgmental way. Lack of safety, isolation, poor self-esteem, and lack of a support network can cause the woman to be afraid to leave the abusive relationship. Counseling and referral to available community resources are essential. The National Domestic Violence Hotline (800-787-7233) provides crisis intervention.

RAPE TRAUMA SYNDROME

Rape is not a sexual experience for a woman, and, in many cases, the male perpetrator does not have a sexual basis for the violent act. The nurse should understand the response of the female rape victim so that he or she can provide caring and comprehensive support.

The victim's immediate response is fear of death or mutilation. After the attack, the woman may appear calm but is focused inward, often not hearing or complying with requests of medical personnel. Anxiety and irritability are primary behavioral responses, which gradually change to shock, disbelief, fear, guilt, and shame. The long-term response can include a change in lifestyle, distrust of men, and development of phobias and fears that interfere with activities of daily living. Posttraumatic stress disorder may be a long-term complication of the experience, and appropriate referrals for psychological help must be initiated as early as possible.

Although specific medical examinations and tests are required, the nurse's primary role is to help the woman regain a feeling of control in the examination setting. Some choices should be made available to the woman. Informed consent is required for examination and collection of evidence. Often, tetanus and antibiotic prophylaxis for sexually transmitted infections may be prescribed. Human immunodeficiency virus (HIV) testing and counseling are provided, and postcoital contraception is offered when appropriate. Psychological referral is highly recommended. The nurse should contact social services to ensure that the woman has transportation to a safe location with friends or relatives and has written appointments for follow-up care and testing.

Nursing Care Plan 20-1 | The Battered Woman

Scenario

A 28-year-old woman has a history of not keeping appointments and providing evasive reasons for the cause of her injuries. Complete physical examination reveals bruises and old injuries to face, chest, and abdomen. The woman verbalizes that her husband frequently tells her she is not worthwhile, "especially when he drinks," and he physically abuses her. The woman's chief symptom is low self-esteem.

Selected Nursing Diagnosis

Situational low self-esteem related to spousal emotional abuse

Expected Outcomes	Nursing Interventions	Rationales
Patient will improve her self-esteem.	Gather information in a nonthreatening and nonjudgmental way.	The woman is dependent on her spouse.
	Ask the woman to express her feelings and concerns.	She (like many women) places blame for abuse on herself.
	Encourage woman to discuss her bruises and old injuries.	Verbalization helps clarify the problem.

Selected Nursing Diagnosis

Ineffective coping related to low self-esteem

Expected Outcomes	Nursing Interventions	Rationales
Patient will increase her self-determination.	Acknowledge her state of confusion in response to questions.	The woman can be assisted in recognizing her self-worth and in developing assertiveness.
	Provide reassurance.	
	Identify supportive counseling for the woman.	

Selected Nursing Diagnosis

Deficient knowledge related to lack of information of available community resources

Expected Outcomes	Nursing Interventions	Rationales
Patient will discuss resources available to her.	Identify support services available to the woman.	She may think she has no options and therefore is trapped in her situation.
	Name available community resources such as safe houses.	She is unaware of community resources.
	Explain the reason for developing an exit plan to protect her from danger.	An exit plan is a way to escape if threatened. It requires advance preparation.
	Provide names and phone numbers of support groups.	Support groups assist the woman in coping without her spouse.

Critical Thinking Question

1. A patient has been admitted to the unit with a diagnosis of rape trauma syndrome. She is irritable and refuses to complete activities of daily living. What is the best response you can provide the patient?

HEPATITIS

Hepatitis is an inflammation of the liver caused by a virus. There are five identified strains of virus causing hepatitis, termed A, B, C, D, and E. Immunizations are available for hepatitis A and B. Hepatitis B may be transmitted by sexual activity, intravenous drug use, or intimate contact with blood and body fluids. In health care workers, exposure may be caused by infected blood from an accidental needle puncture. Vaccination against hepatitis B is advised for all health care workers. Hepatitis A is transmitted by contaminated food and water or the fecal-oral route. Hepatitis B, C, and D are chronic infections. Hepatitis E occurs most often in the Middle East and Asia and is a self-limiting condition.

SEXUALLY TRANSMITTED INFECTIONS

Previously termed *sexually transmitted diseases* (STDs), sexually transmitted infections (STIs) are specific infections that are transmitted primarily during sexual contact. The infection is spread by contact with bodily fluids from the mouth, genitalia, rectum, and blood. STIs during pregnancy can cause spontaneous abortion, preterm birth, intrauterine growth restriction, neonatal death, congenital infection, and postpartum uterine infection (Table 20-2).

Community education, free clinics, disease detection, partner tracing, and improved treatment are goals to reduce the incidence and effects of STIs (Box 20-4 on p. 404). Health care providers must take necessary precautions in caring for individuals with STIs. Rapid diagnosis of

(*Text continued on p. 404*)

Table 20-2   Sexually Transmitted Infections

INFECTION (CAUSATIVE ORGANISM)	SIGNS AND SYMPTOMS	DIAGNOSIS	PREGNANCY, FETAL, AND NEONATAL EFFECTS	TREATMENT	COMMENTS
Candidiasis (yeast) (*Candida albicans*)	Itching and burning on urination, inflammation of vulva and vagina, "cottage cheese" appearance to discharge	Signs and symptoms; identification of spores of the causative fungus	Can infect newborn at birth	Miconazole nitrate (Monistat), clotrimazole (Gyne-Lotrimin), nystatin (Mycostatin), fluconazole (Diflucan)	Medications are available over-the-counter (OTC), but the woman should seek medical attention to diagnose her first infection or if she has persistent or recurrent infections.
Trichomoniasis (*Trichomonas vaginalis*)	Thin, foul-odor, greenish yellow vaginal discharge; vulvar itching; edema; redness	Identification of the organism under microscope in a wet-mount preparation and rapid antibody test; DNA/RNA	Does not cross placenta Can cause postpartum infection	Metronidazole (Flagyl) if not pregnant during first trimester; clotrimazole (Gyne-Lotrimin) for symptom relief during first trimester	Organism thrives in an alkaline environment. Most infections are thought to be transmitted by sexual contact.
Bacterial vaginosis (*Gardnerella vaginalis*)	Thin, grayish white discharge that has a fishy odor	Microscopic evidence of clue cells (epithelial cells with bacteria clinging to their surface) and rapid detection tests	Associated with preterm delivery	Bacteria are normal inhabitants of the vagina, but overgrow. Treatment aims to restore normal balance of vaginal bacterial flora. Metronidazole (Flagyl) may relieve symptoms.	Avoid alcohol during treatment with metronidazole (Flagyl) and for 24 hours after. Flagyl cannot be used during first trimester of pregnancy.
Chlamydia (*Chlamydia trachomatis*)	Yellowish discharge and painful urination Often asymptomatic in women, which delays treatment	Culture, rapid detection tests, DNA probe using urine specimen is noninvasive NAAT	Transmitted via birth canal Causes conjunctivitis and pneumonia in newborn	Azithromycin, doxycycline, erythromycin in pregnancy All newborns have prophylactic eye care.	Untreated infection can ascend into fallopian tubes, causing scarring. Infertility or ectopic pregnancy may result. Can spread to neonate's eyes by contact with infected vaginal secretions.

Continued

Table 20-2 Sexually Transmitted Infections—cont'd

INFECTION (CAUSATIVE ORGANISM)	SIGNS AND SYMPTOMS	DIAGNOSIS	PREGNANCY, FETAL, AND NEONATAL EFFECTS	TREATMENT	COMMENTS
Gonorrhea (*Neisseria gonorrhoeae*)	Purulent discharge, painful urination, dyspareunia	Culture of organism NAAT	Transmitted to newborn's eyes during birth, causing blindness (ophthalmia neonatorum)	Cephalosporin antibiotics (fluoroquinolones are not effective) (CDC, 2006) All newborns have prophylactic eye care	Can result in pelvic inflammatory disease with tubal scarring.
Syphilis (*Treponema pallidum*)	3 stages: *Primary:* painless chancre on genitalia, anus, or lips *Secondary:* 2 months after primary syphilis; enlargement of spleen and liver, headache, anorexia, generalized skin rash, wartlike growths on vulva *Tertiary:* may occur many years after secondary syphilis and cause heart, blood vessel, nervous system damage	*Primary:* examining material scraped from chancre with darkfield microscopy to identify the spirochete organism; serologic tests are not positive this early *Secondary or tertiary:* serologic test (VDRL [less specific], RPR, and FTA-ABS [more specific])	Transmitted across placenta Causes congenital syphilis, stillbirth, spontaneous abortion	Penicillin; doxycycline, tetracycline, or erythromycin if allergic Tetracycline is not recommended during pregnancy; desensitization of the woman is recommended.	Primary and secondary stages are the most contagious. Spread is through sexual contact, by inoculation (sharing needles), or through the placenta from an infected mother.

Disease	Signs and symptoms	Diagnosis	Effect on pregnancy/fetus	Treatment	Comments
Herpes genitalis (herpes simplex virus [HSV], types I and II)	Clusters of painful vesicles (blisters) on the vulva, perineum, and anal areas. Vesicles rupture in 1-7 days and heal in 12 days	By signs and symptoms; confirmed by viral culture antibody or DNA-based rapid test	Can cause spontaneous abortion, stillbirth. Active genital infection requires cesarean delivery. Causes neonatal CNS problems	No cure exists: acyclovir (Zovirax) or valacyclovir (Valtrex) reduces symptoms. Treated with hygiene, sitz baths during pregnancy.	HSV II usually causes genital lesions. The first episode is usually most uncomfortable. The virus "hides" in the nerve cells and can reemerge in later outbreaks that are as contagious as the first.
Condylomata acuminata (human papillomavirus [HPV])	Dry, wart-like growths on the vagina, labia, cervix, and perineum	By typical appearance and location	Growth may obstruct birth canal. Infant may have laryngeal papillomas.	Removal with cryotherapy (cold), electrocautery, laser, or podophyllin applications are alternatives.	Also known as venerea or genital warts; associated with higher rates of cervical cancer. Gardasil is a vaccine that protects against HPV types 6, 11, 16, and 18.
Acquired immunodeficiency syndrome (AIDS) (human immunodeficiency virus [HIV])	Initially, no symptoms; later symptoms include weight loss, night sweats, fever and chills, fatigue, enlarged lymph nodes, skin rashes, diarrhea. Late symptoms include immunosuppression, opportunistic infections, and malignancies	Serologic tests: positive ELISA, followed by positive Western blot test	Avoid breaks in skin to mother and fetus during birth process. Transmitted antepartum to newborn. Drug therapy advised. Infant should be bottle fed.	No cure available yet. Zidovudine (AZT, Retrovir) and didanosine (Videx) may slow progression. Lamivudine and nelfinavir given during pregnancy	Transmitted through contact of nonintact skin or mucous membranes with infectious secretions exposure to blood, and transmission from mother to fetus. Standard precautions reduce risk for caregivers. Condom use reduces risk for sexual transmission.

(handwritten note) ✗ Vaginal birth results in possible risk of baby getting HSV

CNS, central nervous system; DNA/RNA, deoxyribonucleic acid/ribonucleic acid; ELISA, enzyme-linked immunosorbent assay; FTA-ABS, fluorescent treponemal antibody absorption test; NAAT, nucleic acid amplification test; RPR, rapid plasma reagin; VDRL, Venereal Disease Research Laboratory.

Box 20-4	Patient Education for Sexually Transmitted Infections

- Make certain the patient understands what infection he or she has, how it is transmitted, why it must be treated, and when and how to take prescribed medications.
- Impress on the patient the need to take medications as prescribed, even though the symptoms of the disease may have disappeared. Discontinuing antibiotics before the infection is completely gone not only leads to recurrent infection, but also increases the likelihood that drug-resistant strains of pathogen may flourish.
- Prevent reinfection by treating the sexual partner.
- Advise patients to avoid sexual intercourse while completing the full course of therapy.
- Urge the patient to continue to use condoms to prevent repeated infections at all times.
- Help the patient recognize that good health habits require regular assessment of one's body, including genital self-examination.
- Mention that the American Social Health Association maintains a hotline for people to call for current information about sexually transmitted infections (1-800-227-8922).

many STIs is possible in the physician's office, avoiding the need for a waiting period and return visit. *Point of care tests,* which provide rapid test results, are available for herpes simplex virus 2, chlamydia, and gonorrhea. HIV point of care testing is currently used in many delivery rooms for patients who are seen without prenatal care. Point of care HIV testing should be followed by serum testing for secondary confirmation of the rapid test results.

HUMAN PAPILLOMAVIRUS (HPV)

An estimated 11,000 women in the United States were diagnosed with cervical cancer in 2008, and 97% of the cancer specimens showed strains of HPV 16 or 18 and HPV DNA (Klisz & Kaplan, 2009). HPV can also manifest as genital warts caused by HPV strains 6 and 11. The treatment for HPV infection does not necessarily eradicate the virus, and recurrence is common. The goal is to prevent HPV with early vaccination and safe sex education. There are currently two HPV vaccines available and recommended for girls ages 10 to 25:

1. Gardasil—protects against strains 6, 11, 16, and 18.
2. Cervarix—protects against strains 16 and 18.

Gardasil is also recommended for boys and men to prevent genital warts caused by strains 6 and 11 and as a means to prevent cervical cancer in women (Klisz & Kaplan, 2009).

HPV vaccine should be stored in the refrigerator but not frozen.

PREVENTION OF SEXUALLY TRANSMITTED INFECTIONS

Developmentally appropriate education, screening, and immunizations are strategies for preventing STIs. A mutually monogamous relationship with an uninfected partner is best to prevent STIs. With many individuals, this option is not feasible; therefore, they must be aware of how STI transmission takes place. The identification of high-risk behavior, nonjudgmental counseling, diagnosis, treatment, immunization when indicated, and education should be part of every physical checkup.

Safer sex practices, reduction in partners, and avoidance of the exchange of blood and body fluids are all essential components of primary education of STI prevention. Also, critically important is the use of condoms during sexual encounters. Community programs that provide information concerning STIs, their effects, and prevention must start in the public schools and be supported in the home (Table 20-3).

Table 20-3	Principles to Reduce the Risk of Acquiring Sexually Transmitted Infections	
BASIC INFORMATION	**HEALTH PROTECTION AND RATIONALE**	
Know that sexual activity provides potential contact with STIs and that precautions reduce risk.	Practice abstinence or restriction to one partner; increased number of partners increases risk.	
Practice sexual activities that do not cause exchange of bodily fluids with multiple partners.	STI organisms are transmitted by direct contact with mucous surfaces or open skin.	
Understand that barrier forms of contraception such as condoms reduce risk.	Properly used, condoms along with spermicides (contraceptive foam or jelly) reduce risk of many STIs; if an individual's infectious lesions are exposed, the contraceptive devices will not be helpful in preventing STIs.	
Avoid unsafe sex practices.	Avoid practices that may cause skin or mucous membrane injury; avoid unprotected anal contact (e.g., anal intercourse); avoid sexual activities that cause bleeding.	
Recognize importance of periodic screening for STIs.	Individuals at high risk, especially those with more than one sex partner, should be screened or tested often.	
Recognize individuals at high risk for HIV/AIDS.	Recognize those who share intravenous needles; who engage in anal sex, oral-genital sex, or vaginal intercourse without a condom; who have sex with someone who has or who themselves have multiple partners.	
Ask for partner's cooperation.	Recognize that individuals with STIs (e.g., chlamydia, gonorrhea, or HIV infection) may or may not have symptoms.	

AIDS, acquired immunodeficiency syndrome; *HIV,* human immunodeficiency virus; *STIs,* sexually transmitted infections.

Get Ready for the NCLEX® Examination!

Key Points

- TSS is a serious disorder caused by toxins released by a strain of S. aureus or group A streptococci. It is associated with the use of tampons and some barrier methods of contraception. Occluding the cervical os for a prolonged period may allow organisms to reproduce in the vagina and then enter the bloodstream.
- PMS, also called *ovarian cycle syndrome*, involves physical and behavioral symptoms that occur during the luteal phase of the menstrual cycle.
- Dysmenorrhea refers to painful menstrual cramps. Oral contraceptives and prostaglandin inhibitors may provide relief. NSAIDs may lessen discomfort.
- Menopause is the cessation of menses and a time of transition for the woman as a result of lowered estrogen level.
- Osteoporosis results from the loss of bone mass with bones becoming porous, fragile, and susceptible to fracture.
- Disorders of the breasts may be benign, such as fibrocystic breast changes.
- Gardasil, an FDA-approved HPV vaccine, should be part of the regular immunization regimen of young girls. It is also recommended for boys.
- Each year 1 in 8 women in the United States develops breast cancer. Risk factors other than the genes identified include premenopausal breast dysplasia, first-degree relatives (mother or sister) with cancer, and early menarche with late menopause. Lifestyle factors such as smoking, high-fat diet, and consumption of alcohol are also suspected risks.
- Management of breast cancer includes surgical removal of the tumor and varying amounts of surrounding tissue and lymph glands. Adjuvant therapies include radiation, chemotherapy, and hormonal therapy.
- Endometriosis is a condition in which endometrial tissue is present outside of the uterine cavity. Symptoms include dysmenorrhea, deep seated aching pain, dyspareunia, and infertility.
- PID is a condition that results from an infection ascending into the fallopian tubes and sometimes the peritoneal cavity. It can be a contributing cause of ectopic pregnancy and infertility.
- Violence against women is widespread and underreported. It is known by different names, such as battering or intimate partner violence. The violence may start or become worse during pregnancy. It may involve physical, sexual, emotional, social, or financial abuse and involves power and control over the woman.
- STIs are transmitted during sexual contact and with exposure to bodily fluids, including blood.
- Rapid diagnosis of some STIs is available in the health care provider's office.

Additional Learning Resources

SG   Go to your Study Guide on pages 511–512 for additional Review Questions for the NCLEX® Examination, Critical Thinking Clinical Situations, and other learning activities to help you master this chapter content.

 evolve   Go to your Evolve website (http://evolve.elsevier.com/Leifer/maternity) for the following FREE learning resources:

- Animations
- Answer Guidelines for Critical Thinking Questions
- Answers and Rationales for Review Questions for the NCLEX® Examination
- Concept Map Creator
- Glossary with pronunciations in English and Spanish
- Patient Teaching Plans
- Skills Performance Checklists and more!

Online Resources
- www.4women.gov
- www.aarp.org/grandparents
- www.ashastd.org
- www.breastcancer.org/symptoms/types/inflammatory
- www.cancer.gov/cancertopics/factsheet/sites-types/IBC
- ww.cdc.gov/reproductivehealth/unintendedpregnancy/vsmec.htm
- www.cdc.gov/std
- www.hormonecme.org
- www.menopause.org
- www.ndvh.org
- www.niams.nih.gov/boneosteoporosisinfo
- www.preventiveservices.ahrq.gov
- www.quitnet.com

Review Questions for the NCLEX® Examination

1. A woman has been prescribed calcitonin nasal spray to prevent osteoporosis. When explaining potential side effects, the nurse states that the major side effect with use of calcitonin nasal spray is:
   1. Esophageal irritation
   2. Gastric discomfort
   3. Nasal irritation
   4. Headaches

2. Risk factors for the development of breast cancer include: *(Select all that apply.)*
   1. Multigravid status
   2. Age greater than 50 years
   3. Use of alcohol
   4. High-fat diet

3. A patient has returned to the nursing care unit following a surgical procedure that involved removal of the entire right breast, including axillary nodes and the pectoral muscles. The nurse is aware that this surgical procedure is known as a:
   1. Lumpectomy
   2. Simple mastectomy
   3. Modified radical mastectomy
   4. Radical mastectomy

4. It is suspected that a woman has pelvic inflammatory disease (PID). A diagnostic test that would confirm this diagnosis is an elevated:

   1. WBC count
   2. RBC count
   3. Creatinine level
   4. Erythrocyte sedimentation rate (ESR)

5. Toxic shock syndrome (TSS) is a multisystem infection that results from the response of the body to toxins produced by:

   1. *Staphylococcus aureus*
   2. *Chlamydia trachomatis*
   3. *Neisseria gonorrhoeae*
   4. Human papillomavirus

6. What should be included in patient education concerning a breast self-examination (BSE)? *(Select all that apply.)*

   1. Perform a BSE once every 2 months.
   2. A BSE should be performed 1 week after the menstrual period.
   3. Cease BSE after menopause.
   4. A clinical breast examination should be performed every 1 to 3 years for women age 40 and younger.

7. According to the American Psychiatric Association, premenstrual dysphoric disorder (PMDD) is a more severe type of PMS that involves which symptom(s)? *(Select all that apply.)*

   1. Irritability
   2. Dysmenorrhea
   3. Mood swings
   4. Appetite changes

Critical Thinking Question

1. A mother objects to her 10-year-old daughter getting an HPV vaccine. The mother states her daughter is too young to be worried about sexual activity and does not need the vaccine until she is older. What is the best response you can provide?

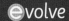
Complementary and Alternative Therapies

Objectives

1. Define key terms listed.
2. Define both complementary and alternative therapies.
3. Review the federal government's involvement in alternative therapies.
4. Discuss the history of complementary and alternative therapies in nursing.
5. List and discuss four complementary and alternative therapies used to relax women in labor.
6. List and discuss three complementary and alternative therapies used to lessen pain during labor.
7. State three herbal products that should be avoided during pregnancy.

Key Terms

acupressure (Ă K-ū-PRĔSH-ŭr, p. 409)
allopathic care (ăl-ō-PĂTH-ĭk, p. 407)
alternative therapy (p. 407)
aromatherapy (p. 410)
biofeedback (p. 411)
complementary therapy (p. 407)
effleurage (ĕf-loo-RĂHZH, p. 414)
holistic health care (hō-lĭs-tĭk, p. 407)
homeopathy (hō-mē-ŎP-ă-thē, p. 414)

hydrotherapy (hī-drō-THĔR-ă-pē, p. 413)
hypnosis (p. 411)
imagery (p. 413)
integrative health care (ĬN-tĕ-GRĀ-tĭv, p. 407)
natural alternative care (NAC) (p. 407)
reflexology (rē-flĕk-SŎL-ŏ-jē, p. 415)
transcutaneous electrical nerve stimulation (TENS) (trăns-kū-TĀ-nē-ŭs, p. 412)

TERMINOLOGY

Traditional Western health care, also known as allopathic care, follows a disease-oriented model that uses technology and bioscience, such as drugs, to treat illness and achieve wellness. The focus is on treatment and cure that are based on evidence provided by research.

Complementary therapy refers to therapy that is used along with conventional treatments. For example, in treatment of hypertension with medication plus relaxation or biofeedback measures, biofeedback assists or complements the medication so that it minimizes the drug's side effects while maximizing treatment effects. Alternative therapy is an unorthodox or unconventional form of therapy. It includes therapies that generally replace or substitute for a traditional or orthodox treatment. Many of the therapies considered complementary and alternative medicine (CAM) in the United States may be traditional therapies in other cultures and have been practiced in other countries for years.

Integrative health care is a blend of the best of both allopathic and CAM therapies. It combines allopathic or traditional Western medical practice with complementary and alternative therapies. Integrative health care focuses on the least invasive, least toxic, least costly methods of patient care, based on an understanding of the individual's physical, emotional, psychological, and spiritual aspects (Rakel, 2007). Integrative health care uses scientific research findings as a basis for care but requires the patient's active participation in designing a comprehensive care plan.

Holistic health care implies a wholeness, or comprehensive care involving physical, mental, and spiritual aspects of care in a healthy environment. Through the years, as technology, managed care systems, and health insurance organizations tended to depersonalize health care, consumers have turned toward self-care and have assumed responsibility for their own health. Health promotion and disease prevention, rather than treatment and cure of disease, became the focus of health care. Changes in lifestyle behaviors, nutrition habits, and the use of mental and spiritual healing powers of the body are important aspects of holistic health care.

Natural alternative care (NAC) refers to practices, including self-care, that may be helpful in providing comfort and healing but are not rooted in evidence-based research. Some NAC practices have not been previously considered as health care practices. NAC care may include bibliotherapy (reading self-help books), journaling (writing private thoughts and reactions), expressions in art, prayer, or affirmations of positive thought. NAC practices are often combined with other CAM therapies and referred to as *NACAM*.

Stress management is an important aspect of wellness, and assisting a patient in coping with or managing stress requires cultural competence, an understanding of and respect for the cultural practices and traditions that influence the patient's responses.

THE CHANGING HEALTH CARE ENVIRONMENT

Mainstream (traditional) medicine follows a disease-oriented model with technology playing an important role in the care, whereas CAM emphasizes prevention, principles of healthy lifestyles, and mental and spiritual healing powers in the body's system. Consumers are becoming increasingly educated and are actively moving toward a holistic or integrative approach to health care. The roles of the physician and hospital are shifting from treating people to helping people treat themselves. The result is a rise in consumer-driven, patient-focused care. The growth of the wellness movement indicates the beginning of a change in health care in the Western model of medicine. Many of the CAM therapies are based on the accepted theories of (1) gate control theory of reduced pain and (2) that natural endorphins control pain and can be stimulated by drugs or alternative means (Box 21-1; see also Chapter 8).

HISTORIC CONTEXT

In ancient China, a system of medical care was developed as part of philosophic teaching. The normal activities of the human body affected the balance of yin and yang, two opposing but complementary principles. A similar but distinct system, Ayurveda, was developed in India centuries ago. Imbalance was the major explanation of disease. Changes to the lifestyle to restore balance included herbs, exercise, and yoga. The Greek physician Galen's ideas influenced what would eventually become the beginning of modern medicine. During the Newtonian era of the eighteenth century, emphasis was placed on

Box 21-1 Pain Management

- Evaluate the patient's pain perceptions.
- Determine the patient's ability to manage her own pain.
- Help the patient recall positive coping techniques.
- Consider cultural factors regarding pain management.
- Empower the patient to make her own decisions concerning pain management.
- Teach pain control techniques to the patient and family.
- Document the responses of the patient and family to interventions and teaching.

objective observations. By the mid-1800s, medicine in the United States was a mixture of many different contributions of philosophies from various countries. Then a great change occurred in medicine with the advent of vaccines and antibiotics.

Traditional Chinese medicine is the basis for many alternative therapies. Popular traditional Chinese medicine practices include:

- **Qigong:** a self-discipline using breathing, meditation, and self-massage practiced daily.
- **Tai chi:** a type of martial art based on physical fitness and also used to improve health (Fontaine, 2005).
- **Moxibustion:** the burning of an herb, called *moxa*, which is then applied to an acupoint, where the heat regulates the flow of *chi* (energy).

FEDERAL REGULATIONS

As a result of the increased interest in CAM, the Office of Alternative Medicine of the National Institutes of Health (NIH) was created in 1992 to evaluate the modalities being used. Since 1998, this office has grown significantly. It was given increased status when it was renamed the National Center for Complementary and Alternative Medicine (NCCAM). The mandate of this federally funded agency is to investigate and evaluate alternative therapies and their effectiveness. NCCAM serves as a public clearinghouse and a research training program. There are 11 institution-affiliated centers of research on alternative medicine throughout the United States.

Botanical (made from living plants) medicines are regulated in the United States as dietary supplements. The Dietary Supplement Health and Education Act (DSHEA) of 1994 clarified marketing regulations for herbal medicines and reclassified them as dietary supplements, distinct from food or drugs. Under DSHEA, dietary supplements that include plant extracts, enzymes, vitamins, minerals, and hormonal products are available to consumers without prescription. The physiologic effects of the product can be noted, but no claims about prevention or cure of specific conditions can be made. Products must display the following disclaimer: "This product has not been evaluated by the Food and Drug Administration." The *Scientific Review of Alternative Medicine* journal is an example of a publication dedicated to evaluating CAM therapy based on reviews of medical research studies.

NURSING ACCEPTANCE OF COMPLEMENTARY AND ALTERNATIVE THERAPY MODALITIES

In the United States, nursing has been promoting self-care for many years through Orem's self-care framework (Orem, 2001) and through Watson's theory of human caring, assessing, and intervening on behalf of the whole person (Watson, 1996). The holistic approach has been a basic part of nursing since the work of Florence Nightingale. Modalities for self-care, such as the use of relaxation and imagery, have increasingly been brought into nursing settings. Touch and massage have been therapeutic modalities of nursing care since the inception of modern nursing. Professional nursing associations, such as the American Holistic Nurses Association, have formed to educate nurses concerning self-care activities and treatment of the whole person.

Many CAM therapies are based upon accepted theories such as the gate control theory of pain relief (see Chapter 8). Nurses use complementary therapies such as imagery, journaling, therapeutic touch, humor, and support groups. In the obstetric unit, guided imagery, prayer, music, massage, storytelling, and aromatherapy are often used by nurses to help women cope with their labor experience. Health consumers expect to be active participants in their own health care, and many use some sort of CAM therapy. Some foods, vitamin and mineral supplements, and herbal therapy are all common forms of CAM therapy practiced in many homes.

The increasing demand by the consumer for CAM therapies makes it imperative that nurses acquaint themselves with types of therapies used by patients at home. In doing so, the nurse can collaborate with the patient, family, community, and multidisciplinary health care team to provide holistic care. These practices enhance rather than inhibit or conflict with nursing care. Many patients from different cultures who have been using home remedies or folk medicine, conventional medicine, or traditional medicine are involved in alternative care. The 2003 social policy statement of the American Nurses Association states, "Nursing helps to serve society's interests in the area of health. The nursing profession has made and continues to make a substantial contribution toward evolution of a health-oriented system of care."

The nurse's role is not to advocate or discourage the use of any CAM therapy but to recognize and respect its use in patients and to use critical thinking skills to determine interactions with traditional therapy, with the patient as a partner.

SELECTED COMPLEMENTARY AND ALTERNATIVE THERAPIES

ACUPRESSURE

Definition
Acupressure is a traditional Chinese therapy that has been used for centuries. It is administered by a variety of practitioners, some of whom combine acupressure with other forms of Asian medicine, such as herbology.

According to traditional Chinese medicine, the body's healing energy flows along an invisible system of energy channels, called *meridians*. Twelve to 14 meridians connect vital organs throughout the body. Chinese practitioners have located hundreds of sensitive *acupoints* along these meridians. They believe that a blockage in the flow of one point on a meridian can cause disease and discomfort in the organ or tissue. Western medical science has since shown that nerve trigger points coincide with these same acupressure points.

How the Therapy Is Performed
Acupressure uses finger, palm, or knuckle pressure at points located along meridians. The Chinese variation involves a massage-like kneading motion. It may be performed on a floor mat or massage table, and the person receiving the treatment usually wears comfortable, loose clothing. Practitioners may administer pressure to various points. Wristbands that apply acupressure to decrease nausea and vomiting during travel and during pregnancy have had positive clinical trials and are widely advertised.

What the Therapy Hopes to Accomplish
Acupressure, as a massage, can be relaxing. It may work by triggering the body to release natural pain-killing compounds such as **endorphins**. It can be regarded as a way of toning the body and promoting general health and well-being. Some studies (Quinlan & Hill, 2003; Cunningham, Simpson, & Brown, 2006) showed a decrease in nausea and vomiting during pregnancy with acupressure.

Contraindications
The massage is administered in a slow and steady manner, although it can involve forceful pressure. Thus, it may not be a choice for a person with brittle bones (osteoporosis) or a history of spinal or other orthopedic injury or those who bruise easily. Acupressure is recommended to ease discomforts of pregnancy and childbirth. However, any pressure near or on the abdominal area should be avoided. Pressure should also be avoided on the legs and feet if the patient has circulation problems or varicose veins.

Possible Side Effects
After an acupressure treatment, some individuals report feeling lightheaded or slightly groggy for a short time. This feeling may be caused by a build-up of endorphins.

ACUPUNCTURE

Definition
Acupuncture is the insertion of slender needles into specific points of the body. It is based on the principle that the body has complex meridians that are pathways to specific organs. Acupuncture points are the

areas of the body in which these meridians surface. Stimulation of these points is thought to influence positive-negative energy (chi) that regulates body function. Acupuncture is a popular pain relief strategy practiced in the United States today.

How the Therapy Is Performed

The "puncture" refers to insertion of tiny needles at specific points on the surface of the body. The insertion of the disposable needles has been described as feeling like a mosquito bite. The needles may be stimulated by twirling them or connecting them to a mild electrical current, which can cause a mild tingling sensation. The needles are left in place up to 20 to 30 minutes.

What the Therapy Hopes to Accomplish

Both acupressure and acupuncture use meridians, and some acupoints have been shown to coincide with nerve trigger points (dermatomes). The basis for the effectiveness of acupressure is the gate control theory (see Chapter 8). Acupuncture may trigger the release of natural pain-killing substances within the body, called *endorphins*, thus blunting the perception of pain. It may also alter the body's output of neurotransmitters, such as serotonin and norepinephrine. According to the NCCAM (2006), well-performed scientific studies have provided evidence of acupuncture reducing nausea and vomiting associated with pregnancy. It is also useful for low back pain, menstrual cramps, and headaches.

Contraindications

People at risk of easy bruising or bleeding and those taking a blood-thinning medication should avoid acupuncture. Pregnant women should avoid needle insertion on or near the abdomen.

Possible Side Effects

Careless application or improperly sterilized needles can cause serious complications if a blood vessel is punctured or injury to organs or nerves occurs. Therefore, acupuncture should be performed by a skilled and reputable practitioner. As with acupressure, individuals may feel lightheaded for a short time after treatment. This is usually attributed to the release of endorphins.

AROMATHERAPY

Definition

Aromatherapy is the use of plant oils to promote wellness. It can improve one's quality of life, whether or not it has other benefits. Improvement is derived from an emotional response to pleasing scents rather than any physiologic effects. It may enhance relaxation and reduce stress; for some people, it has helped lessen insomnia. Aromatherapy is recognized by the NIH as a complementary and alternative therapy (Krebs, 2006).

How the Therapy Is Performed

The therapy relies on the use of concentrated essential oils extracted from various trees and plants. Many oils are used as a form of home remedy. The use of herbal teas and vapors is reported to have good effects on labor and pregnancy for some women. A few drops of lavender oil (diluted in a bathtub of warm water) are sometimes used to promote relaxation (Lowdermilk & Perry, 2007). Inhalation may improve respiratory conditions. Massage and rubbing aromatic oil into the skin may be calming or stimulating and may relieve muscle soreness. Some people have been able to reduce their intake of antiinflammatory drugs with aromatherapy. Essential oils are mixed with a carrier oil, such as vegetable or safflower, to reduce skin irritation (Krebs, 2006).

What the Therapy Hopes to Accomplish

Fragrant oils have been used for thousands of years to lubricate the skin. For some women, scented candles and potpourri have a relaxing effect. Practitioners suggest that the inhaled vapors will have a medicinal and relaxing effect on the body.

Contraindications

Essential oils are very concentrated and extremely potent, and many can be toxic, so they should never be ingested. Some of the well-known oils are contraindicated, such as cedar wood and juniper, in pregnancy (Table 21-1). Also, pregnant women appear to have a particularly sensitive sense of smell; therefore, aromatherapy mixtures, if used, should be well diluted.

Table 21-1	Some Aromatherapy Essential Oils Contraindicated in Pregnancy
OIL	**CONTRAINDICATION**
Pennyroyal	Can cause abortion
Rosemary, sage, thyme, camphor	Hypertensives; can complicate gestational hypertension
Peppermint	Can cause adverse pregnancy outcome
Oils containing citral	Interact with melanocytic hormones; cause photosensitivity
Geranium	Has anticoagulant effect
Black pepper, caraway, cinnamon, hyssop, nutmeg, thyme	Cause cardiovascular adaptations contraindicated in pregnancy
Benzoin, cedarwood, garlic, chamomile, eucalyptus, fennel, lavender, rose, sandalwood	Increase diuresis; contraindicated in severe blood loss

Possible Side Effects

Some essential oils are contraindicated because of a possible increased risk of abortion, gestational hypertension, or hemorrhage; therefore, oils should be administered by trained aromatherapists in collaboration with the obstetrician.

BIOFEEDBACK

Definition

Biofeedback is a technique that allows individuals to gain control over physiologic reactions that are ordinarily unconscious. Malfunctions in these autonomic responses contribute to several medical problems. Biofeedback has the ability to help bring counterproductive reactions back into line, providing significant relief.

Biofeedback requires intensive focused concentration as one learns to control normally involuntary (autonomic) functions such as heart rate, blood pressure, skin temperature, muscle tension, breathing, brain waves, and digestion.

When modern instrumentation made it possible to identify subtle changes in unconscious physical reactions, Western medicine turned its attention to the mind-body connection. Individuals can be educated to recognize their own body responses, learn how to relax, and, through biofeedback, gain control over ordinary physiologic reactions.

How the Therapy Is Performed

Biofeedback therapy involves the application of noninvasive sensors to various points on the body. The location depends on the problem that needs attention. For example, to treat heart problems, the sensors are attached to monitor the heartbeat; to treat muscle tension, the sensors are placed on the skin (electromyelogram). Some biofeedback machines signal changes on a computer display. The therapist teaches the individual mental and physical exercises that can address the function causing the problem. Once the individual has learned the pattern of actions, he or she can assert control without the aid of the feedback device.

What the Therapy Hopes to Accomplish

Biofeedback seeks control over specific, measurable physiologic reactions that have gone astray by aggravated muscular tension or tightening. Through disciplined mental effort, biofeedback can reduce tension and anxiety and combat insomnia and fatigue. It has proved useful for any disorder caused or aggravated by involuntary muscular tension or tightening. Biofeedback is a relaxation technique that can be used for labor. A woman must be educated to become aware of her body and its responses and to relax for biofeedback to be effective.

Contraindications

If a pregnant woman has an implanted medical device, the biofeedback technique that requires an electrical device should not be used to gain control over physiologic reactions.

Possible Side Effects

Like other mind-body forms of therapy, biofeedback is notably free of side effects. Although biofeedback is harmless, it is not a substitute for medical care if a person has a serious medical problem (e.g., diabetes, heart disease, or hypertension).

HYPNOSIS

Definition

Hypnosis is the induction of an altered state of consciousness, somewhat like daydreaming. The brain appears to "switch off" for a time. Hypnosis seems to provide a link with the subconscious mind, including its ability to enhance the power of suggestion. Hypnosis has been found to be effective for a variety of problems that hinge on emotions, habits, and the body's involuntary responses. However, it does not work for everyone. Suggestions refer to the presentation of an idea to a person, and the person accepts the idea (suggestibility), which is influenced by motivation and expectation. The hypnotic state can be self-induced and can be implemented with regular practice. It may take 15 minutes a day to reproduce the feeling and concentrate on the images learned in the sessions with the therapist.

How the Therapy Is Performed

Individuals are usually asked to focus on a point and let their breathing become slow and regular. As the eyelids become heavy, the person is asked to close them and relax. As the individual feels deeply relaxed, the conscious mind will no longer control every thought and emotion as it does when awake. While the person is in a trancelike state (such as a daydream or focused attention), the facilitator (trained therapist) may make suggestions. The facilitator may tell the person how to make an unwanted symptom or habit disappear. A patient may be given a direct suggestion about pain relief, and, on receiving the post-hypnotic suggestion, she may, for example, increase her confidence to accept diminished sensation. Once the woman has been taught how to move into the self-hypnotic state, she can put her self-hypnosis suggestion on tape and respond to her own voice giving commands.

What the Therapy Hopes to Accomplish

Although there seems to be little doubt that hypnosis provides lasting benefits for many of those who try it, no one is quite certain why it works. Some scientists speculate that it prompts the brain to release natural mood-altering substances, enkephalins and endorphins, that can change the way we perceive pain and other physical symptoms. Many believe that hypnotherapy acts through the subconscious (the part of the mind responsible for involuntary reactions that normally are beyond our control), thereby placing reactions under one's control.

One of hypnotherapy's greatest benefits may be its ability to reduce the effects of stress. Psychologists believe that the mind has a direct impact on physical well-being. Hypnosis can allay stress by putting individuals into a relaxed state, offering positive suggestions, and eliminating negative thoughts. As tension in the muscles and blood vessels recedes, the circulation improves and the person's entire body feels healthier. Hypnosis is associated with shorter labors and less need for analgesic medication. Hypnosis techniques used for labor and birth place an emphasis on relaxation. Some women are more susceptible to hypnosis, but it is not effective for everyone.

Contraindications and Possible Side Effects

Hypnosis is considered safe for everyone, although persons with a history of psychosis need careful evaluation. When offered by an appropriately qualified professional, hypnosis is considered safe under most conditions. Many people fear losing control to the therapist; however, the hypnotist is never in control. A hypnotic suggestion works only if the recipient accepts it. The therapist cannot make a person do something that he or she would not consciously do.

TRANSCUTANEOUS ELECTRICAL NERVE STIMULATION

Definition

Transcutaneous electrical nerve stimulation (TENS) is therapy promoted as energy medicine. It is used for all types of localized pain, such as chronic back pain, and can be used in combination with analgesic medication. It is advocated for conditions such as labor contractions, menstrual pain, nausea and vomiting of pregnancy, jaw muscle pain, cancer pain, and nerve damage (Figure 21-1).

How the Therapy Is Performed

TENS is performed with a small electronic unit that sends pulsed currents to a set of electrodes applied to the skin. When used for uterine labor contractions, TENS may involve the placement of two pairs of electrodes from a battery-operated device on either side of the thoracic and sacral spine. Other electrode placement depends on the protocol of the technician or institution. During a contraction, the woman increases the stimulation by turning control knobs on the device. Women describe the sensation as a tingling or buzzing that provides pain relief.

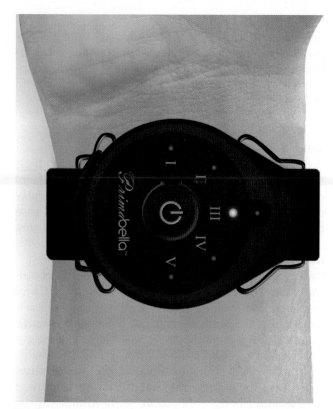

FIGURE 21-1 PrimaBella is a noninvasive transdermal device cleared by the FDA for the treatment of pregnancy-induced nausea and vomiting (morning sickness). The device is applied to the ventral side of the wrist, where the median nerve is closest to the surface of the skin. It emits a programmed pulse that stimulates the nerve to create electrical signals that travel to the central nervous system to restore normal gastric rhythm.

What the Therapy Hopes to Accomplish

The pulsed currents delivered by TENS are believed to drown out pain signals in the affected nerves, thus preventing the pain message from reaching the brain. This effect is based on the hypothesis that pain must pass through a gate in the spinal cord (the gate control theory of pain; see Chapter 8). TENS units are also believed to stimulate the production of endorphins, the body's natural pain killers, thus alleviating the woman's discomfort. TENS is credited with reducing the need for analgesia while increasing the woman's perception of control over the experience.

Contraindications

TENS should be used by women after a full medical consultation only. It should not be used if the individual has poorly controlled epilepsy or an implanted medical device. The therapy should be discontinued if there is skin irritation from the electrode patches. TENS is not used before 37 weeks' gestation.

Possible Side Effects

No harmful side effects have been reported in healthy women in labor; however, approval for its use should be given by the physician. Benzodiazepine drugs and corticosteroids may reduce effectiveness of TENS;

therefore, it is important for the nurse to obtain an accurate medication history. Application of electrodes at appropriate sites must be done by a competent, trained professional.

VISUALIZATION AND GUIDED IMAGERY

Definition
Visualization and guided imagery refer to concentration on images held in the mind's eye. Visualization is a form of mind-to-body technique that has been used extensively in labor. Visualization and guided imagery work in connection between the brain and the involuntary nervous system. Visual images can influence both the voluntary and involuntary nervous system.

How the Therapy Is Performed
Instruments or monitors are not used. Sometimes music is played in the background to aid relaxation. Sessions begin with general relaxation exercises and then move on to a specific visualization. The individual is asked to build a detailed image in her mind using all five senses and may repeat the exercise with a different image. If the person has a specific medical symptom (or discomfort), she will be asked to picture her body away from the problem. She may be asked to picture the affected organ(s) working properly. She may be asked to recall a scene from a book or some peaceful image from the past. Often, guided imagery asks the person to focus on a journey through several visualizations, which may be described as a "focused daydream." Between sessions, the person is asked to use a book or audiotape to practice the visualization.

When TENS is used in preparation for childbirth classes, the woman is asked to focus on a pleasant memory using a favorite object, such as a photograph that she can take with her to the birth facility. During her labor, she can focus her attention on the object, using it as a distraction. This will likely reduce her perception of pain.

What the Therapy Hopes to Accomplish
Studies have confirmed the ability of meditation training to lower blood pressure and control heart rate. Results showed that guided imagery can do so as well (Barnes & Bloom, 2009). One theory proposes that picturing something and actually experiencing it are equivalent as far as brain activity is concerned. Brain scans have verified this effect. Therefore, stimulating the brain through imagery can have a direct effect on both the nervous and endocrine systems, ultimately producing changes in the immune and other body systems.

Contraindications and Possible Side Effects
Guided imagery is generally considered safe for everyone. There are no known side effects unless memory of an unpleasant event occurs.

EXPRESSIVE THERAPY AND SOUND THERAPY

Definition
Expressive therapy is a nonthreatening outlet for people to express feelings that are difficult to put in words and is used as a coping strategy. Expressive therapy includes many forms of expression, such as music, puppetry, and personal diaries. Sound therapy (music) has had an impact on many people. Classical music is soothing to some, soft ballads soothe others, heavy metal music can be both enjoyable or anxiety-provoking, and an anthem sung at the beginning of a ball game can invoke an emotional response. In hospitals, music is used to improve patients' moods, counteract depression, promote rehabilitation, reduce muscle tension, and induce sleep.

What the Therapy Hopes to Accomplish
Sound has a profound influence on the nervous system and a special power to affect consciousness. Music can also enhance relaxation during labor. Women are often encouraged to bring their musical preferences (with an MP3 or CD player) to the hospital and listen to music during their labor. If she has earphones on, the sounds may not be a distraction to others. Although scientific documentation is limited, music is known to decrease the amount of drugs required during labor.

Contraindications and Possible Side Effects
Sound therapy is considered safe. If possible, the patient should select the type of music. The volume should be kept low when using a sound therapy device. With loud music, the patient might incur hearing loss. No other side effects are known.

HYDROTHERAPY

Definition
Hydrotherapy, or warm water therapy with baths, showers, or jet hydrotherapy (whirlpool baths), may be used to promote comfort and relaxation. Water therapy can also reduce anxiety, which triggers a decrease in adrenaline production. This, in turn, can trigger an increase in endorphins, which reduce the pain associated with labor. Pain relief from hydrotherapy has been proposed to be that of a distraction device or stimulation of large-diameter nerve fibers, as mentioned in the gate control theory. The warm water allows local vasodilation and muscle relaxation. The water should be kept at a controlled temperature to prevent hyperthermia or hypothermia.

How the Therapy Is Performed
Water therapy can be accomplished by bathing, showering, or taking whirlpool baths. Jet hydrotherapy or showering can stimulate the nipples and trigger more oxytocin production that results in stimulating labor. If a tub bath is used, it must be extremely clean to prevent infection. If *Escherichia coli* contaminates the water in the tub, the risk for infection is increased.

What the Therapy Hopes to Accomplish
Using warm water can promote comfort and relaxation. Hydrotherapy can trigger an increase in endorphins, which reduce pain in labor and the need for analgesics. If the nipples are stimulated, more oxytocin production can be triggered, which is known to cause the cervix to dilate quicker (stimulating uterine contractions) when the woman is in active labor. Water births are common practice in independent birthing centers (see Chapter 7).

Hydrotherapy is used for relaxation and comfort during labor, soft-tissue injuries, musculoskeletal injuries, back pain, menstrual cramps, and impaired circulation. The application of hot and cold water-soaked compresses to reduce swelling has proven effective in clinical research trials.

Some advocates claim that hydrotherapy can detoxify the system and bring it back into balance. They believe that alternate applications of hot and cold can boost the body's ability to fight infection. The therapy, using warm water, is believed to improve circulation.

Contraindications
Hot-cold hydrotherapy is not advised for patients with asthma, heart disease, or bleeding disorders. Water births are contraindicated in women who have high-risk pregnancies and should be in a hospital-based center where emergency facilities are available.

HOMEOPATHY
Definition
Homeopathy is based on the premise that a small amount of a substance that causes a symptom can actually relieve the symptom. The remedies are diluted solutions of herbs, animal products, or chemicals. Many people tend to think of homeopathic products as herbal remedies, but the products usually contain little of the desired herb.

What the Therapy Hopes to Accomplish
Homeopathy is an approach designed to promote and improve health rather than reverse disease. Remedies are based on individual symptoms rather than disease entities. *Caulophyllum* and *Cimicifuga* are examples of plants, the blue cohosh and black cohosh plants, from which homeopathic medicines are derived and used for inducing and augmenting labor.

Contraindications
Coffee, menthol, and strong flavors such as peppermint should be avoided because they may reduce the effect of the homeopathic product. Many homeopathic tablets contain lactose, which may be contraindicated in diabetic or allergic individuals.

Possible Side Effects
Unlike vitamins and herbal remedies, which are sold as dietary supplements, homeopathic remedies are sold as over-the-counter medications, with an exemption from standard regulatory procedures. The labels do include the ingredients, directions, and dilution. The smallest dose possible to stimulate a reaction is a basic principle of homeopathy, which should be guided by a professional.

MASSAGE AND TOUCH THERAPY
Definition
Effleurage (see Chapter 5) and counterpressure are two methods that have brought relief to many women during labor (see Chapter 8). Massage is not capable of curing any medical disorder, but it can provide relief for tension, anxiety, insomnia, muscle pain, headache, and back pain. It is often recommended for minor sports injuries. Some individuals find that it relieves digestive disorders, such as constipation. Membership and license in the American Massage Therapy Association (AMTA) means that the therapist has graduated from an approved training program and met requirements for membership or passed the national certification examination.

How the Therapy Is Performed
Many massage techniques are practiced, but the most widespread modern variation builds on the basic strokes of Swedish massage. Effleurage is slow, rhythmic, gliding strokes, usually in the direction of blood flow toward the heart. Often the care provider uses the whole hand (palm and fingers), gradually applying an increasing amount of pressure (e.g., during a labor contraction). Variations of effleurage involve strokes applied with the fingertips, heel of the hand, or knuckles. Effleurage is a commonly practiced procedure taught in prenatal classes and is used when the woman is having labor contractions.

What the Therapy Hopes to Accomplish
Massage is an application of pressure and movement to the soft tissues of the body. It encourages healing by promoting the flow of blood and lymph, relieving tension, and loosening muscles and connective tissue. Before physical exercise, massage helps get blood moving to assist in the warm-up. Massage after an exercise workout has been shown to reduce the buildup of waste products (e.g., lactic acid). When these build up in muscles after exercise, they cause cramping and discomfort. An increased fluid intake is encouraged during massage therapy. In addition to general health benefits, massage has shown to be of value in many special problems. During labor, massage provides relaxation, comfort, and relief from painful contractions (see Chapter 8).

Reiki therapy is a type of therapeutic touch involving massage and energy therapy (Kemper & Kelly, 2004). Hand positions correspond with the body's lymphatic and endocrine systems and major body organs. There may be a decrease in pain, anxiety, and a possible biochemical reaction that involves an increase in immunoglobulin A measurements (Wardell & Engebretson, 2001).

Contraindications

Massage is not advised for anyone who has an infectious skin disease, a rash, or an unhealed wound. If the person is prone to blood clots, it is unwise to have the therapy immediately after surgery. Circulatory problems such as varicose veins preclude the use of massage. It should never be performed over bruises, infected wounds, or areas of bleeding or deep tissue damage. Massage should also be avoided over any known tumor. In an unstable pregnancy, abdominal massage should not be performed. It is also not advisable for the woman to have her legs massaged during pregnancy.

Possible Side Effects

Massage can aggravate existing swelling (edema). The pressure on the skin can be painful for someone who has nerve injury. It is advisable to avoid massage immediately after surgery, such as cesarean birth, because of the increased risk of thrombophlebitis or blood clot.

REFLEXOLOGY

Definition

Reflexology has been practiced for thousands of years in China and Egypt. It was introduced in the West at the beginning of the twentieth century. Reflexology suggests that reflexes, zones, or pathways run along the body and terminate in the palms of the hands, soles of the feet, ears, tongue, and head. All systems and organs are said to be reflected on the surface of the skin, in particular, the hands and the feet. Although some studies have been conducted and this therapy often helps with problems such as headaches and bladder control, few major clinical trials verify the theoretic effectiveness.

How the Therapy Is Performed

Unlike massage, which involves a generalized rubbing action, reflexologists use their hands to apply pressure to specific points on the feet and hands (Figure 21-2). The patient usually remains fully clothed, sitting with legs raised or lying on a treatment table. After gently massaging the feet, the reflexologist begins applying pressure to the reflex points thought to correspond to the reported health problems. No instruments are required, but some therapists use devices such as a rubber ball to apply some of the pressure. One can learn to perform reflexology by having the practitioner demonstrate the techniques appropriate to treat the problem.

What the Therapy Hopes to Accomplish

The idea that manipulating the feet can improve health has been an accepted philosophy for many years. Ancient Egyptians massaged feet, and illustrations show that people of many cultures applied massage to their feet to combat illness. Reflexology was originally thought to work in much the same way as acupuncture. Practitioners believed that stimulation of reflex points in the foot could break up blockages in the flow further along the channel. Although few of the theories have been scientifically verified, reflexology appears to produce satisfactory results for a surprising number of people. Reflexology offers women in labor a gentle method of pain control. Gentle pressure applied to the feet and hands may help restore the body's natural equilibrium.

Contraindications

Reflexology has been considered safe; however, if the patient has a foot injury, ulcers, phlebitis, or any other vascular problems in the lower legs, reflexology should be discussed with the physician before providing the treatment. The reflex zone related to the uterus should not have sustained pressure, and reflexology should not be used in unstable pregnancies.

YOGA

Definition

Hatha yoga (one of many types of yoga) is a set of exercises that offers a variety of proven health benefits. It increases the efficiency of the heart and slows the respiratory rate, improves fitness, lowers blood pressure, promotes relaxation, and reduces stress and anxiety. It also serves to improve coordination, range of motion, posture, concentration, sleep, and digestion. Although yoga as we know it today is practiced mainly for health benefits, it is rooted in Hindu religious and mind-body unity principles of some 5000 years ago. *Ayurveda* is based on yoga practices and includes the use of vegetarian diets, exercise, music therapy, aromatherapy, and massage for general health.

How the Therapy Is Performed

Yoga exercises are often conducted in group classes. People are asked to wear loose, comfortable clothing for the class and bring a mat to prevent slipping during the exercises. The typical session includes three disciplines: breathing exercises, body postures, and meditation. Advice about nutrition may also be given. Each session begins with warm-up exercises. Some posture exercises may be complicated and even contorted.

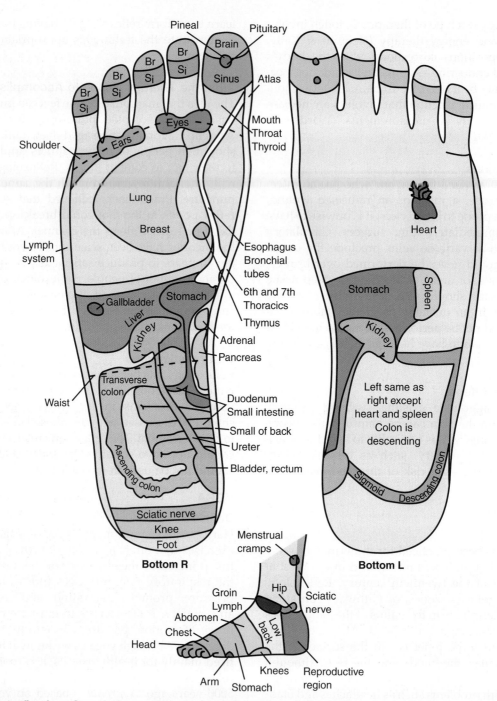

FIGURE 21-2 **Foot reflexology.** General reference points are shown. The opinions of reflexology experts vary slightly on organ or system placement.

What the Therapy Hopes to Accomplish

The exercises are performed to prepare the body by strengthening muscles and by encouraging relaxation and concentration. Through controlled breathing, prescribed postures, and meditation, yoga seeks to enhance the body and achieve a state of balance and harmony between body and mind. Exercises are practiced in prenatal classes to prepare muscles for labor and birth. Regular yoga practice throughout pregnancy will help the pregnant woman to get "in tune" with her body. It can help prevent headaches, morning sickness, fatigue, and back pain and help her be in good physical condition for labor.

Contraindications

Yoga should be avoided in patients who have had a back injury or recent surgery. Individuals should check with their physicians if they have heart disease, arthritis, or hypertension before initiating this treatment. Some postures are not recommended during pregnancy; thus, special classes are often available for expectant mothers. Some suggest that pregnancy is not the ideal time to begin yoga exercises.

Possible Side Effects

In the beginning, stiffness may occur while the body adapts. However, yoga should not be stressful or tiring, and any stiffness should be temporary and minor.

MAGNET THERAPY

Also known as *electromagnetic therapy*, magnet therapy involves placing magnets on the skin. It is thought that magnets stimulate living cells and increase blood flow. This may be beneficial in some conditions and result in the relief of pain and edema. The Reagan Institute has reported that specific electromagnetic fields may disturb calcium ions in the brain cells (Spencer & Jacobs, 2003). Further research is needed to understand side effects and contraindications of magnetic therapy.

HERBAL MEDICINE

Many people use herbal medicine as a treatment of choice. An increasing number of individuals are expressing an interest in herbal medicine to relieve discomforts during pregnancy and for menopause. Herbs can be gentle and healing, but they can also be irritating to the skin and gastrointestinal tract and toxic to the mother or the fetus. It is important for the nurse to be familiar with specific oils and herbs.

Common Herbs Contraindicated in Pregnancy and Lactation

Many pregnant women want to avoid drugs that may interfere with fetal development and therefore often turn to "home remedies" that they think are a "harmless" alternative. Common herbs that are contraindicated in pregnancy and lactation are listed in Table 21-2. Nurses

Table 21-2   Common Herbs Contraindicated in Pregnancy and Lactation

HERB	USE	CONTRAINDICATION
Aloe vera	Prevents constipation Promotes wound healing	Causes engorgement of pelvic vessels that can result in increased bleeding and spontaneous abortion Avoid during pregnancy
Garlic	Decreases cholesterol	Avoid during pregnancy and do not use with other antiplatelet medications Cannot be used with some HIV medications
Ginger	Prevents motion sickness	Increases bleeding times
Ginkgo	Relieves depression	Can cause hemorrhage
St. John's wort	Relieves depression	Avoid exposure to sun; increases tone of uterus; use with caution in pregnancy; interacts with alcohol, cold and flu medications, chocolate, aged cheese, and beer; interacts with oral contraceptives by causing breakthrough bleeding; in high doses is mutagenic to sperm and oocytes, which may result in birth defects
Angelica (dong quai)	Used in gynecologic disorders, menstrual discomfort, and postmenopausal symptoms	Avoid during pregnancy and breastfeeding because of uterine stimulation; prolongs prothrombin time and causes poor glycemic control in women with diabetes
Chamomile	Prevents urinary tract infections and gastrointestinal spasms; also used for sedation	Avoid during pregnancy; may cause abortion and teratogenic effects on fetus
Feverfew	Used as antipyretic for migraine headache and for menstrual problems	Avoid during pregnancy and lactation; can cause withdrawal symptoms
Flax (flaxseed)	Used for bowel problems	Contraindicated in pregnancy; potential for toxicity; must be refrigerated
Ginseng	Relieves stress; increases stamina	Avoid during pregnancy and breastfeeding; may be toxic; central nervous system effects increased when used with coffee or tea; interacts with St. John's wort and monoamine oxidase inhibitors
Kava	Reduces anxiety and stress	Avoid during pregnancy and lactation; may cause nutritional deficiencies or blood dyscrasias
Ma huang (ephedra)	Central nervous system stimulant; appetite suppressant	Avoid during pregnancy; can cause cardiac arrhythmia, urinary retention, and uterine contractions
Nettle	Diuretic	Can cause electrolyte imbalance through diuresis

Data from O'Neil, C., Avilla, J., & Ferroco, C. (1999). Herbal medicine: Getting beyond the hype. *Nursing, 99, 28*(4), 58; Hadley, S., & Petry, J. (1999). Medicinal herbs: A primer for primary care. *Hospital Practice, 34*(6), 105-106, 109-112, 115-116; Spencer, J. W., & Jacobs, J. J. (2003). *Complementary/alternative medicine: An evidence-based approach*. St. Louis: Mosby; Medical Economics. (2005). *PDR for herbal medicines*. Montvale, NJ: Author; Dog, T. (2009). The use of botanicals during pregnancy and lactation. *Alternative Therapies in Health and Medicine, 15*(1), 54-56; and Rakel, D. (2007). *Integrative medicine*. Philadelphia: Saunders.
HIV, human immunodeficiency virus.

need to know the herbal therapies used by their patients and discuss side effects, interactions, advantages, and disadvantages of the herbal therapy.

Many patients believe that because herbs are natural, they are safe. Herbal medicines are consumed in many different forms and can be administered both internally and topically. Some forms are more potent than others, the strongest being tinctures or extracts. Manufacturing quality varies, and safe dosages have not been established by recognized research. More controlled clinical studies are necessary to determine efficacy and safety. A nursing responsibility is to understand interactions and recognize contraindications to the use of specific herbs and oils used during pregnancy and lactation.

Herbs and Menopause

Menopause is a stage of health within the continuum of a woman's life (see Chapter 20). Traditionally, hormone replacement therapy (HRT) has been a popular approach to managing menopausal symptoms. Recently, more natural management techniques have developed, including:

- *Exercise:* weight bearing or water aerobic exercise programs
- *Relaxation techniques:* breathing, biofeedback, and hypnosis
- *Diet:* low fat, high fiber, and soy inclusive
- *Herbs* (Table 21-3)

Future of Herbal Therapy

The NIH Office of Dietary Supplements and the NCCAM have funded the development of research centers to study the physiology, safety, and effectiveness of herbs and supplements. The U.S. Congress has contributed to the funding of this research. The first two centers were established at the University of California at Los Angeles (UCLA) and the University of Illinois at Chicago (UIC). UCLA initially focused on cholesterol-reducing alternative supplements, the treatment of tumors and cancers with soy and green tea extracts, and compounds used to manage depression. UIC initially focused on herbal supplements related to women's health issues and the development of an interactive website (http://nccam.nih.gov) to educate consumers and health professionals.

NUTRITION

Soy

Soy-rich foods have demonstrated lipid-lowering properties, and some labels claim that it "decreases risk of heart disease." However, the long-term effectiveness of nutritional pharmacology and the role of

Table **21-3**	Popular Herbs Used in Menopause
HERB	**USE**
Black cohosh (*Cimicifuga racemosa*)	Diminishes hot flashes by reducing luteinizing hormone Reduces joint pain, vaginal dryness, and other menopausal discomforts
Sage (*Salvia officinalis*)	Contains phytosterol and bioflavonoids Is effective for night sweats and hot flashes and has been used to dry lactating breasts
Dong quai (*Angelica sinensis*)	Contains phytoestrogens Contraindicated with midcycle spotting and fibroids Has synergistic effect when used with other herbs
Chasteberry (*Vitex agnus-castus*	Reduces hot flashes and dizziness caused by high levels of follicle-stimulating hormone Combined with other herbs, balances hormonal fluctuations
Motherwort (*Leonurus cardiaca*)	Relieves hot flashes and moodiness Reduces anxiety and insomnia Lacks research evidence

Data from Learn, C., & Higgins, P. (1999). Harmonizing herbs. *AWHONN Lifelines, 3,* 39-43; Lindsay, S. (1999). Menopause, naturally. *AWHONN Lifelines, 3,* 32-38; Gingrich, P., & Fogel, C. (2003). Herbal therapy use by perimenopausal women. *Journal of Obstetric, Gynecologic, and Neonatal Nursing, 32,* 181-189; Medical Economics. (2005). *PDR for herbal medicines.* Montvale, NJ: Author; and Rakel, D. (2007). *Integrative medicine.* Philadelphia: Saunders.

soy in postmenopausal women is still being studied (Bland, 2008; Bennett, 2009). Soy may also be helpful in preventing bone resorption that occurs in women with estrogen deficiency.

Fish Oil

Omega-3 fatty acids and N-3 polyunsaturated fatty acids have shown positive results in decreasing sudden cardiac death among high-risk patients. Omega-3 fatty acids are important to the developing fetus and are present in most prenatal vitamin supplements. Fish oils found in salmon, herring, albacore, and mackerel are under investigation for evidence of long-term primary prevention of heart disease. However, the mercury levels of the fish selected should be monitored.

Magnesium

Magnesium deficiency in geriatric women may contribute to decreased bone density. Magnesium supplementation may be of value in postmenopausal women because the average U.S. diet does not provide adequate magnesium intake.

Get Ready for the NCLEX® Examination!

Key Points

- Complementary therapies are therapies used in conjunction with traditional medicine.
- Alternative therapies are treatments that replace traditional medical treatments.
- Alternative and complementary methods of self-care have existed for many years.
- The NCCAM of the NIH was created in 1992 to conduct and review research concerning the efficacy and dangers of CAM therapies.
- Types of CAM therapies include acupressure, acupuncture, aromatherapy, biofeedback, hypnotherapy, TENS, guided imagery, expressive therapy, homeopathy, massage, therapeutic touch, reflexology, yoga, and the use of herbs and oils. Many of these therapies are used during pregnancy, labor, and birth as well as with other women's health-related problems in the hospital and in the home.
- Many herbal preparations and oils have not had research-based data to determine safe dosage and use.
- Some commonly used herbal products, such as chamomile, ginseng, and aloe vera, are contraindicated during pregnancy, labor, and delivery.
- Nurses must understand CAM therapies to avoid potentially dangerous interactions and promote positive outcomes.

Additional Learning Resources

SG Go to your Study Guide on pages 513–514 for additional Review Questions for the NCLEX® Examination, Critical Thinking Clinical Situations, and other learning activities to help you master this chapter content.

evolve Go to your Evolve website (http://evolve.elsevier.com/Leifer/maternity) for the following FREE learning resources:

- Animations
- Answer Guidelines for Critical Thinking Questions
- Answers and Rationales for Review Questions for the NCLEX® Examination
- Concept Map Creator
- Glossary with pronunciations in English and Spanish
- Patient Teaching Plans
- Skills Performance Checklists and more!

Online Resources
- www.whattoexpect.com/alternative-medicine-pregnancy.aspx

Review Questions for the NCLEX® Examination

1. Therapies used in conjunction with conventional treatments are referred to as:
   1. Allopathic
   2. Complementary
   3. Alternative
   4. Holistic

2. Acupressure is contraindicated in which condition(s)? *(Select all that apply.)*
   1. Osteoporosis
   2. Pregnancy
   3. Hemophilia
   4. Spinal injury

3. A therapy promoted as energy medicine is:
   1. Transcutaneous electrical nerve stimulation (TENS)
   2. Hypnosis
   3. Aromatherapy
   4. Acupuncture

4. Which therapy is considered safe for everyone?
   1. Yoga
   2. Reiki
   3. Guided imagery
   4. Hot-cold hydrotherapy

5. Rosemary, sage, thyme, and camphor essential oils are contraindicated in pregnancy because they:
   1. Can complicate gestational hypertension
   2. Can cause abortion
   3. Have an anticoagulant effect
   4. Increase diuresis

6. A patient expresses to the health care provider a belief in the use of natural alternative care (NAC) practices to provide comfort and healing. NAC care may include which activity(ies)? *(Select all that apply.)*
   1. Journaling
   2. Prayer
   3. Positive thought
   4. Expressions in art

7. A patient is implementing transcutaneous electrical nerve stimulation (TENS) to help deal with pain secondary to nerve damage. Reduction of the effectiveness of TENS may be caused by which drug(s)? *(Select all that apply.)*
   1. Nonsteroidal analgesics
   2. Benzodiazepine drugs
   3. Corticosteroids
   4. Narcotic drugs

Critical Thinking Questions

1. You are caring for a woman in early labor who appears to be increasingly uncomfortable. Explain how some CAM therapies can be used to help her cope with the labor experience.

2. You are reviewing prenatal class content with a patient who is in late pregnancy. What CAM therapies are routinely taught in prenatal classes that would be helpful to review?

A "minimum list" of dangerous abbreviations, acronyms, and symbols has been approved by The Joint Commission (TJC). The items in Table A-1 must be included on each accredited organization's "Do Not Use" list. The Joint Commission has additional recommendations of terms to avoid (Table A-2).

The Institute for Safe Medication Practices (ISMP) has published a list of dangerous abbreviations (available at www.ismp.org) relating to medication use that it recommends should be explicitly prohibited.

Two nurses must double-check the following before administration: heparin, insulin, parenteral chemotherapeutic agents, patient-controlled analgesia, and epidural pumps.

The Health Insurance Portability and Accountability Act (HIPAA) privacy requirements state that patient information concerning name, age, diagnosis, and other personal information should not be posted. Charts and medication records must be kept in a confidential area.

Table A-1 The Joint Commission Minimum "Do Not Use" List of Abbreviations

DO NOT USE	POTENTIAL PROBLEM	USE INSTEAD
U (unit)	Mistaken for "0" (zero), "4" (four), or cc	Write "unit"
IU (international unit)	Mistaken for IV (intravenous) or the number 10 (ten)	Write "international unit"
Q.D., QD, q.d., qd (daily)	Mistaken for each other	Write "daily"
Q.O.D., QOD, q.o.d., qod (every other day)	Period after the Q mistaken for "I" and the "O" mistaken for "I"	Write "every other day"
Trailing zero (X.0 mg) [NOTE: Prohibited only for medication-related notations] Lack of leading zero (.X mg)	Decimal point is missed	Never write a zero by itself after a decimal point (X mg), and always use a zero before a decimal point (0.X mg)
MS	Can mean morphine sulfate or magnesium sulfate	Write "morphine sulfate" or "magnesium sulfate"
MSO_4 and $MgSO_4$	Confused for one another	

Table A-2 Additional Abbreviations to Avoid

DO NOT USE	POTENTIAL PROBLEM	USE INSTEAD
> (greater than) < (less than)	Misinterpreted as the number "7" (seven) or the letter "L" Confused with one another	Write "greater than" Write "less than"
Abbreviations for drug names	Misinterpreted due to similar abbreviations for multiple drugs	Write drug names in full
Apothecary units	Unfamiliar to many practitioners Confused with metric units	Use metric units
@	Mistaken for the number "2" (two)	Write "at"
cc	Mistaken for U (units) when poorly written	Write "mL" or "ml" or "milliliters" ("mL" is preferred)
µg	Mistaken for mg (milligrams), resulting in 1000-fold dosing overdose	Write "mcg" or "micrograms"

From The Joint Commission. (2009). Official "Do Not Use" list. Oakbrook Terrace, IL: The Joint Commission. Retrieved December 29, 2010, from www.jointcommission.org/Do_Not_Use_List_of_Abbreviations.

Commonly Used Abbreviations in Maternity and Pediatric Nursing

AB	abortion
AC	abdominal circumference
AGA	appropriate for gestational age
AGE	acute gastroenteritis
AROM	artificial rupture of membranes
BCP	birth control pill
BOM	bilateral otitis media
BOW	bag of waters
BPD	biparietal diameter
BPD	bronchopulmonary dysplasia (infants)
bpm	beats per minute
BRP	bathroom privileges
BS	bowel sounds
BSA	body surface area
BSE	breast self-examination
BTB	breakthrough bleeding
BW	birth weight
CAN	child abuse and neglect
cp	cerebral palsy
CNS	central nervous system
CNS	clinical nurse specialist
CPD	cephalopelvic disproportion
CRL	crown-rump length
C/S	cesarean section
CST	contraction stress test
CX	cervix
D&E	dilation and evacuation
DFA	diet for age
DOB	date of birth
EBL	estimated blood loss
EDC	estimated date of confinement
EDD	estimated date of delivery
EFM	electronic fetal monitor
EFW	estimated fetal weight
EGA	estimated gestational age
ENT	ear, nose, and throat
FAS	fetal alcohol syndrome
FB	foreign body
FHR	fetal heart rate
FHS	fetal heart sound
FHT	fetal heart tone
FSH	follicle-stimulating hormone
FTT	failure to thrive
FUO	fever of unknown origin
Fx	fracture
G	gravida (number of pregnancies)
GDM	gestational diabetes mellitus
GER	gastroesophageal reflux
GH	gestational hypertension
GI	gastrointestinal
GIFT	gamete intrafallopian transfer
GnRH	gonadotropin-releasing hormone
GTPAL	gravida, term, premature, abortion, living children
GTT	glucose tolerance test
HBO	hyperbaric oxygen
HC	head circumference
hCG	human chorionic gonadotropin
HELLP	hemolysis, elevated liver enzymes, low platelet count
H&H	hemoglobin and hematocrit
Hib	*Haemophilus influenzae* B conjugate vaccine
H&P	history and physical
hPL	human placental lactogen
HR	heart rate
HRT	hormone replacement therapy
I&D	incision and drainage
IM	intramuscular
I/O	intake and output
IUD	intrauterine device
IUGR	intrauterine growth restriction
IVF	in vitro fertilization
KUB	kidneys, ureters, bladder
KVO	keep vein open
LBW	low birth weight
L&D	labor and delivery
LDR	labor-delivery room
LGA	large for gestational age
LH	luteinizing hormone
LMP	last menstrual period
LMP	left mentoposterior
LNMP	last normal menstrual period
LOM	left otitis media
MAS	meconium aspiration syndrome
MDI	metered dose inhaler
med neb	nebulized medication
mL	milliliter(s)
NCP	nursing care plan
NKDA	no known drug allergies
NPO	nothing by mouth
NST	nonstress test
NSVD	normal spontaneous vaginal delivery
NTT	nasotracheal tube
NV	neurovascular
N/V/D/C	nausea, vomiting, diarrhea, constipation
OB	obstetric
OC	oral contraceptive
OE	otitis externa
ORIF	open reduction internal fixation
OTC	over-the-counter (nonprescription) drug
PAR	postanesthesia recovery
Para	birth of a viable infant
PDA	patent ductus arteriosus
PEG	percutaneous endoscopic gastrostomy
PERRLA	pupils equal, round, reactive to light, and accommodation
PICC	peripherally inserted central venous catheter
PID	pelvic inflammatory disease
PKU	phenylketonuria
PMDD	premenstrual dysphoric disorder
PMS	premenstrual syndrome
PP	postpartum
PPD	purified protein derivative (tuberculin test)
PROM	premature rupture of membranes
PT	prothrombin time
PTT	partial thromboplastin time
RAD	reactive airway disease
RDA	recommended dietary allowance
RDI	recommended daily intake
RDS	respiratory distress syndrome
REM	rapid eye movement
R/O	rule out
ROM	range of motion
ROM	rupture of membranes
SAT	saturation
SGA	small for gestational age
SIDS	sudden infant death syndrome
SL	sublingual (under the tongue)
SOAP	subjective/objective/assessment and planning
SOB	shortness of breath
SPROM	spontaneous premature rupture of membranes
S/S	signs and symptoms
SubQ	subcutaneous
STAT	at once
STI	sexually transmitted infection
TKO	to keep open
TO	telephone order
TPN	total parenteral nutrition
TRA	to run at
TSS	toxic shock syndrome
UC	uterine contractions
VBAC	vaginal birth after cesarean
VDRL	Venereal Disease Research Laboratories
VLBW	very low birth weight
VO	verbal order
W-D	well developed
WIC	Women, Infants, and Children program
WN	well nourished
WNL	within normal limits
y/o	year old
YOB	year of birth
ZIFT	zygote intrafallopian transfer
$\uparrow$	increase
$\downarrow$	decrease
$+$	positive, plus
$<$	less than
$>$	greater than
$\sim$	approximate
Δ	change

Common Phrases for Maternity and Pediatric Nursing with Spanish Translations

ENGLISH	SPANISH TRANSLATION AND PRONUNCIATION
Is there someone with you who speaks English?	¿Hay alguien con usted que hable inglés? *Ah-ee ahl-gee-ehn kohn oos-tehd keh ah-bleh een-glehs?*
I am the nurse.	Soy la enfermera. *Soy lah ehn-fehr-meh-rah.*
Sit down, please.	Siéntese, por favor. *See-ehn-teh-seh, pohr fah-bohr.*
Lie down.	Acuéstese. *Ah-kwehs-teh-seh.*
Turn on your right (left) side.	Voltéese del lado derecho (izquierdo). *Bohl-teh-eh-seh dehl lah-doh deh-reh-choh (ees-kee-her-doh).*
Lie on your back.	Acuéstese boca arriba. *Ah-kwehs-teh-seh boh-kah ah-ree-bah.*
Lie on your stomach.	Acuéstese boca abajo. *Ah-kwehs-teh-seh boh-kah ah-bah-hoh.*
You need to take medicine/medication.	Usted necesita tomar medicina. *Oos-tehd neh-seh-see-tah toh-mahr meh-dee-see-nah.*
Show me with one finger where you have the pain.	Enséñeme con un solo dedo dónde tiene el dolor. *Ehn-seh-nyeh-meh kohn oon soh-loh deh-doh dohn-deh tee-eh-neh ehl doh-lohr.*
Do you have nausea?	¿Tiene náusea? *Tee-eh-neh nah-oo-seh-ah?*
Do you have vomiting?	¿Tiene vómito? *Tee-eh-neh boh-mee-toh?*
When was the last time that you ate?	¿Cuándo fue la última vez que comió? *Kwahn-do fweh lah ool-tee-mah behs keh koh-mee-oh?*
Do you have diarrhea?	¿Tiene diarrea? *Tee-eh-neh dee-ah-reh-ah?*
Are you constipated?	¿Está estreñido/-a? *Ehs-tah ehs-treh-nyee-doh/-dah?*
Are you passing gas?	¿Está pasando gas? *Ehs-tah pah-sahn-doh gahs?*
Does it burn when you urinate?	¿Le arde cuando orina? *Leh ahr-deh kwahn-doh oh-ree-nah?*
Bend your knees.	Doble las rodillas. *Doh-bleh lahs roh-dee-yahs.*
Do you have pain here?	¿Tiene dolor aquí? *Tee-eh-neh doh-lohr ak-kee?*
Breathe deeply.	Respire profundo. *Rehs-pee-reh proh-foon-doh.*
Drink clear liquids.	Tome líquidos claros. *Toh-meh lee-kwee-dohs klah-rohs.*
Can you give us a stool sample?	¿Puede darnos una muestra de excremento?

ENGLISH	SPANISH TRANSLATION AND PRONUNCIATION
	Pweh-deh dahr-nohs oo-nah mwehs-trah deh eks-kreh-mehn-toh?
When was the last time you had a bowel movement?	¿Cuándo fue la última vez que obró (que usó el baño)? *Kwahn-doh fweh lah ool-tee-mah behs keh oh-broh (keh oo-soh ehl bah-nyoh)?*
Drink eight glasses of water a day.	Tome ocho vasos de agua al día. *Toh-meh oh-choh bah-sohs deh ah-gwah ahl dee-ah.*
Do you have sexual relations with men (women, prostitutes)?	¿Tiene usted relaciones sexuales con hombres (mujeres, prostitutas)? *Tee-eh-neh oos-tehd rel-lah-see-oh-nehs sek-soo-ah-lehs kohn ohm-brehs (moo-heh-rehs, prohs-tee-too-tahs)?*
Are you allergic to any medicine or food?	¿Es alérgica a alguna medicina o alimento? *Ehs ah-lehr-hee-kah ah al-goo-nah meh-dee-see-nah oh ah-lee-mehn-toh?*
Do you take medicine?	¿Toma usted medicina? *Toh-mah oos-tehd meh-dee-see-nah?*
Do you have the medicine with you?	¿Trae la medicina con usted? *Trah-eh lah meh-dee-see-na kohn oos-tehd?*
Take your medication.	Tome su medicina. *Toh-meh soo meh-dee-see-nah.*
I am going to give you pain medicine.	Le voy a dar medicina para el dolor. *Leh boy ah dahr med-dee-see-nah pah-rah ehl doh-lohr.*
Do you have shortness of breath?	¿Tiene falta del aire? *Tee-ehn-eh fahl-tah dehl ay-reh?*
We need a urine sample.	Necesitamos una muestra de orina. *Neh-seh-see-tah-mohs oo-nah mwehs-trah deh oh-ree-nah.*
You need a catheter in your bladder.	Usted necesita una sonda en la vejiga. *Oos-tehd neh-seh-see-tah oo-nah sohn-dah ehn lah beh-hee-gah.*
Have you lost weight?	¿Ha perdido peso? *Ah pehr-dee-doh peh-soh?*
How long have you had the discharge?	¿Cuánto tiempo tiene con el deshecho/flujo? *Kwahn-toh tee-ehm-poh tee-eh-neh kohn ehl dehs-eh-choh/ floo-hoh?*
What do you use to prevent pregnancy?	¿Qué clase de anticonceptivo usa para prevenir el embarazo? *Keh klah-seh deh ahn-tee-kohn-sept-tee-boh oo-sah pah-rah preh-beh-neer ehl ehm-bah-rah-soh?*

ENGLISH	SPANISH TRANSLATION AND PRONUNCIATION
When was your last period?	¿Cuándo fue su última regla/menstruación?
	*Kwahn-do fweh soo **ool**-tee-mah **reh**-glah/mehns-troo-ah-see-**ohn?***
Are your periods regular?	¿Sus reglas/menstruaciones son regulares?
	*Soos **rehs**-glahs/mehns-troo-ah-see-**oh**-nehs sohn reh-goo-**lah**-rehs?*
Are you pregnant?	¿Esta embarazada?
	*Ehs-**tah** ehm-bah-rah-**sah**-dah?*
How many times have you been pregnant?	¿Cuántas veces ha esado embarazada?
	*Kwahn-tahs **beh**-sehs ah ehs-**tah**-doh ehm-bah-rah-**sah**-dah?*
How many children do you have?	¿Cuántos hijos tiene?
	*Kwahn-tohs **ee**-hohs tee-eh-neh?*
Have you received prenatal care?	¿Ha recibido cuidado prenatal?
	*Ah reh-see-**bee**-doh kwih-**dah**-doh preh-nah-**tahl?***
When was the last time you visited your doctor?	¿Cuándo fue la última vez que visitó a su médico?
	*Kwahn-doh fweh lah **ool**-tee-mah behs keh bee-see-**toh** ah soo **meh**-dee-koh?*
How long have you had vaginal bleeding?	¿Por cuánto tiempo ha tenido sangrado vaginal?
	*Pohr **kwahn**-toh te-**ehm**-poh ah teh-**nee**-doh sahn-**grah**-doh bah-hee-**nahl?***
How many sanitary pads did you use today?	¿Cuántas toallas femininas usó hoy?
	*Kwhan-tahs toh-**ah**-yahs feh-meh-**nee**-nahs oo-**soh oh**-ee?*
Are you having contractions?	¿Tiene contracciones?
	*Tee-**eh**-neh kohn-trahk-see-**ohn**-ehs?*
How many minutes do the contractions last?	¿Cuántos minutos le duran las contracciones?
	*Kwahn-tohs mee-**noo**-tohs leh **doo**-rahn lahs kohn-trahk-see-**ohn**-ehs?*
Did your bag of waters break?	¿Se le rompió la fuente del agua?
	*Seh leh rohm-pee-**oh** lah **fwehn**-teh dehl **ah**-gwah?*
When did your bag of waters break?	¿Cuándo se le reventó la fuente del agua?
	*Kwahn-doh seh leh reh-behn-**toh** lah **fwehn**-teh dehl **ah**-gwah?*
(Don't) Push.	(No) Empuje.
	*(Noh) Ehm-**poo**-heh.*
I am going to listen to the baby's heartbeat.	Voy a escuchar los latidos del corazón del bebé.
	***Boh**-ee ah ehs-koo-**chahr** lohs lah-**tee**-dohs dehl koh-rah-**sohn** dehl beh-**beh**.*
Do you want me to call a friend or relative for you?	¿Quiere que yo le llame a una amistad o pariente?
	*Kee-**eh**-reh keh yoh leh **yah**-meh ah **oo**-nah ah-mees-**tahd** oh pah-ree-**ehn**-teh?*
I need to comb your hair.	Necesito peinarle el pelo.
	*Neh-seh-**see**-toh peh-ee-**nahr**-leh ehl **peh**-loh.*

ENGLISH	SPANISH TRANSLATION AND PRONUNCIATION
Do you know whether you have diabetes?	¿Usted sabe si tiene diabetes?
	*Oos-**tehd sah**-beh see tee-**eh**-neh dee-ah-**beh**-tehs?*
Do you take insulin (diabetic pills)?	¿Toma insulina (píldoras para la diabetes)?
	***Toh**-mah een-soo-**lee**-nah (**peel**-doh-rahs **pah**-rah lah dee-ah-**beh**-tehs)?*
What type of insulin do you take? Regular? NPH? Humulin 70/30?	¿Qué tipo de insulina toma? ¿Regular? ¿NPH? ¿Humulina 70/30?
	*Keh **tee**-poh deh een-soo-**lee**-nah **toh**-mah? Reh-goo-**lahr?** Eh-neh Peh **Ah**-cheh? Oo-moo-**lee**-nah seh-**tehn**-tah **treh**-een-tah?*
How many units of insulin do you take in the morning (evening)?	¿Cuántas unidades de insulina toma en la mañana (tarde)?
	*Kwahn-tahs oo-nee-**dah**-dehs deh een-soo-**lee**-nah **toh**-mah ehn lah mah-**nyah**-nah (**tahr**-deh)?*
Do you check your blood sugar level at home?	¿Usted revisa en casa el nivel de azúcar de la sangre?
	*Oos-**tehd** reh-**bee**-sah ehn **kah**-sah ehl nee-**behl** deh ah-**soo**-kahr deh lah **sahn**-greh?*
What was the blood sugar when you checked it?	¿Cuánto fue el azúcar cuándo lo revisó?
	*Kwahn-toh fweh ehl ah-**soo**-kahr **kwan**-doh loh reh-bee-**soh?***
When was the last time you took your medicine?	¿Cuándo fue la última vez que tomó su medicina?
	*Kwahn-doh fweh lah **ool**-tee-mah behs keh toh-**moh** soo meh-dee-**see**-nah?*
(X) hours (days, weeks) ago.	(X) horas (días, semanas).
	*(X) **oh**-rahs (**dee**-ahs, seh-**mah**-nahs).*
Have you eaten breakfast?	¿Ha desayunado?
	*Ah dehs-ah-yoo-**nah**-doh?*
Have you eaten lunch?	¿Ha almorzado (merendado, tomado el lonche)?
	*Ah ahl-mohr-**sah**-doh (meh-rehn-**dah**-doh, toh-**mah**-doh ehl **lohn**-cheh)?*
Have you eaten dinner/supper?	¿Ha cenado (tomado la comida)?
	*Ah seh-**nah**-doh (toh-**mah**-doh lah koh-**mee**-dah)?*
When did the accident occur?	¿Cuándo ocurrió el accidente?
	*Kwahn-doh oh-koo-ree-**oh** ehl ak-see-**dehn**-teh?*
Did you lose consciousness?	¿Perdió el conocimiento?
	*Pehr-dee-**oh** ehl koh-noh-see-mee-**ehn**-toh?*
When was the last time you received a tetanus vaccine?	¿Cuándo fue la última vez que recibió una vacuna del tétano?
	*Kwahn-doh fweh lah **ool**-tee-mah behs keh reh-see-bee-**oh oo**-nah bah-**koo**-nah dehl **teh**-tah-noh?*
Does the baby sleep more than usual?	¿El/La bebé duerme más de lo normal?
	*Ehl/Lah beh-**beh dwehr**-meh mahs deh loh nohr-**mahl?***

Continued

ENGLISH	SPANISH TRANSLATION AND PRONUNCIATION
Does the baby cry more than usual?	¿El/La bebé llora más de lo normal? *Ehl/Lah beh-**beh yoh**-rah mahs deh loh nohr-**mahl**?*
Do you have difficulty waking up the child?	¿Tiene dificultad para despertar al niño (a la niña)? *Tee-**eh**-neh dee-fee-kool-**tahd pah**-rah dehs-pehr-**tahr** ahl nee-nyoh (ah lah **nee**-nyah)?*
When was the last time you gave him/her medicine for the fever?	¿Cuándo fue la última vez que le dio medicina para la fiebre? ***Kwahn**-doh fweh lah **ool**-tee-mah behs keh leh dee-**oh** meh-dee-**see**-nah **pah**-rah lah fee-**eh**-breh?*
Be sure he/she drinks plenty of fluids.	Asegure que tome muchos líquidos. *Ah-seh-**goo**-reh keh **toh**-meh **moo**-chohs **lee**-kee-dohs.*
Give him/her Tylenol every 4 hours.	Dele Tylenol cada cuatro horas. ***Deh**-leh **tay**-leh-nohl **kah**-dah koo-**ah**-troh **oh**-rahs.*
Is he/she acting normally?	¿Está actuando normalmente? *Ehs-**tah** ahk-too-**ahn**-doh nohr-mahl-**mehn**-teh?*
When he/she vomits, does the emesis shoot out in projectile form?	Cuándo vomita, ¿sale disparado el vómito en forma proyectil? ***Kwahn**-doh boh-**mee**-tah, **sah**-leh dees-pah-**rah**-doh ehl **boh**-mee-toh en **fohr**-mah proh-yek-**teel**?*
When was the last time he/she vomited?	¿Cuándo fue la última vez que vomitó? ***Kwahn**-doh fweh lah **ool**-tee-mak behs keh boh-mee-**toh**?*
Has the baby lost weight?	¿Ha perdido peso el/la bebé? *Ah pehr-**dee**-doh **peh**-soh ehl/lah beh-**beh**?*
Have you recently traveled outside of the country?	¿Recientemente ha viajado fuera del país? *Reh-see-ehn-teh-**mehn**-teh ah bee-ah-**hah**-doh **fweh**-rah dehl pah-**ees**?*
Have you changed his/her formula?	¿Le ha cambiado la fórmula? *Leh ah kahm-bee-**ah**-doh lah **fohr**-moo-lah?*
What brand of formula does he/she take?	¿Qué marca de fórmula toma? *Keh **mahr**-kah deh **fohr**-moo-lah **toh**-mah?*
Do you give him/her cow's milk?	¿Le da leche de vaca? *Leh dah **leh**-chech deh **bah**-kah?*
Does the baby vomit only when you give him/her milk?	¿El/La bebé vomita solamente cuándo le da leche? *Ehl/Lah beh-**beh** boh-**mee**-tah soh-lah-**mehn**-teh **kwahn**-doh leh dah **leh**-cheh?*
Is there another person in the	¿Hay otra persona en casa con los mismos síntomas?

ENGLISH	SPANISH TRANSLATION AND PRONUNCIATION
house with the same symptoms?	*Ah-ee **oh**-trah pehr-**soh**-nah ehn **kah**-sah kohn lohs **mees**-mohs **seen**-toh-mahs?*
Does he/she have a history of asthma?	¿Tiene una historia de asma? *Tee-**eh**-neh **oo**-nah ees-**toh**-ree-ah deh **ahs**-mah?*
We need to do an x-ray of his/her chest.	Necesitamos hacerle una radiografia del pecho. *Neh-seh-**see**-tah-mohs ah-**sehr**-leh **oo**-nah rah-dee-oh-grah-**fee**-ah dehl **peh**-choh.*
When did the convulsion occur?	¿Cuándo le ocurrió la convulsión? ***Kwahn**-doh leh oh-koo-ree-**oh** lah kohn-bool-see-**ohn**?*
How long did the convulsion last?	¿Cuánto tiempo duró la convulsión? ***Kwahn**-toh tee-**ehm**-poh doo-**roh** lah kohn-bool-see-**ohn**?*
Did the child lose consciousness?	¿Perdió el niño/la niña el conocimiento? *Pehr-dee-oh ehl **nee**-nyoh/lah **nee**-nyah ehl koh-noh-see-mee-**ehn**-toh?*
When did the rash appear?	¿Cuándo empezó la erupción? ***Kwahn**-doh ehm-peh-**soh** lah eh-roop-see-**ohn**?*
Do you have a new dog or cat at home?	¿Tienen un nuevo perro o gato en casa? *Tee-**eh**-nehn oon **nweh**-boh **peh**-roh oh **gah**-toh ehn **kah**-sah?*
Have you used a new soap, shampoo, detergent, or lotion?	¿Ha usado un nuevo jabón, champú, detergente, o loción? *Ah oo-**sah**-doh oon **nweh**-boh hah-**bohn**, chahm-poo, deh-tehr-**hehn**-teh, oh loh-see-**ohn**?*
Are your child's shots up to date?	¿Está al corriente con sus vacunas su hijo/-a? *Ehs-**tah** ahl koh-ree-**ehn**-teh kohn soos bah-**koo**-nahs soo **ee**-hoh/-hah?*
Is he/she teething?	¿Le están saliendo los dientes? *Leh ehs-**tahn** sah-lee-**ehn**-doh lohs dee-**ehn**-tehs?*
Does he/she have problems swallowing?	¿Tiene problemas al tragar? *Tee-**eh**-neh proh-**bleh**-mahs ahl trah-**gahr**?*
How long has he/she had trouble walking?	¿Cuánto tiempo lleva con dificultad al caminar? ***Kwahn**-toh tee-**ehm**-poh **yeh**-bah kohn dee-fee-kool-**tad** ahl kah-mee-**nahr**?*
Did he/she fall?	¿Se cayó? *Seh kah-**yoh**?*

Modified from Nasr, I., & Cordero, M. (1996). *Medical Spanish: An instant translator.* Philadelphia: Saunders.

Multilingual Glossary of Symptoms

glossary of **Symptoms**

Symptom	Definition	
Abnormal Bleeding	Unusual loss of blood from stools, urine, bleeding gums, internal organs.	
Chills	A feeling of being cold and shivering, usually with pale skin and a high temperature.	
Cough	Rapid expulsion of air from the lungs in order to clear fluid, mucous, or phlegm.	
Diarrhea	Having loose and watery stools (bowel movements) often.	
Disorientation	To lose a sense of time, place, and one's personal identity.	
Dizziness	A feeling of unsteadiness.	
Dyspnea	Shortness of breath or difficulty breathing.	
Fever	A rise in the temperature of the body above normal, usually when the body has an infection. (A temperature taken by mouth greater than 100.4° Fahrenheit means you have a fever.)	
Headache	A pain located in the head, as over the eyes, at the temples, or at the bottom of the skull.	
Hemoptysis	Coughing up blood (or bloody mucous).	
Jaundice	Yellowing of eyes, skin.	
Loss of Appetite	No desire to eat.	
Loss of Consciousness (Unconscious)	Not responsive, not aware, not feeling, not thinking (sometimes as a result of fainting).	
Malaise	Feeling generally weak and tired, and bodily discomfort.	
Nausea	An unpleasant feeling in the stomach, with an urge to vomit (throw up).	
Pain	An unpleasant feeling in the body that can range from being mild to extremely painful. The pain can be physical or emotional. Body pain is physical pain, usually due to tissue damage.	
Rash	Red bumps (or flaky patches) on the body that are sometimes itchy.	
Sore Throat	Pain or discomfort in swallowing.	
Tremor	An uncontrollable trembling, shaking, or quivering from physical weakness, emotional stress, or disease.	
Vomiting	To throw up what is inside the stomach through the mouth.	

Division of Communicable Disease Control — IMM-835 (3/05)

glossary of **Symptoms**

Symptom	Spanish	Chinese	Korean	
Abnormal Bleeding	Sangrado anormal	異常出血	비정상 출혈	
Chills	Escalofrío	寒顫	오한	
Cough	Tos	咳嗽	기침	
Diarrhea	Diarrea, excrementos líquidos	腹瀉	설사	
Disorientation	Desorientación, confusión mental	定向障礙	방향 감각 상실	
Dizziness	Sentirese desmayado	頭暈	현기증	
Dyspnea	Dificultad de respirar	呼吸困難	호흡 곤란	
Fever	Fiebre	發燒	열	
Headache	Dolor de cabeza intenso	頭痛	두통	
Hemoptysis	Tos con sangre	咯血	객혈	
Jaundice	Piel y ojos de color amarillo (ictericia)	黃疸	황달	
Loss of Appetite	Pérdida del apetito	食欲不振	식욕 부진	
Loss of Consciousness (Unconscious)	Desmayarse	失去知覺	무의식	
Malaise	Indisposción o malestar	不舒服	권태감	
Nausea	Ganas de vomitar o náuseas	噁心	메스꺼움	
Pain	Dolor	疼痛	통증	
Rash	Erupción o sarpullido	皮疹	발진	
Sore Throat	Dolor de garganta	喉嚨痛	목앓이	
Tremor	Temblor continuo	震顫	떨림	
Vomiting	Vómito	嘔吐	구토	

Division of Communicable Disease Control — IMM-835 (3/05)

Continued

glossary of Symptoms

Symptom	Japanese	Tagalog	Cambodian
Abnormal Bleeding	異常出血	Di-normal na Pagdugo	ឈាមហូរខុសធម្មតា
Chills	悪寒	Ginaw	ត្រើងជោរ
Cough	咳	Ubo	ក្អក
Diarrhea	下痢	Pagtatae	ជម្ងឺរាក
Disorientation	方向感覚の喪失	Pagkalito	វង្វេងស្មារតី
Dizziness	めまい	Pagkahilo	វិលមុខ
Dyspnea	呼吸困難	Pangangapos ng Hininga	ពិបាកដកដង្ហើម
Fever	発熱	Lagnat	គ្រុន
Headache	頭痛	Sakit ng Ulo	ឈឺក្បាល
Hemoptysis	血を吐く	Pag-ubo ng Dugo	ក្អកផ្លាក់ឈាម
Jaundice	黄疸	Paninilaw ng Mata at Balat	ជម្ងឺខាន់លឿង
Loss of Appetite	食欲不振	Pagkawala ng Ganang Kumain	មិនឃ្លានអាហារ
Loss of Consciousness (Unconscious)	意識不明	Pagkawala ng Malay	ផ្ដច់ដង្ហើមខូន
Malaise	倦怠感	Panlulupaypay	ឈ្លើកឈ្លេ
Nausea	吐き気	Nasusuka	ចង់ក្អួត
Pain	痛み	Masakit	ឈឺ
Rash	発疹	Singaw sa Balat	កន្ទួលឡើងស្បែក
Sore Throat	喉の痛み	Masakit na Lalamunan	ឈឺបំពង់ក
Tremor	震え	Pangangatal	ញ័រញ្ញោក
Vomiting	嘔吐	Pagsusuka	ក្អួត

Division of Communicable Disease Control   IMM-835 (3/05)

glossary of Symptoms

Symptom	Hmong	Laotian	Vietnamese
Abnormal Bleeding	Los ntshav	ເລືອດອອກຜິດປົກກະຕິ	Chảy Máu Bất Thường
Chills	No	ໜາວໄຂ້ສັ່ນ	Ớn Lạnh
Cough	Hnoos	ອາການໄອ/ໄອ	Ho
Diarrhea	Thoj plab	ທ້ອງຮ່ວງ	Tiêu Chảy
Disorientation	Feeb tsis meej	ສັບສົນ	Bối Rối Mất Định Hướng
Dizziness	Kiv taubhau	ຮູ້ສຶກວິນຫົວ	Chóng mặt
Dyspnea	Txog Siav	ຫາຍໃຈຍົກ	Hụt Hơi Khó Thở
Fever	Kub cev	ເປັນໄຂ້	Sốt
Headache	Mob taubhau	ເຈັບຫົວ	Nhức Đầu
Hemoptysis	Hnoos tau ntshav	ໄອອອກເລືອດ	Ho Khạc Ra Máu
Jaundice	Daj ntseg	ເປັນຂີ້ຫຍາກເຫລືອງ	Vàng Da
Loss of Appetite	Tsis qab los	ກິນເຂົ້າບໍ່ແຊບ	Biếng ăn
Loss of Consciousness (Unconscious)	Looj lawm	ໝົດສະຕິ (ສະຫລົບ)	Bất Tỉnh
Malaise	Nkees	ອາການບໍ່ສະບາຍ	Mệt Mỏi Uể Oải
Nausea	Xeev siab	ປວດຮາກ	Buồn Nôn
Pain	Mob	ເຈັບ/ປວດ	Đau Nhức
Rash	Ua xua	ຜື່ນແດງ	Da nổi mụn đỏ
Sore Throat	Mob cajpas	ເຈັບຄໍ	Đau Cổ Họng
Tremor	Tshee	ສັ່ນ	Run Rẩy
Vomiting	Ntuav	ຮາກ	Ói Mửa

Division of Communicable Disease Control   IMM-835 (3/05)

glossary of Symptoms

Symptom	Arabic	Farsi	Armenian	
Abnormal Bleeding	نزيف شديد غير طبيعي	خونریزی غیرعادی (اَب نُرمال بلیدینگ)	Արտասովոր Արյունահոսություն	
Chills	قشعريرة	لرز (چیلز)	Սարսռություն	
Cough	سعال / كحة	سرفه (کاف)	Հազ	
Diarrhea	إسهال	اسهال (دایریا)	Լուծ	
Disorientation	توهان	اختلال در جهت یابی (دیس اَرینتیشن)	Ապակողմնորոշում	
Dizziness	دوخة/دوار	سرگیجه	Գլխապտույտ	
Dyspnea	ضيق نفس / صعوبة في التنفس	تنگی نفس (دیسپنیا)	Աշխատավոր Շնչառություն	
Fever	سخونة شديدة	تب (فیور)	Ջերմություն	
Headache	صداع	سردرد (هد اِک)	Գլխացավ	
Hemoptysis	سعال مع بصق الدم / كحة مع بصق الدم	خلط خونی (هِمُپتیا یسبس)	Արյունախառն Հազ	
Jaundice	الصفراء	یرقان . زردی (جاندیس)	Դեղնախտ	
Loss of Appetite	فقدان الشهية/عدم الرغبة في الطعام	بی اشتهایی	Ախորժակի Կորուստ	
Loss of Consciousness (Unconscious)	فقدان الوعي (فاقد الوعي)	ناهوشیاری (آنکانشِس نس)	Ուշաթափություն (Ուշակորույս լինել)	
Malaise	تعب في الجسم كله	احساس بیحالی و ناخوشی. کوفتگی (مَیلِز)	Թուլություն	
Nausea	ميل للتقيؤ/ غثيان	حال بهم خوردگی. تهوع (نازیا)	Սրտախառնություն	
Pain	ألم	درد (پین)	Ցավ	
Rash	طفح	جوش و دانه های قرمز روی پوست (رَش)	Ցան	
Sore Throat	ألم في الزور	گلو درد (سُرتُرُت)	Կոկորդի Բորբքում	
Tremor	رعشة	لرزش و تكان غیر ارادی (تِرمُر)	Դող	
Vomiting	تقيؤ	استفراغ (وامیتینگ)	Փսխումներ	

Division of Communicable Disease Control   IMM-835 (3/05)

glossary of Symptoms

Symptom	Russian	Punjabi	
Abnormal Bleeding	Кровотечение в брюшную полость	ਬਹੁਤ ਖੂਨ ਪੈਣਾ	
Chills	Озноб	ਪਾਲਾ	
Cough	Кашель	ਖੰਘ	
Diarrhea	Понос	ਟੱਟੀਆਂ ਲੱਗਣਾ	
Disorientation	Дезориентация	ਬੌਂਦਲਣਾ	
Dizziness	Головокружение	ਚੱਕਰ ਆਉਣੇ	
Dyspnea	Одышка	ਸਾਹ ਲੈਣ ਵਿਚ ਮੁਸ਼ਕਲ	
Fever	Жар	ਬੁਖਾਰ	
Headache	Головная боль	ਸਿਰਦਰਦ	
Hemoptysis	Кровохарканье	ਖੰਘ ਨਾਲ ਖੂਨ ਆਉਣਾ	
Jaundice	Желтуха	ਪੀਲੀਆ	
Loss of Appetite	Потеря аппетита	ਭੁੱਖ ਨਾ ਲੱਗਣਾ	
Loss of Consciousness (Unconscious)	Потеря сознания	ਬੇਹੋਸ਼ੀ	
Malaise	Недомогание	ਕਮਜ਼ੋਰੀ	
Nausea	Тошнота	ਜੀਅ ਕੱਚਾ ਹੋਣਾ	
Pain	Боль	ਦਰਦ	
Rash	Сыпь	ਧੱਫੜ	
Sore Throat	Больное горло	ਗਲਾ ਦੁਖਣਾ	
Tremor	Дрожь	ਕੰਬਣਾ	
Vomiting	Рвота	ਉਲਟੀਆਂ	

Division of Communicable Disease Control   IMM-835 (3/05)

This glossary includes only the most common signs and symptoms of most communicable diseases. Disease investigators can use this as a supplement when interviewing non-English speaking clients. Languages included are the most common ones in California. A phonetic pronunciation supplement is available online for download at *www.cdlhn.com*.

Conversion Tables

Table E-1 Conversion of Pounds and Ounces to Grams for Newborn Weights*

POUNDS	OUNCES															
	0	1	2	3	4	5	6	7	8	9	10	11	12	13	14	15
0	—	28	57	85	113	142	170	198	227	255	283	312	336	369	397	425
1	454	482	510	539	567	595	624	652	680	709	737	765	794	822	850	879
2	907	936	964	992	1021	1049	1077	1106	1134	1162	1191	1219	1247	1276	1304	1332
3	1361	1389	1417	1446	1474	1503	1531	1559	1588	1616	1644	1673	1701	1729	1758	1786
4	1814	1843	1871	1899	1928	1956	1984	2013	2041	2070	2098	2126	2155	2183	2211	2240
5	2268	2296	2325	2353	2381	2410	2438	2466	2495	2523	2551	2580	2608	2637	2665	2693
6	2722	2750	2778	2807	2835	2863	2892	2920	2948	2977	3005	3033	3062	3090	3118	3147
7	3175	3203	3232	3260	3289	3317	3345	3374	3402	3430	3459	3487	3515	3544	3572	3600
8	3629	3657	3685	3714	3742	3770	3799	3827	3856	3884	3912	3941	3969	3997	4026	4054
9	4082	4111	4139	4167	4196	4224	4252	4281	4309	4337	4366	4394	4423	4451	4479	4508
10	4536	4564	4593	4621	4649	4678	4706	4734	4763	4791	4819	4848	4876	4904	4933	4961
11	4990	5018	5046	5075	5103	5131	5160	5188	5216	5245	5273	5301	5330	5358	5386	5415
12	5443	5471	5500	5528	5557	5585	5613	5642	5670	5698	5727	5755	5783	5812	5840	5868
13	5897	5925	5953	5982	6010	6038	6067	6095	6123	6152	6180	6209	6237	6265	6294	6322
14	6350	6379	6407	6435	6464	6492	6520	6549	6577	6605	6634	6662	6690	6719	6747	6776
15	6804	6832	6860	6889	6917	6945	6973	7002	7030	7059	7087	7115	7144	7172	7201	7228
	0	1	2	3	4	5	6	7	8	9	10	11	12	13	14	15

Ounces

*To convert the weight known in grams to pounds and ounces, for example, of a baby weighing 3317 g, glance down columns to find the figure closest to 3317, which is 3714. Refer to the number to the far left or right of the column for pounds and the number at the top or bottom for ounces to get 8 pounds, 3 ounces.

Conversion formulas:
Pounds × 453.6 = grams
Ounces × 28.35 = grams
Grams ÷ 453.6 = pounds
Grams ÷ 28.35 = ounces

Table E-2 Conversion of Fahrenheit to Celsius

FAHRENHEIT (°)	CELSIUS (°)	FAHRENHEIT (°)	CELSIUS (°)	FAHRENHEIT (°)	CELSIUS (°)
96.1	35.6	99.3	37.4	102.6	39.2
96.4	35.8	99.7	37.6	102.9	39.4
96.8	36.0	100.0	37.8	103.3	39.6
97.2	36.2	100.4	38.0	103.6	39.8
97.5	36.4	100.8	38.2	104.0	40.0
97.9	36.6	101.1	38.4	104.4	40.2
98.2	36.8	101.5	38.6	104.7	40.4
98.6	37.0	101.8	38.8	105.2	40.6
99.0	37.2	102.2	39.0		

Conversion formulas:
Fahrenheit to Celsius: $(°F - 32) \times (5/9) = °C$
Celsius to Fahrenheit: $(°C) \times (9/5) + 32 = °F$

Selected Maternal and Newborn Laboratory Values

Table F-1 Normal Maternal Laboratory Range and Abnormal Findings

LABORATORY TEST	NONPREGNANT VALUES	PREGNANT VALUES	ABNORMAL FINDINGS
Hemoglobin (Hb)	12-16 g/dL	11-12 g/dL	Decreased levels may indicate anemia.
Hematocrit (Hct)	37%-48%	33%-46%	Decreased levels may indicate anemia.
White blood cell total (WBCs)	5000-10,000/mm^3	5000-15,000/mm^3	Increased levels may indicate compromise in immune system.
Red blood cell total (RBCs) (million/mm^3)	3.8-5.1 g/dL	Decreased levels may indicate anemia.	Increased levels may indicate polycythemia (can occur in dehydration).
Platelets	150,000-350,000/mm^3	May have significant increase 3-5 days after birth	Increase predisposes to thrombosis.
Partial thromboplastin time (PTT)	21-35 seconds	Slight decrease in pregnancy and in labor	Allows placental site clotting.
Fibrinogen	200-400 mg/dL	300-600 mg/dL	
Lymphocytes	38%-46%	15%-40%	
Polymorphonuclear cells	54%-62%	60%-85%	
Total protein	6.7-8.3 g/dL	5.5-7.5 g/dL	
Glucose serum Fasting 2 hours Postprandial	70-80 mg/dL 60-110 mg/dL	65 mg/dL 140 mg/dL considered normal	

Table F-2 Normal Newborn Laboratory Values

LABORATORY TEST	NORMAL TERM VALUES
Hemoglobin	14.5-22.5 g/dL (cord blood)
Hematocrit	44%-64%
Platelets	150,000-300,000/mm^3
White blood cells	9000-30,000/mm^3
Lymphocytes	30%
Serum glucose	40-65 mg/dL
Bilirubin, total serum	1 day full-term <6 mg/dL 1 day preterm <8 mg/dL

Modified from Behrman, R. E., Kliegman, R. M., Jenson, H. B., & Stanton, B. (2007). *Nelson textbook of pediatrics* (18th ed.). Philadelphia: Saunders.

Answers to Review Questions for the NCLEX® Examination

CHAPTER 1

1. 3
2. 1
3. 3
4. 1, 4, 3, 5, 2
5. 1
6. 2, 4, 5

CHAPTER 2

1. 3
2. 3
3. 3
4. 2
5. 2
6. 2, 3, 4
7. 2, 5
8. 2, 3, 1, 4

CHAPTER 3

1. 2
2. 2
3. 3
4. 4
5. 1
6. 1, 2, 3, 4, 5
7. 3, 4
8. 2, 1, 4, 5, 3

CHAPTER 4

1. 2
2. 3
3. 4
4. 1
5. 3
6. 1
7. 2, 3, 4
8. 3, 1, 4, 2

CHAPTER 5

1. 2
2. 4
3. 2
4. 2
5. 1, 5
6. 4
7. 3
8. 4

CHAPTER 6

1. 4
2. 3
3. 3
4. 1
5. 2, 3, 4
6. 3
7. 1, 2, 3
8. 2, 1, 6, 5, 3, 4

CHAPTER 7

1. 3
2. 1
3. 4
4. 3
5. 1
6. 2, 3, 4
7. 2, 3, 4

CHAPTER 8

1. 2
2. 1
3. 1, 3, 4
4. 2
5. 2
6. 1, 2, 3, 5

CHAPTER 9

1. 2
2. 3
3. 1
4. 2
5. 4
6. 1
7. 1, 2, 4, 5

CHAPTER 10

1. 2
2. 4
3. 1
4. 2
5. 1, 4, 5
6. 1

CHAPTER 11

1. 2
2. 1
3. 3
4. 2
5. 1, 2, 3, 4
6. 4
7. 3
8. 2, 3, 5

CHAPTER 12

1. 3
2. 1, 3, 4
3. 4
4. 1
5. 3
6. 1, 3, 4
7. 4, 1, 2, 3

CHAPTER 13

1. 1, 3, 4
2. 4
3. 4
4. 1
5. 2
6. 2
7. 1
8. 2

CHAPTER 14

1. 2
2. 3
3. 1
4. 2
5. 3
6. 3
7. 1, 2, 4

CHAPTER 15

1. 3
2. 1, 2, 3
3. 1
4. 3
5. 2
6. 4
7. 1, 2, 4

CHAPTER 16

1. 4
2. 4
3. 4

4. 1
5. 1
6. 1
7. 1, 2, 3, 4, 5

CHAPTER 17

1. 3
2. 4
3. 2
4. 2
5. 1, 2, 3
6. 3, 4
7. 1, 3, 4

CHAPTER 18

1. 3
2. 1
3. 2
4. 4
5. 2, 3, 4
6. 1, 2, 3, 5

CHAPTER 19

1. 2
2. 3
3. 2, 3, 4
4. 3
5. 4
6. 3
7. 2, 3, 4, 5

CHAPTER 20

1. 3
2. 2, 3, 4
3. 4
4. 4
5. 1
6. 2, 3, 5
7. 1, 3, 4, 5

CHAPTER 21

1. 2
2. 1, 4
3. 1
4. 3
5. 1
6. 1, 2, 3, 4, 5
7. 2, 3

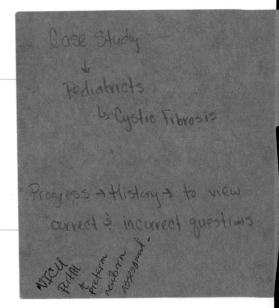

Case Study
↓
Pediatrics
↳ Cystic Fibrosis

Progress → History → to view
correct & incorrect questions

NICU
Rectal
& preterm
newborn
assessment

Bibliography and Reader References

CHAPTER 1

Alfaro-LeFevre, R. (2008). *Critical thinking and clinical judgment: A practical approach to outcome-focused thinking* (4th ed.). St. Louis: Saunders.

Callister, L. C. (2006). Global health and nursing. *MCN. The American Journal of Maternal Child Nursing, 31*(3), 202.

Carey, W., Crocker, A., Elias, E., Feldman, H., & Coleman, W. (2009). *Developmental-behavioral pediatrics* (4th ed.). Philadelphia: Saunders.

Cumming, A., Simpson, K., & Brown, D. (2006). *Complementary and alternative medicine.* London: Churchill Livingstone.

D'Avanzo, C. (2007). *Mosby's pocket guide to cultural health assessment* (4th ed.). St. Louis: Mosby.

Ernst, E., Pittler, M., & Wider, B. (2006). *The desktop guide to complementary and alternative medicine: An evidence-based approach* (2nd ed.). St. Louis: Mosby.

Gabbe, S., Niebyl, J., & Simpson, J. (2007). *Obstetrics: Normal and problem pregnancies* (5th ed.). New York: Churchill Livingstone.

Joint Commission on Accreditation of Health Care Organizations (2010). *Comprehensive accreditation manual for hospitals.* Chicago: Author.

Kliegman, R., Behrman, R., Jenson, H., & Stanton, B. (2007). *Nelson textbook of pediatrics* (18th ed.). Philadelphia: Saunders.

Leifer, G. (2010). *Introduction to maternity and pediatric nursing* (6th ed.). Philadelphia: Saunders.

Leifer, G., & Hartston, H. (2004). *Growth and development across the lifespan: A health promotion focus.* Philadelphia: Saunders.

Levine, M., Carey, W., & Crocker, A. (1999). *Developmental behavioral pediatrics.* Philadelphia: WB Saunders.

London, M., Ladewig, P., Ball, J., & Bindler, R. (2006). *Maternal & child nursing care* (2nd ed.). Upper Saddle River, NJ: Prentice-Hall Health.

Lowdermilk, D. L., & Perry, S. E. (2007). *Maternity and women's health care* (9th ed.). St. Louis: Mosby.

McCartney, P. (2006). Using technology to provide perinatal patient safety. *Journal of Obstetric, Gynecologic, and Neonatal Nursing: JOGNN/NAACOG, 35*(3), 424–431.

Murray, S. S., & McKinney, E. S. (2010). *Foundations of maternal-newborn and women's health nursing* (5th ed.). Philadelphia: Saunders.

NLN (2008). *Preparing the next generation of nurses to practice in a technology rich environment.* New York: NLN Press.

North American Nursing Diagnosis Association (2006). *Nursing diagnosis: Definitions and classifications.* Philadelphia: Author.

Perry, S. (2010). *Maternal child nursing care.* St. Louis: Mosby.

Rajecki, R. (2009). National patient safety goals: Changing, but the same. *RN, 72*(8), 30–35.

Rakel, D. (2007). *Integrative medicine* (2nd ed.). Philadelphia: Saunders.

Schneiderman, J. U. (1998). Rituals of placenta disposal. *MCN. The American Journal of Maternal Child Nursing, 23*(3), 142–143.

Shu-Hsin Lee, S. H., & Kuo, B. J. (2000). Chinese traditional childbearing attitudes and infertile couples in Taiwan. *Journal of Nursing Scholarship, 32*(1), 54.

Wolraich, M., Perrin, E., Dworkin, P., & Drotar, D. (2007). *Developmental-behavioral pediatrics: Evidence and practice.* St. Louis: Mosby.

CHAPTER 2

Blackburn, S. (2007). *Maternal, fetal, and neonatal physiology: A clinical perspective* (3rd ed.). Philadelphia: Saunders.

Creasy, R., Resnik, R., Iams, J., Lockwood, C., & Moore, T. (2008). *Creasy & Resnik's maternal-fetal medicine* (6th ed.). Philadelphia: Saunders.

Gabbe, S., Niebyl, J., & Simpson, J. (2007). *Obstetrics: Normal and problem pregnancies* (5th ed.). New York: Churchill Livingstone.

Leifer, G. (2010). *Introduction to maternity and pediatric nursing* (6th ed.). Philadelphia: Saunders.

Leifer, G., & Hartston, H. (2004). *Growth and development across the lifespan: A health promotion focus.* Philadelphia: Saunders.

London, M., Ladewig, P., Ball, J., & Bindler, R. (2006). *Maternal & child nursing care* (2nd ed.). Upper Saddle River, NJ: Prentice-Hall Health.

Lowdermilk, D. L., & Perry, S. E. (2007). *Maternity and women's health care* (9th ed.). St. Louis: Mosby.

Murray, S. S., & McKinney, E. S. (2005). *Foundations of maternal-newborn nursing* (4th ed.). Philadelphia: Saunders.

Oats, J., & Abraham, S. (2010). *Llewellyn-Jones fundamentals of obstetrics and gynecology* (9th ed.). St. Louis: Mosby.

CHAPTER 3

AWHONN, Mattson, S., & Smith, J. E. (2010). *Core curriculum for maternal-newborn nursing* (4th ed.). Philadelphia: Saunders.

Blackburn, S. (2007). *Maternal, fetal, and neonatal physiology: A clinical perspective* (3rd ed.). Philadelphia: Saunders.

Creasy, R., Resnik, R., Iams, J., Lockwood, C., & Moore, T. (2008). *Creasy & Resnik's maternal-fetal medicine* (6th ed.). Philadelphia: Saunders.

Gabbe, S., Niebyl, J., & Simpson, J. (2007). *Obstetrics: Normal and problem pregnancies* (5th ed.). New York: Churchill Livingstone.

London, M., Ladewig, P., Ball, J., & Bindler, R. (2006). *Maternal & child nursing care* (2nd ed.). Upper Saddle River, NJ: Prentice Hall Health.

Lowdermilk, D. L., & Perry, S. E. (2007). *Maternity and women's health care* (9th ed.). St. Louis: Mosby.

Moore, K. L., & Persaud, T. V. N. (2007). *Before we are born: Essentials of embryology and birth defects* (7th ed.). Philadelphia: Saunders.

Murray, S. S., & McKinney, E. S. (2010). *Foundations of maternal-newborn and women's health nursing* (5th ed.). Philadelphia: Saunders.

CHAPTER 4

Gordon, M. (2007). Maternal physiology. In S. Gabbe, J. Niebyl, & J. Simpson (Eds.), *Obstetrics: Normal and problem pregnancies.* (5th ed.). New York: Churchill Livingstone.

Creasy, R., Resnik, R., Iams, J., Lockwood, C., & Moore, T. (2008). *Creasy & Resnik's maternal-fetal medicine* (6th ed.). Philadelphia: Saunders.

Driscoll, J. (2008). Psychosocial adaptation to pregnancy and postpartum. In K. Simpson & P. Creehan (Eds.), *AWHONN Perinatal nursing.* Philadelphia: Lippincott Williams & Wilkins.

Gabbe, S., Niebyl, J., & Simpson, J. (2007). *Obstetrics: Normal and problem pregnancies* (5th ed.). New York: Churchill Livingstone.

Hacker, N., Gambone, J., & Hobel, C. (2009). *Hacker & Moore's essentials of obstetrics and gynecology* (5th ed.). Philadelphia: Saunders.

Kliegman, R., Behrman, R., Jenson, H., & Stanton, B. (2007). *Nelson textbook of pediatrics* (18th ed.). Philadelphia: Saunders.

Leifer, G. (2010). *Introduction to maternity and pediatric nursing* (6th ed.). Philadelphia: Saunders.

Leifer, G., & Hartston, H. (2004). *Growth and development across the lifespan: A health promotion focus.* Philadelphia: Saunders.

London, M., Ladewig, P., Ball, J., & Bindler, R. (2006). *Maternal & child nursing care* (2nd ed.). Upper Saddle River, NJ: Prentice Hall Health.

Lowdermilk, D. L., & Perry, S. E. (2007). *Maternity and women's health care* (9th ed.). St. Louis: Mosby.

Murray, S., & McKinney, E. (2010). *Foundations of maternal-newborn and women's health nursing* (5th ed.). Philadelphia: Saunders.

Stables, D., & Rankin, J. (2005). *Physiology in childbearing with anatomy and related biosciences* (2nd ed.). London: Balliere-Tindall.

CHAPTER 5

Alex, M. (2011). Occupational hazards for pregnant nurses. *American Journal of Nursing, 111*(1), 28–37.

American Academy of Pediatrics (2008). *Guidelines for perinatal care* (6th ed.). Elk Grove Village, IL: Author.

American College of Obstetrics and Gynecology (ACOG) (2004). ACOG (American College of Obstetrics and Gynecology) Practice Bulletin: Nausea and vomiting of pregnancy. *Obstetrics and Gynecology, 103,* 803–815.

American Dietary Association (2008). Position of the American Dietary Association on nutrition and lifestyle for a healthy pregnancy outcome. *Journal of the American Dietetic Association, 108*(3), 553–561.

AWHONN, Mattson, S., & Smith, J. E. (2010). *Core curriculum for maternal-newborn nursing* (4th ed.). Philadelphia: Saunders.

AWHONN, Simpson, K., & Creehan, P. (2007). *Perinatal nursing* (3rd ed.). Philadelphia: Lippincott Williams & Wilkins.

Berry, R., Baily, L., Mulinare, J., & Bower, C. (2010). Fortification of flour with folic acid. *Food and Nutrition Bulletin, 31* (Suppl. 1), S32–S35.

Blackburn, S. (2007). *Maternal, fetal, and neonatal physiology: A clinical perspective* (3rd ed.). Philadelphia: Saunders.

Carroll, I. (2005). Avoiding travel related infections during pregnancy. *Contemporary Obstetrics/Gynecology, 55,* 34–48.

Centers for Disease Control and Prevention (2006). *Immunizations for the pregnant woman.* www.cdc.gov/vaccines/pubs/downloads/f_preg_chart.pdf.

Centers for Disease Control and Prevention (2010). Grand Rounds: Opportunities to prevent neural tube defects with folic acid fortification. *MMWR. Morbidity and Mortality Weekly Report, 59*(31), 980–984. www.cdc.gov/about/grandrounds.

Colombio, J., Carlson, S., & Levine, B. (2004). Pregnant? Omega-3 essential for baby's brain. *Child Development, 275,* 1254–1267.

Cox, J., & Phelan, S. (2009). Prenatal nutrition: special considerations. *Minerva Ginecologica, 61*(5), 373–400.

Creasy, R., Resnik, R., Iams, J., Lockwood, C., & Moore, T. (2008). *Creasy & Resnik's maternal-fetal medicine* (6th ed.). Philadelphia: Saunders.

Dugan-Kim, M., Connell, S., Stitka, C., Wong, C., & Gossett, D. (2009). Epistaxis during pregnancy and association with postpartum hemorrhage. *Journal of Obstetric, Gynecologic, and Neonatal Nursing: JOGNN/NAACOG, 114*(6), 1322–1325.

Gabbe, S., Niebyl, J., & Simpson, J. (2007). *Obstetrics: Normal and problem pregnancies* (5th ed.). New York: Churchill Livingstone.

Hacker, N. F., & Moore, J. G. (2009). *Hacker & Moore's essentials of obstetrics and gynecology* (5th ed.). Philadelphia: Saunders.

Institute of Medicine (2010). *Vitamin A and pregnancy.* Retrieved July 10, 2010, from www.iom.edu/~/media/files/activity%20files/nutrition/dris/dri_vitamins.ashx.

Kinser, P. (2008). Prenatal yoga: guidance for providers and patients. *Advance for Nurse Practitioners, 16*(1), 59–60.

Kliegman, R., Behrman, R., Jensen, H., & Stanton, B. (2007). *Nelson textbook of pediatrics* (18th ed.). Philadelpha: Saunders.

Leifer, G. (2010). *Introduction to maternity and pediatric nursing* (6th ed.). Philadelphia: Saunders.

London, M., Ladewig, P., Ball, J., & Bindler, R. (2006). *Maternal & child nursing care* (2nd ed.). Upper Saddle River, NJ: Prentice Hall Health.

Lowdermilk, D. L., & Perry, S. E. (2007). *Maternity and women's health care* (9th ed.). St. Louis: Mosby.

Mahan, L. K., & Escott-Stump, S. (2007). *Krause's food & nutrition therapy* (12th ed.). Philadelphia: Saunders.

Murray, S., & McKinney, E. (2010). *Foundations of maternal-newborn and women's health nursing* (5th ed.). Philadelphia: Saunders.

Oepkes, D., Seaward, P., & Vandenbussche, F. (2006). Doppler ultrasonography versus amniocentesis to predict fetal anemia. *The New England Journal of Medicine, 355*(2), 156–164.

Steffen, R., DuPont, H., & Wilder-Smith, A. (2007). *Manual of travel medicine and health* (3rd ed.). Hamilton, ON: BC Decker.

Taylor, K. (2010). What not to eat and how not to sleep: Common myths about pregnancy. *The Nurse Practitioner, 18*(3), 46.

Thiroux, R. (2008). Caffeine during pregnancy: How much is safe? *Nursing for Women's Health, 12*(3), 240–242.

Zeisel, S., & da Costa, K. (2009). Choline: an essential nutrient for public health. *Nutrition Reviews, 67*(11), 615–623.

CHAPTER 6

American Academy of Pediatrics (2008). *Guidelines for perinatal care* (6th ed.). Elk Grove Village, IL: Author.

AWHONN (2008). *Nursing care and management of second stage of labor: Evidence-based procedure guidelines* (2nd ed.). Washington, DC: Author.

AWHONN, Mattson, S., & Smith, J. E. (2010). *Core curriculum for maternal-newborn nursing* (4th ed.). Philadelphia: Saunders.

AWHONN, Simpson, K., & Creehan, P. (2007). *Perinatal nursing* (3rd ed.). Philadelphia: Lippincott Williams & Wilkins.

Blackburn, S. (2007). *Maternal, fetal, neonatal physiology: A clinical perspective* (3rd ed.). Philadelphia: Saunders.

Creasy, R., Resnik, R., Iams, J., Lockwood, C., & Moore, T. (2008). *Creasy & Resnik's maternal-fetal medicine* (6th ed.). Philadelphia: Saunders.

Gabbe, S., Niebyl, J., & Simpson, J. (2007). *Obstetrics: Normal and problem pregnancies* (5th ed.). New York: Churchill Livingstone.

Hacker, N., Gambone, J., & Hobel, C. (2009). *Hacker & Moore's essentials of obstetrics and gynecology* (5th ed.). Philadelphia: Saunders.

Institute of Medicine (2009). *Weight gain during pregnancy: Re-examining the guidelines.* Washington, DC: National Academy Press.

Kliegman, R., Behrman, R., Jensen, H., & Stanton, B. (2007). *Nelson textbook of pediatrics* (18th ed.). Philadelphia: Saunders.

Leifer, G. (2010). *Introduction to maternity and pediatric nursing* (6th ed.). Philadelphia: Saunders.

London, M., Ladewig, P., Ball, J., & Bindler, R. (2006). *Maternal & child nursing care* (2nd ed.). Upper Saddle River, NJ: Prentice Hall Health.

Lowdermilk, D. L., & Perry, S. E. (2007). *Maternity and women's health care* (9th ed.). St. Louis: Mosby.

MacDorman, M., & Kirmeyer, S. (2009). Fetal and perinatal mortality in the United States, 2005. *National Vital Statistics Report, 57*(8). Hyattsville, MD: National Center for Health Statistics.

Murray, S. S., & McKinney, E. (2010). *Foundations of maternal-newborn and women's health nursing* (5th ed.). Philadelphia: Saunders.

Oepkes, D., Seaward, P., & Vandenbussche, F. (2006). Doppler ultrasonography vs. amniocentesis to predict fetal anemia. *The New England Journal of Medicine, 355*(2), 156–164.

Patton, K., & Thibodeau, G. (2009). *Anatomy and physiology* (7th ed.). St. Louis: Mosby.

Vande Vusse, L. (1999). The essential forces of labor revisited: 13 P's reported in women's stories. *MCN. The American Journal of Maternal Child Nursing, 24*(4), 176–184.

CHAPTER 7

Adams, E., & Bianchi, A. (2008). A practical approach to labor support. *Journal of Obstetric, Gynecologic, and Neonatal Nursing: JOGNN/NAACOG, 37*(1), 106–115.

American Academy of Pediatrics (2008). *Guidelines for perinatal care* (6th ed.). Elk Grove, IL: Author.

Apgar, V. (1966). The newborn (Apgar) scoring system: Reflections and advice. *Pediatric Clinics of North America, 13*(3), 645–650.

AWHONN (2008). *Nursing care and management of second stage of labor: Evidence-based practice guidelines* (2nd ed.). Washington, DC: Author.

AWHONN, Mattson, S., & Smith, J. E. (2010). *Core curriculum for maternal-newborn nursing* (4th ed.). Philadelphia: Saunders.

AWHONN, Simpson, K., & Creehan, P. (2007). *Perinatal nursing* (3rd ed.). Philadelphia: Lippincott Williams & Wilkins.

Bianchi, A., & Adams, E. (2009). Labor support during second stage labor for women with epidurals. *Nursing for Women's Health, 13*(1), 38–47.

Blackburn, S. (2007). *Maternal, fetal, and neonatal physiology: A clinical perspective* (3rd ed.). Philadelphia: Saunders.

Bowes, W., & Thorp, J. (2007). Clinical aspects of normal and abnormal labor. In R. Creasy & R. Resnik (Eds.), *Maternal-fetal medicine.* (6th ed.). Philadelphia: Saunders.

CDC (2010). Yellow book: CDC health information for international travel. In *Chapter 9: Planning for a healthy pregnancy while travelling.* U.S. Government.

Chermont, A. (2009). Skin-to-skin contact and/or oral 25% dextrose for procedural pain relief for term newborn infants. *Pediatrics, 124*(6), e1101.

Creasy, R., Resnik, R., Iams, J., Lockwood, C., & Moore, T. (2008). *Creasy & Resnick's maternal-fetal medicine* (6th ed.). Philadelphia: Saunders.

Feinstein, N., Sprague, A., & Trepanier, M. (2008). *Fetal heart auscultation* (2nd ed.). Washington, DC: AWHONN.

Gabbe, S., Niebyl, J., & Simpson, J. (2007). *Obstetrics: Normal and problem pregnancies* (5th ed.). New York: Churchill Livingstone.

Hacker, N., Gambone, J., & Hobel, C. (2009). *Hacker & Moore's essentials of obstetrics and gynecology* (5th ed.). Philadelphia: Saunders.

Institute of Medicine (2009). *Weight gain during pregnancy: Re-examining the guidelines.* Washington, DC: National Academy Press.

Lewis, B., Avery, M., Jennings, E., Sherwood, N., Martinson, N., & Crain, L. (2008). The effect of exercise during pregnancy on maternal outcomes: Practical implications for practice. *American Journal of Lifestyle Medicine, 2*(5), 441–445.

London, M., Ladewig, P., Ball, J., & Bindler, R. (2006). *Maternal & child nursing care* (2nd ed.). Upper Saddle River, NJ: Prentice Hall Health.

Lowdermilk, D. L., & Perry, S. E. (2007). *Maternity and women's health care* (9th ed.). St. Louis: Mosby.

MacDorman, M., & Kirmeyer, S. (2009). Fetal and perinatal mortality in the United States, 2005. *National Vital Statistics Report, 57*(8). Hyattsville, MD: National Center for Health Statistics.

Miller, D. (2010). Intrapartum fetal monitoring. *Contemporary Obstetrics/Gynecology, 55*(2), 26–41.

Murray, S. S., & McKinney, E. (2010). *Foundations of maternal-newborn and women's health nursing* (5th ed.). Philadelphia: Saunders.

Newton, P. (2004). The doula's role during labor and delivery. *RN, 67*(3), 34–38.

Oats, J., & Abraham, S. (2010). *Llewellyn-Jones fundamentals of obstetrics and gynecology* (9th ed.). St. Louis: Mosby.

Palmer, L., & Carty, E. (2006). Deciding when it's labor: The experience of women who have received antepartum care at home for preterm labor. *Journal of Obstetric, Gynecologic, and Neonatal Nursing: JOGNN/NAACOG, 35*(4), 509–515.

Patton, K., & Thibodeau, G. (2009). *Anatomy and physiology* (7th ed.). St. Louis: Mosby.

Schuman, A. (2006). When parents ask about water birth. *Contemporary Pediatrics, 23*(11), 84–90.

Vande Vusse, L. (1999). The essential forces of labor revisited: 13 P's reported in women's stories. *MCN. The American Journal of Maternal Child Nursing, 24*, 176–184.

CHAPTER 8

AWHONN, Mattson, S., & Smith, J. E. (2010). *Core curriculum for maternal-newborn nursing* (4th ed.). Philadelphia: Saunders.

Blackburn, S. (2007). *Maternal, fetal, and neonatal physiology: A clinical perspective* (3rd ed.). Philadelphia: Saunders.

Bowes, W., & Thorp, J. (2004). Clinical aspects of normal and abnormal labor. In R. Creasy, R. Resnick, & J. Iams (Eds.), *Maternal-fetal medicine.* Philadelphia: Saunders.

Bricker, L., & Lavender, T. (2002). Parenteral opiods for labor pain relief: A systematic review. *American Journal of Obstetrics and Gynecology, 186*(5), S94–S109.

Creasy, R., Resnik, R., Iams, J., Lockwood, C., & Moore, T. (2008). *Creasy & Resnick's maternal-fetal medicine* (6th ed.). Philadelphia: Saunders.

Gabbe, S., Niebyl, J., & Simpson, J. (2007). *Obstetrics: Normal and problem pregnancies* (5th ed.). New York: Churchill Livingstone.

Green, C., & Wilkinson, J. (2004). *Maternal newborn nursing care plans.* St. Louis: Mosby.

Leifer, G. (2010). *Introduction to maternity and pediatric nursing* (6th ed.). Philadelphia: Saunders.

London, M., Ladewig, P., Ball, J., & Bindler, R. (2006). *Maternal & child nursing care* (2nd ed.). Upper Saddle River, NJ: Prentice Hall Health.

Lowdermilk, D. L., & Perry, S. E. (2007). *Maternity and women's health care* (9th ed.). St. Louis: Mosby.

Murray, S. S., & McKinney, E. S. (2010). *Foundations of maternal-newborn and women's health nursing* (5th ed.). Philadelphia: Saunders.

Newton, P. (2004). The doula's role during labor and delivery. *RN, 67*(3), 34–38.

Semenic, S., Callister, L., & Feldman, P. (2004). Giving birth: The voices of Orthodox Jewish women living in Canada. *Journal of Obstetric, Gynecologic, and Neonatal Nursing: JOGNN/NAACOG, 33*(1), 80–87.

CHAPTER 9

AWHONN, Mattson, S., & Smith, J. E. (2010). *Core curriculum for maternal-newborn nursing* (4th ed.). Philadelphia: Saunders.

Blackburn, S. (2007). *Maternal, fetal, and neonatal physiology: A clinical perspective* (3rd ed.). Philadelphia: Saunders.

Brown, L., Thoyre, S., Pridham, K., & Schubert, C. (2009). The mother-infant feeding tool. *Journal of Obstetric, Gynecologic, and Neonatal Nursing: JOGNN/NAACOG, 38*(4), 491–503.

Gabbe, S., Niebyl, J., & Simpson, J. (2007). *Obstetrics: Normal and problem pregnancies* (5th ed.). New York: Churchill Livingstone.

Hockenberry, M., & Wilson, D. (2006). *Wong's nursing care of infants and children* (8th ed.). St. Louis: Mosby.

Kenner, C., & Lott, J. W. (2007). *Comprehensive neonatal care* (4th ed.). Philadelphia: Saunders.

Kiesler, J., & Ricer, R. (2003). The abnormal fontanel. *American Family Physician, 67*(12), 2547–2552.

Kliegman, R., Behrman, R., Jenson, H., & Stanton, B. (2007). *Nelson textbook of pediatrics* (18th ed.). Philadelphia: Saunders.

London, M., Ladewig, P., Ball, J., & Bindler, R. (2006). *Maternal & child nursing care* (2nd ed.). Upper Saddle River, NJ: Prentice Hall Health.

Lowdermilk, D. L., & Perry, S. E. (2007). *Maternity and women's health care* (9th ed.). St. Louis: Mosby.

Murray, S. S., & McKinney, E. (2010). *Foundations of maternal-newborn and women's health nursing* (5th ed.). Philadelphia: Saunders.

Spahis, J., & Bowers, N. (2006). Navigating the maze of newborn screening. *MCN. The American Journal of Maternal Child Nursing, 31*(3), 190–196.

CHAPTER 10

American Academy of Pediatrics (2007). *Guidelines for perinatal care* (6th ed.). Elk Grove Village, IL: Author.

American Academy of Pediatrics (2009). *AAP report on committee for infectious diseases.* Elk Grove, IL: Author.

Amy, E. (2001). Reflections on the interactive newborn bath demonstration. *MCN. The American Journal of Maternal Child Nursing, 26*(6), 320–322.

AWHONN, Mattson, S., & Smith, J. E. (2010). *Core curriculum for maternal-newborn nursing* (4th ed.). Philadelphia: Saunders.

Brady, M. (2010). Newborn circumcision: Routine or not routine, that is the question. *Archives of Pediatrics & Adolescent Medicine, 164*(1), 94–96.

Byers, J., & Thornley, K. (2004). Cueing into infant pain. *MCN. The American Journal of Maternal Child Nursing, 29*(2), 84–90.

Camile, C., Kuo, R., & Wiener, J. (2002). Caring for the uncircumcised penis: What parents (and you) should know. *Contemporary Pediatrics, 19*, 61–73.

Chermont, A. (2009). Skin-to-skin contact and/or oral 25% oral dextrose for procedural pain relief for term newborn infants. *Pediatrics, 124*(6), e1101.

Creasy, R., Resnik, R., Iams, J., Lockwood, C., & Moore, T. (2008). *Creasy & Resnik's maternal-fetal medicine* (6th ed.). Philadelphia: Saunders.

Gabbe, S., Niebyl, J., & Simpson, J. (2007). *Obstetrics: Normal and problem pregnancies* (5th ed.). New York: Churchill Livingstone.

Galligan, M. (2006). Proposed guidelines for skin-to-skin treatment of neonatal hypothermia. *MCN. The American Journal of Maternal Child Nursing, 31*(5), 298–305.

Harrison, D., Stevens, B., Bueno, M., Yamada, J., Adams-Webber, T., Beyene, J., et al. (2010). Efficacy of sweet solutions for analgesia for infants between 1 and 12 months of age: A systematic review. *Archives of Disease in Childhood, 95*(5), 20–31.

Hockenberry, M., & Wilson, D. (2006). *Wong's nursing care of infants and children* (8th ed.). St. Louis: Mosby.

Jackson, P. (2010). Diaper dermatitis. *Protecting the bottom line. Advance for Nurse Practitioners, 18*(3), 35–41.

Karl, D. J. (1999). The interactive newborn bath. *MCN. The American Journal of Maternal Child Nursing, 24*, 280–286.

Kenner, C., & Lott, J. W. (2007). *Comprehensive neonatal care* (4th ed.). Philadelphia: Saunders.

Kliegman, R., Behrman, R., Jenson, H., & Stanton, B. (2007). *Nelson textbook of pediatrics* (18th ed.). Philadelphia: Saunders.

Langan, R. (2006). Discharge procedures for healthy newborns. *American Family Physician, 73*(5), 849–852.

Leifer, G. (2010). *Introduction to maternity and pediatric nursing* (6th ed.). Philadelphia: Saunders.

Lewis, J. A. (2003). Jewish perspectives on pregnancy and childbearing. *MCN. The American Journal of Maternal Child Nursing, 28*(5), 306–312.

Li, M., Sun, G., & Neubauer, H. (2004). Change in body temperature in newborn healthy term infants over first 72 hours after birth. *Journal of Zhejiang University. Science, 5*(4), 486–493.

Lowdermilk, D. L., & Perry, S. E. (2007). *Maternity and women's health care* (9th ed.). St. Louis: Mosby.

Moyer, V. (2006). Effective guidelines for counseling parents before discharging a newborn. *American Family Physician, 75*(3), 771.

Murray, S. S., & McKinney, E. (2010). *Foundations of maternal-newborn and women's health nursing* (5th ed.). Philadelphia: Saunders.

Northam, S., & Knapp, T. (2006). The reliability and validity of birth certificates. *Journal of Obstetric, Gynecologic, and Neonatal Nursing: JOGNN/NAACOG, 35*(1), 3–11.

Simpson, K. (2006). Circumcision pain management. *MCN. The American Journal of Maternal Child Nursing, 31*(4), 276.

Spahis, J., & Bowers, N. (2006). Navigating the maze of newborn screening. *MCN. The American Journal of Maternal Child Nursing, 31*(3), 190–196.

Tobian, A. (2010). Male circumcision for the prevention of acquisition and transmission of sexually transmitted infections: The case for neonatal circumcision. *Archives of Pediatrics & Adolescent Medicine, 164*(1), 78–84.

Vural, G., & Kisa, S. (2006). Umbilical cord care: A pilot study comparing topical human milk, providone-iodine, and dry care. *Journal of Obstetric, Gynecologic, and Neonatal Nursing: JOGNN/NAACOG, 35*(1), 123–128.

CHAPTER 11

American Academy of Pediatrics. (2007). *Guidelines for perinatal care* (6th ed.). Elk Grove, IL: Authors.

Bhatia, J., & Greer, F. (2008). The use of soy protein-based formula in infant feeding. *Pediatrics, 121*(5), 1062–1068.

Blanchard, D. (2006). Omega-3 fatty acid supplementation in perinatal settings. *MCN. The American Journal of Maternal Child Nursing, 31*(4), 250–255.

Centers for Disease Control and Prevention (2005). *Breastfeeding data and statistics from 2004 national immunization survey.* Retrieved December 20, 2006, from www.cdc.gov/breastfeeding/nis_data/.

Centers for Disease Control and Prevention (2006). Recommendations on immunizations: Recommendation of advisory committee on immunization practices and the American Academy of Family Practice. *MMWR. Morbidity and Mortality Weekly Report, 55*(RR15).

Chang, K., & Spatz, D. (2006). The family and breastfeeding laws: What nurses need to know. *MCN. The American Journal of Maternal Child Nursing, 31*(4), 224–230.

Chertok, I. (2009). Reexamination of ultra-thin nipple shield use, infant growth and maternal satisfaction. *Journal of Clinical Nursing, 18*(21), 2949–2955.

Eby, A. (2009). Metabolic alkalosis after using enhanced water to dilute powdered formula. *MCN. The American Journal of Maternal Child Nursing, 34*(5), 290–294.

Gabbe, S., Niebyl, J., & Simpson, J. (2007). *Obstetrics: Normal and problem pregnancies* (5th ed.). New York: Churchill Livingstone.

Green, C., & Wilkinson, J. (2004). *Maternal newborn nursing care plans.* St. Louis: Mosby.

Huber, C., Blanco, M., & Davis, M. (2009). Expressed breast milk: Safety in the hospital. *Pediatrics, 118*(1), 110–112.

Jenik, A., Vain, N., Gorestein, A., & Jacobi, N. (2009). Does the recommendation to use a pacifier influence the prevalence of breastfeeding? *The Journal of Pediatrics, 115*(3), 350.

Kenner, C., & Lott, J. W. (2007). *Comprehensive neonatal care* (4th ed.). Philadelphia: Saunders.

Kleigman, R., Behrman, R., Jenson, H., & Stanton, B. (2007). *Nelson textbook of pediatrics* (18th ed.). Philadelphia: Saunders.

Langan, R. (2006). Discharge procedures for healthy newborns. *American Family Physician, 73*(5), 849–852.

Lawrence, R. (2010). *Breastfeeding: A guide for the medical professional* (7th ed.). Philadelphia: Saunders.

Leifer, G. (2010). *Introduction to maternity and pediatric nursing* (6th ed.). Philadelphia: Saunders.

Lowdermilk, D. L., & Perry, S. E. (2007). *Maternity and women's health care* (9th ed.). St. Louis: Mosby.

Morin, K. (2009). Preparing infant formula: Increasing caregiver knowledge. *MCN. The American Journal of Maternal Child Nursing, 34*(6), 387.

Morrow, C., Hidinger, A., & Wilkinson-Faulk, D. (2010). Reducing neonatal pain during routine heel lance procedures. *MCN. The American Journal of Maternal Child Nursing, 35*(6), 346–353.

National Conference of State Legislatures (2010). *Breastfeeding state laws*. Retrieved January 2011, from www.ncsl.org/programs/health/breast50.htm.

Ouwehand, A. (2007). Antibacterial effects of probiotics. *The Journal of Nutrition, 137*(1), 7945–7975.

Skidmore-Roth, L. (2009). *Mosby's handbook of herbs and natural supplements* (4th ed.). St. Louis: Mosby.

Wawer, M., Tobian, A., Kigozi, G., Kong, X., Gravitt, P., Serwadda, D., et al. (2011). The effect of circumcision on HIV-negative men on transmission of HPV to HIV-negative women: A randomized trial. *Lancet, 377*(9761), 209–218.

Weber, B., Derrico, D., Yoon, S., & Sherwill-Navarro, P. (2010). Educating patients to evaluate web-based health care information. *Journal of Clinical Nursing, 19*(9), 1371–1377.

Weil, V. (2010). Optimum nutrition for babies. *Advance for Nurse Practitioners, 18*(3), 22–26.

WHO (2007). *Safe preparation, storage, and handling of powdered infant formula: Guidelines*. Geneva, Switzerland: Author.

CHAPTER 12

AWOHNN, Mattson, S., & Smith, J. E. (2010). *Core curriculum for maternal-newborn nursing* (4th ed.). Philadelphia: Saunders.

Blackburn, S. (2007). *Maternal, fetal, and neonatal physiology: A clinical perspective* (3rd ed.). Philadelphia: Saunders.

Centers for Disease Control and Prevention & American Advisory Committee on Immunization Practice (2008). *Recommended immunization schedules*. Retrieved December 2010, from www.cdc.gov/vaccines/pubs/preg-guide.htm.

Chertok, I. (1999). Relief of breast engorgement for the Sabbath-observant Jewish woman. *Journal of Obstetric, Gynecologic, and Neonatal Nursing: JOGNN/NAACOG, 28*(4), 365–369.

Dodd, V., & Chalmers, C. (2003). Comparing the use of hydrogel dressings to lanolin ointment with lactating mothers. *Journal of Obstetric, Gynecologic, and Neonatal Nursing: JOGNN/NAACOG, 32*(4), 486–494.

Gabbe, S., Niebyl, J., & Simpson, J. (2007). *Obstetrics: Normal and problem pregnancies* (5th ed.). New York: Churchill Livingstone.

Kim-Godwin, Y. S. (2003). Postpartum beliefs and practices among non-Western cultures. *MCN. The American Journal of Maternal Child Nursing, 28*(2), 74–78.

Leifer, G. (2010). *Introduction to maternity and pediatric nursing* (6th ed.). Philadelphia: Saunders.

Leifer, G., & Hartston, H. (2004). *Growth and development across the lifespan: A health promotion focus*. Philadelphia: Saunders.

Lowdermilk, D. L., & Perry, S. E. (2007). *Maternity and women's health care* (9th ed.). St. Louis: Mosby.

Murray, S. S., & McKinney, E. (2010). *Foundations of maternal-newborn and women's health nursing* (5th ed.). Philadelphia: Saunders.

Oats, J., & Abraham, S. (2010). *Llewellyn-Jones fundamentals of obstetrics and gynecology* (9th ed.). St. Louis: Mosby.

Rubin, R. (1984). *Maternal identity and the maternal experience*. New York: Springer.

CHAPTER 13

American College of Obstetricians and Gynecologists (ACOG) (2001). ACOG Practice Bulletin. Clinical management guidelines for obstetrician-gynecologists. Number 30, September 2001. Gestational diabetes. *Obstetrics and Gynecology, 98*(3), 525–538.

American College of Obstetricians and Gynecologists (ACOG) (2002). ACOG Practice Bulletin. Diagnosis and management of preeclampsia and eclampsia. Number 33, January 2002. *International Journal of Gynaecology and Obstetrics, 77*(1), 67–75.

American College of Obstetricians and Gynecologists (ACOG) (2005). ACOG Practice Bulletin. Clinical management guidelines for obstetrician–gynecologists. Number 60, March 2005. Pregestational diabetes mellitus, *Obstetrics and Gynecology, 105*(3), 675–685.

American Heart Association (2006). *BLS for Health Care Providers*. Author.

AWOHNN, Mattson, S., & Smith, J. E. (2010). *Core curriculum for maternal-newborn nursing* (4th ed.). Philadelphia: Saunders.

Callaghan, W. (2010). Delivery is not the end of the story: Follow-up of women with GDM. *Contemporary Obstetrics/Gynecology, 55*(4), 40–43.

Centers for Disease Control and Prevention (2009). National Center for Health Statistics: Final data for 2006. *National Vital Statistic Report, 57*(14).

Cono, J., Cragan, J., Jamieson, D., & Rasmussen, S. (2006). Prophylaxis and treatment of pregnant women for emerging infections and bioterrorism emergencies. *Emerging Infectious Diseases, 12*(11), 1631–1636.

Creasy, R., Resnik, R., Iams, J., Lockwood, C., & Moore, T. (2008). *Creasy & Resnik's maternal-fetal medicine* (6th ed.). Philadelphia: Saunders.

Criddle, L. (2009). Trauma in pregnancy. *American Journal of Nursing, 109*(11), 41–47.

Crider, K., Cleves, M., Reefhuis, J., Berry, R., Hobbs, C., & Hu, D. (2009). Antibacterial medication use during pregnancy and risk of birth defects. *Archives of Pediatrics & Adolescent Medicine, 163*(11), 978–985.

Dugan-Kim, M., Connell, S., Stitka, C., Wong, C., & Gossett, D. (2009). Epistaxis of pregnancy and association with postpartum hemorrhage. *Obstetrics and Gynecology, 114*(6), 1322–1325.

Emad, A., & Gardner, M. (2007). CPR in pregnancy. *Obstetrics and Gynecology Clinics of North America, 34*(3), 585–597.

Gabbe, S., Niebyl, J., & Simpson, J. (2007). *Obstetrics: Normal and problem pregnancies* (5th ed.). New York: Churchill Livingstone.

Goldstein, G., Baron, E., & Berkowitz, R. (2010). Managing molar pregnancy. *Contemporary Obstetrics/Gynecology, 55*(4), 48–51.

James, A., Kouides, P., Abdul-Kadir, R., Edlund, M., Federici, A., Halimeh, S., et al. (2009). Von Willebrand disease and other bleeding disorders in women. *American Journal of Obstetrics and Gynecology, 201*(1), 12.

Keough, V. (2009). Emergency care of the pregnant patient. *Journal of Obstetric, Gynecologic, and Neonatal Nursing: JOGNN/NAACOG, 38*(6), 703.

Kuo, C., Jamieson, D., McPheeters, M., Meikle, S., & Posner, S. (2007). Injury hospitalizations of pregnant women in the United States, 2002. *American Journal of Obstetrics and Gynecology, 196*(2), 161.

London, M., Ladewig, P., Ball, J., & Bindler, R. (2006). *Maternal & child nursing care* (2nd ed.). Upper Saddle River, NJ: Prentice Hall Health.

Lowdermilk, D. L., & Perry, S. E. (2007). *Maternity and women's health care* (9th ed.). St. Louis: Mosby.

Lykke, J., Dideriksen, K., Lidegaard, O., & Langhoff-Roos, J. (2009). First-trimester vaginal bleeding and complications later in pregnancy. *Obstetrics and Gynecology, 115*(5), 935.

Major, C. (2010). Using oral hypoglycemics in pregnancy to manage type 2 and gestational diabetes. *Contemporary Obstetrics/Gynecology, 55*(4), 34.

Maughan, K., Heim, S., & Galazka, S. (2006). Preventing postpartum hemorrhage. *American Family Physician, 73*(6), 1025–1028.

McQuillan, K. (2009). *Trauma nursing: From resuscitation through rehabilitation* (4th ed.). Philadelphia: Saunders.

Meroz, Y., Elchalal, U., & Ginsonar, U. (2007). Initial trauma management in advanced pregnancy. *Anesthesiology Clinics, 25*(1), 117–129.

Moise, K., Jr., (2004). RH disease: It's still a threat. *Contemporary Obstetrics/Gynecology, 49*(5), 34–38.

Oats, J., & Abraham, S. (2010). *Llewellyn-Jones fundamentals of obstetrics and gynecology* (9th ed.). St. Louis: Mosby.

Oepkes, D., Seaward, P., & Vandenbussche, F. (2006). Doppler ultrasonography vs. amniocentesis to predict fetal anemia. *The New England Journal of Medicine, 355*(2), 156–164.

Pasternak, B., & Hviid, A. (2010). Use of proton-pump inhibitors in early pregnancy and risk of birth defects. *The New England Journal of Medicine, 363*(22), 2114–2123.

Perry, S., Hockenberry, M., Lowdermilk, D., & Wilson, D. (2009). *Maternal-child nursing* (4th ed.). St. Louis: Mosby.

Ruffolo, D. (2009). Trauma care and managing the injured pregnant patient. *Journal of Obstetric, Gynecologic, and Neonatal Nursing: JOGNN/NAACOG, 38*(6), 704–709.

Tan, P., Khine, P., Vallikkannu, N., & Omar, S. (2010). Promethazine compared with metoclopramide for hyperemesis gravidarum: A randomized control trial. *Journal of Obstetrics and Gynaecology (Tokyo, Japan), 115*(5), 975–981.

Villar, J., Merialdi, M., Gulmezoglu, A., Abalos, E., Carrol, G., Kulier, R., et al. (2003). Nutritional interventions during pregnancy for the prevention or treatment of maternal morbidity and preterm delivery: An overview of randomized controlled trials. *The Journal of Nutrition, 133*(5 Suppl 2), 1606S–1625S.

Williams, J., Lyss, S., & Cragan, J. (2003). Your pregnant or lactating patient has been exposed to anthrax: Now what? *Contemporary Obstetrics/Gynecology, 48*(9), 84–90.

CHAPTER 14

American College of Obstetricians and Gynecologists (ACOG) (2003). ACOG Committee Opinion. Use of progesterone to reduce preterm birth. *Obstetrics and Gynecology, 102*(5 Pt 1), 1115–1116.

American College of Obstetricians and Gynecologists (ACOG) (2003). ACOG practice bulletin. Management of preterm labor. Number 43, May 2003. *International Journal of Gynaecology and Obstetrics, 82*(1), 127–135.

American College of Obstetricians and Gynecologists (ACOG) (2003). ACOG Practice Bulletin Number 49, December 2003: Dystocia and augmentation of labor. *Obstetrics and Gynecology, 102*(6), 1445–1454.

American College of Obstetricians and Gynecologists (ACOG) (2006). *Induction of labor with misoprostol.* Committee opinion, #228. Washington, DC: Author.

American College of Obstetricians and Gynecologists (ACOG) (2007). *Guidelines for perinatal care.* Elk Grove Village, IL: Author.

American College of Obstetricians and Gynecologists (ACOG) (2010). ACOG Practice bulletin no. 115: Vaginal birth after previous cesarean delivery. *Obstetrics and Gynecology, 116* (2), 450–463.

AWOHNN, Mattson, S., & Smith, J. E. (2010). *Core curriculum for maternal-newborn nursing* (4th ed.). Philadelphia: Saunders.

Barclay, L. (2010). ACOG issues less restrictive guidelines for vaginal birth after cesarean section. *Journal of Obstetrics and Gynaecology (Tokyo, Japan), 116*, 450–463.

FDA (2011). US Department of Health and Human Services: FDA drug safety communication. In *New warnings against use of terbutaline to treat preterm labor.* Safety Labeling Change Information Press Release, February 17, 2011.

Gabbe, S., Niebyl, J., & Simpson, J. (2007). *Obstetrics: Normal and problem pregnancies* (5th ed.). New York: Churchill Livingstone.

Hacker, N., Gambone, J., & Hobel, C. (2009). *Hacker & Moore's essentials of obstetrics and gynecology* (5th ed.). Philadelphia: Saunders.

Iams, J., Romero, R., & Creasy, R. (2009). Preterm labor and birth. In Creasy & Resnik (Eds.), *Maternal-fetal medicine: Principles and practice.* (6th ed.). Philadelphia: Saunders.

Kamath, B., Todd, J., Glazner, J., Lezotte, D., & Lynch, A. (2009). Neonatal outcomes after elective cesarean section. *Journal of Obstetrics and Gynaecology (Tokyo, Japan), 113*(6), 1231.

London, M., Ladewig, P., Ball, J., & Bindler, R. (2006). *Maternal & child nursing care* (2nd ed.). Upper Saddle River, NJ: Prentice Hall Health.

Lowdermilk, D. L., & Perry, S. E. (2007). *Maternity and women's health care* (9th ed.). St. Louis: Mosby.

Menacker, F., & Hamilton, B. (2010). *Recent trends in cesarean section deliveries in the United States.* NCHS data brief, March 2010. Retrieved July 2010, from www.cdc.gov/nchs/databriefs/db35.pdf.

Murray, S. S., & McKinney, E. S. (2010). *Foundations of maternal-newborn and women's health nursing* (5th ed.). Philadelphia: Saunders.

Neri, I., Airola, G., Contu, G., Allais, G., Facchinetti, F., & Benedetto, C. (2004). Acupuncture plus moxibustion to resolve breech presentation: A randomized controlled study. *The Journal of Maternal-Fetal & Neonatal Medicine, 15*(4), 247–252.

NIH (2006). NIH State-of-the-Science Conference Statement on cesarean delivery on maternal request. *NIH Consensus and State-of-the-Science Statements, 23*(1), 1–29.

Tournaire, M., & Theau-Yonneau, A. (2007). Complementary and alternative approaches to pain relief during labor. *Evidence-Based Complementary and Alternative Medicine, 4*(4), 409–417.

US Department of Health and Human Services (2010). *Healthy People 2020 National Health Promotion and Disease Prevention Objectives.* Washington, DC: US Government Printing Office.

Werner, E., Han, C., & Pettker, C. (2010). *Universal cervical length screening to prevent preterm birth: A cost-effective analysis.* Presented at the Society for Maternal-Fetal Medicine, 30th annual meeting, Chicago, February 1, 2010. Retrieved June 10, 2010, from http://opa.yale.edu/news/article.aspx?id=7262.

CHAPTER 15

AWOHNN, Mattson, S., & Smith, J. E. (2010). *Core curriculum for maternal-newborn nursing* (4th ed.). Philadelphia: Saunders.

Blackburn, S. (2007). *Maternal, fetal, and neonatal physiology* (3rd ed.). Philadelphia: Saunders.

Centers for Disease Control and Prevention (2010). Births: Preliminary data for 2008. *National Vital Statistics Reports, 58*(16), 1–17.

Creasy, R., Resnik, R., Iams, J., Lockwood, C., & Moore, T. (2008). *Creasy & Resnick's maternal-fetal medicine* (6th ed.). Philadelphia: Saunders.

Davidoff, M., Dias, T., Damus, K., Russell, R., Bettegowda, V., Dolan, S., et al. (2006). Changes in the gestational age distribution among U.S. singleton births: Impact on rates of late preterm births 1992 to 2002. *Perinatology, 30*(1), 8–15.

Engle, W. (2006). Recommendations for definition of "late preterm" (near term) and birth weight-gestational age classification system. *Perinatology, 30*(1), 2–7.

Engle, W., Tomashek, K., & Wallman, C. (2007). "Late preterm" infants: A population at risk. *Pediatrics, 120*(6), 1390–1398.

Gabbe, S., Niebyl, J., & Simpson, J. (2007). *Obstetrics: Normal and problem pregnancies* (5th ed.). New York: Churchill Livingstone.

Giarratano, G. (2006). Genetic influences on preterm birth. *MCN. The American Journal of Maternal Child Nursing, 31*(3), 169–175.

Hacker, N., Gambone, J., & Hobel, C. (2009). *Hacker & Moore's essentials of obstetrics and gynecology* (5th ed.). Philadelphia: Saunders.

Huber, C., Blanco, M., & Davis, M. (2009). Expressed breast milk: Safety in the hospital. *American Journal of Nursing, 109*(2), 54–55.

Kenner, C., & Lott, J. W. (2007). *Comprehensive neonatal care* (4th ed.). Philadelphia: Saunders.

Kenner, C., & McGrath, J. (2004). *Developmental care of the newborn and infant.* St. Louis: Mosby.

Kliegman, R., Behrman, R., Jenson, H., & Stanton, B. (2007). *Nelson textbook of pediatrics* (18th ed.). Philadelphia: Saunders.

Lasky, R., & Von Drongelen, W. (2010). Is sucrose as an effective analgesic for newborn babies? *Lancet, 376*, 1201.

Lee, K. (2008). Identifying the high risk newborn and evaluating gestational age, prematurity, postmaturity, LGA, and SGA infants. In J. Cloherty, E. Eichenwald, & A. Stark (Eds.), *Manual of neonatal care.* (6th ed.). Philadelphia: Lippincott Williams & Wilkins.

Leifer, G. (2010). *Introduction to maternity and pediatric nursing* (6th ed.). Philadelphia: Saunders.

London, M., Ladewig, P., Ball, J., & Bindler, R. (2006). *Maternal & child nursing care* (2nd ed.). Upper Saddle River, NJ: Prentice Hall Health.

Lowdermilk, D. L., & Perry, S. E. (2007). *Maternity and women's health care* (9th ed.). St. Louis: Mosby.

McIntire, D., & Leveno, K. (2008). Neonatal mortality and morbidity rates in late preterm births compared with births at term. *Obstetrics and Gynecology, 111*(1), 35–41.

Murray, S. S., & McKinney, E. (2010). *Foundations of maternal-newborn and women's health nursing* (5th ed.). Philadelphia: Saunders.

National Center for Health Statistics (NCHS) (2010). *Final mortality data prepared by March of Dimes.* Perinatal Data Center.

Resnik, J., & Resnik, R. (2009). Postterm pregnancy. In Creasy & Resnik (Eds.), *Maternal fetal medicine.* (6th ed.). St. Louis: Mosby.

Saniski, D. (2005). Neonatal pain relief protocols in their infancy. *Nebraska Nurse, 38*(2), 24.

Slater, R., Cornelissen, L., Fabrisi, L., Patten, D., Yoxen, J., Worley, A., et al. (2010). Oral sucrose as an analgesic drug for procedural pain in newborn infants: A randomized controlled trial. *Lancet, 376*, 1225.

Urso, A. (2007). The reality of neonatal pain and resulting effects. *Journal of Neonatal Nursing, 13*(6), 236–238.

Vohr, B., Poindexter, B., Dusick, A., McKinley, L., Wright, L., Langer, J., et al. (2006). Beneficial effects of breast milk in the neonatal intensive care unit on the developmental outcome of extremely low birth weight infants at 18 months of age. *Pediatrics, 118*(1), 115–123.

CHAPTER 16

American Academy of Pediatrics, Subcommittee on Hyperbilirubinemia (2004). Clinical practice guidelines: Management of hyperbilirubinemia in the newborn infant of 35 weeks' gestation. *Pediatrics, 114*, 297–316. www.aap.org/jaundiceguidelines.

AWOHNN, Mattson, S., & Smith, J. E. (2010). *Core curriculum for maternal-newborn nursing* (4th ed.). Philadelphia: Saunders.

Bauchner, H. (2010). Universal predischarge bilirubin screening. *Pediatrics, 124*, 1031.

Bhutani, V., Johnson, L., Schwoebel, A., & Gennaro, S. (2006). A systems approach for neonatal hyperbilirubinemia in term and near-term newborns. *Journal of Obstetric, Gynecologic, and Neonatal Nursing: JOGNN/NAACOG, 35*(4), 444–455.

Cicero, S., Avgidou, K., Rembouskos, G., Kagan, K., & Nicolaides, K. (2006). Nasal bone in first trimester screening for trisomy 21. *American Journal of Obstetrics and Gynecology, 195*(1), 109–114.

Creasy, R., Resnik, R., Iams, J., Lockwood, C., & Moore, T. (2008). *Creasy & Resnick's maternal-fetal medicine* (6th ed.). Philadelphia: Saunders.

Gabbe, S., Niebyl, J., & Simpson, J. (2007). *Obstetrics: Normal and problem pregnancies* (5th ed.). New York: Churchill Livingston.

Hacker, N., Gambone, J., & Hobel, C. (2009). *Hacker & Moore's essentials of obstetrics and gynecology* (5th ed.). Philadelphia: Saunders.

Kenner, C., & Lott, J. W. (2007). *Comprehensive neonatal care* (4th ed.). Philadelphia: Saunders.

Kliegman, R., Behrman, R., Jenson, H., & Stanton, B. (2007). *Nelson textbook of pediatrics* (18th ed.). Philadelphia: Saunders.

Leifer, G. (2010). *Introduction to maternity and pediatric nursing* (6th ed.). Philadelphia: Saunders.

London, M., Ladewig, P., Ball, J., & Bindler, R. (2006). *Maternal & child nursing care* (2nd ed.). Upper Saddle River, NJ: Prentice Hall Health.

Lowdermilk, D. L., Perry, S. E., & Bobak, I. M. (2007). *Maternity nursing* (6th ed.). St. Louis: Mosby.

Mah, M., Clark, S., Akhigbe, E., Englebright, J., Frye, D., Meyers, J., et al. (2010). Reduction of severe hyperbilirubinemia after institution of predischarge bilirubin screening. *Pediatrics, 125*(5), 1143.

Maisels, J. (2006). Jaundice in the newborn. *Contemporary Pediatrics, 22*(5), 34–40.

March of Dimes, (2007). *Prematurity campaign.* Retrieved December 8, 2010, from www.marchofdimes.com/prematurity/prematurity.asp.

Moise, K., Jr., (2004). RH disease: It's still a threat. *Contemporary Obstetrics/Gynecology, 49*(5), 34–38.

National Collaborating Center for Women's and Children's Health (2010). *Neonatal jaundice: Clinical guidelines.* Retrieved August 20, 2010, from www.nice.org.uk/nicemedia/live/12986/48678/48678.pdf.

National Institute of Health and Clinical Excellence (NICE) (2010). *Neonatal jaundice: Clinical guidelines.* Retrieved July 2010, from www.nice.org.uk/nicemedia/live/129861 48678/48678.pdf.

Palma-Sisto, P. (2004). Endocrine disorders in the neonate. *Pediatric Clinics of North America, 51*(4), 1141–1168.

Rennie, J. (2010). Neonatal jaundice: Summary of NICE guidance. *BMJ (Clinical Research ed.), 340*, c2409. Retrieved August 20, 2010, from http://dx.doi.org/10.1136/bmj.c2409.

Tarini, B., & Freed, G. (2007). Keeping up with the newborn screening revolution. *Contemporary Pediatrics, 24*(4), 36–49.

Trahms, C. (2008). *Cristine M. Trahms Program for Phenylketonuria,* Seattle. Retrieved May 20, 2011, from http://depts.washington.edu/pku/.

CHAPTER 17

American College of Obstetricians and Gynecologists (ACOG) (2006). ACOG Practice Bulletin: Clinical Management Guidelines for Obstetrician–Gynecologists, Number 76, October 2006: Postpartum hemorrhage. *Obstetrics and Gynecology, 108*(4), 1039–1047.

American College of Obstetricians and Gynecologists (ACOG) (2009). ACOG Committee Opinion No. #435: postpartum screening for abnormal glucose tolerance in women who had gestational diabetes mellitus. *Obstetrics and Gynecology, 113*(6), 1419–1421.

AWHONN, Mattson, S., & Smith, J. E. (2010). *Core curriculum for maternal-newborn nursing* (4th ed.). Philadelphia: Saunders.

Beck, C. (2008). *Postpartum mood and anxiety disorders. Case studies, research and nursing care.* Washington, DC: AWHONN.

Beck, C. (2008). State of science on postpartum depression: what nurses and research have contributed - Part 2. *MCN. The American Journal of Maternal Child Nursing, 33*(3), 151–156.

Callaghan, W. (2010). Delivery is not the end of the story: Follow-up of women with GDM. *Contemporary Obstetrics/Gynecology, 55*(4), 40–43.

Callister, L., Beckstrand, R., & Corbett, C. (2010). Postpartum depression and culture. *MCN. The American Journal of Maternal Child Nursing, 35*(5), 254–260.

Creasy, R., Resnik, R., Iams, J., Lockwood, C., & Moore, T. (2008). *Creasy & Resnick's maternal-fetal medicine* (6th ed.). Philadelphia: Saunders.

Douglas, M., Pierce, J., Rosenkoetter, M., Callister, L., Hattar-Pollara, M., Lauderdale, J., Miller, J., Milstead, J., Nardi, D. A., & Pacquiao, D. (2009). Standards of practice for culturally competent nursing care. *Journal of Transcultural Nursing, 203*(3), 257–269.

Driscoll, J. (2008). Psychosocial adaptation to pregnancy and postpartum. In K. Simpson, & P. Creehan (Eds.), *Perinatal Nursing, AWHONN.* (3rd ed.). Philadelphia: Lippincott Williams & Wilkins.

Dugan-Kim, M., Connell, S., Stika, C., Wong, C., & Gossett, D. (2009). Epistaxis of pregnancy and association with postpartum hemorrhage. *Journal of Obstetrics and Gynaecology (Tokyo, Japan), 114*(6), 1322–1325.

Gabbe, S., Niebyl, J., & Simpson, J. (2007). *Obstetrics: Normal and problem pregnancies* (5th ed.). New York: Churchill Livingstone.

Hacker, N., Gambone, J., & Hobel, C. (2009). *Hacker & Moore's essentials of obstetrics and gynecology* (5th ed.). Philadelphia: Saunders.

Karrie, F. (2006). Managing uterine atony and hemorrhagic shock. *MCN. The American Journal of Maternal Child Nursing, 51*(2), 52–55.

Katz, A. (2010). Sexually speaking: Sexual changes during and after pregnancy. *American Journal of Nursing, 110*(8), 50–52.

Kim, M., Hayashi, R., & Gambone, J. (2009). Obstetric hemorrhage and puerperal sepsis. In *Hacker & Moore's essentials of obstetrics and gynecology.* (5th ed.). Philadelphia: Saunders.

London, M., Ladewig, P., Ball, J., & Bindler, R. (2006). *Maternal & child nursing care* (2nd ed.). Upper Saddle River, NJ: Prentice Hall Health.

Lowdermilk, D. L., & Perry, S. E. (2007). *Maternity and women's health care* (9th ed.). St. Louis: Mosby.

Murray, S. S., & McKinney, E. (2010). *Foundations of maternal-newborn and women's health nursing* (5th ed.). Philadelphia: Saunders.

Oats, J., & Abraham, S. (2005). *Llewellyn-Jones fundamentals of obstetrics and gynecology,* (9th ed.). St. Louis: Mosby.

Pauleta, J., Pereira, N., & Graça, L. (2010). Sexuality during pregnancy. *The Journal of Sexual Medicine, 1*(Pt 1), 142–144.

Simpson, K. R. (2010). Postpartum hemorrhage. *MCN. The American Journal of Maternal Child Nursing, 35*(2), 124.

Simpson, K. R. (2006). Venous thromboembolism during pregnancy and postpartum: An inherited risk. *MCN. The American Journal of Maternal Child Nursing, 31*(3), 208.

WHO (2009). *WHO guidelines for management of postpartum hemorrhage and retained placenta.* Geneva, Switzerland: Author.

CHAPTER 18

Anderson, S., Schoechter, J., & Brassco, J. (2006). Adolescents, patients, and their confidentiality: Staying within legal bounds. *Contemporary Obstetrics/Gynecology, 51*(5), 53–64.

Cavazos-Rehg, P., Krauss, M., Spitznagel, E., Schootman, M., Bucholz, K., Peipert, J., et al. (2009). Age of sexual debut among U.S. adolescents. *Contraception, 80*(2), 158.

Centers for Disease Control and Prevention (2006). *MMWR. Morbidity and Mortality Weekly Report, 55*(No SS-5).

Centers for Disease Control and Prevention (2006). *Recent trends in teenage pregnancy in the United States, 1990–2002.* Retrieved December 2010, from www.cdc.gov/nchs/products/pubs/pubd/hestats/teenpreg1990-2002/teenpreg1990-2002.htm.

Epstein, J. (2006). Does abstinence-only education put adolescents at risk? *MCN. The American Journal of Maternal Child Nursing, 31*(6), 348.

Gabbe, S., Niebyl, J., & Simpson, J. (2007). *Obstetrics: Normal and problem pregnancies* (5th ed.). New York: Churchill Livingstone.

Glasier, A., Cameron, S., Fine, P., Logan, S., Casale, W., Van Horn, J., et al. (2010). Ulipristal acetate versus levonorgestrel for emergency contraception: A randomized trial. *Lancet, 375,* 555–562.

Guttmacher Institute (2006). *U.S. teen pregnancy statistics: National and state trends by race and ethnicity.* New York: Guttmacher Institute.

Hamilton, B., Martin, J., & Ventura, S. (2006). Preliminary data for 2005: Health e-stats, released November 21, 2006.

Jemmott, J. B. III, Jemmott, L., & Fong, G. (2010). Efficacy of theory-based abstinence-only intervention over 24 months: A randomized controlled trial with young adolescents. *Archives of Pediatrics & Adolescent Medicine, 164*(2), 152.

Kliegman, R., Behrman, R., Jenson, H., & Stanton, B. (2007). *Nelson textbook of pediatrics* (18th ed.). Philadelphia: Saunders.

Leifer, G., & Hartston, H. (2004). *Growth and development across the lifespan: A health promotion focus.* Philadelphia: Saunders.

March of Dimes Birth Defect Foundation (2007). *Teen pregnancy.* Retrieved May 2010, from www.modimes.com.

Nelson, L. (2010). The menstrual cycle: A vital sign of bone health. *Contemporary Pediatrics, 27*(5), 52–55.

Oski, J. (2010). Then and now: Counseling adolescents in contraceptive choices. *Contemporary Pediatrics, 26*(7), 28–30.

Robbins, C., & Shew, M. (2010). Urinary tract infections in adolescents. *Contemporary Pediatrics, 26*(7), 31–35.

Sadler, L., Dynes, M., Daley, A., Ickovics, J., Leventhal, J., & Reynolds, H. (2004). Use of home pregnancy tests among adolescent women. *MCN. The American Journal of Maternal Child Nursing, 29*(1), 50–55.

Ventura, S., Abma, J., Mosher, W., & Henshaw, S. (2008). Estimated pregnancy rate outcomes for US, 1990–2004. *National Vital Statistics Report, 56*(15), Table 2.

WHO (2001). *54th WHO Assembly. Global strategy for infant and young child feeding: The optimal duration of exclusive breastfeeding.* Geneva: WHO. A54/inf.doc/4 Paragraph 10 Professional Agenda Item #13.1.

CHAPTER 19

American College of Obstetrics and Gynecology (ACOG) (2007). ACOG releases guidelines on hormonal contraceptives in women with coexisting medical conditions. *American Family Physician, 75*(8), 1252–1258.

American College of Obstetrics and Gynecology (ACOG) (2010). ACOG Practice Bulletin No. 112: Emergency contraception. *Obstetrics and Gynecology, 115*(5), 1100–1109.

American College of Obstetrics and Gynecology (ACOG) (2010). ACOG Practice Bulletin No. 110: Noncontraceptive uses of hormonal contraceptives. *Obstetrics and Gynecology, 115*(1), 206–218.

ASRM (2008). Definition of infertility and recurrent pregnancy loss. *Fertility and Sterility, 90*(Suppl. 3), S60.

Association of Reproductive Health Professionals (2007). *Choosing a birth control method.* Retrieved February 2011, *from* www.arhp.org/patienteducation/interactivetools/choosing/index.cfm?id=275.

AWHONN, Mattson, S., & Smith, J. E. (2010). *Core curriculum for maternal-newborn nursing* (4th ed.). Philadelphia: Saunders.

AWHONN, Simpson, K., & Creehan, P. (2007). *Perinatal nursing* (3rd ed.). Philadelphia: Lippincott Williams & Wilkins.

Bennington, L. (2010). Can complementary/alternative medicine be used to treat infertility? *MCN. The American Journal of Maternal Child Nursing, 35*(3), 140–143.

Centers for Disease Control and Prevention (2010). U.S. medical eligibility criteria for contraceptive use. Adapted from the *WHO medical eligibility criteria for contraceptive use* (4th ed.). *MMWR. Morbidity and Mortality Weekly Report, 18* (59), RR–4:1.

Dassow, P., & Bennet, J. (2006). Vasectomy: An update. *American Family Physician, 74*(12), 2069–2074.

DeFleurian, G., Perrin, J., Ecochard, R., Dantony, E., Lanteaume, A., Achard, V., et al. (2009). Occupational exposures obtained by questionnaire in clinical practice and their association with semen quality. *Journal of Andrology, 30*(9), 566.

Fantasia, H. (2010). Options for intrauterine contraception. *Journal of Obstetric, Gynecologic, and Neonatal Nursing: JOGNN/NAACOG, 37*(3), 375–380.

Ficorelli, C., & Weeks, B. (2007). Untangling the complexities of male infertility. *Nursing, 37*(1), 24–26.

Fontenot, H., & Harris, A. (2008). The latest advances in hormonal contraception. *Journal of Obstetric, Gynecologic, and Neonatal Nursing: JOGNN/NAACOG, 37*(3), 369–374.

Gabbe, S., Niebyl, J., & Simpson, J. (2007). *Obstetrics: Normal and problem pregnancies* (5th ed.). New York: Churchill Livingstone.

Glasier, A., Cameron, S., Fine, P., Logan, S., Casale, W., Van Horn, J., et al. (2010). Ulipristal acetate versus levonorgestrel for emergency contraception: A randomized trial. *Lancet, 375*, 555–562.

Hacker, N., Gambone, J., & Hobel, C. (2009). *Hacker & Moore's essentials of obstetrics and gynecology* (5th ed.). Philadelphia: Saunders.

Hatcher, R., Trussell, J., & Nelson, A. (2008). *Contraceptive technology* (19th ed.). New York: Ardent Media.

Johnson, B. (2006). Insertion and removal of intrauterine devices. *American Family Physician, 71*(1), 95–102.

Lowdermilk, D. L., & Perry, S. E. (2007). *Maternity and women's health care* (9th ed.). St. Louis: Mosby.

Morin, K. (2010). Nutrition and infertility. *MCN. The American Journal of Maternal Child Nursing, 35*(3), 172–173.

Murray, S. S., & McKinney, E. S. (2010). *Foundations of maternal-newborn and women's health nursing* (5th ed.). Philadelphia: Saunders.

NIH, National Center for CAM, NIH NCCAM (2009c). *What is CAM?* Retrieved November 9, 2010, from http://nccam.nih.gov/health/whatiscam/overview.htm.

Noe, G., Croxatto, H., Salvatierra, A., Reyes, V., Villarroel, C., Muñoz, C., Morales, G., & Retamales, A. (2009). Contraceptive efficacy of emergency contraception with levonorgestrel given before or after ovulation. *Contraception, 81*(5), 414.

Oats, J. K., & Abraham, S. (2010). *Llewellyn-Jones fundamentals of obstetrics and gynecology* (9th ed.). St. Louis: Mosby.

Oski, J. (2010). Then and now: Counseling adolescents in contraceptive choices. *Contemporary Pediatrics, 26*(7), 28–30.

Scoccia, B. (2006). Leveling with patients about the risks of ART. *Contemporary Obstetrics/Gynecology, 51*(11), 90–96.

Simon, H. (2006). An update on hysteroscopic tubal sterilization. *Contemporary Obstetrics/Gynecology, 51*(8), 43–48.

Torske, B. (2010). A fresh look at natural family planning. *Advance for Nurse Practitioners, 18*(4), 35.

U.S. Department of Health and Human Services (2010). *OASH Press Office: HHS announces the nation's new health promotion and disease prevention agenda: Healthy People 2020.* Retrieved January 10, 2011, from www.hp.gov/2020/about/default pressrelease.pdf.

White, A. (2003). A review of control trials of acupuncture for women's reproductive health care. *The Journal of Family Planning and Reproductive Health Care, 29*(4), 233–236.

WHO (2001). *54th WHO Assembly. Global strategy for infant and young child feeding: The optimal duration of exclusive breast feeding.* Geneva: WHO. A54/inf.doc/4 Paragraph 10 Professional Agenda Item #13.1.

Yranski, P., & Gamache, M. (2008). New options for barrier contraception. *Journal of Obstetric, Gynecologic, and Neonatal Nursing: JOGNN/NAACOG, 37*(3), 384–386.

CHAPTER 20

American Cancer Society (2009). *Cervical cancer: Prevention and early detection.* www.cancer.org/docroot/cri/content/cri_2_6x_ cervical_cancer_prevention_and_early_detection_8.asp?sitearia=ped.

American College of Obstetrics and Gynecology (ACOG) (2009). ACOG Practice Bulletin No. 109: Cervical cytology screening. *Obstetrics and Gynecology, 114*(6), 1409–1420.

American Psychiatric Association (2000). *Diagnostic and statistical manual of mental disorders* (4th ed.). Washington, DC: Author.

Ayers, D., & Montgomery, M. (2009). Putting a stop to dysfunctional uterine bleeding. *Nursing, 39*(1), 45.

Blackwell, J., & Burns, R. (2010). Nutrition and breast cancer. *Advance for Nurse Practitioners, 16*(10), 55–57.

Bonnick, S. (2010). Position statement: Management of osteoporosis in postmenopausal women: 2010 Position statement of the National Menopause Society. *Menopause (New York, N. Y.), 17*(1), 25.

Buzek, N. (2009). Breast tomosynthesis. *Advance for Nurse Practitioners, 17*(10), 25.

Ceballos, S. (2009). HPV vaccination for adolescents. *Advance for Nurse Practitioners, 17*(11), 31–33.

Cedars, M., & Evans, M. (2008). Menopause. In R. Gibbs, B. Karlan, A. Q. Haney, & I. Nygaard (Eds.), *Danforth's obstetrics and gynecology* (10th ed., pp. 725–741). Philadelphia: Lippincott Williams & Wilkins.

Centers for Disease Control and Prevention (CDC) (2006). Update to CDC's sexually transmitted diseases treatment guidelines, 2006: Fluoroquinolones no longer recommended for treatment of gonococcal infections. *MMWR. Morbidity and Mortality Weekly Report, 56*(14), 332–336.

Chiarelli, A., Majpruz, V., Brown, P., Thériault, M., Shumak, R., & Mai, V. (2009). The contribution of clinical breast examination to accuracy of breast screening. *Journal of the National Cancer Institute, 101*(18), 1236.

Cottrell, B. (2010). An updated review of evidence to discourage douching. *MCN. The American Journal of Maternal Child Nursing, 35*(2), 102–107.

Creasy, R., Resnik, R., Iams, J., Lockwood, C., & Moore, T. (2008). *Creasy & Resnick's maternal-fetal medicine* (6th ed.). Philadelphia: Saunders.

Elmore, G., & Li, A. (2010). Statins and cancer: What we know and what we don't. *Contemporary Obstetrics/Gynecology, 55*(1), 24–32.

Flowers, J. (2008). Uterine fibroids: Presentation, diagnosis, and treatment. *Advance for Nurse Practitioners, 16*(10), 36–38.

Freeman, S. (2010). Stuck in between: A closer look at perimenopause. *Advance for Nurse Practitioners, 16*(10), 43–45.

Hatcher, R. A., Trussell, J., & Nelson, A. (2008). *Contraceptive technology* (19th ed.). New York: Ardent Media.

Holmes, M., Chen, Y., Li, L., Hertzmark, E., Spiegelman, D., & Hankinson, S. (2010). Aspirin intake and survival after breast cancer. *Journal of Clinical Oncology, 28*(9), 1467–1472.

Katipamula, R., Degnim, A., Hoskin, T., Boughey, J., Loprinzi, C., Grant, C., et al. (2009). Trends in mastectomy rates at Mayo Clinic, Rochester: Effect of surgical year and preoperative magnetic resonance imaging. *Journal of Clinical Oncology, 27*(25), 4082.

Klisz, C., & Kaplan, N. (2009). HPV prevention update. *Advance for Nurse Practitioners, 17*(11), 28–29.

Leifer, G., & Hartston, H. (2004). *Growth and development across the lifespan: A health promotion perspective.* Philadelphia: Saunders.

Lowdermilk, D. L., & Perry, S. E. (2007). *Maternity and women's health care* (9th ed.). St. Louis: Mosby.

Morris, L. (2010). Targeting the red-hot danger of inflammatory breast cancer. *Nursing, 40*(9), 58–63.

Morrow, M., & Harris, J. (2009). More mastectomies: Is this what patients really want? *Journal of Clinical Oncology, 27*(25), 4038.

NAMS (2008). *North American Medical Society hormone treatment position statement.* Retrieved December 5, 2009, from www.menopause.org/aboutmeno/consensus.aspx.

NAMS (2010). Estrogen and progesterone use in postmenopausal women: Position statement of the National Menopause Society. *Menopause (New York, N Y), 17*, 242.

Patel, D., & Pearlman, M. (2006). Point of care diagnosis of STIs in women. *Contemporary Obstetrics/Gynecology, 51*(11), 69–74.

Saraiya, M. (2010). Cervical cancer screening with both HPV and Pap testing vs. Pap testing alone: What screening intervals are physicians recommending? *Archives of International Medicine, 170*(11), 977.

Sheffler, S. (2010). Uterine cancer. *Nursing, 40*(1), 31–34.

USFDA (2010). FDA approves Lysteda to treat heavy menstrual bleeding. *Contemporary Obstetrics/Gynecology, 54*(12), 12.

Weaver, C. (2009). Caring for a patient after mastectomy. *Nursing, 39*(5), 44–48.

Wysocki, S. (2010). Vaginitis assessment with vaginal pH. *Advance for Nurse Practitioners, 17*(10), 29–30.

CHAPTER 21

Barnes, M., & Bloom, B. (2009). *CAM use among adults and children in the United States in 2007.* National Health Statistics Report, Retrieved February 2010, from www.cdc.gov.

Bennett, D. (2009). Alternate therapies/integrated medicine. *RN, 72*(3), 38–41.

Bland, J. (2008). The future of nutritional pharmacology. *Alternative Therapies in Health and Medicine, 14*(5), 12–16.

Cumming, A., Simpson, K., & Brown, D. (2006). *Complementary and alternative medicine.* Philadelphia: Churchill Livingstone.

Diamond, J., & Diamond, W. (2005). CAM for common bowel problems. *Advance for Nurse Practitioners, 13*(5), 31–34.

Edwards, Q., Colquist, S., & Maradiegue, A. (2005). What's cooking with garlic? Is this complementary and alternative medicine for hypertension? *Journal of the American Academy of Nursing Practitioners, 19*(9), 381–385.

Ernst, E., Pittler, M., & Wider, B. (2006). *The desktop guide to complementary and alternative medicine: An evidence-based approach,* (2nd ed.). St. Louis: Mosby.

Fontaine, K. (2005). *Healing practices, alternative therapies for nursing practice* (2nd ed.). Upper Saddle River, NJ: Prentice Hall Health.

Gardner, P., & Kemper, K. (2005). For GI complaints, which herbs and supplements spell relief? *Contemporary Pediatrics, 22*(8), 51–55.

Guthrie, C. (2005). Alternative medicine cabinet. *Alternative Medicine,* April, 59–61.

Kemper, K., & Kelly, E. (2004). Treating children with therapeutic and healing touch. *Pediatric Annals, 33*(4), 248–252.

Krebs, M. (2006). The sweet smell of healing: Promoting wellness with aromatherapy. *Advance for Nurse Practitioners, 14*(5), 41–44.

Leifer, G. (2010). *Introduction to maternity and pediatric nursing* (6th ed.). Philadelphia: Saunders.

Low Dog, T. (2009). The use of botanicals during pregnancy and lactation. *Alternative Therapies in Health and Medicine, 15*(1), 54–56.

Lowdermilk, D. L., & Perry, S. E. (2007). *Maternity and women's health care* (9th ed.). St. Louis: Mosby.

Mancho, P., & Edwards, Q. (2005). Chaste tree for PMS. *Advance for Nurse Practitioners, 13*(5), 43–45.

Mantle, F., & Tiran, D. (2007). *A-Z of complementary and alternative medicine therapy for health professionals.* Philadelphia: Saunders.

Medical Economics Company (2005). *Physician's desk reference for herbal medicines.* Montvale, NJ: Medical Economics Company.

Micozzi, M. (2006). *Fundamentals of complementary and integrative medicine* (3rd ed.). Philadelphia: Saunders.

National Center for Complementary and Alternative Medicine. NCCAM (2004). *Herbal supplements.* Retrieved December 8, 2008, from http://nccam.nih.gov/health/supplements/index.htm.

National Center for Complementary and Alternative Medicine (2006). *Acupuncture: get the facts.* Retrieved June 10, 2009, from http://nccam.nih.gov/health/acupuncture.

Orem, D. E. (2001). *Nursing: Concepts of practice* (6th ed.). Philadelphia: Saunders.

Pettigrew, A., King, M., & McGee, K. (2005). CAM therapy use by women's health clinic clients. *Alternative Therapies in Health and Medicine, 10*(6), 50–54.

Quinlan, J., & Hill, D. (2003). Nausea and vomiting in pregnancy. *American Family Physician, 68*, 121–128.

Rakel, D. (2007). *Integrative medicine* (2nd ed.). Philadelphia: Saunders.

Rankin-Box, D., & Williamson, E. (2007). *Complementary medicine.* Philadelphia: Saunders.

Reilly, A. (2005). The role of massage therapy in patient care. *Advance for Nurse Practitioners, 13*(5), 37–42.

Schultz, V., Hansel, R., Blumenthal, M., & Tyler, V. (2004). *Rational phytotherapy: A reference guide for physicians and pharmacists* (5th ed.). Berlin: Springer.

Sierpina, V., Wallschlaeger, B., & Blumenthal, M. (2004). Ginkgo biloba. *American Family Physician, 68*(5), 923–927.

Spencer, J., & Jacobs, J. (2003). *Complementary and alternative medicine: An evidence-based approach* (2nd ed.). St. Louis: Mosby.

Wardell, D., & Engebretson, J. (2001). Biological correlates of Reiki Touch healing. *Journal of Advanced Nursing, 33*(4), 439–445.

Watson, J. (1996). Watson's theory of transpersonal caring. In P. Walker, & B. Bewman (Eds.), *Blueprints for Use as Nursing Models: Education, Research, Practice, and Administration.* New York: NLN Press (classic reference).

Illustration Credits

CHAPTER 1

1-1: From Harrison, M. R., Globus, M. S., & Gilly, R. A. (Eds.). (1991). *The unborn patient: Prenatal diagnosis and treatment* (2nd ed.). Philadelphia: Saunders.

CHAPTER 2

2-1, 2-2, 2-7: From Lowdermilk, D. L., Perry, S. E., Cashion, M. C. (2012). *Maternity & women's health care* (10th ed.). St. Louis: Mosby; **2-3:** Oats, J., & Abraham, S. (2005). *Llewellyn-Jones fundamentals of obstetrics and gynaecology* (8th ed.). Philadelphia: Elsevier; **2-4, 2-8:** From Patton, K. T. & Thibodeau, G. A. (2010). *Anatomy and physiology* (7th ed.). St. Louis: Mosby; **2-5:** From Lowdermilk, D. L., & Perry, S. E. (2004). *Maternity and women's health care* (8th ed.). St. Louis: Mosby; **2-9:** From Herlihy, B. (2011). *The human body in health and illness* (4th ed.). Philadelphia: Saunders.

CHAPTER 3

3-2: From Leifer, G. (2011). *Introduction to maternity and pediatric nursing* (6th ed.). Philadelphia: Saunders; **3-3:** From Herlihy, B. (2010). *The human body in health and illness* (4th ed.). Philadelphia: Saunders; **3-4, 3-5, 3-8, Unn 3-1, 3-2:** From Moore, K. L., & Persaud, T. V. N. (2008). *The developing human: Clinically oriented embryology* (8th ed.). Philadelphia: Saunders; **3-6:** Creasy, R. K., Resnik, R., Iams, J., Lockwood, C., Moore, T., & Greene, M. (2009). Creasy & Resnick's *Maternal-fetal medicine* (6th ed.). Philadelphia: Saunders; **3-9:** From Patton, K. T., & Thibodeau, G. A. (2010). *Anatomy and physiology* (7th ed.). St. Louis: Mosby; **Unn 3-3, 3-4, 3-5, 3-6:** From Moore, K. L., Persaud, T. V. N., & Shiota, K. (2000). *Color atlas of clinical embryology* (2nd ed.). Philadelphia: Saunders.

CHAPTER 4

4-1: Courtesy Cooper Surgical, Inc., Turnbull, Connecticut; **4-2:** From Swartz, M. H. (2010). *Textbook of physical diagnosis: History and examination* (6th ed.). Philadelphia: Saunders; **4-3:** From Matteson, P. (2001). *Women's health during the childbearing years: A community-based approach*. St. Louis: Mosby; **4-4:** From Moore, K. L., & Persaud, T. V. N. (2008). *The developing human: Clinically oriented embryology* (8th ed.). Philadelphia: Saunders; **4-6:** Courtesy Pat Spier, RN-C and Loma Linda University Medical Center, Loma Linda, California.

CHAPTER 5

5-3, *A*: From Murray, S. S., & McKinney, E. S. (2010). *Foundations of maternal-newborn and women's health nursing* (5th ed.). Philadelphia: Saunders; **5-3, *B*:** Courtesy Pat Spier, RN-C; **5-5:** From Moore, K. L., & Persaud, T. V. N. (2008). *The developing human: Clinically oriented embryology*. (8th ed.). Philadelphia: Saunders; **5-6:** Creasy, R. K., Resnik, R., Iams, J., Lockwood, C., Moore, T., & Greene, M. (2009). Creasy & Resnick's *Maternal-fetal medicine* (6th ed.). Philadelphia: Saunders; **5-10:** From Leifer, G. (2010). *Introduction to maternity & pediatric nursing* (6th ed.). Philadelphia: Saunders; **5-11:** Courtesy U.S. Department of Agriculture; **5-12:** From Painter, J., Rah, J., & Lee, Y. (2002). Comparison of international food guide pictorial representations. *Journal of the American Dietetic Association, 102*, 483–489; **5-15:** Courtesy Pat Spier, RN-C and Loma Linda University Medical Center, Loma Linda, California.

CHAPTER 6

6-1, 6-2: From Murray, S. S., & McKinney, E. S. (2010). *Foundations of maternal-newborn and women's health nursing* (5th ed.). Philadelphia: Saunders; **6-3:** From McKinney, E. S., James, S. R., Ashwill, J. W., & Murray, S. S. (2009). *Maternal-child nursing* (3rd ed.). Philadelphia: Saunders; **6-4:** Perry, S. E., Hockenberry, M. J., Lowdermilk, D. L., & Wilson, D. (2009). *Maternal child nursing care* (4th ed.). St. Louis: Mosby; **6-5:** Lowdermilk, D. L., Perry, S. E., & Cashion M. C. (2012). *Maternity & women's health care* (10th ed.). St. Louis: Mosby; **6-6:** Lowdermilk, D. L., Perry, S. E., & Cashion M. C. (2011). *Maternity nursing* (8th ed.). St. Louis: Mosby; **6-7:** From Matteson, P. (2001). *Women's health during the childbearing years: A community-based approach*. St. Louis: Mosby.

CHAPTER 7

7-1: Courtesy Hill-Rom Services, Inc., Batesville, Indiana; **7-2:** From Matteson, P. (2001). *Women's health during the childbearing years: A community-based approach*. St. Louis: Mosby; **7-3:** From Hacker, N. F., Gambone, J. C., & Hobel, C. T. (2010). *Hacker and Moore's Essentials of obstetrics and gynecology* (5th ed.). Philadelphia: Saunders; **7-4:** Courtesy GE Healthcare, Milwaukee, Wisconsin; **7-6, 7-9:** From Lowdermilk, D. L., Perry, S. E., Cashion, M. C. (2012). *Maternity & women's health care* (10th ed.). St. Louis: Mosby; **7-7:** From Gabbe, S.,

Simpson, J., Niebyl, J., & Galan, H. (2007). *Obstetrics: Normal and problem pregnancies* (5th ed.). Philadelphia: Churchill Livingstone; **7-8:** From Tucker, S. (2000). *Mosby's pocket guide to fetal monitoring and assessment.* (4th ed.). St. Louis: Mosby; **7-10, 7-11, 7-14, 7-15, Unn 7-2, 7-7:** Courtesy Pat Spier, RN-C and Loma Linda University Medical Center, Loma Linda, California; **Unn 7-1:** Courtesy Pat Spier, RN-C; **7-12:** From Nichols, F. H., & Humenick, S. S. (2000). *Childbirth education: Practice, research, and theory* (2nd ed.). Philadelphia: Saunders.

CHAPTER 8

8-1, *A*, 8-2: Courtesy Pat Spier, RN-C and Loma Linda University Medical Center, Loma Linda, California; **8-3:** From Moore, S. (1997). *Understanding pain and its relief in labor.* New York: Churchill Livingstone.

CHAPTER 9

9-8: From Beischer, N. A., Mackay, E. V., & Colditz, P. B. (1997). *Obstetrics and the newborn* (3rd ed.) Philadelphia: Saunders; **9-9:** From McKinney, E. S., James, S.R., Murray, S. S., & Ashwill, J. W. (2009). *Maternal-child nursing* (3rd ed.). Philadelphia: Saunders; **9-10:** From Thureen, P. J., Deacon, J., Hernandez, J. A. , & Hall, D. (2004). *Assessment and care of the well newborn* (2nd ed.). Philadephia: Saunders; **9-11, 9-13:** (1978). Courtesy Ross Laboratories, Columbus, Ohio; **9-14, *B*:** Courtesy Loma Linda University Medical Center, Loma Linda, California; **9-15, *A*, Unn 9-1:** From Murray, S. S., & McKinney, E. S. (2010). *Foundations of maternal-newborn nursing and women's health nursing* (5th ed.). Philadelphia: Saunders; **9-15 *B*, Unn 9-5, 9-8:** From Zitelli, B. J., & Davis, H. W. (2007). *Atlas of pediatric physical diagnosis* (5th ed.). St. Louis: Mosby; **9-18, *B*:** Courtesy Natus Medical, Inc., San Carlos, California; **Unn 9-2, 9-3, 9-4, 9-7:** From Eichenfield, L. F., Frieden, I. J., & Esterly, N. B. (2008). *Textbook of neonatal dermatology* (2nd ed.). Philadelphia: Saunders; **Unn 9-9:** From Murray, S. S., McKinney, E. S., & Gorrie, T. M. (2002). *Foundations of maternal-newborn nursing* (3rd ed.). Philadelphia: Saunders; **Unn 9-10:** From Swartz, M. H. (2010). *Textbook of physical diagnosis: History and examination* (6th ed.). Philadelphia: Saunders.

CHAPTER 10

10-1, *B*, Unn 10-3: Courtesy Pat Spier, RN-C and Loma Linda University Medical Center, Loma Linda, California; **Unn 10-1:** Courtesy Pat Spier, RN-C.

CHAPTER 11

11-2, 11-3, *B*, 11-3, *C*, 11-4: Courtesy Pat Spier, RN-C; **11-5, 11-8:** Courtesy Medela Inc., McKenry, Illinois.

CHAPTER 12

12-1: From Oats, J., & Abraham, S. (2005). *Llewellyn-Jones fundamentals of obstetrics and gynaecology* (8th ed.). Philadelphia: Elsevier; **12-2:** From Lowdermilk, D. L., Perry, S. E., & Cashion, M. C. (2010). *Maternity & women's health care* (10th ed.). St. Louis: Mosby; **12-3:** From Matteson, P. (2001). *Women's health during the childbearing years: A community-based approach.* St. Louis: Mosby; **Unn 12-1:** Courtesy Pat Spier, RN-C; **Unn 12-3:** From Murray, S. S., & McKinney, E. S. (2010). *Foundations of maternal-newborn nursing and women's health nursing* (5th ed.). Philadelphia: Saunders; **Unn 12-4:** Courtesy Carex Health Brands.

CHAPTER 13

13-2: From Moore, K. L., & Persaud, T. V. N. (2008). *The developing human: Clinically oriented embryology* (8th ed.). Philadelphia: Saunders; **13-3:** From Oats, J., & Abraham, S. (2005). *Llewellyn-Jones fundamentals of obstetrics and gynaecology* (8th ed.). Philadelphia: Elsevier; **13-4:** From Matteson, P. (2001). *Women's health during the childbearing years: A community-based approach.* St. Louis: Mosby; **13-5:** From Murray, S. S., & McKinney, E. S. (2010). *Foundations of maternal-newborn and women's health nursing* (5th ed.). Philadelphia: Saunders; **13-6:** From Thibodeau, G. A., & Patton, K. T. (2008). *Structure and function of the body* (13th ed.). St. Louis: Mosby; **13-7:** From Dickason, E. J., & Schultz, M. O. (1998). *Maternal-infant nursing care* (3rd ed.). St. Louis: Mosby.

CHAPTER 14

14-1, 14-3: From Gabbe, S., Niebyl, J., & Simpson, J. (2007). *Obstetrics: Normal and problem pregnancies.* (5th ed.). Philadelphia: Churchill Livingstone; **14-10:** From Murray, S. S., & McKinney, E. S. (2010). *Foundations of maternal-newborn and women's health nursing* (5th ed.). Philadelphia: Saunders; **14-11:** From Lowdermilk, D. L., & Perry, S. E. (2004). *Maternity and women's health care* (8th ed.). St. Louis: Mosby; **14-12, *A-H, J, K*:** Courtesy Pat Spier, RN-C.

CHAPTER 15

15-1: Modified from Klaus, M. H., & Fanaroff, A. A. (2001). *Care of the high risk neonate* (5th ed.). Philadelphia: Saunders; **15-2, 15-4, *C, E*:** From Zitelli, B. J., & Davis, H. W. (2007). *Atlas of pediatric physical diagnosis* (5th ed.). St. Louis: Mosby; **15-7:** Reprinted by permission of Nellcor Puritan Bennett Incorporated, Pleasanton, California; **15-8:** Courtesy Pat Spier, RN-C; **Unn 15-1, 15-2:** Courtesy Pat Spier, RN-C and Loma Linda University Medical Center, Loma Linda, California.

CHAPTER 16

16-1: From Zitelli, B. J., & Davis, H. W. (2007). *Atlas of pediatric physical diagnosis* (5th ed.). St. Louis: Mosby; **16-2:** From Herlihy, B. (2010). *The human body in health and illness* (4th ed.). Philadelphia: Saunders; **16-3:** Courtesy Natus Medical Inc., San Carlos, California; **16-4:** Courtesy Medela Labs, Inc. McHenry, Illinois; **16-5, 16-8:** From Leifer, G. (2007). *Introduction to maternity and pediatric nursing* (5th ed.). Philadelphia: Saunders; **16-6,** *A:* From McKinney, E. S., James, S. R., Murray, S. S., & Ashwill, J. W. (2009). *Maternal-child nursing* (3rd ed.). Philadelphia: Saunders; **16-6,** *B:* From McKinney, E. S., James, S. R., Murray, S. S., & Ashwill, J. W. (2008). *Maternal-child nursing* (2nd ed.). Philadelphia: Saunders; **16-7:** From Silverman, W., & Andersen, D. (1956). A controlled clinical trial of effects of water mist on obstructive respiratory signs, death rate, and necropsy findings among premature infants. *Pediatrics, 17*(4), 1–9; **16-9:** Courtesy Pat Spier, RN-C; **Unn 16-5:** From Thureen, P. J., Deacon, J., Hall, D., & Hernandez, J. A. (2005). *Assessment and care of the well newborn* (2nd ed.). Philadephia: Saunders.

CHAPTER 17

17-1: From McKinney, E. S., James, S. R., Murray, S. S., & Ashwill, J. W. (2009). *Maternal-child nursing* (3rd ed.). Philadelphia: Saunders; **17-2:** From Murray, S. S., & McKinney, E. S. (2010). *Foundations of maternal-newborn and women's health nursing* (5th ed.). Philadelphia: Saunders; **17-3:** From Swartz, M. H. (2010). *Textbook of physical diagnosis: History and examination* (6th ed.). Philadelphia: Saunders.

CHAPTER 18

18-1, 18-4: Courtesy Pat Spier, RN-C; **18-3:** Courtesy GE Healthcare, Milwaukee, Wisconsin.

CHAPTER 19

19-1: From Leifer, G. (2011). *Introduction to maternity & pediatric nursing* (6th ed.). Philadelphia: Saunders.

CHAPTER 20

Unn 20-4: From Grimes, D. E., & Grimes, R. M. (1994). *AIDS and HIV infection.* St. Louis: Mosby; **Unn 20-5, 20-6:** From Jarvis, C. (2000). *Physical examination and health assessment* (3rd ed.). Philadelphia: Saunders; **Unn 20-7:** From Callen, J. P., Greer, K. E., Paller, A. S., & Swinyer, L. J. (2000). *Color atlas of dermatology* (2nd ed.). Philadelphia: Saunders; **Unn 20-8:** From Swartz, M. H. (2009). *Textbook of physical diagnosis: History and examination* (6th ed.). Philadelphia: Saunders.

CHAPTER 21

21-1: Courtesy Neurowave Technologies; **21-2:** Redrawn from Breslin, E. T., & Lucas, V. A. (Eds.). (2003). *Women's health nursing.* Philadelphia: Saunders.

Glossary

A

abortion Termination of pregnancy before viability of a fetus (approximately 20 weeks' gestation). *Miscarriage* is the lay term for spontaneous abortion.

abruptio placentae Premature separation of a normally implanted placenta from the uterine wall.

abstinence Refraining from having sexual intercourse.

acceleration Periodic increase in the baseline fetal heart rate.

acidosis Excessive acidity of body fluids caused by the accumulation of acids or the loss of bicarbonate, resulting in lowered pH.

acini cells Milk-producing cells of the breast.

acme Peak, or period of greatest strength, of a uterine contraction.

acquired immunodeficiency syndrome (AIDS) Disease that destroys the body's natural immune system, resulting in the loss of defense against malignancies and opportunistic infections.

acrocyanosis Cyanosis of hands and feet seen in most newborns.

active acquired immunity Formation of antibodies in response to immunization or illness.

acupressure Finger, palm, or knuckle pressure at points located along an invisible system of energy channels, called *meridians*, for the purpose of relaxation, pain relief, and promotion of general health.

acupuncture A Chinese medical technique that involves inserting needles on the surface of the body at specific points; aims to promote health by stimulating the body's self-healing powers.

adolescence Period of development between puberty and adulthood.

advice telephone line A telephone number usually staffed by nurses that is given to patients on hospital discharge to foster communication, answer questions, and reinforce discharge teaching instructions.

afterbirth Placenta and membranes that are expelled after the birth of a newborn.

afterpains Cramping pain after childbirth resulting from alternating relaxation and contraction of the uterine muscles.

agonist An agent that activates something.

albuminuria Presence of albumin, a protein, in the urine.

allopathic care Traditional Western health care, which follows a disease-oriented model that uses technology and bioscience to treat illness and promote wellness.

alpha-fetoprotein (AFP) An antigen present in the human fetus. Elevated levels in amniotic fluid or adult serum during pregnancy may indicate a neural tube defect; decreased levels may indicate Down syndrome.

alternative therapies Forms of therapy that generally replace or substitute for a traditional treatment.

alveoli Small air sacs present in the lungs.

amenorrhea Absence of menstruation.

amniocentesis Removal of amniotic fluid by insertion of a needle into the amniotic sac. Amniotic fluid is obtained to assess fetal health and maturity.

amnioinfusion Infusion of warmed isotonic saline or Ringer's lactate solution into the uterine cavity to reduce umbilical cord compression; also performed to flush meconium out of the cavity to reduce risk of fetal meconium aspiration.

amnion The inner of two membranes that form a sac containing the fetus and the amniotic fluid. (The outer membrane is the chorion.)

amnionitis Inflammation of the amnion, occurring most commonly after prolonged rupture of membranes.

amniotic fluid Fluid that surrounds the fetus within the amniotic sac and permits fetal movement, absorbs shocks, and prevents heat loss.

amniotomy Artificial rupture of the fetal membranes (AROM).

analgesic Drug used to relieve pain.

androgen Male hormone that stimulates the development of secondary male characteristics.

anemia Condition caused by a decrease in erythrocytes, hemoglobin, or both.

anesthesia Use of an agent that causes partial or complete loss of sensation, with or without loss of consciousness.

anoxia Deficiency of oxygen.

antagonist An agent that blocks something.

antepartum Occurring before birth; prenatal.

antibody Protein substance (immunoglobulins) made by the body that exerts restrictive or destructive action on specific antigens (e.g., bacteria, dust, Rh factor).

antigen Protein foreign to the body that stimulates the immune system to form antibodies.

anuria Failure of the kidney to produce urine.

Apgar score Numeric evaluation of the newborn obtained at 1 minute and 5 minutes after birth.

apnea Cessation of respirations for more than 20 seconds.

appropriate-for-gestational-age (AGA) newborn A neonate who weighs less than the heaviest 10% and more than the lightest 10% of neonates of the same gestational age.

AquaMEPHYTON Phytonadione; a fat-soluble vitamin K liquid necessary for formulation of coagulation factors.

areola Pigmented ring surrounding the nipple of the breast.

aromatherapy A form of treatment using essential plant oils that may be inhaled or massaged into the skin for therapeutic effects.

asphyxia A condition in which there is deficient oxygen in the blood and excess carbon dioxide in the blood and tissues.

assisted reproductive technology (ART) Techniques used to treat infertility; may include ovulation induction, in vitro fertilization, GIFT, and IV-ET.

asymptomatic Without symptoms.

ataractic Drug that promotes tranquility; a tranquilizer.

atelectasis Incomplete expansion of the lung or portion of the lung.

atony Lack of normal muscle tone or strength.

attachment A bond or relationship of affection between persons.

attitude The relation of the fetal parts to one another. *See also* fetal attitude.

augmentation of labor The enhancement of labor after it has begun through use of an oxytocic drug.

autoimmune disease A state in which the body produces antibodies against itself, causing cell damage.

autoimmunization Development of antibodies against constituents of one's own tissues (e.g., a man may develop antibodies against his own sperm); an immune response to the body's own tissues.

autolysis A self-digestive process by which cells are destroyed by enzymes.

autosomal inheritance The process by which characteristics are transmitted by genes on the autosomes, not the sex chromosomes.

autosome A chromosome that is not a sex chromosome.

B

bag of waters The membranes containing the amniotic fluid and the fetus; also called *amniotic sac.*

Bartholin's glands Small, mucus-secreting glands located on either side of the base of the vagina.

basal body temperature (BBT) Body temperature at rest.

baseline fetal heart rate (FHR) Average fetal heart rate observed within a 10-minute period of monitoring.

biischial diameter Distance between the inner surfaces of the ischial tuberosities of the pelvic outlet.

bilirubin Yellowish pigment of bile produced from the hemoglobin of the red blood cells.

bilirubinemia Presence of abnormal amount of bilirubin in the blood when red blood cells are broken down or destroyed from a pathologic cause.

Billings method A technique for checking cervical mucus for elasticity, stickiness, wetness, and lubrication to provide information about the menstrual cycle; also called *cervical mucus method.*

biofeedback A method of training designed to enable an individual to control involuntary bodily functions.

birth The process of being born.

birthing centers Locations outside of the traditional hospital setting that provide comprehensive perinatal care, typically with midwives.

Bishop score A scoring system to determine whether labor can be safely induced.

blastocyst Stage of development of the embryo that follows the morula; the outer layer of the trophoblast to which is attached an inner cell mass.

blastula Stage of the fertilized ovum in which the cells are arranged in a hollow ball.

blood patch A small amount of a woman's blood injected into the epidural space in the area of a spinal puncture that forms a seal and stops spinal fluid leakage that may be causing headache or discomfort.

bonding A process by which parents, over time, form an emotional relationship with their newborn.

bradycardia Slow heart rate (< 110 beats per minute in a fetus).

Braxton Hicks contractions Intermittent, painless uterine contractions that occur during pregnancy. They become stronger and more evident in the last trimester and are sometimes mistaken for true labor signs.

breasts Mammary glands.

breech presentation A situation when the fetus is turned so that the buttocks or feet (instead of the head) lead into the birth canal, nearest the cervical opening.

bronchopulmonary dysplasia (BPD) Pulmonary condition affecting preterm newborns who have had respiratory failure and have been oxygen-dependent for several days.

brown adipose tissue (BAT) Fat deposits that provide greater heat-generating activity than usual fat in neonates; found around the neck, between the scapulas, around the kidneys and adrenal glands, and behind the sternum; also called *brown fat.*

C

calendar method The timing of sexual intercourse to avoid the fertile period associated with ovulation.

caput succedaneum Swelling or edema occurring under the fetal scalp (or presenting part) during labor.

carpal tunnel syndrome Pressure on the median nerve at the point where it goes through the carpal tunnel of the wrist. The result is soreness and weakness of muscles in the area of the median nerve.

CDC Centers for Disease Control and Prevention; collects statistics of diseases and deaths in the United States.

cephalhematoma Accumulation of blood under the periosteum of the newborn's skull; caused by trauma of blood vessels during birth.

cephalic Pertaining to the head.

cephalopelvic disproportion (CPD) A condition in which the fetal head is of a shape, size, or position that prevents it from passing through the maternal pelvis.

cerclage *See* cervical cerclage.

certified nurse-midwife A registered nurse who has received special education to care for the family during the normal pregnancy, labor, delivery, and postpartum periods.

cervical cap Pliable contraceptive device that fits over the cervix.

cervical cerclage The use of sutures to close an incompetent cervix to prevent it from opening as the growing fetus presses against it.

cervical mucus method *See* Billings method.

cervix Lower portion of the uterus extending into the vagina.

cesarean birth Birth of the fetus (placenta and membranes) through an incision made into the abdominal wall and the uterus.

chemical predictor test An over-the-counter test kit for determining pregnancy.

Chlamydia **infection** A sexually transmitted infection with purulent vaginal discharge, burning on urination, and lower abdominal discomfort. It may cause sterility.

chloasma gravidarum Increased pigmentation of the face during pregnancy that fades after delivery; also known as the "mask of pregnancy" or melasma.

chorioamnionitis Inflammation of the fetal membranes.

chorion Outer membrane of the amniotic sac that is formed from the trophoblast.

chorionic villi Root-like, branching projections of the chorion containing capillaries that are the means by which substances (gases, nutrients, waste products) are exchanged between the maternal and fetal circulations.

chromosome Thread of deoxyribonucleic acid (DNA) that carries the genetic code for each unique individual. There are 23 pairs in each soma cell; one chromosome in each pair is from each parent.

circumcision Surgical removal of part or all of the prepuce (foreskin) of the penis.

cleansing breath A deep breath taken at the beginning and end of each labor contraction.

cleft lip Congenital separation of one or both sides of the upper lip.

cleft palate Congenital incomplete closure of the roof of the mouth.

climacteric The physiologic and psychological alterations that occur around the time of menopause.

clinical pathway A multidisciplinary care plan for a specific diagnosis.

clitoris A female organ that is homologous to the penis of the male and made up of erectile tissue situated at the anterior junction of the vulva.

cognitive stimulation Activation of the conscious mind.

coitus Sexual intercourse.

coitus interruptus Removal of the penis from the vagina during sexual intercourse before ejaculation occurs.

cold stress Environmental chilling that causes increased metabolism and increased oxygen consumption in the body.

collaborative care Cooperative care between members of the multidisciplinary health care team and the patient.

collaborative practice A partnership with health professions other than medicine that uses a multidisciplinary team to provide care with parent participation.

colostrum Yellowish secretion from the breasts before the onset of true lactation.

colposcopy Examination of the vagina and cervix with a colposcope to identify neoplastic or other changes.

complementary therapy A nontraditional therapy that is used along with conventional therapy.

conception Union of the sperm and ovum resulting in fertilization; formation of the one-celled zygote.

conceptus Product of fertilization.

conditioning A process in which a person learns to modify behavior when certain stimuli are applied.

condom A soft, flexible latex sheath covering the penis or lining of the vagina to prevent sperm from entering the cervix and to prevent infection.

conduction The transfer of heat to a cooler surface, resulting in loss of body heat and chilling.

condyloma Sexually transmitted, viral, wart-like growth on the skin of genitalia.

congenital Present at birth.

conjunctivitis Inflammation of the mucous membrane lining of the eyelids.

contraception Prevention of conception or pregnancy.

contraction stress test (CST) Test to stimulate uterine contractions for the purpose of assessing the fetal heart rate in relation to uterine contractions.

convection Loss of heat from warm body surface to cooler air currents.

Coombs' test Test used to detect sensitized red blood cells. The indirect test determines the presence of Rh+ antibodies in maternal blood; the direct test determines the presence of maternal Rh+ antibodies in fetal cord blood.

cord care Technique of preventing infection and promoting healing of the umbilical cord of the newborn.

corpus luteum Solid, yellow body that develops within a ruptured follicle; an endocrine structure that secretes primarily progesterone.

cotyledon Segment or subdivision of the uterine surface of the placenta.

crepitation Crackling sound of fractured bone ends rubbing against each other; frequently noted in fractured clavicle of the newborn.

crowning Visibility of the fetal head in the birth canal before delivery.

culdocentesis Aspiration of fluid from the cul-de-sac by puncture of the vaginal vault in the posterior fornix of the vagina.

culture An individual's and family's beliefs, attitudes, practices, and actions that direct their socialization within a specific group and in relations with others outside of the group.

cutaneous stimulation Activation of skin sensation.

cyanosis Blueness of the skin caused by a lack of oxygenation of the blood.

cytomegalovirus (CMV) A viral infection that may result in fetal anomalies.

D

deceleration Decrease in the fetal heart rate. *See also* early deceleration, late deceleration, and variable deceleration.

decidua The endometrium, or lining of the uterus, that thickens during pregnancy and is shed after delivery.

decrement Decrease of intensity (strength) of uterine contraction.

deep tendon reflexes A deep stretch reflex within the body often used to detect central nervous system irritability in women with eclampsia.

dehiscence Rupture of a surgical wound or scar.

deoxyribonucleic acid (DNA) Intracellular complex protein that carries genetic information, consisting of two purines (adenine and guanine) and two pyridines (thymine and cytosine).

diagonal conjugate Distance between the sacral promontory and the lower border or the symphysis pubis; may be obtained by manual measurement.

diaphoresis Profuse sweating.

diaphragm A contraceptive device consisting of a latex dome that covers the cervix and prevents the entrance of sperm.

diastasis recti abdominis A separation of the rectus abdominis muscles in the midline.

dilation of cervix Stretching of the cervical canal to a size of opening large enough to allow the passage of a newborn.

disproportion Lack of normal relationship, in which the fetus is too large or the pelvis is too small for a normal vaginal birth.

disseminated intravascular coagulation (DIC) Coagulation disorder in which clotting factors are consumed and maternal blood does not clot.

diuresis Passage of large amounts of urine.

dizygotic twins Twins that develop from two separate fertilized ova and have different genetic constitutions; also known as fraternal twins.

documentation Verification of details of patient care given by writing in a permanent record.

dorsiflexion Movement of a body part backward (e.g., upward flexion of wrist).

doula A trained person who is a supportive partner during labor and delivery.

Down syndrome A congenital abnormality with specific physical characteristics and mental retardation; also referred to as *trisomy 21*.

ductus arteriosus A fetal vessel connecting the pulmonary artery with the aorta; transports oxygenated blood for distribution to the body.

ductus venosus A fetal vessel that connects the umbilical vein and the inferior vena cava; transports blood to the portal vein of the liver and the inferior vena cava.

Duncan mechanism Delivery of the placenta with the maternal side expelled first.

duration of contraction The length of a contraction, measured from the beginning to its completion.

dysfunctional labor Abnormally painful or prolonged labor.

dysmenorrhea Painful menstrual cramps.

dyspareunia Painful intercourse.

dyspnea Difficult or labored breathing.

dystocia Difficult or slow labor and delivery, or both; also known as dysfunctional labor.

E

early deceleration Periodic change in fetal heart rate pattern caused by head compression. Deceleration has a uniform appearance and early onset in relation to the maternal contraction.

ecchymosis A bluish black area on the skin associated with bleeding into that area.

eclampsia Severe form of gestational hypertension accompanied by convulsions.

ectopic pregnancy Implantation of the fertilized ovum outside of the uterus.

effacement Thinning and shortening of the cervix before and during labor.

effleurage A slight stroking movement of the fingertips over the abdomen during labor; used as a distraction for pain relief during contractions.

electronic fetal monitoring (EFM) Electronic surveillance of fetal heart rate by external and internal methods.

emancipated minor An independent person younger than 18 years who may be married and living away from family.

embryo Stage of human development occurring between the ovum and fetal stages, or from 2 to 8 weeks' gestation.

endometriosis Endometrium located outside of the uterus.

en face A position in which parent and newborn have eye-to-eye contact within a 9- to 10-inch distance.

endometritis Infection of the endometrium.

endometrium Mucous lining of the uterus.

endorphins Endogenous opioids (morphine-like substance) secreted by the pituitary gland that act on the central and peripheral nervous systems to reduce pain.

engagement Descent of the fetal presenting part to at least a zero station (the level of the ischial spines in the maternal pelvis).

engorgement Vascular congestion and distention resulting in swelling of the breast tissue, brought about by an increase of blood and lymph supply to the breasts.

epididymis Coiled, oblong canal where the sperm mature and increase their motility.

epidural block Injection of local anesthetic into the epidural space of the spinal column.

episiotomy Surgical incision of the perineum before birth to permit delivery of newborn without lacerations to the area.

epispadias A congenital anomaly in which the urethral meatus is located on the dorsal surface of the penis.

Epstein's pearls Small, white blebs found on the gums and at the junction of the soft and hard palates; commonly seen in newborns.

erythema Inflammation of the skin or mucous membranes.

erythroblastosis fetalis Hemolytic disease of the newborn usually caused by isoimmunization resulting from Rh incompatibility or ABO incompatibility.

estrogen Female sex hormone secreted by ovaries and placenta.

evaporation Conversion from liquid to vapor, resulting in loss of body heat when wet skin is exposed to the air.

evidence-based practice Practice based on scientific studies.

exfoliation The scaling off of tissues in layers.

expected date of delivery (EDD) Approximate date of birth (due date); usually determined by calculation using Nägele's rule.

expiratory grunting An audible noise heard during each exhalation, often indicative of respiratory distress.

expulsion Pushing out or expelling.

extension Part of the birth process in which the fetal head changes position from chin on the chest to chin away from the chest (extension), enabling the infant's head and face to emerge onto the perineum during the normal birth process.

external fetal monitoring Monitoring of the fetal heart by placing a monitor on the external surface of the maternal abdomen. *See also* electronic fetal monitoring.

external rotation The realignment of the fetal head with the shoulders after the head is delivered, and the alignment of the fetal shoulders with the mother's pelvis before delivery of the newborn.

external version Changing the fetal presentation in the uterus, usually from breech to cephalic, by pressing on the woman's abdomen.

extracorporeal membrane oxygenation (ECMO) Heart-lung machine that provides a cardiopulmonary bypass for newborns with disorders such as meconium aspiration syndrome.

F

fallopian tubes (uterine tubes) Tubes extending laterally from each side of the uterus to the ovary, through which the ovum travels, after ovulation, to the uterus.

false labor Irregular uterine contractions that do not result in cervical dilation. They do not get longer or become stronger.

family A social group composed of parents and children living together and sharing common interests.

female condom *See* condom.

ferning (fern test) Formation of a palm-leaf pattern of cervical mucus as it dries at midmenstrual cycle.

fertility Quality of being able to reproduce, of being fertile.

fertilization Penetration of one ovum (single pregnancy) by a sperm.

fetal alcohol syndrome (FAS) Disorder resulting from maternal alcohol consumption during pregnancy. It is characterized by physical deficits and mental retardation.

fetal attitude Relation of the fetal parts to one another. Normal attitude is one of flexion of arms and legs.

fetal blood sampling Sample of blood drawn from the presenting part (usually the head) of the fetus during labor.

fetal heart rate (FHR) Rate of fetal heart beats per minute. Normal FHR is 110 to 160 beats per minute.

fetal heart rate fluctuations Tachycardia, bradycardia, accelerations, decelerations, or changes in fetal heart rate variability.

fetal lie Relation of the long axis of the fetus to the long axis of the woman. Fetal lie may be longitudinal, transverse, or oblique.

fetal lung fluid Fluid that fills the lungs during prenatal life, expanding the alveoli and promoting normal development of the lungs.

fetal position Relation of presenting fetal part to the front, sides, and back of the maternal pelvis.

fetal presentation The fetal body parts that enter the maternal pelvis first. Three potential presentations are cephalic, breech, and shoulder.

fetal pulse oximetry Fetal oxygen saturation measured by a transcervical catheter positioned against the fetal cheek; used when the amniotic membranes are ruptured and the cervix is at least 2 cm dilated.

fetoscope A stethoscope specially adapted for listening to fetal heart tones.

fetus Undelivered baby after the embryonic period of development.

fibrinogen A blood constituent necessary for the formation of clots.

fibrocystic breast disorder Benign breast disorder characterized by the formation of cysts.

fimbriae Finger-like projections at the end of the fallopian tube.

flexion Normal bending forward of the fetal head (with the chin on the chest) in the uterus and uterine canal during the birth process.

floating A term used to describe the level of the fetal head (or presenting part) in the pelvis when it is above the level ischial spines.

fluctuate To move up or down, as a wave.

follicle-stimulating hormone (FSH) Hormone produced by the anterior pituitary gland during the first half of the menstrual cycle, stimulating development of the graafian follicle.

fontanelle Unfused areas between fetal skull bones covered with strong connective tissue; allows for movement of bones and molding during birth.

foramen ovale Opening between the right and left atria in the fetal heart.

forceps A pincer instrument that is used to assist in rotating and extracting the fetal head in the second stage of labor.

foremilk Milk obtained at the beginning of each breastfeeding session. *See also* hindmilk.

foreskin (prepuce) Fold of skin covering the glans penis; removed during circumcision.

frequency of contractions Period from the beginning of one uterine contraction until the beginning of the next.

functional residual capacity (FRC) The amount of air that remains in the lung after a normal expiration.

fundus Upper portion of the uterus.

G

galactogogue An agent that promotes the flow of human breast milk.

galactosemia An increase of galactose in the blood from a congenital inability to metabolize galactose into glucose.

gamete Reproductive cell. The female gamete is an ovum; the male gamete is a spermatozoon.

gametogenesis The development of a sex cell such as an ovum or sperm.

gate control theory Theory explaining the neurophysical mechanism underlying the perception of pain, whereby the travel of the pain message to the brain is blocked by distraction or drugs.

gavage Feeding of liquid nutrients through a tube passed into the stomach through the nose or mouth.

gene Deoxyribonucleic acid (DNA) component on the chromosome that determines inherited characteristics from parents.

genetic code The information system in the cells that determines the amino acid sequence in polypeptides. This system specifies all of the genetic information transmitted to an offspring.

genotype Genetic makeup of an individual.

gestation Time from conception to birth; approximately 280 days.

gestational age Number of completed weeks of fetal development; calculated from the first day of the last normal menstrual period.

gestational diabetes mellitus (GDM) Diabetes of variable severity with the onset or first recognition during pregnancy (usually first noticed because of altered carbohydrate metabolism).

gestational hypertension (GH) A hypertensive disorder of pregnancy or the puerperium, characterized by hypertension, proteinuria, and edema. It includes preeclampsia and eclampsia.

gestational trophoblastic disease Disorder classified as two types: benign and malignant (hydatidiform mole).

GIFT (gamete intrafallopian transfer) A type of assisted reproductive technology.

glomerular filtration rate (GFR) Amount of plasma filtered by the glomeruli of both kidneys per minute.

glucosuria Presence of glucose in the urine.

gonads Male and female sex organs (testes and ovaries).

graafian follicle A mature follicle (containing a near-mature ovum) of the ovary to be released; secretes estrogen.

grasp reflex The newborn's response of grasping lightly when the palms of hands are stimulated (by pressure).

gravida Woman who is or has been pregnant, regardless of outcome.

guided imagery A form of mind-body therapy that seeks to make beneficial changes in the body by repeatedly visualizing them; a technique that uses the imagination to think of a pleasant experience as a distraction to labor pains.

gynecoid pelvis A female pelvis in which the inlet is round.

gynecology The art and science of caring for a woman with a disorder of the female reproductive tract and associated structures.

H

habituation The newborn's natural ability to diminish responses to specific repeated stimuli.

heel stick A method for obtaining a blood specimen by puncturing a small capillary in the newborn's heel with a sharp microlancet.

HELLP syndrome An acronym for a variant of gestational hypertension involving *H*emolysis, *E*levated *L*iver Enzymes, and *L*ow *P*latelet count.

hematoma A collection of clotted blood in a confined space usually caused by breakage of a blood vessel.

hemolysis The abnormal destruction of a red blood cell and liberation of its hemoglobin.

hemorrhage An abnormally excessive loss of blood.

herbal medicine The use of plant material to promote healing and recovery from disease.

herpesvirus A virus that causes an infection and is spread by sexual contact.

hindmilk The milk an infant obtains after initial minutes of breastfeeding; contains a higher fat content than foremilk and is most hunger relieving.

holistic health care The comprehensive physical, emotional, spiritual, social, and economic care of a person.

Homans' sign Pain or tenderness in the calf of the leg on dorsiflexion of the foot; an indicator of thrombosis or thrombophlebitis.

homeopathy Health care practice based on the premise that illness is an energy imbalance; uses plants, herbs, and minerals that are thought to stimulate the immune system to deal with specific health problems.

hormone A chemical substance originating in a gland or organ that is carried by the blood or lymph to another organ or tissue where it acts as a stimulator or accelerator.

hormone replacement therapy (HRT) Use of estrogen and progestin to decrease the symptoms of menopause and help prevent osteoporosis.

hot flashes Vasomotor changes related to menopause, resulting in feeling warm or sweating.

hotlines Telephone lines used to help in emergency maternal or infant care.

human immunodeficiency virus (HIV) Virus that causes acquired immunodeficiency syndrome (AIDS).

hydatidiform mole A gestational trophoblastic disease that occurs when the chorionic villi form grapelike clusters and pregnancy does not progress; may be precancerous; also known as a molar pregnancy.

hydramnios Excessive amounts of amniotic fluid; also known as polyhydramnios.

hydrocephalus An abnormal condition in which there is an excessive amount of cerebral fluid within the brain cavities or surrounding the brain, or both.

hydrops fetalis Massive edema of the fetus caused by hyperbilirubinemia.

hydrotherapy Therapeutic use of water to promote relaxation.

hyperbilirubinemia Excessive amount of bilirubin in the blood; indicative of hemolytic disorder caused by blood incompatibility, intrauterine infection, septicemia, and other disorders.

hyperemesis gravidarum Excessive vomiting during pregnancy.

hyperglycemia An excess amount of glucose in the blood.

hypertonic uterine dysfunction Uterine contractions during labor that are frequent, painful, but poorly coordinated and nonproductive. Uterus may remain tense between contractions.

hyperventilation Decrease of carbon dioxide in the blood as a result of rapid and deep breathing. Relief may result from rebreathing in a paper bag or into one's cupped hands to replace the carbon dioxide "blown off" during hyperventilation.

hypnosis An induced state of sleep involving an enhanced state of suggestibility.

hypocalcemia Low calcium level in the blood.

hypoglycemia Low glucose level in the blood.

hypospadias A congenital anomaly in which the urethra opens on the lower surface of the penis.

hypotension Low blood pressure.

hypothermia Below normal body temperature.

hypotonic uterine dysfunction Contractions of the uterus during labor that are too weak to be effective; often occurs with uterine overdistention.

hypoxia Reduced availability of oxygen to the body tissues.

hysterectomy Surgical removal of the uterus.

I

icterus neonatorum Physiologic jaundice of the newborn.

immune response Reaction of the body to foreign substances or substances the body interprets as being foreign.

immunodeficiency Decreased or compromised ability to respond to antigenic stimuli by production of antibodies.

immunoglobulin Closely related, although not identical, proteins capable of acting as antibodies.

implantation Process by which the conceptus attaches to the uterine wall.

impotence Inability of the male to achieve or maintain an erection.

inborn error of metabolism A hereditary deficiency of a specific enzyme needed for normal metabolism of specific chemicals.

incompetent cervix A cervix that is unable to remain closed during pregnancy, resulting in spontaneous abortion.

increment Increased intensity of a uterine contraction.

induction of labor Artificial initiation of labor.

infant mortality rate Number of deaths per 1000 live births that occur within the first 12 months of life.

infants of diabetic mothers (IDMs) Infants born to mothers who have diabetes. They often have health problems such as macrosomia and hypoglycemia and require close observation after birth.

infertility Diminished ability or inability to conceive.

integrative health care A combination of complementary and alternative therapy with traditional medicine to facilitate healing.

intensity (of contractions) Strength of contractions.

internal fetal monitoring *See* electronic fetal monitoring.

internal os An inside opening; the opening between the cervix and uterus.

internal rotation The turning of the fetal head until the occiput is directly under the maternal symphysis pubis in preparation for birth of the head.

intrapartum The time from the onset of true labor until the birth of the newborn and delivery of the placenta.

intrauterine device (IUD) A mechanical device inserted in the uterus to prevent pregnancy.

intrauterine growth restriction (or retardation) (IUGR) Failure of a fetus to grow at the expected rate.

intraventricular hemorrhage (IVH) Bleeding within the ventricles of the brain.

involution Return of the reproductive organs to the nonpregnant state after the termination of pregnancy.

isoimmunization The phenomenon in which the Rh-negative woman develops antibodies against the Rh-positive fetus she is carrying

IVF (in vitro fertilization) A type of assisted reproductive technology.

J

jaundice Yellow pigmentation of the skin in response to excessive bilirubin in the blood.

K

kangaroo care A method of care that uses skin-to-skin contact of the newborn and parent to warm and calm the newborn and promote bonding.

karyotype An arrangement of a set of chromosomes in a standard order.

Kegel exercises Conscious tightening and relaxing of the pubococcygeal muscles, which strengthens the vagina and perineum.

kernicterus Accumulation of unconjugated bilirubin in the brain, resulting in brain damage.

kilogram (kg) 1000 g or 2.2 lbs.

L

labor Process by which the fetus, placenta, and membranes are expelled from the maternal uterus; also called *parturition* and *childbirth.*

laceration Tearing of tissue; during labor, tearing of vulvar, vaginal, and possibly rectal tissue as newborn is born.

lactation Process of producing and supplying breast milk.

lactose intolerance Inherited absence of the enzyme lactase, resulting in the inability to digest milk and milk products.

Lamaze technique A technique taught in childbirth education classes that teaches women ways to decrease their perception of pain during the childbirth experience.

lanugo Fine, downy hair found on the fetus and parts of the newborn after birth.

large-for-gestational-age (LGA) newborn Newborn of any weight who falls above the 90th percentile on the intrauterine growth curve.

latch-on technique The grasping of the entire areola of the nipple in the newborn's mouth to enable effective breastfeeding.

late deceleration A decrease in the fetal heart rate that occurs after the acme of a uterine contraction.

lecithin/sphingomyelin ratio (L/S ratio) Chemical component of surfactant. A 2:1 ratio determines the maturity of fetal lungs.

leiomyoma A benign uterine fibroid tumor.

Leopold's maneuvers A series of four maneuvers (abdominal palpation) designed to provide a systematic approach to determine fetal presentation and position.

let-down reflex Release of milk into the breasts in response to stimulation.

letting go A phase of maternal adaptation that involves assumption of a new role as a parent.

libido Sexual drive.

lie Relation of the long axis of the fetus to the long axis of the pregnant woman. The fetal lie may be longitudinal, transverse, or oblique.

lightening Moving of the fetus and uterus downward into the pelvic cavity; engagement.

local infiltration Insertion of a local anesthetic agent to numb the area before performing an episiotomy or suturing a laceration.

lochia Uterine (vaginal) discharge after delivery, typically lasting 3 to 6 weeks.

lochia alba Whitish yellow discharge, typically seen 10 to 21 days postpartum.
lochia rubra Bright red vaginal discharge, typically seen 1 to 3 days postpartum.
lochia serosa Pinkish vaginal discharge, typically seen 4 to 10 days postpartum.
lordosis Abnormal anterior curvature of the lumbar spine.
lunar month A period of 28 days (4 weeks).
luteinizing hormone (LH) One of the gonadotropic hormones produced by the anterior pituitary gland that stimulates development of the corpus luteum.

M

macrosomia Abnormally large fetal size; newborn weighing more than 4000 g (8 lbs, 13 oz).
male condom *See* condom.
managed care A system of health care delivery that has contracted services and cost containment with prescribed membership.
massage Therapeutic stroking of the body.
mastectomy Surgical removal of the breast.
mastitis Acute inflammation of the breast.
maternal mortality rate Number of maternal deaths within 42 days after giving birth per 100,000 live births.
maternity care Care of the childbearing family.
mechanism of labor A series of passive movements undergone by the fetus in passing through the birth canal.
meconium First greenish black, viscid stool of newborns; contains mucus, bile, and epithelial shreds.
meconium aspiration syndrome (MAS) Aspiration of meconium by the fetus in utero or during the birth process.
meiosis Reduction cell division in gametes (ova and sperm) that halves the number of chromosomes in each cell.
menopause The permanent cessation of menses.
menorrhagia Excessive bleeding during menses.
menses *See* menstruation.
menstruation A cyclic sloughing of uterine lining.
meridians Conceptual channels along which chi energy flows in the body; used in acupuncture and acupressure.
metrorrhagia Bleeding from the uterus between menstrual cycles.
microcephaly A congenital anomaly in which the head of the newborn is abnormally small.
milia Tiny white papules or cysts that disappear in a few weeks, commonly over the bridge of the nose, chin, and cheeks of newborns.
miliaria Small red papules on the skin caused by obstruction of the sweat glands.
milk-ejection reflex Release of milk from the alveoli into the ducts; also known as let-down reflex.
miscarriage A lay term for spontaneous abortion.
mitosis Type of cell division in somatic cells in which each daughter cell contains the same number of chromosomes as the parent cell. It is the process by which the body grows and by which cells are replaced.
mittelschmerz Abdominal pain occurring at the time of ovulation.
molding Shaping the fetal head by overlapping of the cranial bones to facilitate movement through the birth canal during labor.
mongolian spots Benign bluish pigmentation over the lower back and buttocks that may be present at birth, especially in dark-skinned newborns.
monozygotic twins Twins who develop from one fertilized ovum; identical twins.
Montgomery's tubercles Small glands situated on the areola around the nipple.

morbidity The state of being sick or diseased.
mortality Pertains to death rate.
morula Development stage of the fertilized ovum in which there is a solid mass of cells.
multifetal pregnancy Pregnancy involving more than one fetus (e.g., twins); also called *multiple pregnancy.*
multigravida A woman who has been pregnant two or more times.
multipara A woman who has delivered two or more babies after the period of viability, regardless of whether the babies were alive or stillborn.
mutation A permanent and transmissible change in a gene.
MyPyramid A guide for healthy daily food choices. Specific information is available at http://www.mypyramid.gov.

N

Nägele's rule Method to calculate the expected date of birth; count back 3 months from the first day of the last menstrual cycle, and add 7 days.
narcotic antagonist A compound, such as naloxone (Narcan), that is used to reverse the effects of narcotics.
nares Nostrils.
nasal flaring Widening of the nares on inspiration.
natural alternative care Practices, including self-care, journaling, and prayer, that may promote health but are not rooted in evidence-based research.
necrotizing enterocolitis (NEC) Acute inflammation of the bowel that leads to necrosis.
neonatal sepsis An infection that spreads from a local site to the bloodstream, initiating a systemic response in a newborn younger than 1 month.
neonate Newborn from birth through the first 28 days of life.
nesting Enclosure of newborn in a blanket roll to increase feeling of security.
neutral thermal environment Environment in which the body temperature is maintained without an increase in oxygen consumption or metabolic rate.
Nitrazine paper test Use of Nitrazine paper to measure pH in assessing the presence of amniotic fluid.
nonnutritive sucking Sucking activity that is not related to the intake of nutrients.
nonreassuring heart rate pattern A fetal heart rate pattern that indicates fetal distress, such as late decelerations, bradycardia, or absence of variability.
nonshivering thermogenesis Heat production without shivering by oxidation of brown fat.
nonstress test (NST) A test used to assess the response of fetal heart rate to movement.
nuchal cord Term used to describe the umbilical cord when it is wrapped around the fetal neck.
nuclear family Family consisting of parents (husband and wife) and their dependent children.
nursing care plan A care plan containing specific patient data that is designed to identify, prioritize, and manage problems encountered with nursing interventions.
nursing process A series of steps describing a problem-solving approach nurses use to identify, prevent, or treat actual or potential patient problems. It includes assessment, nursing diagnosis, planning, implementation, and evaluation.

O

obstetrics The art and science of caring for a woman during pregnancy, labor, and puerperium.
occiput The back part of the head.
oligohydramnios A decreased amount of amniotic fluid.

ophthalmia neonatorum Purulent infection of the eye or conjunctiva of the newborn, most often caused by gonococci or *Chlamydia* organisms.

opisthotonos Extension of the neck with an arched back, associated with central nervous system problems in the newborn.

opportunistic infection Infection in which organisms that do not usually cause disease become pathogenic (such as *Pneumocystis carinii* pneumonia).

oral contraceptives (OCs) Birth control pills that inhibit ovulation and contain progestins alone or in combination with estrogen.

Orem's theory A self-care theory of nursing that emphasizes purposeful actions to promote life and well-being.

orgasm The climax of sexual intercourse.

orthostatic hypotension Decrease in blood pressure when shifting to sitting or standing from a lying down position.

Ortolani's maneuver An assessment maneuver that is performed on the newborn to detect congenital hip dysplasia.

osteoporosis Increased spaces (porosity) in bone. The process greatly accelerates after menopause.

ovarian cycle Depicts the changes the follicle undergoes. There are two phases in the 28-day cycle: the follicular phase (days 1 to 14) and the luteal phase (days 15 to 28).

ovulation The maturation and release of the ovum from the ovary.

ovum (pl. ova) Female gamete, or sex cell.

oxytocin Hormone produced by the posterior pituitary that stimulates uterine contractions and the release of milk in the mammary gland by the let-down reflex.

P

paced breathing Learned breathing technique used during labor contractions to promote relaxation and increase pain tolerance.

palpation Examination performed by touching and exploring with the hands.

Papanicolaou (Pap) test (smear) Cytologic test of cervical cells used as a screening test for cervical cancer.

para The number of pregnancies that have reached the age of viability.

paracervical block Injection of local anesthetic into the lower uterine segment near the outer rim of the cervix.

parametritis An inflammation of tissue adjacent to the uterus.

parity (para) Number of pregnancies reaching viability regardless of the outcome.

parturition Childbirth.

passive acquired immunity Transfer of antibodies (immunoglobulin G) from the mother to the fetus in utero.

patent ductus arteriosus Congenital heart disease resulting when the opening between the pulmonary artery and the aorta does not close after birth.

pelvic inflammatory disease (PID) Infection of internal reproductive structures and adjacent tissues usually caused by a sexually transmitted infection.

pelvic tilt exercise An exercise to strengthen abdominal muscles and reduce backache; often used during pregnancy.

penis The male organ of copulation and reproduction.

perinatal mortality rate The number of neonatal and fetal deaths per 1000 live births.

perineum Floor of the pelvis; area of tissue between the anus and vagina in the woman and between the anus and scrotum in the man.

periodic abstinence Refraining from sexual intercourse at specified intervals of time.

peristalsis Wavelike progression of muscular contraction and relaxation, propelling the contents through a tubular organ.

phenylketonuria (PKU) A metabolic disorder caused by an inborn error of metabolism of the amino acid phenyl-alanine. If PKU remains untreated, mental retardation occurs.

phimosis Tightening or narrowing of the foreskin on the penis.

phototherapy Treatment of jaundice by exposure to light rays; used to aid bilirubin clearance.

pica Consumption of substances ordinarily considered inedible (e.g., laundry starch or red clay).

placenta Flat, vascular structure that connects the fetus to the uterine wall for gas and nutrient exchange; also known as the afterbirth.

placenta accreta A placenta that is embedded into the uterine muscle, resulting in failure to separate and be expelled during the third stage of labor.

placenta previa Abnormal implantation of the placenta in the lower uterine segment.

placental separation A disconnection of the placenta from the uterine decidua in the third stage of labor.

polycythemia An excess of red blood cells.

polydactyly Presence of extra fingers or toes.

polyhydramnios Excessive amount of amniotic fluid; also called *hydramnios.*

position *See* fetal position.

postpartum After childbirth or delivery.

postpartum blues A nonpsychotic depression occurring within 2 weeks of delivery.

postpartum fatigue A weakened condition of the mother after the birth of her infant because of the failure to rest and adjust to the postpartum phase.

postpartum hemorrhage Loss of 500 mL or more of blood after vaginal birth.

postterm newborn A newborn who has completed 42 weeks' gestation or more.

precipitate labor A rapid progression of labor that lasts less than 3 hours.

preconception care Health care and screening before pregnancy; can identify medical risks or lifestyle behaviors that can be managed before conception.

preeclampsia Hypertensive disorder of pregnancy or the puerperium with the three cardinal signs of hypertension, edema, and proteinuria.

pregestational diabetic A woman who had diabetes before conception occurred.

premature rupture of membranes Rupture of amniotic sac that occurs 42 hours or more before the onset of labor.

premenstrual dysphoric disorder (PMDD) A more severe type of premenstrual syndrome.

premenstrual syndrome (PMS) Cluster of symptoms experienced by some women. It typically occurs from a few days to 2 weeks before onset of menses.

prenatal Occurring before birth.

presentation *See* fetal presentation.

presenting part That part of the fetus lying closest to the internal os of the cervix.

preterm labor The onset of labor between 20 and 37 weeks' gestation.

preterm newborn Newborn born before the end of 37 weeks' gestation; also called *premature newborn.*

primigravida A woman pregnant for the first time.

primipara A woman giving birth to her first child at age of viability.

progesterone A hormone produced by the corpus luteum, adrenal cortex, and placenta that stimulates the growth of the endometrium for implantation, develops mammary glands, and maintains the pregnancy.

prolactin A hormone secreted by the anterior pituitary that stimulates and sustains lactation.

prolapsed umbilical cord Umbilical cord that becomes trapped in the vagina before the fetus is delivered. The cord is beside or ahead of the presenting part.

prophylactic eye care Eye medication administered to the newborn at birth to prevent ophthalmia neonatorum.

prophylaxis Protection from or prevention of a disease.

prostaglandin (PGE$_2$) Substance present in many body tissues that has a role in many reproductive tract functions.

prostate gland A gland that surrounds the urethra of the male and contributes to semen secretion.

proteinuria Presence of protein in the urine.

psychoprophylactic method *See* Lamaze technique.

puberty Period of sexual maturation accompanied by the development of secondary sex characteristics.

pudendal block Anesthesia injected around the pudendal nerve for pain relief.

puerperal fever A maternal temperature of 38° C (100.4° F) or higher on any 2 of the first 10 postpartum days, excluding the first 24 hours.

puerperium The period after delivery until complete involution of organs (e.g., uterus); usually 6 weeks; also called *postpartum period*.

pulmonary embolism A blood clot that obstructs a vessel in the lung.

pulmonary vascular resistance Opposition (resistance) to blood flow in the blood vessels of the fetal lungs.

pulse oximeter Equipment that measures the level of blood oxygen saturation by a sensor placed on the skin.

Q

quickening The first fetal movements felt by the mother, usually between 16 and 20 weeks of pregnancy.

R

radiant warmer A newborn bed that supplies overhead heat to provide a stable thermal environment while providing open access for care.

radiation Heat loss that occurs when heat transfers to cooler surfaces and objects not in direct contact with the body.

radioimmunoassay A very sensitive method of determining the concentration of substances (hormones) in blood plasma.

reassuring heart rate pattern A fetal heart rate that reflects adequate fetal oxygenation.

REEDA scale A mnemonic used in assessing wound healing or inflammation. It includes *Redness, Edema, Ecchymosis, Discharge,* and *Approximation.*

reflexology A treatment that applies varying degrees of pressure to different parts of the body, commonly the hands and feet. Practitioners believe that zones (of organs and systems) used to promote body function run along the body and terminate in the hands and feet.

respiratory distress syndrome (RDS) Inability of newborn, especially preterm newborn, to maintain adequate respiratory effort, resulting from insufficient surfactant in the lungs.

retinopathy of prematurity (ROP) Retinal damage and blindness in the preterm neonate resulting from exposure to high oxygen concentrations; also known as retrolental fibroplasia.

retraction Abnormal "sucking in" of the chest wall during inspiration; also, the pulling back of the foreskin over the glans penis to expose the urinary meatus.

Rh factor An inherited antigen present on erythrocytes. The individual with the factor is referred to as *Rh positive (Rh+),* and an individual without the factor is called *Rh negative (Rh−).*

RhoGAM Rh (D) immune globulin given after delivery to an Rh(−) mother of an Rh(+) fetus to prevent the maternal Rh immune response.

rhythm method *See* calendar method.

rooting reflex An infant's reflex to turn head and open lips to suck when one side of the mouth or cheek is touched.

rubella (German measles) An acute infection that can cause serious anomalies in the developing fetus.

rugae Folds of mucous membranes on internal surfaces such as the vagina.

S

sacral pressure A complementary therapeutic technique that involves massage or pressure on the sacral area to aid in pain management during labor.

salpingitis Infection of the fallopian tubes.

satiety A feeling of being full to satisfaction.

Schultze mechanism Delivery of the placenta in which the fetal side of the placenta is expelled first.

screening Multiple tests performed to rule out common abnormalities known to cause physical or mental disability.

semen Thick, whitish fluid ejaculated by the male during orgasm and containing spermatozoa; the transporting medium for sperm.

sex chromosomes Chromosomes responsible for sex determination. Females have two X chromosomes, and males have one X and one Y.

sexuality Refers to sexual behaviors and attitudes in the male and female.

sexually transmitted infections (STIs) Infections usually transmitted by direct contact (ordinarily by sexual activity) with an infected person.

show Vaginal discharge during the first stage of labor.

sickle cell anemia Inherited disorder caused by abnormal hemoglobin, resulting in a sickling of red blood cells.

sitz bath A warm water bath that covers the buttocks and perineal area only.

Skene's glands Two glands opening near the meatus of the female urethra.

small-for-gestational-age (SGA) newborn Newborn whose weight falls below the 10th percentile of the intrauterine growth curve.

smegma An accumulation of cheese-like secretions that may be found under the foreskin of the penis and around the labia minora.

soma cells Body cells.

spermatogenesis Formation of male gametes (sperm) in the testes.

spermatozoon (pl. spermatozoa) The male reproductive cell (sperm) consisting of a head, or nucleus, and a flagellum, or tail.

spermicide An agent that kills sperm.

spina bifida A congenital defect involving failure in closure of the bony spinal canal.

spinal block Injection of a local anesthetic agent directly into the spinal fluid in the spinal canal; used in vaginal and cesarean births.

spinnbarkeit Refers to the elasticity of the cervical mucus that is present at the time of ovulation.

spontaneous abortion An abortion that occurs naturally; also called a *miscarriage.*

standards of care A statement of minimum safe care or conduct expectations determined by a professional organization.

station Relation of the presenting fetal part to the pelvic ischial spines of the birth canal.

sterility Inability to conceive.

sterilization A process of permanently removing the ability to reproduce.

stillbirth The birth of a dead newborn.

strabismus A turning inward (crossing) or outward of the eyes.

stress incontinence Involuntary loss of urine that occurs in situations such as sneezing or coughing. May be indicative of pelvic floor dysfunction.

striae gravidarum Irregular pinkish or purplish streaks (stretch marks) resulting from the stretching and tearing of connective tissue during pregnancy. They generally appear on the abdomen, breasts, and thighs.

subinvolution Delay of a structure (e.g., the uterus) to return to its normal size after enlargement (e.g., pregnancy).

supine hypotensive syndrome Lowered blood pressure and decreased pulse in the supine position resulting from compression of the inferior vena cava by pressure of the gravid uterus.

surfactant A substance formed in the lungs that reduces surface tension and helps keep the alveoli (air sacs) expanded and not collapsed.

suture Junction of the cranial bones.

symptothermal method A contraceptive technique that combines basal body temperature with the cervical mucus method.

syndactyly Webbing between two fingers or toes so that they are attached.

systemic vascular resistance Opposition to blood flow in the various vessels of the body.

T

tachycardia (fetal) Rapid fetal heart rate (above 160 beats per minute).

tachypnea Rapid respiration.

taking hold Second phase of maternal adaptation during which the mother assumes some independence in control over her body and some responsibility for newborn care.

taking in First phase of maternal adaptation during which the mother passively accepts care (dependency) for herself and her newborn.

teratogen (teratogenic agent) An agent or substance that causes abnormal development of an embryo.

term newborn A newborn born between 38 and 42 weeks' gestation.

testosterone A male hormone.

therapeutic insemination A technique used to promote pregnancy in an otherwise infertile couple.

thermoregulation Maintenance of body temperature within normal limits.

thrombophlebitis Inflammation of a vein related to the formation of the thrombus (clot).

thrombus Blood clot obstructing a blood vessel. If detached, it becomes an embolus and can occlude a vessel at a distance from the original site.

tocolytic agent Drug that inhibits uterine contractions; commonly used with labor involving preterm newborns.

tocotransducer Electronic device used for measuring uterine contractions.

TORCH An acronym that refers to a group of infections that represent potentially severe problems during pregnancy: *Toxoplasmosis*, "*Other*" infections, *Rubella*, *Cytomegalovirus*, and *Herpesvirus*.

toxic shock syndrome (TSS) Infection predominantly caused by *Staphylococcus aureus*; found primarily in women of reproductive age who use tampons.

toxoplasmosis A parasitic infection acquired by contact with cat feces and transmitted through the placenta, causing fetal abnormalities.

transcutaneous electrical nerve stimulation (TENS) A form of energy therapy that emits low-level current to a body area; used to prevent nausea and other problems.

transition The last phase of active labor, from 8 to 10 cm cervical dilation, which is usually characterized by intense maternal discomfort.

translocation Alteration of a chromosome by transfer of a portion of it either to another chromosome or to another portion of the same chromosome.

transplacental Across the placenta, such as the exchange of nutrients, waste products, and hormones between mother and fetus. Drugs can also cross the placenta and be harmful to the fetus.

trial of labor A period of labor under close monitoring for complications in high-risk pregnancies.

trimester A 3-month period representing one third of the gestational time.

trophoblast The outer layer of the blastoderm that will establish the nutrient relation with the uterine endometrium.

true labor Uterine contractions with the intensity to cause effacement and dilation of the cervix.

tubal ligation Permanent blocking of the fallopian tube for purpose of sterilization.

tympanic membrane sensor A device used to measure temperature by inserting a covered plastic probe into the auditory canal.

U

ultrasound Use of high-frequency sound waves that may be directed, through use of a transducer, into the maternal abdomen; used in fetal assessment.

umbilical cord Cord containing two arteries and one vein that connects the fetus with the placenta.

umbilicus The navel.

uterine dysfunction A labor pattern that interferes with the normal progress of cervical dilation.

uterine rupture A tear in the uterine wall.

V

vagina The canal from the vulva to the cervix of the uterus.

vaginal birth after cesarean (VBAC) A labor management approach of providing close monitoring and support to encourage vaginal delivery and reduce the rate of cesarean births.

Valsalva's maneuver Increasing pressure within the abdomen and thorax by holding one's breath and pushing against the glottis.

variable deceleration A transient decrease in the fetal heart rate before, during, or after a uterine contraction. It is usually associated with a heart acceleration before and/or after the deceleration.

variability Normal irregularity of fetal cardiac rhythm; short-term beat-to-beat changes; long-term rhythmic changes or waves from the baseline (usually 3 to 5 beats per minute).

variances Deviations from an expected outcome in the expected clinical pathway of a medical diagnosis.

vas deferens Duct that transports sperm from the testes to the urethra.

vasectomy Tying or ligating of the vas deferens to prevent passage of sperm, thereby preventing pregnancy.

vasoconstriction Narrowing of the blood vessels.

vernix caseosa A protective, cheese-like, whitish coating found in varying quantities on the skin of the newborn.

vertex The top of the fetal head, between the anterior and posterior fontanelles.

viability Ability to live outside of the uterus. The minimum age of viability of a fetus is designated as 20 weeks' gestation.

viscosity State of being thick and slow flowing, or thin and runny; compares the rate of flow of liquid through a tube, such as blood through blood vessels.

vulva The external female genitalia lying below the mons pubis.

W

warm lines Telephone advice lines that provide communication with the patient at home in non-urgent situations.

Watson's theory A theory emphasizing the importance of caring and a holistic approach.

Wharton's jelly Yellow-white gelatinous material surrounding the vessels in the umbilical cord.

womb Lay term for the uterus.

Z

zygote A fertilized ovum (egg); cell produced by union of two gametes.

Index

b indicates boxes, f indicates illustrations, and t indicates tables.

assessment

The Newborn at Risk: Conditions Associated with Gestational Age and Development

Name _____   Date _____

Multiple Choice

1. The newborn born at 38 weeks and assessed by the nurse to be in the 7th percentile for weight would be classified as: (p. 303)
    1. SGA, preterm
    2. AGA, term
    3. SGA, term
    4. AGA, preterm

2. The nurse should observe the newborn with intrauterine growth restriction for what nutritional problem? (p. 306)
    1. Hypoglycemia
    2. Obesity
    3. Excess glycogen reserve
    4. Anemia

3. Inadequate surfactant may cause a newborn to have respiratory distress because: (p. 309)
    1. Excess lung fluid accumulates in the air sacs, reducing oxygen and carbon dioxide exchange.
    2. Mucus becomes thick and sticky, adhering to the smaller airways in the respiratory tract.
    3. It allows solid material to remain in the airways, where it tends to cause infection.
    4. It reduces the ability of the alveoli to remain slightly open during expiration.

4. Periodic breathing is defined as: (p. 310)
    1. Cessation of breathing for 15 seconds or more
    2. An irregular pattern to the respirations
    3. Occasional grunting sounds with expirations
    4. Inadequate brown fat to fuel respiratory effort

5. To reduce the preterm newborn's risk for developing retinopathy of prematurity, the nurse should: (pp. 313–314)
    1. Closely monitor the oxygen content of the blood
    2. Provide supplemental oxygen with an Oxyhood only
    3. Minimize the disturbances of the newborn
    4. Limit formula or breast milk feedings in the first week

6. The ideal feeding for a preterm newborn is: (p. 313)
    1. Commercial preterm newborn formula
    2. Human breast milk
    3. Regular newborn formula
    4. Breast milk, diluted half strength

7. The nurse should suspect development of necrotizing enterocolitis in the gavage-fed preterm newborn if: (pp. 314–315)
    1. The newborn has overactive bowel sounds
    2. Bowel movements are absent for 1 day
    3. Radiographs show an absence of air in the bowel
    4. Gastric residuals increase over several feedings

8. What result will a patent ductus arteriosus have on the pulmonary circulation? (p. 314)
    1. It will reduce circulation to the lungs initially and then increase circulation.
    2. It will cause congestion in the lungs and reduce body oxygenation.
    3. It will cause a right-to-left shunting of blood through the foramen ovale.
    4. It will reduce the total area in the lungs available for oxygen and carbon dioxide exchange.

9. Nursing care that may reduce the risk for an intracranial hemorrhage in the preterm newborn is to: (p. 315)
    1. Provide continuous noninvasive oxygen monitoring
    2. Teach parents how to gently handle their preterm newborn
    3. Avoid giving the newborn too much formula or breast milk
    4. Limit the use of analgesics such as morphine

10. The nurse is assisting the mother of a preterm newborn in performing kangaroo care for the first time with her intubated newborn. Select the best teaching by the nurse related to this type of care. (pp. 316–317)
    1. "Kangaroo care helps reduce the incidence of infections and brain hemorrhage in very preterm newborns."
    2. "Kangaroo care gives you a chance to feel important to your baby and reduces the baby's risk for infection."
    3. "Kangaroo care will make it much easier for you when you take your baby home from the hospital."
    4. "Kangaroo care can facilitate parent-newborn attachment and help stabilize the newborn."

Clinical Situations

1. A mother and father are entering the special care nursery for the first time to see their preterm newborn girl born earlier in the day by cesarean birth. What would be a good nursing approach to the first visit by these new parents and the rationale for each action?

2. The mother of a preterm newborn girl, 32 weeks' gestation, says that she is disappointed that she cannot breastfeed her baby as she planned. How should the nurse respond to this mother?

Group Internet Activities

1. Access the Merck Manual website to find the signs, symptoms, and complications of prematurity.

2. Access the websites in the list of Online Resources on p. 318 and discuss information concerning topics in this chapter.

The Newborn at Risk: Acquired and Congenital Conditions

chapter

16

STUDY GUIDE

Name _____ Date _____

Multiple Choice

1. A trisomy is best described as the: (p. 321)
   1. Absence of a gene on the X chromosome
   2. Rearrangement of genetic material in the ovum
   3. Presence of an extra chromosome in each body cell
   4. Absence of an entire chromosome in each ovum

2. Parents of a child with Down syndrome will need to take extra steps to reduce the incidence of: (p. 322)
   1. Unintended impregnation of a female by their male child
   2. Excessive problems with respiratory tract infections
   3. Hearing difficulties and deafness
   4. Poor eye and hand coordination

3. What discharge teaching is essential related to the phenylketonuria screening test? (p. 323)
   1. Normal screening results reassure the parents that their baby does not have this uncommon genetic disorder.
   2. The parents should feed their baby a low-phenylalanine formula until the screening results are complete.
   3. Results from the screening will be known in approximately 3 weeks when they visit their pediatrician.
   4. They should return to the pediatrician as recommended in approximately 3 weeks for a follow-up phenylketonuria test.

4. Which condition increases the newborn's risk for excessive jaundice? (p. 324)
   1. Neonatal anemia
   2. Cephalhematoma
   3. Hypothyroidism
   4. Early passage of meconium

5. To reduce the likelihood that an Rh-negative newborn will be affected by the development of maternal antibodies to Rh-positive blood, the mother should receive: (p. 329)
   1. Indirect Coombs' factor within 72 hours of birth
   2. Limited amounts of Rh-positive blood to reduce her sensitivity
   3. A blood transfusion to replace destroyed erythrocytes
   4. Rho(D) immune globulin after each Rh-positive pregnancy or as indicated

6. When a newborn is receiving phototherapy, the nurse must pay special attention to: (p. 330)
   1. Fluid balance
   2. Glucose level
   3. Respiratory function
   4. Mouth care

7. Meconium aspiration syndrome may be prevented by the use of _____ at birth. (p. 335)
   1. Artificial surfactant
   2. Extracorporeal membrane oxygenation
   3. Amniocentesis
   4. Immediate upper airway suctioning

8. A common manifestation of neonatal sepsis is: (p. 337)
   1. Hypoglycemia
   2. A low and unstable temperature
   3. Hypertension and a red skin color
   4. Abdominal distention

9. One sign of neonatal hypoglycemia is: (p. 332)
   1. Hypertonicity
   2. Fever
   3. Jitteriness
   4. Tachycardia

10. The best environment for the newborn who is withdrawing from maternal substance exposure is in: (p. 339, Table 16-3)
    1. A rocking swing in a quiet, cool, well-lit room
    2. The main nursery to facilitate observation
    3. A darkened, quiet area with few disturbances
    4. An incubator to reduce infection risk

Clinical Situations

1. A newborn of a diabetic mother has a glucose level of 38 mg/dL on a routine screen. According to hospital policy, the nurse has the laboratory draw a stat venous sample for glucose level, which has just been done. What are the next steps that are appropriate for this newborn?

2. Check your clinical facility's policies regarding steps taken when a woman who abuses substances is admitted. These policies may include both the woman and her newborn. Are there safeguards in place to ensure the safety of the newborn on discharge?

Group Internet Activities

1. Access the National Association for Down Syndrome website and discuss services available to the public.

2. Access the websites in the list of Online Resources on p. 342 and discuss information concerning topics in this chapter.

The Pregnant Adolescent and Maternity Nursing in the Community

Name _____   Date _____

Multiple Choice

1. When providing health counseling to an adolescent, the nurse must realize that one of the most important influences in a girl's life is her: (pp. 356, 357, Table 18-2)
   1. Siblings
   2. Peer group
   3. Teachers
   4. Boyfriend

2. The nurse should remember that young adolescent parents may need added support in caring for their newborn because: (p. 356)
   1. Teen parents are unable to learn what should be done in the care of a newborn.
   2. Teens can handle only one or two care tasks at a time rather than multiple tasks.
   3. They are more interested in further sexual encounters than in caring for their newborn.
   4. Their behavior is self-centered, and they cannot easily face their responsibilities as parents.

3. In their efforts to develop emotional intimacy, adolescents are often confused by: (p. 357, Table 18-2)
   1. Peers who expect them to retell everything that happens after an encounter
   2. Parents who send mixed messages that sex before marriage is acceptable if no pregnancy results
   3. Limits placed on their behaviors by parents who try to prevent a premature pregnancy
   4. Misinterpretation of sexual relationships as commitment or intimacy by the partner

4. Nutritional concerns during the adolescent's pregnancy include: (p. 359, Table 18-3)
   1. Reduced vitamin C absorption because of immature uptake
   2. Excessive iron absorption related to high calcium intake
   3. Consumption of empty-calorie foods and fad diets
   4. Increased incidence of gestational diabetes mellitus

5. Although contraceptives are available to adolescents, they may not use them because adolescents tend to: (p. 362)
   1. Fear the contraceptives' adverse effects on their sexual function
   2. Think that the contraceptives interfere with spontaneity of sex
   3. Expect their parents to disapprove of their sexual activity
   4. Set limits of responsibility for their own behavior

6. A common reason the adolescent girl delays prenatal care is: (p. 360, Table 18-4)
   1. Denial that the pregnancy actually exists
   2. Belief that she does not really need medical care
   3. A lack of understanding of the benefits of prenatal care
   4. A desire to avoid being told what she should eat or do

7. Professional negligence occurs when a patient: (p. 365)
   1. Is not given care in the time frame prescribed by a critical pathway
   2. Has an injury or dies as a direct result of the nurse's action
   3. Has care provided by nonlicensed assistants, such as aides
   4. Declines the services of a professional nurse in the outpatient setting

8. A common prenatal test for fetal health that the nurse would teach a woman to perform in her home is the: (p. 366)
   1. Kick count
   2. Biophysical profile
   3. Amniocentesis
   4. Nonstress test

9. A cause for a positive home pregnancy test other than a normal intrauterine pregnancy is: (p. 365)
   1. Hydatidiform mole
   2. Uterine fibroid tumors
   3. Diabetes mellitus
   4. Group B Streptococcus infection

10. Home prenatal visits for low-risk women are primarily aimed at: (p. 366)
    1. Explaining how to obtain governmental aid for medical and nutritional care during pregnancy
    2. Increasing the number of women who breastfeed their newborns for at least 6 months
    3. Reducing barriers that prevent the woman from obtaining early and regular prenatal care
    4. Giving poor women free or low-cost care that they cannot obtain from physicians

11. The nurse is making a home visit 3 days after birth. The newborn has been nursing poorly and is jaundiced. His bilirubin level is slightly elevated. What action should the nurse expect based on this information? (p. 368)
   1. The pediatrician will recommend that the parents change the newborn to formula rather than breast milk.
   2. The newborn will probably be readmitted to the hospital for intravenous fluids and antibiotics.
   3. The newborn will need to have added water fed by syringe rather than by bottle.
   4. Phototherapy in the form of a BiliBlanket will be prescribed to bring the level down.

12. A vital nursing role when a newborn is discharged with an apnea monitor is to: (pp. 368–369)
   1. Verify the parents' ability to perform newborn cardiopulmonary resuscitation (basic life support)
   2. Teach the mother to breastfeed the newborn without causing the monitor alarm to sound
   3. Determine whether the parents have a pharmacy within easy walking distance
   4. Emphasize to the parents that one of them must always be with the baby

Clinical Situations

1. An adolescent mother seems impatient when her newborn has difficulty feeding and soils his diaper. The mother watches TV and talks with her friends on the phone while the baby cries. What is an approach the nurse might take to address this situation?

2. If you have an antepartal unit in your clinical facility, talk with women who have been hospitalized about their feelings about being unable to go home. What facilities and activities does the facility provide to help the women pass the time? Do they have occupational or physical therapy activities?

3. Discuss public health policies related to screening pregnant women for depression or other problems in the community.

Group Internet Activities

1. Access the Planned Parenthood website (www.plannedparenthood.org) and discuss the mission statement regarding adolescent reproductive health care services.

2. Access the Johns Hopkins Children's Center website (www.hopkinschildrens.org) and report on the parenting resources section.

3. Access the following websites for additional support groups and bulletin boards for pregnant women on bed rest and for parents-to-be. How does their information compare with your text? Is it accurate and generally current?

www.sidelines.org
www.babycenter.com
www.cdc.gov/nccdphp/drh

Complementary and Alternative Therapies

Name   Date

Multiple Choice

1. Which change in health consumerism has increased the use of complementary and alternative therapies? (p. 408)
   1. Distrust in medical professionals
   2. Growth of the wellness movement
   3. Increasing limitations of insurance
   4. Reduced access to traditional medicine

2. The Dietary Supplement Health and Education Act of 1994 was passed to: (p. 408)
   1. Require prescriptions for herbal medicines
   2. Evaluate the effectiveness of alternative therapies
   3. Determine whether plant-source products are safe
   4. Provide marketing regulations for botanical medicines

3. An elderly neighbor with osteoporosis asks whether acupressure might ease her persistent back pain. As a nurse, you should initially tell her that: (p. 409)
   1. Acupressure can promote general relaxation but may be too forceful for someone with osteoporosis.
   2. Aromatherapy is likely to have a stronger pain-relieving effect than acupressure for osteoporosis.
   3. Acupuncture is likely to have a more positive effect for osteoporosis.
   4. She might like to try some homeopathic remedies in addition to her physician's prescription.

4. Biofeedback is defined as: (p. 411)
   1. Inducing an altered state of consciousness that is similar to daydreaming
   2. Applying very light electrical currents to electrodes applied to the skin
   3. Introducing tiny disposable needles into meridians in the body to alter function
   4. Training a person to gain control over bodily functions that are normally subconscious

5. People who should not use a transcutaneous electrical nerve stimulation include those who: (p. 412)
   1. Are in term labor
   2. Have a heart pacemaker
   3. Have dysmenorrhea
   4. Are undergoing chemotherapy

6. How can hydrotherapy increase the speed of labor? (pp. 413–414)
   1. Distraction from the pain of labor allows the cervix to dilate more quickly.
   2. Relaxation of the smooth muscle of the cervix and vagina causes these structures to open.
   3. Stimulation of the nipples causes oxytocin release, increasing contractions.
   4. Vasodilation improves blood flow to the uterus and placenta, thus improving contractions.

7. A safety problem that often occurs with herbal medicines is that patients often: (p. 413)
   1. List only food supplements on history forms
   2. Believe herbs are better than other medicine
   3. Do not take the medicines as directed
   4. Equate natural products with safety

8. A friend who takes several herbal supplements regularly wants to become pregnant soon. As a nurse, you should tell her to: (pp. 417–418)
   1. Stop all herbal medicines before she becomes pregnant
   2. Consult a physician because not all herbal medicines are safe during pregnancy
   3. Avoid the herbal and all other medicines for the first 3 months of pregnancy
   4. Continue the herbal supplements because these are organic compounds rather than drugs

9. A patient is interested in some herbal medicines that she found on the Internet and asks for your opinion. As a nurse, you should reply that: (p. 418)
   1. As long as a specific dose range is given for the medication on its container, the herbal medicine should be safe.
   2. Because the botanical medicines are natural, they are usually safer than manufactured medications that have similar effects.
   3. Most herbal medicines have well-established safety records, although some aromatherapy oils have been questioned.
   4. More controlled research studies are needed to determine the efficacy and safety of most of these medicines.

10. An herb that may be used to reduce the hot flashes of menopause is: (p. 418, Table 21-3)
    1. Black cohosh
    2. Feverfew
    3. Nettle
    4. Ginseng

Clinical Situation

1. A young woman enters the hospital in early labor and is tense and uncomfortable. Write some sample guided imagery or visualization statements that you might use with her to help her relax and cope with labor.

Group Internet Activities

1. Access the website, http://nccam.nih.gov/health/webresources, and review 10 Things to Know About Evaluating Medical Resources on the Web. Discuss the information provided.

2. Access a website that focuses on complementary or alternative therapies. Discuss whether the website is focused on "selling" one product or service (i.e., an infomercial) or the information is presented by unbiased experts.

3. Access the websites in the list of Online Resources on p. 419 and discuss information concerning topics in this chapter.

- anemia
  beets, dark leafy green
  veg + vit. C, beans, kelp
  (tomatoes/OJ)

Nerve pain, hypertension.

- migraines: tea.
  └ ginger, tumerik
  ↑ fluid intake,
  eucaliptis, peppermint oil
  eucaliptis (essential oil)

↑
Wt loss
- water portion, Mg+
  control, sea weed,
  guggul, ↑ thyroid function,

Asthma
- rosemary, eucaliptis
  (oil) (essential oil)
  messaging pressure point
  on feet.

• Raspberry leaf tea
  - helps body go into
    labor & prevent
    hemorrhage
  - good for menstrual
    cramps

• Ginger - for morning
  sickness & peppermint
  gas relief.

• Alphalpha leafe
  improves kidney
  function & hemroids

• Camamill tea, lavender
  oil (scent.
  anxiety, restlessness

• Omega 3, 6, 9
  are very essensial
  as well as vit. D

• message sacral
  point to help for
  labor pains

• Blood cleaning, bowels
  - detox ↗

→ Look up holistic
  nursing classess.

⬯ grape seed oil
  BAD !!

↑ fertility.
Vitex, acupuncture
Chase tree

doctorax

Arthritis
- essential oils
- glucocadamine, cintradine, MSN (vasuela)
  (joint formula)
high uromic acid

- anti-inflammatory
  tumerick. frankansis
- ↑ fluids
- coconut /olive/
  avocado oil